D0105183

PROFESSIONAL GUIDE TO
Assessment

PROFESSIONAL GUIDE TO Assessment

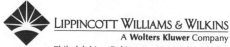

LIPPINCOTT WILLIAMS & WILKINS
A **Wolters Kluwer** Company
Philadelphia • Baltimore • New York • London
Buenos Aires • Hong Kong • Sydney • Tokyo

STAFF

Executive Publisher
Judith A. Schilling McCann, RN, MSN

Editorial Director
H. Nancy Holmes

Clinical Director
Joan M. Robinson, RN, MSN

Senior Art Director
Arlene Putterman

Editorial Project Manager
Jennifer P. Kowalak

Clinical Project Manager
Beverly Ann Tscheschlog, RN, BS

Editor
Julie Munden

Clinical Editor
Maryann Foley, RN, BSN

Copy Editors
Kimberly Bilotta (supervisor), Scotti Cohn, Heather Ditch, Judith Orioli, Carolyn Petersen, Irene Pontarelli, Kelly Taylor, Dorothy P. Terry, Pamela Wingrod

Designer
Linda Jovinelly Franklin (project manager)

Digital Composition Services
Diane Paluba (manager), Joyce Rossi Biletz, Donna S. Morris

Manufacturing
Patricia K. Dorshaw (director), Beth J. Welsh

Editorial Assistants
Megan L. Aldinger, Karen J. Kirk, Linda K. Ruhf

Indexer
Barbara Hodgson

The clinical treatments described and recommended in this publication are based on research and consultation with nursing, medical, and legal authorities. To the best of our knowledge, these procedures reflect currently accepted practice. Nevertheless, they can't be considered absolute and universal recommendations. For individual applications, all recommendations must be considered in light of the patient's clinical condition and, before administration of new or infrequently used drugs, in light of the latest package insert information. The authors and publisher disclaim any responsibility for any adverse effects resulting from the suggested procedures, from any undetected errors, or from the reader's misunderstanding of the text.

PGASS – D N O S A J J M A M

07 06 05 10 9 8 7 6 5 4 3 2 1

Library of Congress Cataloging-in-Publication Data

Professional guide to assessment.
p. ; cm.
Includes bibliographical references and index.
1. Diagnosis — Handbooks, manuals, etc. 2. Nursing assessment — Handbooks, manuals, etc. 3. Physical diagnosis — Handbooks, manuals, etc. I. Lippincott Williams & Wilkins.
[DNLM: 1. Physical Examination — Handbooks. 2. Laboratory Techniques and Procedures — Handbooks. 3. Medical History Taking — Handbooks. WB 39 P9625 2006]
RC71.P758 2006
616.07'5 — dc22
ISBN 1-58255-403-X (alk. paper) 2004028714

Contents

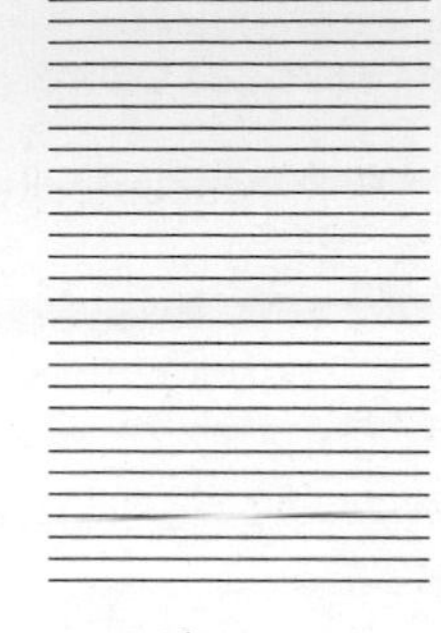

Contributors and consultants

Deborah A. Andris, RN-CS, MSN, APNP
Nurse Practitioner, Bariatric Surgery Program
Medical College of Wisconsin
Milwaukee

Jemma Bailey-Kunte, APRN-BC, MS, FNP
Clinical Lecturer
Binghamton (N.Y.) University
Nurse Practitioner
Lourdes Hospital
Binghamton, N.Y.

Cheryl A. Bean, APRN,BC, DSN, ANP, AOCN
Associate Professor
Indiana University School of Nursing
Indianapolis

Natalie Burkhalter, RN, MSN, ACNP, CS, FNP
Associate Professor
Texas A&M International University
Laredo

Shelba Durston, RN, MSN, CCRN
Nursing Instructor
San Joaquin Delta College
Stockton, Calif.
Staff Nurse
San Joaquin General Hospital
French Camp, Calif.

Tamara D. Espejo, RN, MS
RN/Clinical Educator
Aurora Behavioral Healthcare-Charter Oak
Covina, Calif.

Michelle L. Foley, RN,C, MA
Director, Nursing Education
Charles E. Gregory School of Nursing
Raritan Bay Medical Center
Perth Amboy, N.J.

Catherine B. Holland, RN, PhD, ANP, BC-APRN, CNS
Associate Professor
Southeastern Louisiana University
Baton Rouge

Julia Anne Isen, RN, MS, FNP-C
Nurse Practitioner – Internal Medicine
Veterans Administration Medical Center
San Francisco
Assistant Clinical Professor
University of California at San Francisco School of Nursing

Nancy Banfield Johnson, RN, MSN, ANP (inactive)
Nurse Manager
Kendal at Ithaca (N.Y.)

Gary R. Jones, RN, MSN, CNS, FNP
ARNP, Disease Management Program
Mercy Health Center
Fort Scott, Kans.

Vanessa C. Kramasz, RN, MSN, FNP-C
Nursing Faculty & Family Nurse Practitioner
Gateway Technical College
Kenosha, Wis.

Priscilla A. Lee, MN, FNP
Instructor in Nursing
Moorpark (Calif.) College

Susan Luck, RN, MS, CCN
Director of Nutrition
Biodoron Immunology Center
Hollywood, Fla.

Ann S. McQueen, RNC, MSN, CRNP
Family Nurse Practitioner
Healthlink Medical Center
Southampton, Pa.

Dale O'Donnell, RN, BSN
Administrator Community Surgery Center
Community Hospital
Munster, Ind.

William J. Pawlyshyn, RN, MS, MN, APRN,BC
Nurse Practitioner Consultant
New England Geriatrics
West Springfield, Mass.

Catherine Pence, RN, MSN, CCRN
Assistant Professor
Good Samaritan College of Nursing
Cincinnati

Abby Plambeck, RN, BSN
Freelance Writer
Milwaukee

Theresa Pulvano, RN, BSN
Nursing Educator
Ocean County Vocational Technical School
Lakehurst, N.J.

Monica Narvaez Ramirez, RN, MSN
Faculty
University of the Incarnate Word
San Antonio, Tex.

Regina Reed, RN, MSN, FNP
Associate Professor
Washington State Community College
Marrietta, Ohio

Foreword

Physical assessment skills and accurate interpretation of assessment findings are the foundation for the implementation of safe, competent care to individuals across all levels of care delivery. As the cornerstone of the health care process, assessment assists in identifying health status, health needs, and problems in order to provide timely, evidence-based, effective care.

Today, more than ever, health care professionals face multiple challenges in their daily practice including performing the assessments, recording the findings, and making the decisions — always under constant cognizance of time. The ultimate challenge is balancing these tasks with total competence and accuracy, while keeping patient care in the forefront.

Professional Guide to Assessment aims to enhance and refine your knowledge base and skill proficiency level, permitting an accurate, reliable, and thorough health assessment. Indeed, it's imperative that as a health care professional, you have this streamlined resource available to meet the needs of a growing, ever-changing, multiproblem patient population.

Professional Guide to Assessment provides the latest on taking a thorough patient history and performing the right physical assessment techniques. Eye-catching icons highlight racial and age-related differences in assessments and findings as well as special assessment points or emergency situations that may be revealed during an assessment. Additionally, abundant tables and illustrations help to highlight key topics and illustrate expert techniques.

The first four chapters are devoted to a detailed collection of subjective and objective data, including health history, assessment techniques, mental health status, and nutritional assessment. Thereafter, each chapter focuses on assessment for an individual body system. Each body system chapter covers anatomy and physiology; health history, which includes chief complaing, current and past health, and family and psychosocial history; physical assessment, and normal and abnormal findings in an easy-to-follow format. Further, chapters include a quick-scan chart that helps interpret abnormal findings and differentiate among possible causes. Appendices provide valuable information about head-to-toe assessment, laboratory test results, and resources for the health care professional, for the patients you care for, and for their caregivers.

In these times of increasing multiproblem patients in a complex health care environment, *Professional Guide to Assessment* provides you with the right questions and the best techniques to perform a complete patient history and expert physical examination in any clinical setting.

Mario R. Ortiz, RN, PhD
Assistant Professor
Family & Community Nursing
School of Nursing
University of Portland (Ore.)

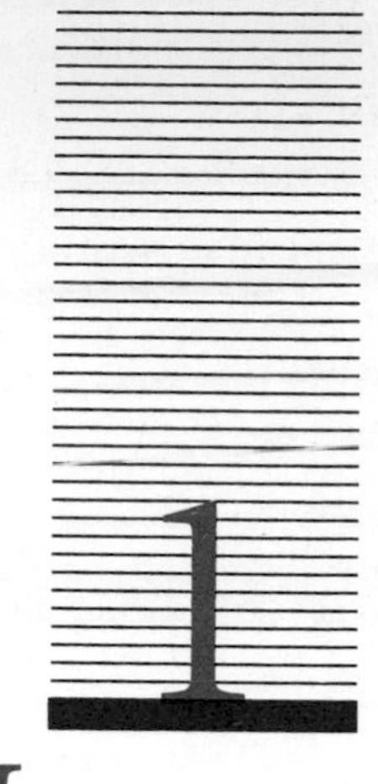

1 Health history

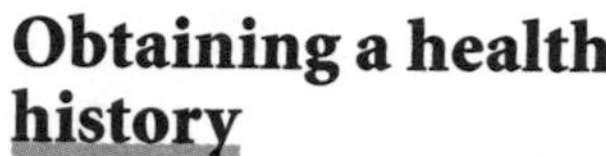

Obtaining a health history

Obtaining a health history and performing a physical assessment are the essential steps of the assessment process. Although these steps can be time-consuming, it's important to complete them accurately and thoroughly. Doing so will help you uncover significant problems and establish an appropriate care plan for your patient.

The health history organizes physiologic, psychological, cultural, and psychosocial information. It relates to the patient's current health status and accounts for such influences as lifestyle, family relationships, and cultural influences. This chapter will tell you what you need to know to get the most out of an assessment interview and what to look for when collecting health history data.

Preparing to take the history

Before beginning the assessment interview, take time to self-reflect, review the patient's chart, and set goals.

Self-reflecting

Health care providers have the unique opportunity to develop relationships with people from a broad spectrum of ages, classes, races, and ethnicities. It can be challenging at times to be respectful of individual differences. Self-reflection can help to deepen your own personal awareness and allow you to be open to these differences.

Reviewing the chart

Before speaking with the patient, review his medical chart. This will allow you to gather information and develop ideas of what to focus on during your interview. Remember, however, that data may not be complete and

CONSIDERING COMMUNICATION BARRIERS

This diagram shows the components of health care provider-patient communication. Note the influences that affect communication, such as orientation, preconceptions, and language. To avoid communication barriers, your sensitivity to these influences can make the difference between effective and ineffective communication with your patient.

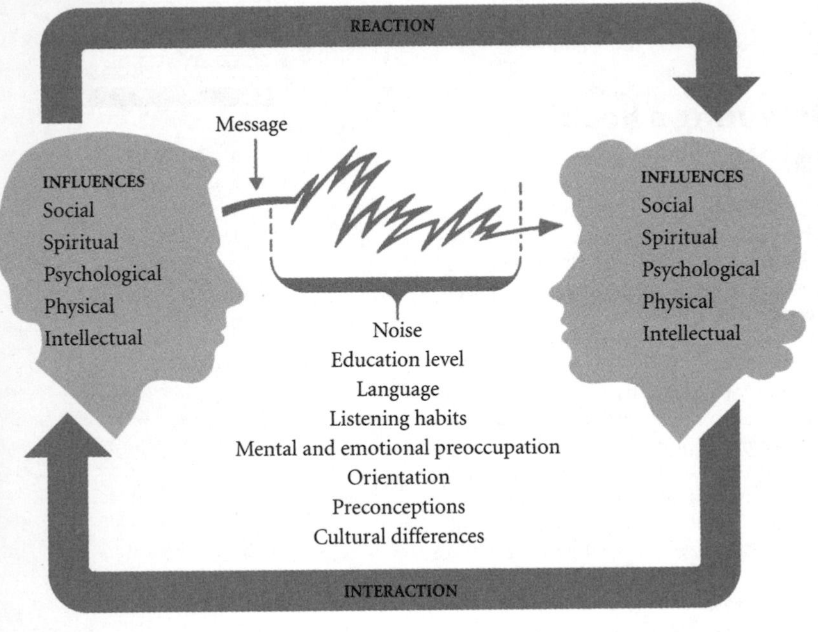

that information comes from different observers. Don't let the chart prevent you from developing new ideas or approaches.

Setting goals

Before the interview, clarify and set your own goals. You may need to complete a certain form for insurance purposes, or you may want to validate the information in the patient's medical chart. Your goals will differ from patient to patient. Setting goals before beginning the interview will help you to stay focused and organized.

The accuracy and completeness of the patient's answers largely depend on your skill as an interviewer. Before you start asking questions, review the communication guidelines in the following sections.

Communicating effectively

Effective health interviews require good communication and interpersonal skills. The interview is a dialogue with the patient, not a simple question-and-answer session. An effective communication style helps eliminate mannerisms—yours or the patient's—that may hinder the candid exchange of information. By developing self-awareness and acceptance of different lifestyles, you can overcome barriers to effective communication, such as emotional or cultural biases. (See *Considering communication barriers.*)

Communication skills

Effective interview skills rely on verbal and nonverbal communication. The patient can manipulate conversation to create a desired impression but rarely can manipulate nonverbal communication. Observe his body language for clues to unstated feelings or behaviors. In addition, be aware of your own body language to ensure optimal communication. Your posture, gestures, eye contact, and tone of voice can express interest and understanding. Your appearance also can affect your relationship with the patient. A patient is reassured by a health care provider who's clean, neat, and wearing conservative clothes and a name tag.

Interpersonal skills

Therapeutic use of self is an interpersonal skill that you can use to help the patient in a healing way. Three important techniques enhance therapeutic use of self, including exhibiting empathy, demonstrating acceptance, and giving recognition.

To show empathy, use phrases that address the patient's feelings such as "That must have upset you." To demonstrate acceptance, use neutral statements such as "I hear what you're saying" and "I see." Nonverbal behaviors, such as nodding or making momentary eye contact, also provide encouragement without indicating agreement or disagreement. To give recognition, listen actively to what the patient says, occasionally providing verbal or nonverbal acknowledgment to encourage him to continue speaking.

Clarifying expectations

Personal values and previous experiences with the health care system can affect the patient's health history expectations. Help him clarify expectations, concerns, and questions. If possible, provide answers that appropriately address the patient's misconceptions. A patient may be uncomfortable providing personal information; reassure him that the information is confidential and accessible only to authorized health care professionals.

Taking notes

No one can remember all the details of a health history without taking notes, although you'll remember more as your experience increases. During the interview, write down short phrases, dates, and words, rather than trying to write a narrative. Don't let note taking distract you from the patient, and put down your pen when a sensitive subject is being discussed.

INTERVIEWING TIPS

Before you perform a patient interview, keep these tips in mind:

- Select a quiet, private setting.
- Choose terms carefully and avoid using jargon.
- Use appropriate body language.
- Confirm the patient's statements to avoid misunderstanding.
- Utilize open-ended questions.

Collecting objective and subjective data

An assessment involves collecting two kinds of data: objective and subjective.

Objective data is obtained through observation and is verifiable. For instance, a red, swollen arm in a patient who's complaining of arm pain is an example of data that can be seen and verified by someone other than the patient. Subjective data, on the other hand, can't be verified by anyone other than the patient; it's based solely on the patient's own account — for example, "My head hurts" or "I have trouble sleeping at night."

A health history is used to gather subjective data about the patient and to explore past and present problems. First, ask the patient about his general physical and emotional health, and then ask him questions about specific body systems and structures.

Interviewing the patient

Physical surroundings, psychological atmosphere, interview structure, and questioning style can affect the interview flow and outcome; so can your ability to adopt a communication style to fit each patient's needs and situation. Before asking your first question, you'll need to set the stage, explain what you'll cover during the interview, and establish rapport with the patient. (See *Interviewing tips.*) In addition, take these steps when interviewing a patient:

TYPES OF INTERVIEW QUESTIONS

Interview questions can be characterized as either open-ended or closed.

Open-ended questions

Open-ended questions require the patient to express feelings, opinions, and ideas. They also help you gather more information than can be gathered with closed questions. Open-ended questions encourage a good rapport with your patient because they show that you're interested in what the patient has to say. Examples of such questions include:

- Why did you come to the hospital tonight?
- How would you describe the problems you're having with your breathing?
- What lung problems, if any, do other members of your family have?

Closed questions

Closed questions elicit yes-or-no answers or one- or two-word responses. They limit the development of rapport with your patient. Closed questions can help you "zoom in" on specific points, but they don't provide the patient the opportunity to elaborate. Examples of closed questions include:

- Do you ever get short of breath?
- Are you the only one in your family with lung problems?

- Choose a quiet, private, well-lit interview setting away from distractions. Such a setting will ease interaction between you and the patient. Take time before beginning the interview to make adjustments to the location and seating as needed.
- Make sure that the patient is comfortable. Sit facing him, 3′ to 4′ (1 to 1.5 m) away.
- Introduce yourself, and explain that the purpose of the health history and assessment is to identify the patient's problem and provide information for planning his care.
- Reassure the patient that everything he says will be kept confidential.
- Tell the patient how long the interview will last, and ask him what he expects from the interview. Identifying the patient's concerns and goals at the beginning of the interview will help you to use time effectively and address all of the issues.
- Use touch sparingly. Many people aren't comfortable with strangers hugging, patting, or touching them.
- Assess the patient to see if language barriers exist. For instance, does he speak and understand English?

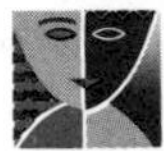

CULTURAL INSIGHT *If the patient doesn't speak English, your facility may have language interpreters you can call on for help. A trained medical interpreter would be ideal, one who's familiar with medical terminology, knows interpreting techniques, and understands patient rights. Simply tell the interpreter to translate the patient's speech verbatim. Avoid using one of the patient's family members or friends as an interpreter. Doing so would violate the patient's right to confidentiality.*

- Assess the patient's hearing ability. Make sure that he can hear you clearly.

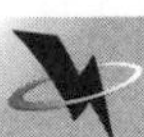

CRITICAL POINT *If your patient is hearing impaired, make sure the interviewing area is well lit and that you face him and speak clearly so that he can read your lips. If needed, have the patient use an assistive device, such as a hearing aid or an amplifier. If the patient uses sign language, you'll need to check with your facility for a sign-language interpreter.*

- Speak slowly and clearly, using easy-to-understand language. Avoid using medical terms and jargon.
- Address the patient by his surname, for example, "Good afternoon, Mr. Jones." Don't call him by his first name unless he asks you to. Avoid using terms of endearment such as "honey" or "sweetie." Treating the patient with respect encourages him to trust you and to provide more accurate and complete information.
- Listen attentively and make eye contact frequently.

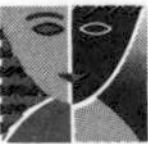

CULTURAL INSIGHT *Remember that the patient's cultural behaviors and beliefs may differ from your*

own. Be aware that people in many cultures — including Native Americans, Asians, and those from Arab-speaking countries — may find eye contact disrespectful or aggressive.

- Use reassuring gestures, such as nodding your head, to encourage the patient to keep talking.
- Watch for nonverbal clues that indicate the patient is uncomfortable or unsure about how to answer a question. For example, he might lower his voice or glance around uneasily.
- Be aware of your own nonverbal behaviors that might cause the patient to clam up or become defensive. For example, if you cross your arms, you might appear closed off from him. If you stand while he's sitting, you might appear superior. If you glance at your watch, you might appear to be bored or rushed, which could keep the patient from answering questions completely.

Asking questions

During the interview, observe the patient closely to see if he understands each question. If he doesn't appear to understand, repeat the question using different words or familiar examples. For instance, instead of asking, "Did you have respiratory difficulty after exercising?" ask, "Did you have to sit down after walking around the block?"

You might also use a different type of question. An open-ended question such as "How did you fall?" lets the patient respond more freely. His response can provide answers to many other questions.

For instance, from the patient's answer, you might learn that he has fallen before, he was unsteady on his feet, and he fell before dinner. Armed with this information, you might deduce that he had a syncopal episode caused by hypoglycemia.

You also can ask closed questions, which are unlikely to provide extra information but might encourage the patient to give clear, concise feedback. (See *Types of interview questions.*)

Using communication strategies

In addition to the steps listed above, some special communication techniques — silence, active listening, adaptive questioning, facilitation, confirmation, reflection, clarification, observation, validation, highlighting transitions, summary, and conclusion — can help you make the most of your patient's assessment interview. Remember, however, that successful techniques in one situation may not be effective in another. Your attitude and the patient's interpretation of your questions can vary. So be sure to individualize your interviewing style for each patient as needed. (See *Establishing effective communication.*)

ESTABLISHING EFFECTIVE COMMUNICATION

Communicating effectively can make or break an interview. Follow these tips:

- Use silence effectively.
- Encourage responses.
- Use repetition and reflection to help clarify meaning.
- Use clarification to make ambiguous information clearer.
- Summarize and conclude with "Is there anything else?"

Silence

Moments of silence during the interview encourage the patient to continue talking and give you a chance to assess his ability to organize thoughts. You may find this technique difficult (most people are uncomfortable with silence), but the more often you use it, the more comfortable you'll become.

Active listening

Active listening involves:

- fully attending to the patient
- being aware of the patient's emotional state
- using verbal and nonverbal communication to encourage the patient to continue to speak.

Active listening takes practice. It's easy to become distracted and begin to think ahead to your next question or something else. You must concentrate and focus your attention on what's being communicated by the patient.

Adaptive questioning

A goal of the interview process is to facilitate the flow of the interview while asking the right questions to add detail to the patient's story. Use the following adaptive questioning techniques to help you do this:

- directed questioning
- questioning to elicit a graded response
- asking a series of questions, one at a time
- offering multiple-choice answers.

Directed questioning should flow from the general to the specific. Directed questions shouldn't be leading questions that require a yes-or-no answer. Examples include:

- "Tell me about your chest pain."
- "Where did you feel it?"
- "Did you feel pain anywhere else?"
- "Where?"

Questions that require a graded response rather than a single answer will allow you to elicit more information from the patient. For example, instead of asking "Do you get short of breath while climbing stairs?" ask "What physical activities make you short of breath?" Also, be sure to ask questions one at a time. When asking "Do you have a history of asthma, hypertension, diabetes, or heart disease?" the patient may become confused. Instead, ask, "Do you have a history of any of the following?" and then list them one at a time, pausing after each problem to give the patient time to think and respond.

Sometimes it's difficult for patients to respond to questions without some guidance. Offer multiple choices in order to limit bias. "Is your pain aching, dull, throbbing, pressing, burning, or what?" This gives the patient an idea of what you're looking for, and gives permission to describe the pain in his own words.

Facilitation

Facilitation encourages the patient to continue with his story. Using such phrases as "please continue," "go on," or even "uh-huh" shows him that you're interested in what he's saying. Leaning forward and maintaining eye contact are also examples of facilitation.

Confirmation

Confirmation ensures that both you and the patient are on the same track. You might say, "If I understand you correctly, you said. . . ," and then repeat the information the patient gave. This technique helps to clear up misconceptions you or the patient might have.

Reflection

Reflection — repeating something that the patient has just said — can help you obtain more specific information. For example, a patient with a stomachache might say, "I know I have an ulcer." You might repeat, "You know you have an ulcer?" And the patient might then say, "Yes. I had one before and the pain is the same."

When appropriate, give him an opportunity to reconsider a response and to add information. For example, if the patient says he has provided complete information about his meals, a question that encourages reflection is, "Do you think you've covered all the important things about your nutrition?"

Stating what's implied or unspoken sometimes helps interpret a patient's statement accurately or yields additional insight into the patient's symptoms or concerns. Start by asking, "What events led to this?"

Clarification

Clarification is used to clear up confusing, vague, or misunderstood information. For example, if your patient says, "I can't stand this," your response might be, "What can't you stand?" or "What do you mean by 'I can't stand this?'" This gives the patient an opportunity to explain his statement.

Observation

Observe the patient to interpret and validate nonverbal behavior. For example, the statement, "I notice that you're rubbing your eyes a lot. Do they bother you?" may lead to a discussion of other health concerns.

Validation

Validating the patient's emotional experiences will make him feel accepted and more willing to communicate openly with you. A patient who has been involved in a trauma may experience distress even if no physical injuries occurred. Stating "A car accident can remind us of our own mortality. That must have been scary for you." helps the patient feel that his emotions are legitimate.

Utilizing transitions

Be sure to tell the patient when you're changing directions during the interview. It allows the patient to feel more in control. Use transitional phrases such as "Now I'd like to ask you some questions about your family history." Make clear what the patient should expect or do next.

Summarization

Summarizing is restating the information the patient gave you. It ensures that the data you've collected is accurate and complete. Summarizing also signals that the interview is about to end. You can also use summarization at different points in the interview to structure the interview and aid with transitions. It also allows you to organize your thinking and convey it to the patient. This technique adds to a more collaborative relationship.

Conclusion

Signaling the patient that you're ready to conclude the interview provides him the opportunity to gather his thoughts and make any final statements. You can do this verbally by saying, "I think I have all the information I need now. Is there anything you'd like to add?"

Techniques to avoid

Some interview techniques create communication problems between the health care provider and the patient. Techniques to avoid include asking "why" or "how" questions, asking probing or persistent questions, using inappropriate language, giving advice, giving false reassurance, and changing the subject or interrupting. Also avoid using clichés or stereotyped responses, giving excessive approval or agreement, jumping to conclusions, and using defensive responses.

Specific questions to ask

Asking the right questions is a critical part of an interview. Be sure to routinely document the date and time that the interview is occurring. To obtain a complete health history, gather information by asking questions from each of the following categories, in sequence:

1. biographic data
2. chief complaint
3. medical history
4. family history
5. psychosocial history
6. activities of daily living (ADLs).

Biographic data

Begin the health history by obtaining biographic information from the patient. Do this first before you become involved in details of the patient's health. Ask the patient for his name, address, telephone number, birth date, age, marital status, religion, and nationality. Find out whom he lives with and the name and telephone number of a person to contact in case of an emergency.

Also ask the patient about his health care, including who his primary health care provider is and how he gets to the health care provider's office. Ask if he has ever been treated before for his present problem. Ask if he has an advance directive in place. (See *Understanding an advance directive,* page 8.)

Your patient's answers to basic questions can provide important clues about his personality, medical problems, and reliability. If he can't give accurate information, ask him for the name of a relative or friend who can. Document who gave you the information. Also document if the use of an interpreter was necessary.

Chief complaint

Try to pinpoint why the patient is seeking health care at this time. Document this information in the patient's exact words to avoid misinterpretation. Ask how and when the symptoms developed, what led the patient to seek medical attention, and how the problem has affected his life and ability to function.

To ensure you don't omit pertinent data, use the PQRSTU mnemonic device, which provides a systematic approach to obtaining information. (See *Using the PQRSTU device,* page 9.)

The patient may present for health maintenance assessment, health counseling, or health education. In this case, ask the patient about recent minor illnesses or health concerns.

Medical history

Ask the patient about current and past medical problems, such as hypertension, dia-

UNDERSTANDING AN ADVANCE DIRECTIVE

The Patient Self-Determination Act allows a patient to prepare an advance directive — a written document that states his wishes regarding health care in the event he becomes incapacitated or incompetent to make decisions. Elderly patients in particular may be interested in an advance directive because they tend to be concerned with end-of-life issues.

Providing direction

If a patient doesn't have an advance directive in place, your health care facility must provide him with information about it and how to establish one.

An advance directive may include:

- the name of the person authorized by the patient to make medical decisions if the patient can no longer do so
- specific medical treatment the patient wants or doesn't want
- instructions regarding pain medication and comfort; specifically, whether the patient wishes to receive certain treatment even if it may hasten his death
- information the patient wants to relay to his loved ones
- name of the patient's primary health care provider
- any other wishes.

betes, or back pain. Typical questions include:

- Are you allergic to anything in the environment or to any medications or foods? If so, what kind of allergic reaction do you have?
- Are you taking medications, including over-the-counter preparations, such as aspirin, vitamins, and cough syrup? If so, how much do you take and how often do you take it? Do you use home remedies such as homemade ointments? Do you use herbal preparations or take dietary supplements? Do you use other alternative therapies, such as acupuncture, therapeutic massage, or chiropractic therapy?
- Are you under treatment for any problem? If so, for what reason?
- Have you ever been hospitalized? If so, when and for what reason?
- What childhood illnesses did you have? Did you receive all of your childhood immunizations?
- Have you ever had surgery? If so, when and for what reason?

Family history

Questioning the patient about his family's health is a good way to uncover his risk of having certain illnesses. Some diseases may be genetically linked, such as cardiovascular disease, alcoholism, depression, and cancer. Others, such as hemophilia, cystic fibrosis, sickle cell anemia, and Tay-Sachs disease are genetically transmitted. Typical questions include:

- Are your mother, father, and siblings living? If not, how old were they when they died? What was the cause of death?
- If they're alive, do they have diabetes, high blood pressure, heart disease, asthma, cancer, sickle cell anemia, hemophilia, cataracts, glaucoma, or any other illnesses?

Use a genogram to organize your patient's family data. (See *Developing a genogram,* page 10.)

Psychosocial history

Find out how the patient feels about himself, his place in society, and his relationships with others. Ask about his occupation (past and present), education, economic status, and responsibilities. Typical questions include:

- How have you coped with medical or emotional crises in the past? (See *Asking about abuse,* page 11.)
- Has your life changed recently? What changes in your personality or behavior have you noticed?
- How adequate is the emotional support you receive from family and friends?
- How often do you exercise? What types of activities do you do to exercise? Do you walk, use a stationary bike, or lift weights? How often do you eat a healthful diet?

EXPERT TECHNIQUE

USING THE PQRSTU DEVICE

Use the PQRSTU mnemonic device to fully explore your patient's chief complaint. When you ask the questions below, encourage him to describe his symptoms in greater detail.

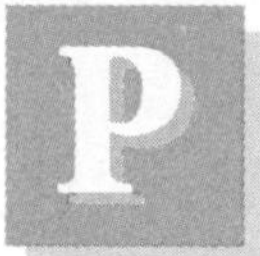

Provocative or palliative
- What provokes or relieves the symptom?
- Do stress, anger, certain physical positions, or other events trigger the symptom?
- What makes the symptom worsen or subside?

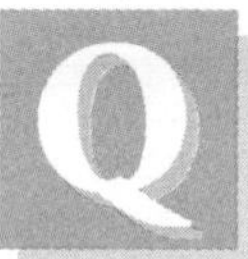

Quality or quantity
- What does the symptom feel, look, or sound like?
- Are you having the symptom right now? If so, is it more or less severe than usual?
- To what degree does the symptom affect your normal activities?

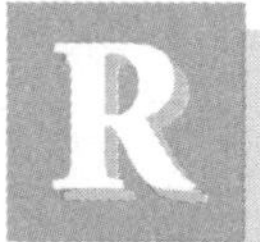

Region or radiation
- Where in the body does the symptom occur?
- Does the symptom appear in other regions? If so, where?

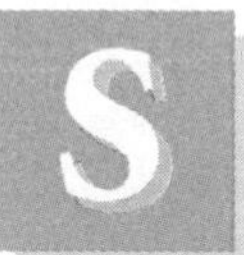

Severity
- How severe is the symptom? How would you rate it on a scale of 1 to 10, with 10 being the most severe?
- Does the symptom seem to be diminishing, intensifying, or staying about the same?

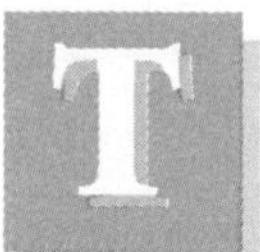

Timing
- When did the symptom begin?
- Was the onset sudden or gradual?
- How often does the symptom occur?
- How long does the symptom last?

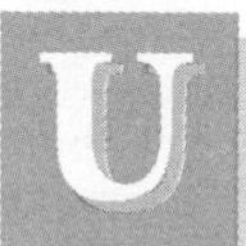

Understanding
- What do you think caused the symptom?
- How do you feel about the symptom? Do you have fears associated with it?
- How is the symptom affecting your life?
- What are your expectations of the health care team?

- How close do you live to health care facilities, and can you get to them easily?
- Do you have health insurance?
- Are you on a fixed income with no extra money for health care?

Stress level. Emotional, social, and physical demands on the body cause stress. The amount of stress the patient experiences affects physiologic and psychological health. These questions can help assess stress and coping strategies:

DEVELOPING A GENOGRAM

A genogram provides a visual family health summary. It includes the patient and his spouse, children, and parents. To develop a genogram, first draw the relationships of family members to the patient, as shown in the diagram below. Then fill in the ages of living members, noting deceased members and the ages at which they died. Also, record diseases that have a familial tendency (such as Huntington's disease) or an environmental cause (such as lung cancer from exposure to coal tar).

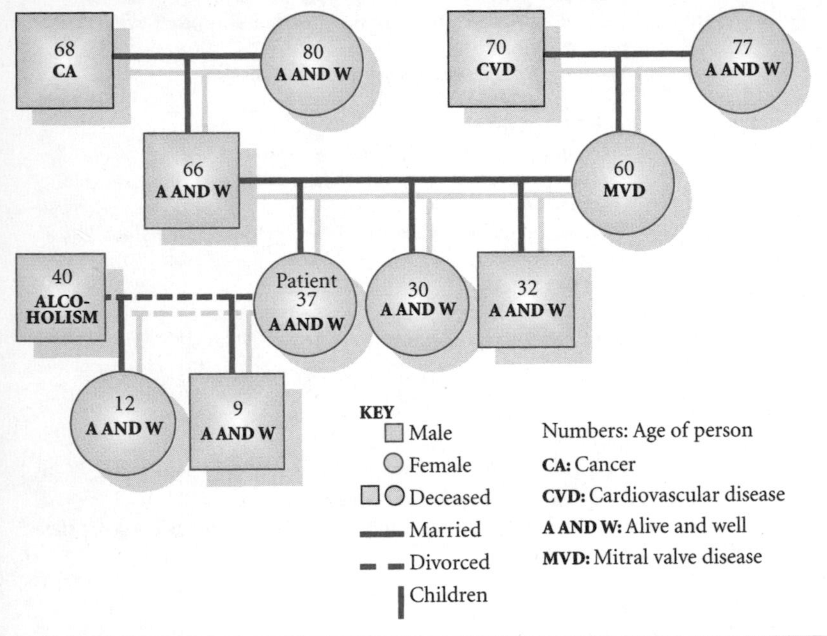

- How do you know when you're feeling stressed?
- What situations are stressful to you?
- How do you respond physically to stress? For example, do you sweat, get butterflies in your stomach, develop a headache, or become nauseated?
- What do you do when you're feeling stressed?
- Does stress ever affect your family relationships or your work? If so, how?
- What stresses have you experienced during the past year?
- How did you deal with these stresses?
- Did these stresses cause significant changes for you?
- Do you think stress affects your health?

ADLs

Find out what's normal for the patient by asking him to describe his typical day. Areas to include in your assessment are diet and elimination; exercise and sleep; work and leisure; use of tobacco, alcohol, and other drugs; and religious observances.

Diet and elimination. Ask the patient about his appetite, special diets, and food allergies. Can he afford to buy enough food? Who cooks and shops at his house? Ask about the frequency of bowel movements and laxative use.

Exercise and sleep. Ask the patient if he has a special exercise program and, if so, why?

Have him describe it. What activities does he perform and for how long? Is he satisfied with his current activity and exercise levels? Ask how many hours he sleeps at night, what his sleep pattern is like, and whether he feels rested after sleep. Ask him if he has any difficulties with sleep.

Work and leisure. Ask the patient what he does for a living and how many hours he spends working. Ask him what he does during his leisure time. Does he have hobbies?

Use of tobacco, alcohol, and other drugs. Ask the patient if he smokes cigarettes. Also, inquire about use of other forms of tobacco, such as pipes, cigars, and chewing tobacco. How much tobacco does he consume daily? How long has he used tobacco? Does he drink alcohol? If so, what kind and how much each day? How long has he consumed alcohol? Ask if he uses illicit drugs, such as marijuana or cocaine. If so, how often?

Be aware that patients may understate the amount they drink because of embarrassment. If you're having trouble getting what you believe are honest answers to such questions, you might try overestimating the amount. For example, you might say, "You told me you drink beer. Do you drink about a six-pack per day?" The patient's response might be, "No, I drink about half that."

Religious observances. Ask the patient if he has religious beliefs that affect diet, dress, or health practices. Patients will feel reassured when you make it clear that you understand these points.

ASKING ABOUT ABUSE

Abuse is a sensitive subject. Anyone can be a victim of abuse: a boyfriend or girlfriend, a spouse, an elderly patient, a child, or a parent. Also, abuse can come in many forms: physical, psychological, emotional, and sexual. When taking a patient's health history, ask two open-ended questions: When do you feel safe at home? When don't you feel safe?

Observe the reaction

Even when you don't immediately suspect an abusive situation, be aware of how your patient reacts to these open-ended questions. Is the patient defensive, hostile, confused, or frightened? Assess how he interacts with you and others. Does he seem withdrawn or frightened or show other inappropriate behavior? Keep his reactions in mind while you perform the physical assessment.

Remember, if the patient reports abuse of any kind to you, you're a mandated reporter. Inform the patient that you're obligated to report the abuse to the appropriate authorities.

Adapting to specific situations

Your skills at handling difficult interviews will evolve throughout your professional career. The following patient situations may be especially challenging.

The silent patient

Periods of silence may be uncomfortable, especially for the novice interviewer. Try not to feel obligated to keep the conversation going. Silence has many meanings and purposes. It allows the patient to collect thoughts, remember details, and decide whether he would like to discuss certain information with you. You should appear attentive and give encouragement when appropriate. Watch the patient closely for nonverbal cues.

Silence could be a response to your approach to asking questions. Could the patient be overwhelmed or even offended? Ask the patient directly if something is wrong by saying, "Have I done something to upset you?"

Some patients are just naturally quiet. Be accepting and ask the patient for other ways that you can gather the necessary information. Perhaps he'll give you permission to talk with family or friends or access other sources of information.

The talkative patient

The patient who rambles can be just as difficult. You typically have limited time to conduct the interview and need to gather much information during that time. Several techniques can be helpful in this situation.

Give the patient 5 to 10 minutes of free rein and listen closely to what he says. What clues is the patient giving you? Perhaps he has lacked a good listener in the past and is expressing pent-up concerns. Does he seem anxious or display disorganized thought processes?

Try to focus on what seems most important to the patient. Show your interest in those areas. Interrupt if needed, but do so courteously. It's acceptable to be direct and set limits if needed. Use the techniques of transitioning and summarization to help you do this.

If possible, set up a time for a second interview. Say "I know we have much more to talk about. Can you come in again next week?"

The anxious patient

Anxiety is an emotion commonly experienced during sickness, treatment, or in reaction to the health care system itself. Watch for verbal and nonverbal clues of anxiety. These may include:

- sitting tensely
- fidgeting
- sighing frequently
- licking lips
- sweating
- trembling
- silence.

When you detect anxiety, express your impressions to the patient, and encourage him to talk about any underlying concerns. Be cautious not to transmit your own anxiety about completing the interview.

The crying patient

Crying is usually therapeutic and can signal strong emotions, such as sadness, anger, or frustration. Allow the patient to cry and respond with empathy. If the patient is on the verge of tears, pausing or gentle probing may give the signal that it's okay to cry. Offer a tissue and wait while the patient composes himself. Use supportive remarks, such as "I'm glad you got that out," to put the patient at ease. It's unusual for crying to escalate and become uncontrollable.

The confusing patient

Patients with multiple symptoms can add confusion to the interview. Focus on the meaning or the function of the symptoms and guide the interview appropriately.

In some instances, you may become confused by the patient. This may occur if the history is vague and difficult to understand, if language is hard to follow, or ideas are poorly related to one another. Use appropriate communication strategies to get the information you're looking for.

If you suspect a psychiatric or neurologic disorder, don't spend too much time trying to get a detailed history. Shift to the mental status examination and focus on level of consciousness, orientation, and memory.

The angry patient

Encounters with an angry or hostile patient occur occasionally. To maintain control of the interview, don't waste time or energy arguing with the patient or feeling insulted. Rather, listen without showing disapproval. Try to relax. Speak in a firm, quiet voice, and use short sentences. A composed, unobtrusive, and nonthreatening manner usually soothes the patient. However, if this technique fails, postpone the interview and, if necessary, call for assistance.

The patient with a language barrier

When the patient speaks a different language, make every attempt to get an interpreter. The ideal interpreter is an objective person who's familiar with the language and culture of the patient. Beware of using family members or friends as interpreters; confidentiality may be violated or meanings may be distorted.

Establish a rapport with the interpreter, and review what information would be most useful. Tell the interpreter that you need her to interpret exactly what you're saying. Seat the interpreter next to you and allow the patient to establish a rapport with her as well. Address the patient directly and keep sentences short and simple. Be patient and allow more time for this type of interview.

The patient with difficulty reading

Always assess the patient's reading ability before giving written instructions. Ask "I understand this may be difficult for you to discuss, but do you have problems reading?" Respond sensitively and remember that illiteracy isn't synonymous with lack of intelligence.

The patient with impaired hearing

Communicating with a hearing-impaired patient presents many of the same challenges as communicating with those who speak a different language. Ask the patient what his preferred method of communication is. If he prefers sign language, make every effort to find an interpreter.

If the patient can read lips, follow these guidelines:

- face him directly, in good light
- speak at a normal tone and rate
- don't let your voice trail off at the ends of sentences
- avoid covering your mouth or looking down
- have him repeat what you said back to you.

If the patient has unilateral hearing loss, sit on his hearing side. If he has a hearing aid, make sure he's using it and that it's functioning properly. Eliminate background noise as much as possible. Supplement instructions with written copies.

The patient with impaired vision

Use the following suggestions, when interviewing a blind patient:

- shake hands to establish contact
- explain who you are and why you're there
- orient him to the room and tell him if anyone else is present
- remember to respond with words because postures and gestures are unseen.

Maintaining a professional outlook

Don't let your personal opinions interfere with your assessment. Maintain a professional, neutral approach and don't offer advice. For example, don't suggest that the patient enter a drug rehabilitation program. That type of response puts him on the defensive and may make him reluctant to answer subsequent questions honestly.

Also, avoid making statements such as, "I know what's best for you." This type of statement makes the patient feel inferior and breaks down communication. Finally, don't use leading questions such as "You don't do drugs, do you?" to get the answer you're looking for. This type of question, based on your own value system, will make the patient feel guilty and might prevent him from responding honestly.

Reviewing body structures and systems

The last part of the health history is a systematic assessment of the patient's body structures and systems. Always start at the top of the head and work your way down the body. This avoids skipping any areas. When questioning an elderly patient, remember that he may have difficulty hearing or communicating.

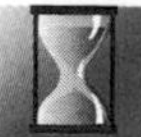

AGE ISSUE *An elderly patient might have sensory or memory impairment or a decreased attention span. If your patient is confused or has trouble communicating, you may need to rely on a family member for some or all of the health history.*

Asking the right questions

Information gained from a health history forms the basis for your care plan and enables you to distinguish physical changes and devise a holistic approach to treatment. As with other nursing skills, the only way you can improve your interviewing technique is with practice, practice, and more practice. (See *Evaluating a symptom,* pages 14 and 15.)

Body structure

Here are some key questions to ask your patient about each body structure.

General health. What's your usual weight? Have you noticed that your clothes fit more loosely or tightly than usual? Do you suffer from excessive fatigue? How many colds or other minor illnesses do you have each year? Do you ever have unexplained episodes of fever, weakness, or night sweats? Do you ever have trouble carrying out ADLs?

Skin, hair, and nails. Do you have any known skin diseases such as psoriasis? Do you have rashes, scars, sores, or ulcers? Do you have any skin growths, such as warts, moles, tumors, or masses? Do you experience skin reactions to hot or cold weather?

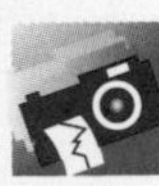

CLINICAL PICTURE

EVALUATING A SYMPTOM

In the following interview situation, the patient is vague in describing his chief complaint. Using your interviewing skills, you discover his problem is related to abdominal distention. Now what? This flowchart will help you decide what to do next, using abdominal distention as the patient's chief complaint.

Ask the patient to identify the symptom that's bothering him. He tells you, "My stomach gets bloated."

↓

Form a first impression. Does the patient's condition alert you to an emergency? For example, does he say the bloating developed suddenly? Does he mention that other signs or symptoms occur with it, such as sweating or light-headedness? (Both are indicators of hypovolemia.)

YES ↓

Take a brief health history to gather more clues. For example, ask the patient if he has severe abdominal pain or difficulty breathing or if he ever had an abdominal injury.

↓

Perform a focused physical examination to quickly determine the severity of the patient's condition. Check for bruising, lacerations, changes in bowel sounds, or abdominal rigidity.

↓

Evaluate your findings. Are emergency signs or symptoms present, such as abdominal rigidity or abnormal bowel sounds?

YES ↓

Based on your findings, intervene appropriately to stabilize the patient. Immediately notify the health care provider, place the patient in a supine position, administer oxygen, and start an I.V. line. GI or nasogastric tube insertion and emergency surgery may be needed.

↓

After the patient's condition is stabilized, review your findings to consider possible causes, such as trauma, large-bowel obstruction, mesenteric artery occlusion, or peritonitis.

NO ↓

Review your findings to consider possible causes, such as cancer, bladder distention, cirrhosis, heart failure, or gastric dilation.

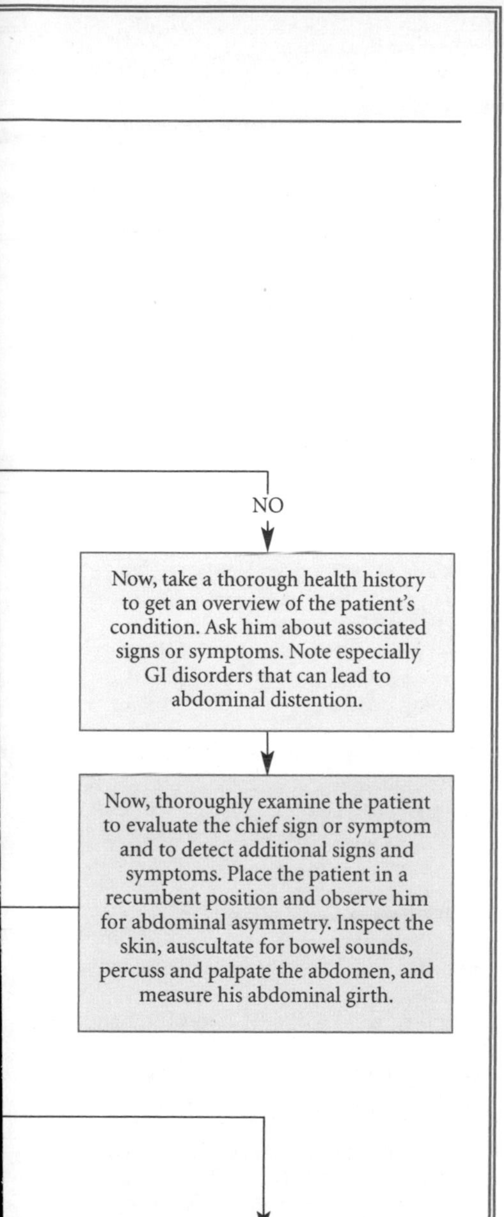

NO

Now, take a thorough health history to get an overview of the patient's condition. Ask him about associated signs or symptoms. Note especially GI disorders that can lead to abdominal distention.

Now, thoroughly examine the patient to evaluate the chief sign or symptom and to detect additional signs and symptoms. Place the patient in a recumbent position and observe him for abdominal asymmetry. Inspect the skin, auscultate for bowel sounds, percuss and palpate the abdomen, and measure his abdominal girth.

Evaluate your findings and devise an appropriate care plan. Position the patient comfortably, administer analgesics, and prepare him for diagnostic tests.

Have you noticed any changes in the amount, texture, or character of your hair? Have you noticed any changes in your nails? Do you have excessive nail splitting, cracking, or breaking?

Head. Do you get headaches? If so, where are they and how painful are they? How often do they occur, and how long do they last? What triggers them, and how do you relieve them? Have you ever had a head injury? If so, how and when did it occur? Do you have lumps or bumps on your head?

Eyes, ears, and nose. When was your last eye examination? Do you wear glasses? Do you have glaucoma, cataracts, or color blindness? Does light bother your eyes? Do you have excessive tearing; blurred vision; double vision; or dry, itchy, burning, inflamed, or swollen eyes?

Do you have loss of balance, ringing in your ears, deafness, or poor hearing? Have you ever had ear surgery? If so, why and when? Do you wear a hearing aid? Are you having pain, swelling, or discharge from your ears? If so, has this problem occurred before and how frequently?

Have you ever had nasal surgery? If so, why and when? Have you ever had sinusitis or nosebleeds? Do you have nasal problems that cause breathing difficulties, frequent sneezing, or discharge or that impair your ability to smell?

Mouth and throat. Do you have mouth sores, a dry mouth, loss of taste, a toothache, or bleeding gums? Do you wear dentures and, if so, do they fit well?

Do you have a sore throat, fever, or chills? How often do you get a sore throat, and have you seen a health care provider for this?

Do you have difficulty swallowing? If so, is the problem with solid foods or liquids? Is it a constant problem, or does it accompany a sore throat or another problem? What, if anything, makes it go away?

Neck. Do you have swelling, soreness, lack of movement, stiffness, or pain in your neck? If so, did something specific cause it to happen such as too much exercise? How long have you had this symptom? Does anything relieve it or aggravate it?

ASSESSING SEVERELY ILL PATIENTS

When the patient's condition doesn't allow for a full assessment—for instance, if he's in severe pain—get as much information as possible from other sources. With severely ill patients, keep these key points in mind:

- Identify yourself to the patient and his family.
- Stay calm to gain their confidence and allay anxiety.
- Pay close attention to revealing information. For example, if a patient seeks help for a ringing in his ears, don't overlook his casual mention of a periodic "racing heartbeat."
- Avoid making quick conclusions. Don't assume the patient's chief complaint is related to his admitting diagnosis. Use a systematic approach, and collect the appropriate information; then draw your own conclusions.

Body systems

Here are some key questions to ask your patient about each body system. For techniques to use when examining patients with severe illnesses, see *Assessing severely ill patients.*

Respiratory system. Do you have shortness of breath on exertion or while lying in bed? How many pillows do you use at night? Does breathing cause pain or wheezing? Do you have a productive cough? If so, do you cough up blood-tinged sputum? Do you have night sweats?

Have you ever been treated for pneumonia, asthma, emphysema, or frequent respiratory tract infections? Have you ever had a chest X-ray or tuberculin skin test? If so, when and what were the results?

Cardiovascular system. Do you have chest pain, palpitations, irregular heartbeat, fast heartbeat, shortness of breath, or a persistent cough? Have you ever had an electrocardiogram? If so, when?

Do you have high blood pressure, peripheral vascular disease, swelling of the ankles and hands, varicose veins, cold extremities, or intermittent pain in your legs?

Breasts. Ask your female patients these questions: Do you perform monthly breast self-examinations? Have you noticed a lump, a change in breast contour, breast pain, or discharge from your nipples? Have you ever had breast cancer? If not, has anyone else in your family had it? Have you ever had a mammogram? When and what were the results?

Ask your male patients these questions: Do you have pain in your breast tissue? Have you noticed lumps or a change in contour?

GI system. Have you had nausea, vomiting, loss of appetite, heartburn, abdominal pain, frequent belching, or passing of gas? Have you lost or gained weight recently? How often do you have a bowel movement, and what color, odor, and consistency are your stools? Have you noticed a change in your regular elimination pattern? Do you use laxatives frequently?

Have you had hemorrhoids, rectal bleeding, hernias, gallbladder disease, or liver disease?

Urinary system. Do you have urinary problems, such as burning during urination, incontinence, urgency, retention, reduced urinary flow, and dribbling? Do you get up during the night to urinate? If so, how many times? What color is your urine? Have you ever noticed blood in it? Have you ever been treated for kidney stones?

Reproductive system. Ask your female patients these questions: How old were you when you started menstruating? How often do you get your periods, and how many days do they usually last? Do you have pain or pass blood clots? If you're postmenopausal, at what age did you stop menstruating? If you're in the transitional stage, what perimenopausal symptoms are you experiencing? Have you ever been pregnant? If so, how many times? What was the method of delivery? How many pregnancies resulted in live births? How many resulted in miscarriages? Have you had an abortion?

What's your method of birth control? Are you involved in a long-term, monogamous relationship? Have you had frequent vaginal infections or a sexually transmitted disease? When was your last gynecologic examination and Papanicolaou test? What were the results?

Ask your male patients these questions: Do you perform monthly testicular self-examinations? Have you ever had a prostate examination and, if so, when? Have you noticed penile pain, discharge, or lesions or testicular lumps? Which form of birth control do you use? Have you had a vasectomy? Are you involved in a long-term, monogamous relationship? Have you ever had a sexually transmitted disease?

Musculoskeletal system. Do you have difficulty walking, sitting, or standing? Are you steady on your feet, or do you lose your balance easily? Do you have arthritis, gout, a back injury, muscle weakness, or paralysis?

Neurologic system. Have you ever had seizures? Do you ever experience tremors, twitching, numbness, tingling, or loss of sensation in a part of your body? Are you less able to get around than you think you should be?

Endocrine system. Have you been unusually tired lately? Do you feel hungry or thirsty more often than usual? Have you lost weight for unexplained reasons? How well can you tolerate heat or cold? Have you noticed changes in your hair texture or color? Have you been losing hair? Do you take hormone medications?

Hematologic system. Have you ever been diagnosed with anemia or blood abnormalities? Do you bruise easily or become fatigued quickly? Have you ever had a blood transfusion? If so, did you have any reaction to it?

Emotional status. Do you ever experience mood swings or memory loss? Do you ever feel anxious, depressed, or unable to concentrate? Are you feeling unusually stressed? Do you ever feel unable to cope?

After you've obtained the health history, you're ready to move on to the next essential step in the assessment process — performing the physical assessment.

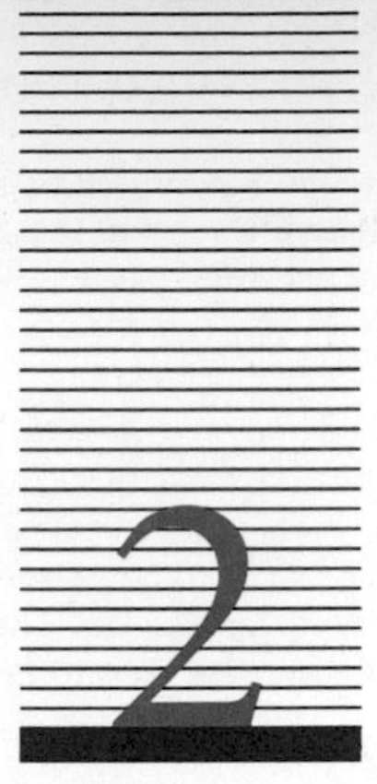

Fundamental physical assessment techniques

Looking at physical assessment

After you've taken the patient's health history, proceed to the hands-on part of the assessment. During the physical assessment, you'll use all of your senses and a systematic approach to collect information about your patient's health. A complete physical examination — appropriate for periodic health checks — includes a general survey, vital sign measurements, height and weight measurements, and assessment of all organs and body systems. At times, a modified physical examination, based on the patient's history and complaints, may be warranted.

As you proceed through the physical examination, you also can teach your patient about his body. For instance, you can explain how to do a testicular self-examination or why the patient should monitor the appearance of a mole.

More than any other skill, successful assessment requires critical thinking. How does one finding fit in with the big picture? An initial assessment will help guide your entire care plan.

Preparing for the examination

Take the time to prepare for the examination before you begin. Think about how you'll approach the patient, your demeanor, and how you'll make the patient comfortable. Make sure you wash your hands and that you do this in front of the patient — it's a subtle way to show concern for his welfare.

Approaching the patient

When first examining a patient, feelings of anxiety are inevitable. Let the patient know if you're new at doing physical assessments and try to appear calm, competent, and organized. You may need to go back and assess certain parts of the interview that you may have forgotten. This isn't uncommon. Even though you may be performing certain steps out of order, try to do so smoothly, without causing too much discomfort to the patient.

If you're a beginner at physical assessments, certain tasks may take you longer than experienced clinicians. Explain to the patient ahead of time if you anticipate taking a long time for certain aspects of the examination. State "I'll be spending a little extra time listening to your lungs, but this doesn't mean that I hear anything wrong."

Over time, as you become more comfortable performing physical assessments, you'll become quicker and more efficient. You may begin sharing your findings with the patient as you go along. Be selective, however, of what you share. You may want to finish your complete assessment before making any conclusions. If you find an unexpected abnormality, such as a suspicious lesion or a wound, avoid showing alarm or other negative reaction.

Conducting a complete examination

How complete should your assessment be? This question has no definitive answer. As a rule, a new patient should always have a complete physical examination, regardless of his chief complaint or the type of setting in which you practice. A more limited or problem-focused assessment may be appropriate for the patient requiring urgent care or a patient you know well.

A comprehensive physical examination is more than an assessment of body systems. It also:

- provides a source of knowledge about the patient
- helps to identify or rule out physical cause for the patient's concerns
- serves as a baseline for future comparisons
- allows for important opportunities for health promotion
- increases the credibility of your reassurance and advice.

Scope of the examination. If you'll be performing a focused examination, choose the methods for assessing the problem carefully. The scope of your examination should be determined by:

- the patient's symptoms
- the patient's age
- the patient's health history
- your knowledge of disease patterns.

For example, if a patient presents with a sore throat, you'll need to decide if he needs careful palpation of the liver and spleen to assess for mononucleosis or if he has a cold and this examination isn't necessary.

Periodic physical assessment for screening and prevention is recommended for several areas. These include:

- blood pressure measurement
- cardiac assessment
- breast examination
- assessment for splenic and hepatic enlargement
- pelvic examination with a Papanicolaou test.

Planning logistics

The physical examination sequence should be planned to maximize patient comfort, avoid frequent position changes, and enhance your efficiency. As a rule, move from "head to toe." (See *Suggested physical examination sequence,* page 20.)

It's recommended that you perform the physical assessment while standing at the patient's right side and moving to different positions as necessary. This technique has several advantages compared with the left side:

- It's more reliable to assess jugular vein distention from the right.
- The palpating hand rests easier on the apical impulse.
- The right kidney can be palpated more easily than the left kidney.

Adjusting the environment

The reliability of your assessment depends on several factors, including your comfort, lighting, and noise. Take the time to adjust the examination area for your comfort. Raise the bed or table, if needed, being sure to lower it again at the end of the examination. You may need to ask the patient to move closer to you at times to make it easier for you to reach certain areas of the body. Awkward positions will impair the quality of your assessments.

SUGGESTED PHYSICAL EXAMINATION SEQUENCE

You'll develop your own personal sequence for physical assessments as you gain more experience. Use the suggested sequence below as a guide.

With the patient in the sitting position:

- General survey
- Vital signs
- Skin of upper torso (anterior and posterior)
- Head and neck, including thyroid and lymph nodes
- Mental status, cranial nerves, upper extremity strength and tone, cerebellar function
- Thorax and lungs
- Breasts
- Musculoskeletal assessment of upper extremities

With the patient in the supine position, with the head of the bed raised 30 degrees, and then turned to left side:

- Cardiovascular assessment

With the patient sitting, leaning forward:

- Cardiovascular assessment (for murmur of aortic insufficiency)

With the patient lying supine:

- Thorax and lungs
- Breasts and axillae
- Abdomen
- Peripheral vascular and skin of the lower extremities and lower torso
- Lower extremity strength and tone, reflexes

With the patient sitting or standing:

- Gait
- Musculoskeletal examination

With the patient in the lithotomy position:

- Pelvic and rectal examinations (women)

With the patient supine and turned to left side:

- Prostate and rectal examinations (men)

Good lighting is important for the inspection aspect of your assessment. When a light source is perpendicular to the patient, shadows are minimized and subtle changes in the surface you're examining may be lost. Tangential lighting casts light across the surfaces of the body and will make contours, elevations, and depressions easier and sharper to visualize. Using tangential lighting for evaluating the jugular venous pulse, the thyroid gland, and the apical impulse is optimal.

A quiet environment is vital during the assessment. Background noise can interfere with auscultation and can be distracting throughout the examination. Try to adjust the environment as best you can. Ask those nearby to lower the volume on their televisions or radios or to lower their voices. Be courteous and thank them when the examination is completed.

Promoting comfort

Remain professional during the entire examination and show concern for the patient's privacy and modesty. This will help the patient to feel respected and more at ease. Close doors and curtains before beginning the examination.

You'll learn the methods for draping the patient with a gown or sheet as you assess each of the different organ systems. Indeed, the goal should be to visualize only one area of the body at a time. This preserves the patient's modesty and allows you to better focus on what you're doing. For example, during the abdominal examination, only the abdomen should be exposed. Cover the patient's chest with his gown, and place a sheet or drape over the inguinal area and lower extremities.

Before beginning parts of the assessment that may be awkward or stressful for the patient, briefly tell the patient what you'll be doing. Keep the patient informed as you proceed.

Be clear in your instructions at each step of the examination. Say "I'd like to listen to your heart now. Please lie down." Be sensitive to his feelings and comfort. Assess nonverbal cues such as facial expression. Ask "Are you okay?" Rearrange pillows or blankets as needed for comfort and warmth throughout the assessment.

When you're finished, tell the patient your impressions as appropriate. Tell him what to expect next, whether it will be making a follow-up appointment (for an outpatient), or assessing laboratory values (for an inpatient). Leave the hospitalized patient in a comfortable and safe position, with the bed in the low position and the side rails raised.

Collecting the tools

Generally, for a physical examination, you'll need a thermometer, stethoscope, sphygmomanometer, visual acuity chart, penlight or flashlight, measuring tape and pocket ruler, marking pencil, and a scale.

A complete collection of equipment also will include:

- wooden tongue blade to help assess the gag reflex and reveal the pharynx
- safety pins to test how well a patient differentiates between dull and sharp pain
- cotton balls to check fine-touch sensitivity
- test tubes filled with hot and cold water to assess temperature sensitivity
- common, easily identified substances, such as ground coffee and vanilla extract, to evaluate smell and taste sensations
- a water-soluble lubricant and disposable gloves for rectal and vaginal examinations.

Certain steps in the physical examination may require such equipment as an ophthalmoscope, a nasoscope, an otoscope, and a tuning fork. Other equipment may include a reflex hammer, skin calipers, vaginal speculum, goniometer, and transilluminator.

Performing a general survey

After assembling the necessary equipment, begin the first part of the physical assessment: forming your initial impressions of the patient, preparing him for the assessment, and obtaining his baseline data, including height, weight, and vital signs. This information will direct the rest of your assessment.

During your first contact with the patient, be prepared to receive a steady stream of impressions, mostly visual. The patient's gender, race, and approximate age will be obvious. Because some health concerns may relate to these visual impressions, be sure to note them. Also be sure to note less obvious visual signs that can contribute to an overall impression, including obvious distress; facial characteristics; body type, posture, and movements; speech; dress, grooming, and personal hygiene; and psychological state. (See *Observing the patient,* page 22.)

Preparing the patient

If possible, introduce yourself to the patient before you begin the physical assessment, preferably when he's dressed. Meeting him under less-threatening circumstances will decrease his anxiety when you perform the assessment. (See *Tips for assessment success,* page 22.)

Keep in mind that the patient may be worried that you'll find a problem. He also may consider the assessment an invasion of his privacy because you're observing and touching sensitive, private and, perhaps, painful body areas.

Before you start, briefly explain what you're planning to do, why you're doing it, how long it will take, what position changes it will require, and what equipment you'll use. As you perform the assessment, explain each step in detail. A well-prepared patient won't be surprised or feel unexpected discomfort, so he'll trust you more and cooperate better.

Put your patient at ease but know where to draw the line. Maintain professionalism during the examination. Humor can help put the patient at ease, but make sure you avoid sarcasm and keep jokes in good taste.

When you're finished with your assessment, allow the patient to get dressed. Document your findings in a short, concise paragraph. Include only essential information that communicates your overall impression of the patient. For example, if your patient has a lesion, simply note it now. You'll describe the lesion in detail when you complete the physical assessment.

OBSERVING THE PATIENT

A patient's behavior and appearance can offer subtle clues about his health. Carefully observe him for unusual behavior or signs of illness. Use this mnemonic checklist—SOME TEAMS—to help you remember what to look for.

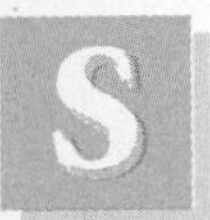

Symmetry—Are his face and body symmetrical?

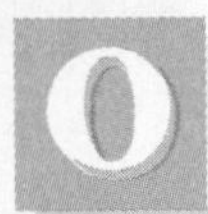

Old—Does he look his age?

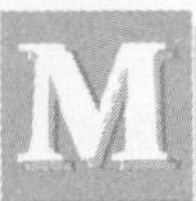

Mental acuity—Is he alert, confused, agitated, or inattentive?

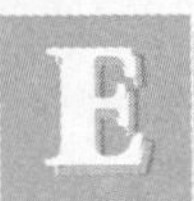

Expression—Does he appear ill, in pain, or anxious?

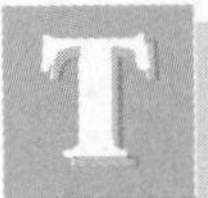

Trunk—Is he lean, stocky, obese, or barrel-chested?

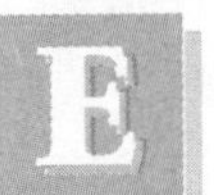

Extremities—Are his fingers clubbed? Does he have joint abnormalities or edema?

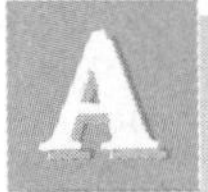

Appearance—Is he clean and appropriately dressed?

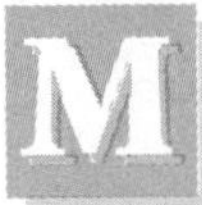

Movement—Are his posture, gait, and coordination normal? Does he move around in a normal fashion?

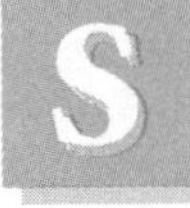

Speech—Is his speech relaxed, clear, strong, understandable, and appropriate? Does it sound stressed?

TIPS FOR ASSESSMENT SUCCESS

Before starting the physical assessment, review this checklist.

- Eliminate as many distractions and disruptions as possible.
- Ask your patient to void.
- Wash your hands before and after the assessment—preferably in the patient's presence.
- Have all the necessary equipment on hand and in working order.
- Make sure the examination room is well lit and warm.
- Warm your hands and equipment before touching the patient.
- Be aware of your nonverbal communication and of possible negative reactions from the patient.

Obtaining baseline data

Accurate measurements of your patient's height, weight, and vital signs provide critical information about his body functions.

The first time you assess a patient, record his baseline vital signs and statistics. Afterward, take measurements at regular intervals, depending on the patient's condition and your facility's policy. A series of readings usually provides more valuable information than a single set. If you obtain an abnormal value, take the vital sign again to make sure it's accurate. Remember that normal readings vary with the patient's age and from patient to patient (an abnormal value for one patient may be a normal value for another).

Height and weight

For every patient in any setting, record height and weight (anthropometric measurements) as part of your assessment profile. Although the general survey gives an overall impression of body size and type, height and weight measurements provide more specific information about a patient's general health and nutritional status. These measurements should be taken periodically throughout the patient's life to help evaluate normal growth and development and to identify abnormal patterns of weight gain or loss (usually an early sign of acute or chronic illness). (See *Obtaining pediatric measurements,* page 24.)

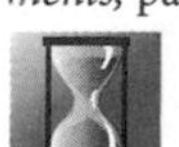

AGE ISSUE *Accurate height and weight measurements also serve other important purposes. In children, they guide dosage calculations for various drugs; in adults, they help guide cancer chemotherapy and anesthesia administration, and they help evaluate the response to I.V. fluids, drugs, or nutritional therapy.*

Vital signs

Assessing vital signs — blood pressure, pulse rate, respirations, and temperature — is a basic, yet important method, for monitoring essential body functions. Vital signs give insight into the function of specific organs — especially the heart and the lungs — as well as entire body systems. You obtain vital signs to establish baseline measurements, observe for trends, identify physiologic problems, and monitor a patient's response to therapy.

When assessing a patient's vital signs, keep in mind that a single measurement usually proves far less valuable than a series of measurements, which can help to substantiate a trend. In most cases, look for a change — from the normal range, from the patient's normal measurement or from previous measurements. Because vital signs reflect basic body functions, significant changes warrant further investigation.

Blood pressure. Blood pressure measurements are helpful in evaluating cardiac output, fluid and circulatory status, and arterial resistance. Blood pressure measurements consist of systolic and diastolic readings. The systolic reading reflects the maximum pressure exerted on the arterial wall at the peak of left ventricular contraction. Normal systolic pressure ranges from 100 to 140 mm Hg.

The diastolic reading reflects the minimum pressure exerted on the arterial wall during left ventricular relaxation. This reading is generally more significant than the systolic reading because it evaluates arterial pressure when the heart is at rest. Normal diastolic pressure ranges from 60 to 90 mm Hg.

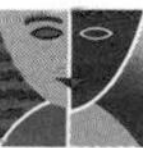

CULTURAL INSIGHT *When taking the patient's blood pressure, know that it may vary depending on the patient's race or sex. For example, Black women tend to have higher systolic blood pressures than White women do, regardless of age. Furthermore, after age 45, the average blood pressures of Black women are almost 16 mm Hg higher than those of White women in the same age-group. With this in mind, carefully monitor the blood pressures of your Black female patients, being alert for signs of hypertension. Early detection and treatment — combined with lifestyle changes — can help prevent such complications as stroke and kidney disease.*

The sphygmomanometer, a device used to measure blood pressure, consists of an inflatable cuff, a pressure manometer, and a bulb with a valve. To obtain a blood pressure measurement, center the cuff over an artery, inflate the cuff, and then deflate it. (See *Obtaining blood pressure readings,* page 25.)

As the cuff deflates, listen with a stethoscope for Korotkoff sounds, which indicate the systolic and diastolic pressures. Blood pressure can be measured from most extremity pulse points. The brachial artery is used for most patients because of its accessibility.

When assessing a patient's blood pressure for the first time, take measurements in both arms. Consider a slight pressure difference (5 to 10 mm Hg) between arms to be normal; a difference of 15 mm Hg or more may indicate cardiac disease, especially

EXPERT TECHNIQUE

OBTAINING PEDIATRIC MEASUREMENTS

Infants and young children require alternative methods to obtain accurate height and weight. Head circumference is an additional measurement that's part of the routine assessment during infancy and early childhood.

Height

Up to age 3, height is measured in the supine position, from the top of the head to the bottom of the heel. When taken in this recumbent position, height is more commonly referred to as length. Here are some tips for measuring infant length more accurately:

- Hold the infant's head in the midline position.
- Then, hold his knees together with your other hand, and gently press them down toward the table until fully extended.
- Take the length measurement.

Weight

Those infants and young children whose length is measured recumbently are typically weighed on an infant scale. The scale may be digital or balanced. Remember, never turn away from or leave a child unattended while on a scale. After age 3, the child may be weighed on an adult scale.

Head circumference

Measured routinely until age 3, head circumference reflects the growth of the cranium and its contents. To obtain this measurement, place a flexible measuring tape around the largest diameter of the head from the frontal bone of the forehead to the occipital prominence at the back of the head.

coarctation of the aorta or arterial obstruction.

In some cases, you may want to assess orthostatic (postural) blood pressure by taking readings with the patient lying down, sitting, and standing, then checking for differences with each position change. Normally, blood pressure rises or falls slightly with a position change. A drop of 20 mm Hg or more, however, indicates orthostatic hypotension.

In a patient with venous congestion or hypertension, you may detect a silent period between systolic and diastolic sounds, when you can't hear intervening pulse sounds. Known as the *auscultatory gap,* this phenomenon may cause you to underestimate the systolic or overestimate the diastolic significantly. To avoid either error, be sure to inflate the blood pressure cuff at least 20 mm Hg over the point at which the palpated pulse first disappeared. (See *Assessing for hypertension,* page 26.)

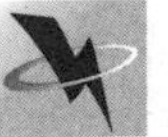

CRITICAL POINT *When measuring blood pressure in obese patients and those with anxiety, special considerations must be kept in mind. Because high blood pressure is commonly caused by anxiety, try to relax the patient and repeat the procedure later in the examination. For obese patients, it's important to use a wide cuff; for patients with an arm circumference greater than 16″ (40.6 cm), use a thigh cuff.*

To assess the blood pressure in the leg, use a wide, long thigh cuff that has a bladder size of 7″ × 16½″ (17.5 × 42 cm), and apply it to the midthigh. Center the bladder over the posterior surface, and listen over the popliteal artery. Ideally, the patient should be in a prone position, but you can also do this with the patient in a supine position with his leg flexed slightly and his heel resting on the bed or table. When an appropriate-sized cuff is used for the arm and leg, blood pressure measurements should be equal.

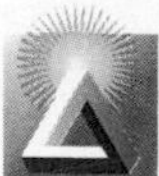

EXPERT TECHNIQUE

OBTAINING BLOOD PRESSURE READINGS

When choosing a blood pressure cuff for your patient, keep these points in mind:

- The width of the cuff's bladder should be about 40% of the circumference of the patient's upper arm.
- The length of the cuff's bladder should be about 80% of the circumference of the patient's arm.
- A cuff that's too short or too narrow will give a false-high reading.

Follow the guidelines below to use a sphygmomanometer properly:

- For accuracy and consistency, position your patient with his upper arm at heart level and his palm turned up.
- Apply the cuff snugly, 1″ (2.5 cm) above the brachial pulse, as shown in the photo below.

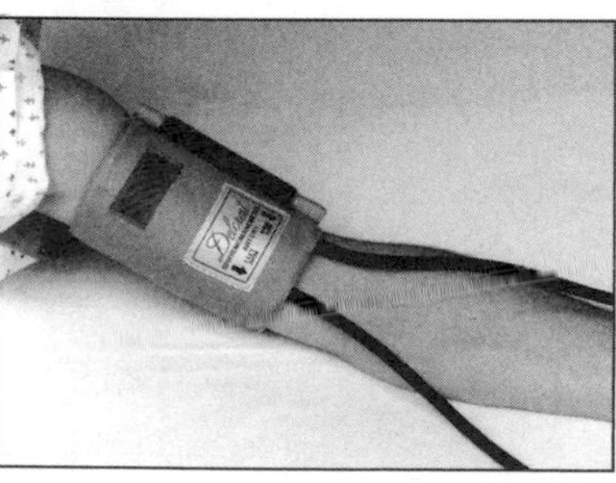

- Position the manometer in line with your eye level.
- Palpate the brachial or radial pulse with your fingertips while inflating the cuff.
- Inflate the cuff to 30 mm Hg above the point where the pulse disappears.
- Place the bell of the stethoscope over the point where you felt the pulse, as shown in the top right photo. Using the bell will help you better hear Korotkoff sounds, which indicate pulse.

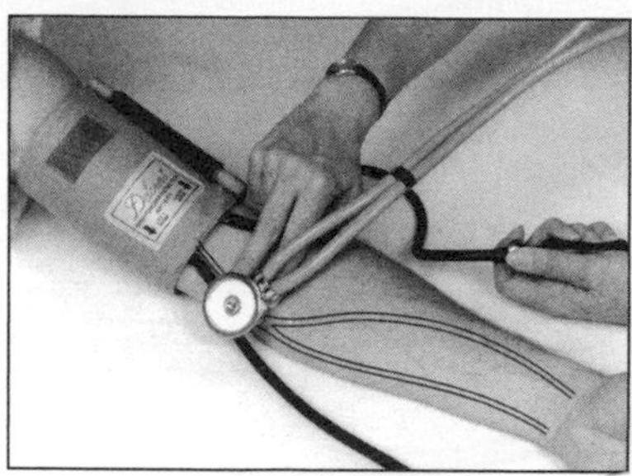

- The sounds will become muffled and then disappear. The last Korotkoff sound you hear is the diastolic pressure.

If you have difficulty hearing Korotkoff sounds, try to intensify them by increasing vascular pressure below the cuff. Here are two techniques you can use.

Have the patient raise his arm
Palpate the brachial pulse and mark its location with a pen to avoid losing the pulse spot. Apply the cuff and have the patient raise his arm above his head. Then inflate the cuff about 30 mm Hg above the patient's systolic pressure. Have him lower his arm until the cuff reaches heart level, deflate the cuff, and take a reading.

Have the patient make a fist
Position the patient's arm at heart level. Inflate the cuff to 30 mm Hg above the patient's systolic pressure and ask him to make a fist. Have him rapidly open and close his hand about 10 times; then deflate the cuff and take the reading.

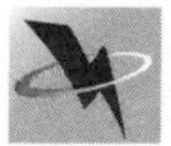

CRITICAL POINT *To rule out coarctation of the aorta, the following two assessments should be performed for every patient with hypertension:*

- *Comparison of the strength and timing of the radial and femoral pulses*
- *Comparison of the blood pressures in the arm and leg.*

Coarctation of the aorta or occlusive aortic disease is suggested by a femoral pulse that's weaker and later than the radial pulse. Also, blood pressure is lower in the legs than in the arms in these conditions.

ASSESSING FOR HYPERTENSION

The seventh report of the Joint National Committee on Detection, Evaluation, and Treatment of High Blood Pressure recommends that hypertension be diagnosed when a higher than normal level has been found on at least two or more readings after initial screening. The chart below outlines the classification for adults age 18 and older.

Category	Systolic blood pressure (mm Hg)		Diastolic blood pressure (mm Hg)
Normal	< 120	and	< 80
Prehypertension	120 to 139	or	80 to 89
Stage 1 hypertension	140 to 159	or	90 to 99
Stage 2 hypertension	≥ 160	or	≥ 100

Pulse. The patient's pulse reflects the amount of blood ejected with each heartbeat. To assess the pulse, palpate one of the patient's arterial pulse points, and note the rate, rhythm, and amplitude (strength) of the pulse. By assessing heartbeat characteristics, you can determine how well the heart handles its blood volume and, indirectly, how well it perfuses organs with oxygenated blood. A normal pulse for an adult is between 60 and 100 beats/minute.

The radial pulse is the most easily accessible. However, in cardiovascular emergencies, you may palpate for the femoral or carotid pulse. The vessels where you palpate for these pulses are larger and closer to the heart and more accurately reflect the heart's activity. (See *Locating pulse sites.*)

To palpate for a pulse, use the pads of your index and middle fingers. Press the area over the artery until you feel pulsations. If the rhythm is regular, count the beats for 30 seconds and then multiply by two to get the number of beats per minute.

If the pulse rhythm is irregular or the patient has a pacemaker, count the beats for 60 seconds. If an irregular pattern is palpated, atrial fibrillation should be suspected. Irregular rhythms should be investigated using an electrocardiogram (ECG).

When taking the patient's pulse for the first time (or when obtaining baseline data) count the beats for 1 minute.

Avoid using your thumb to count the pulse because the thumb has a strong pulse of its own. If you need to palpate the carotid artery, avoid exerting a lot of pressure, which can stimulate the vagus nerve and cause reflex bradycardia. Also, don't palpate both carotid pulses at the same time. Putting pressure on both sides of the patient's neck can impair cerebral blood flow and function.

When you note an irregular pulse, take these steps:

- Evaluate whether the irregularity follows a pattern.
- Auscultate the apical pulse while palpating the radial pulse. You should feel the pulse every time you hear a heartbeat.
- Measure the difference between the apical pulse rate and radial pulse rate, a measurement called the *pulse deficit.*

A pulse deficit occurs when a premature heartbeat can't produce the wave of blood needed to fill the arteries; thus, peripheral radial artery pressure is too low to palpate every heartbeat. To calculate a pulse deficit, have another health care provider record one pulse rate while you record the other for 60 seconds. Usually, you must obtain an ECG to confirm findings.

You also need to assess the pulse amplitude. To do this, use a numerical scale or a descriptive term to rate or describe the strength. Numerical scales differ slightly

LOCATING PULSE SITES

This illustration shows the locations of the major peripheral arterial pulses and the apical pulse.

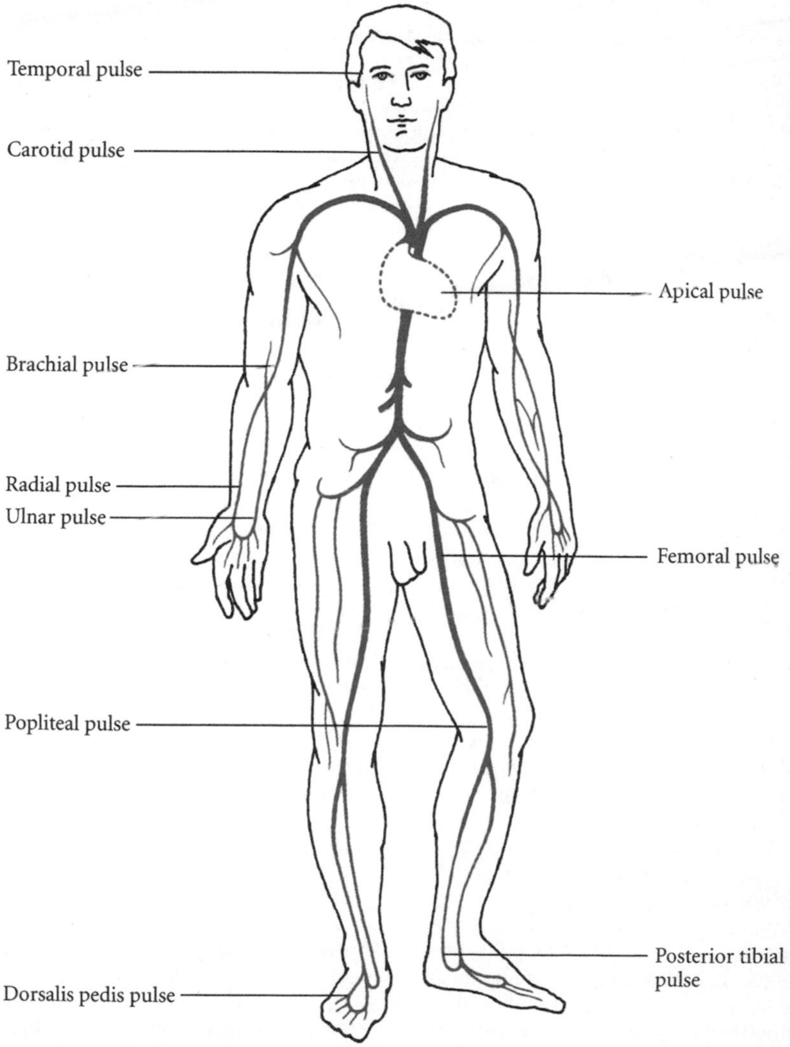

Temporal pulse
Carotid pulse
Apical pulse
Brachial pulse
Radial pulse
Ulnar pulse
Femoral pulse
Popliteal pulse
Posterior tibial pulse
Dorsalis pedis pulse

among health care facilities, but the following scale is commonly used.

- Absent pulse — not palpable, measured as 0.
- Weak or thready pulse — difficult to feel, easily obliterated by slight finger pressure, measured as +1.
- Normal pulse — easily palpable, obliterated by strong finger pressure, measured as +2.
- Bounding pulse — readily palpable, forceful, not easily obliterated by pressure from the fingers, measured as +3.

HOW TEMPERATURE READINGS COMPARE

You can take the patient's temperature four different ways. The chart below compares each route.

Route	Normal temperature	Used for
Oral	97.7° to 99.5° F (36.5° to 37.5° C)	Adults and older children who are awake, alert, oriented, and cooperative
Axillary (armpit)	96.7° to 98.5° F (35.9° to 36.9° C)	Neonates and patients with impaired immune systems when infection is a concern; less accurate because it can vary with blood flow to the skin
Rectal	98.7° to 100.5° F (37° to 38° C)	Infants, young children, and confused or unconscious patients; wear gloves and lubricate the thermometer
Tympanic (ear)	98.2° to 100° F (36.8° to 37.8° C)	Adults and children, conscious and cooperative patients, and confused or unconscious patients; provides automatic timing through a push-button device

You can also evaluate a patient's heart rate by auscultating at the heart's apex with a stethoscope. This method is superior for assessing heart rhythm (regularity).

Respirations. Along with counting respirations, be aware of the depth and rhythm of each breath. To determine the respiratory rate, count the number of respirations for 60 seconds. A rate of 16 to 20 breaths/minute is normal for an adult. If the patient knows you're counting how often he breathes, he may subconsciously alter the rate. To avoid this, count his respirations while you take his pulse.

Pay attention as well to the depth of the patient's respirations by watching his chest rise and fall. Is his breathing shallow, moderate, or deep? Observe the rhythm and symmetry of his chest wall as it expands during inspiration and relaxes during expiration. If respirations are too shallow to see a rise and fall of the chest wall, hold the back of your hand next to the patient's nose and mouth to feel expirations. Be aware that skeletal deformity, broken ribs, and collapsed lung tissue can cause unequal chest expansion.

Use of accessory muscles can enhance lung expansion when oxygenation drops. Patients with chronic obstructive pulmonary disease (COPD) or respiratory distress may use neck muscles, including the sternocleidomastoid muscles, and abdominal muscles for breathing. The patient's position during normal breathing may also suggest problems such as COPD. Prolonged expiration suggests narrowing in the bronchioles. Normal respirations are quiet and easy, so note abnormal sounds, such as wheezing or stridor.

Body temperature. Temperature can be measured and recorded in degrees Fahrenheit (° F) or degrees Celsius (° C). You can take a patient's temperature by several routes, including tympanic (infrared), oral, rectal, or axillary. Unless a specific route is ordered, choose the one that seems most appropriate for the patient's age and physical condition. Whichever route you choose, be sure to document it on the patient's chart.

Use of the tympanic (infrared) thermometer has become increasingly popular. There's little or no discomfort when it's placed in the ear canal, and the results are obtained in a matter of seconds. Follow the manufacturer's directions for the most accurate results.

EFFECTS OF AGE ON VITAL SIGNS

Vital-sign ranges vary from neonate to older adult, as shown in the chart below.

Age (years)	Temperature	Pulse rate (beats/ minute)	Respiratory rate (breaths/ minute)	Blood pressure (mm Hg)
Neonate	98.6° to 99.8° F (37° to 37.7° C)	110 to 160	30 to 40	Systolic: 64 to 96 Diastolic: 30 to 62
3 to 9	98.5° to 99.5° F (36.9° to 37.5° C)	80 to 125	20 to 30	Systolic: 78 to 114 Diastolic: 46 to 78
10 to 15	97.5° to 98.6° F (36.4° to 37° C)	70 to 110	16 to 22	Systolic: 90 to 132 Diastolic: 56 to 86
16 to 18	97.6° to 98.8° F (36.4° to 37.1° C)	55 to 100	15 to 20	Systolic: 104 to 142 Diastolic: 60 to 92
Adult (19 to 65)	96.8° to 99.5° F (36° to 37.5° C)	60 to 100	12 to 20	Systolic: 95 to 140 Diastolic: 60 to 90
Older adult (over 65)	96.5° to 97.5° F (35.8° to 36.4° C)	60 to 100	15 to 25	Systolic: 140 to 160 Diastolic: 70 to 90

The oral route is another convenient method. Ideal for an alert adult, make sure the patient doesn't breathe through his mouth and hasn't had a hot or cold beverage or smoked a cigarette in the past 15 minutes; these events can cause an inaccurate reading. Avoid taking an oral temperature in a patient who has an oral deformity or who has undergone recent oral surgery.

When absolute accuracy is required, such as with hypothermic patients or with children after febrile seizures, take a temperature rectally. Avoid the rectal route in a patient with anal lesions, bleeding hemorrhoids, or history of recent rectal surgery. Also avoid the rectal route in a patient with a cardiac disorder because it may stimulate the vagus nerve, possibly leading to vasodilation and a decreased heart rate.

You can also measure a temperature by the axillary route if a tympanic thermometer is unavailable. You can use this technique with an alert patient who has had oral surgery, a patient who can't close his lips around a thermometer because of a deformity, or a patient who's wearing an oxygen mask.

Normal body temperature ranges from about 96.8° F to 99.5° F (36° C to 37.5° C). When evaluating temperature, keep in mind that some people have a higher or lower baseline temperature.

Hyperthermia describes an oral temperature above 106° F (41.1° C). Causes of hyperthermia include:

- infection
- trauma
- malignancy
- blood disorders
- drug reactions
- immune disorders.

Hypothermia describes a rectal temperature below 95° F (35° C). The main cause of hypothermia is exposure to cold.

To convert Celsius to Fahrenheit, multiply the Celsius temperature by 1.8 and add 32. To convert Fahrenheit to Celsius, subtract 32 from the Fahrenheit temperature and divide by 1.8. (See *How temperature readings compare* and *Effects of age on vital signs.*)

Using physical assessment techniques

During the physical assessment, use drapes so only the area being examined is exposed. Develop a pattern for your assessment, starting with the same body system and proceeding in the same sequence. Organize your steps to minimize the number of times the patient needs to change position. By using a systematic approach, you'll also be less likely to forget an area.

No matter where you start your physical assessment, you'll use four techniques: inspection, palpation, percussion, and auscultation. The techniques are used in sequence, except when performing an abdominal assessment. Because palpation and percussion can alter bowel sounds, the sequence for assessing the abdomen is: inspection, auscultation, percussion, and palpation.

Inspection

Critical observation or inspection is the most commonly used assessment technique. It begins when you first meet the patient and continues throughout the health history and physical examination. Performed correctly, it also reveals more than the other techniques. However, an incomplete or hasty inspection may neglect important details or even yield false or misleading findings. To ensure accurate, useful information, approach inspection in a careful, unhurried manner, pay close attention to details, and try to draw logical conclusions from your findings.

Inspection can be direct or indirect. During direct inspection, rely totally on sight, hearing, and smell. During indirect inspection, use equipment such as a nasal or vaginal speculum or an ophthalmoscope to expose internal tissues or to enhance the view of a specific body area.

To inspect a specific body area, first make sure the area is sufficiently exposed and adequately lit. Then survey the entire area, noting key landmarks and checking the overall condition. Next, focus on specifics, such as color, size, location, movement, texture, symmetry, odor, and sound.

Palpation

Palpation requires you to touch the patient with different parts of your hand, using varying degrees of pressure. To do this properly, make sure your fingernails are short and your hands are warm. Palpation involves touching the patient's body to feel pulsations and vibrations, to locate body structures (particularly in the abdomen), and to assess such characteristics as size, texture, warmth, mobility, and tenderness. It allows you to detect a pulse, muscle rigidity, enlarged lymph nodes, skin or hair dryness, organ tenderness, or breast lumps as well as measure the chest's expansion and contraction with each respiration. Always palpate tender areas last. Tell the patient the purpose of your touch and what you're feeling with your hands.

Usually, palpation follows inspection. For example, if a rash is present on inspection, determine through palpation if the rash has a raised surface or feels tender or warm. However, during an abdominal or urinary system examination, palpation should be performed last to avoid causing the patient discomfort and stimulating peristalsis (smooth-muscle contractions that force food through the GI tract, bile through the bile duct, and urine through the ureters).

Correct palpation requires a highly developed sense of touch. Learn to use the various parts of the fingers and hands for different purposes; also expect to learn several palpation techniques. (See *Understanding palpation techniques.*)

Don't forget to wear gloves when palpating, especially when palpating mucous membranes or other areas where you might come in contact with body fluids.

As you palpate each body system, evaluate these features:

- *texture* — rough or smooth
- *temperature* — warm, hot, or cold
- *moisture* — dry, wet, or moist
- *motion* — still or vibrating
- *consistency of structures* — solid or fluid-filled.

The patient may react to palpation with anxiety, embarrassment, or discomfort. This, in turn, can lead to muscle tension or guarding, possibly interfering with palpation and causing misleading results. To put the patient at ease and thus enhance the ac-

EXPERT TECHNIQUE

UNDERSTANDING PALPATION TECHNIQUES

To perform thorough physical assessments, you'll need to learn several palpation techniques as described below. Light palpation involves using the tips and pads of the fingers to apply light pressure to the skin surface. Deep palpation requires the use of both hands and heavier pressure. Light ballottement involves gentle, repetitive bouncing of tissues against the hand (think of bouncing a small ball gently). Deep ballottement requires heavier pressure to assess deeper structures.

Light palpation

For light palpation, press gently on the skin, indenting it ½″ to ¾″ (1 to 2 cm). Use the lightest touch possible because too much pressure blunts your sensitivity. To concentrate on what you're feeling, close your eyes.

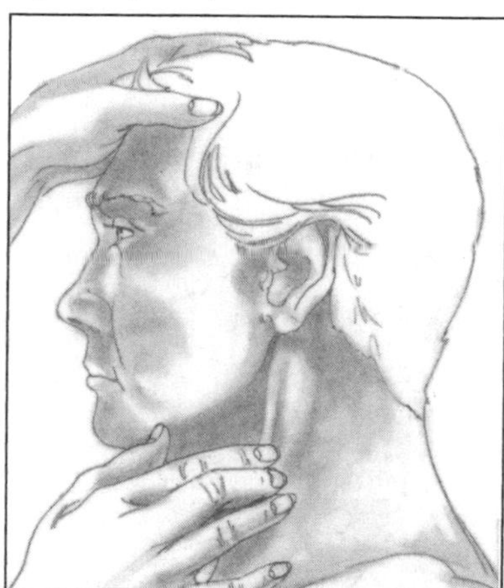

Deep palpation (bimanual palpation)

For deep palpation, increase your fingertip pressure, indenting the skin about 1½″ (3.8 cm). Place your other hand on top of the palpating hand to control and guide your movements. To perform a variation of deep palpation that allows pinpointing an inflamed area, press firmly with one hand, and then lift your hand away quickly. If the patient complains of increased pain as you release the pressure, you've identified rebound tenderness. (Suspect peritonitis if you elicit rebound tenderness when examining the abdomen.)

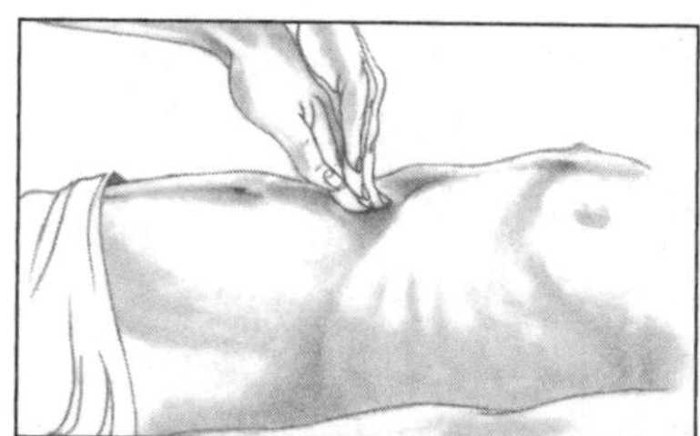

Light ballottement

To perform light ballottement, apply light, rapid pressure from quadrant to quadrant on the patient's abdomen. Keep your hand on the skin surface to detect any tissue rebound.

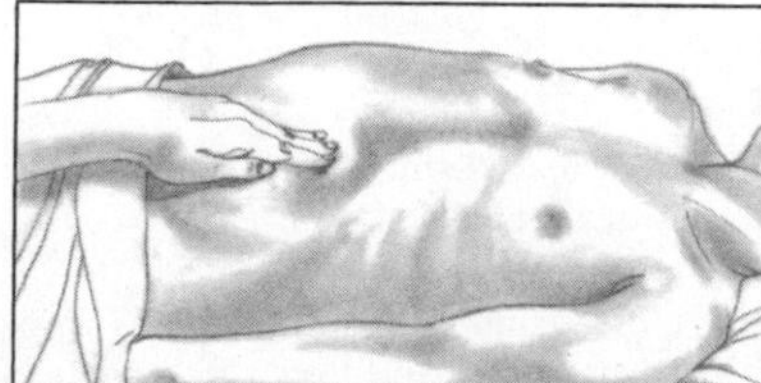

Deep ballottement

To perform deep ballottement, apply abrupt, deep pressure, then release the pressure, but maintain fingertip contact with the skin.

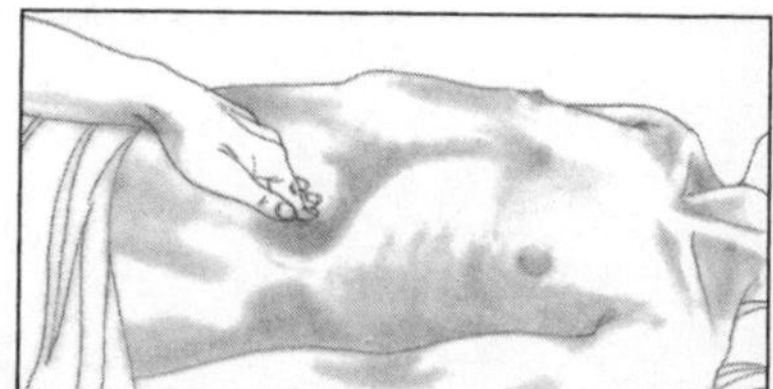

EXPERT TECHNIQUE

USING PERCUSSION TECHNIQUES

To assess a patient completely, you'll need to use three percussion techniques: indirect, direct, and blunt.

Indirect percussion

To perform indirect percussion, use the second finger of your nondominant hand as the pleximeter (the mediating device used to receive the taps) and the middle finger of your dominant hand as the plexor (the device used to tap the pleximeter). Place the pleximeter finger firmly against a body surface such as the patient's upper back. With your wrist flexed loosely, use the tip of your plexor finger to deliver a crisp blow just beneath the distal joint of the pleximeter. Be sure to hold the plexor perpendicular to the pleximeter. Tap lightly and quickly, removing the plexor as soon as you have delivered each blow.

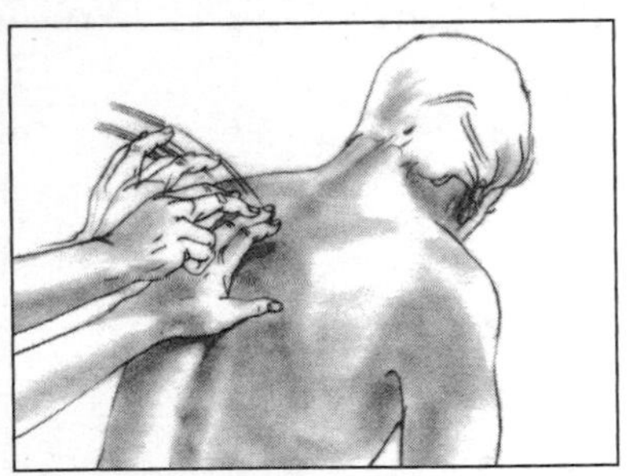

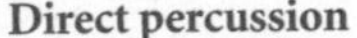

Direct percussion

To perform direct percussion, tap your hand or fingertip directly against the patient's body surface. This method helps assess an adult's sinuses for tenderness or elicit sounds in a child's thorax.

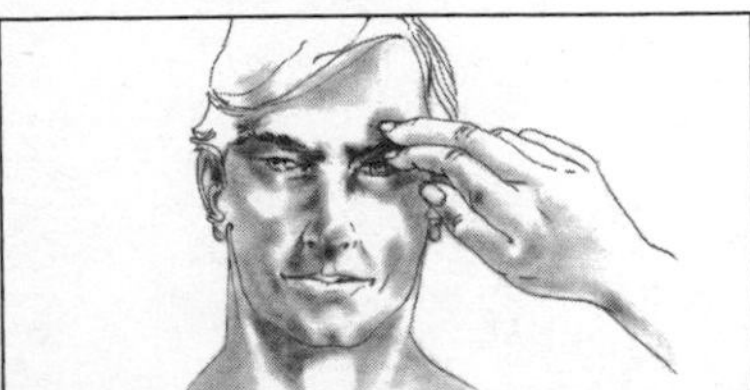

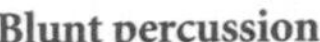

Blunt percussion

To perform blunt percussion, strike the ulnar surface of your fist against the patient's body surface. Alternatively, you may use both hands by placing the palm of one hand over the area to be percussed, then making a fist with the other hand and using it to strike the back of the first hand. Both techniques aim to detect tenderness — not to create a sound — over such organs as the kidneys, gallbladder, or liver. (Another blunt percussion method, used in a neurologic examination, involves tapping a rubber-tipped reflex hammer against a tendon to create a reflexive muscle contraction.)

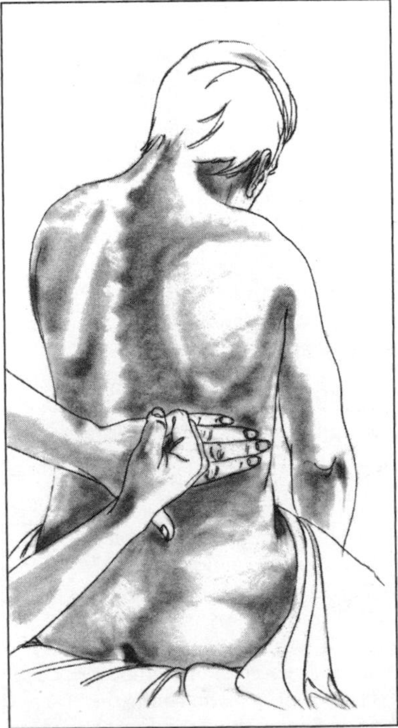

RECOGNIZING PERCUSSION SOUNDS

Percussion produces sounds that vary according to the tissue being percussed. This chart shows important percussion sounds along with their characteristics and typical sources.

Sound	Intensity	Pitch	Duration	Quality	Source
Resonance	Moderate to loud	Low	Long	Hollow	Normal lung
Tympany	Loud	High	Moderate	Drumlike	Gastric air bubble; intestinal air
Dullness	Soft to moderate	High	Moderate	Thudlike	Liver; full bladder; pregnant uterus
Hyper-resonance	Very loud	Very Low	Long	Booming	Hyperinflated lung (as in emphysema)
Flatness	Soft	High	Short	Flat	Muscle

curacy of palpation findings, follow these guidelines:

- Warm your hands before beginning.
- Explain what you'll do and why, and describe what the patient can expect, especially in sensitive areas.
- Encourage the patient to relax by suggesting that he take several deep breaths while concentrating on inhaling and exhaling.
- Stop palpating immediately if the patient complains of pain.

Percussion

Percussion involves tapping the fingers or hands quickly and sharply against body surfaces (usually the chest and abdomen) to produce sounds, to detect tenderness, or to assess reflexes. Percussing for sound (the most common percussion goal) helps locate organ borders, identify shape and position, and determine if an organ is solid or filled with fluid or gas.

Three basic percussion methods include indirect (mediate), direct (immediate), and blunt (fist) percussion. In indirect percussion, the examiner taps one finger against an object — usually the middle finger of the other hand — held against the skin surface. Although indirect percussion commonly produces clearer, crisper sounds than direct or blunt percussion, this technique requires practice to achieve good sound quality. (See *Using percussion techniques.*)

Percussing for sound — perhaps the most difficult assessment method to master — requires a skilled touch and an ear trained to detect slight sound variations. Organs and tissues produce sounds of varying loudness, pitch, and duration, depending on their intensity. For instance, air-filled cavities, such as the lungs, produce markedly different sounds from those produced by the liver and other dense tissues.

When percussing for sound with the direct or indirect method, use quick, light blows to create vibrations that penetrate about 1½″ to 2″ (4 to 5 cm) under the skin surface. The returning sounds reflect the contents of the percussed body cavity. (See *Recognizing percussion sounds.*)

Normal percussion sounds over the chest and abdomen include:

USING A STETHOSCOPE

Even if using a stethoscope is second nature to you, it might still be a good idea to brush up on your technique. For starters, your stethoscope should have these features:

- snug-fitting ear plugs, which you'll position toward your nose
- tubing no longer than 15″ (38.1 cm) and an internal diameter not greater than ⅛″ (0.3 cm)
- a diaphragm and bell.

How to auscultate

Hold the diaphragm firmly against the patient's skin, enough to leave a slight ring afterward. Hold the bell lightly against the patient's skin, just enough to form a seal. Don't hold the bell too firmly, or it will cause the skin to act as a diaphragm, obliterating low-pitched sounds.

Hair on the patient's chest may cause friction on the end piece, which can mimic abnormal breath sounds such as crackles. You can minimize this problem by lightly wetting the hair before auscultating.

Additional steps

- Provide a quiet environment.
- Make sure the area to be auscultated is exposed. Don't try to auscultate over a gown or bed linens because they can interfere with sounds.
- Warm the stethoscope head in your hand.
- Close your eyes to help focus your attention.
- Listen to and try to identify the characteristics of one sound at a time.

- *resonance*—the long, low, hollow sound heard over an intercostal space lying above healthy lung tissue
- *tympany*—the loud, high-pitched, drumlike sound heard over a gastric air bubble or gas-filled bowel
- *dullness*—the soft, high-pitched thudding sound normally heard over more solid organs, such as the liver and heart.

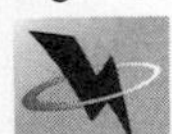

CRITICAL POINT *Dullness heard in a normally resonant or tympanic area signals the need for further investigation.*

Abnormal percussion sounds may be heard over body organs. Consider hyperresonance—a long, loud, low-pitched sound—to be a classic sign of lung hyperinflation, which can occur in emphysema. Flatness, similar to dullness but shorter in duration and softer in intensity, may also be heard over pleural fluid accumulation or pleural thickening.

To enhance percussion technique and improve results, keep your fingernails short and warm your hands before starting. Have the patient void before you begin; otherwise, you could mistake a full bladder for a mass or cause the patient discomfort. Make sure the examination room is quiet and distraction-free. Remove any jewelry or other items that could clatter and interfere with the ability to hear returning sounds.

Before performing percussion, briefly explain to the patient what you'll do and why. This technique may startle and upset an unprepared patient. In an obese patient, expect percussion sounds to be muffled by a thick subcutaneous fat layer. To help overcome this problem, use the lateral aspect of the thumb as the pleximeter and tap sharply on the last thumb joint with your plexor finger.

As you percuss, move gradually from areas of resonance to those of dullness and then compare sounds. Also compare sounds on one side of the body with sounds on the other side.

Auscultation

Auscultation—usually the last step—involves listening for various breath, heart, and bowel sounds with a stethoscope. Most auscultated sounds result from air or fluid movement, such as the rush of air through respiratory pathways, the turbulent flow of blood through blood vessels, and the movement of gas (agitated by peristalsis) through the bowels.

You can hear pronounced body sounds, such as the voice, loud wheezing, or stomach growls, fairly easily, but you'll need a stethoscope to hear softer sounds. Use the diaphragm of the stethoscope to detect high-pitched sounds, such as breath sounds and bowel sounds, and use the bell side to listen to low-pitched sounds, such as abnormal heart sounds and bruits (abnormal blowing sound heard when auscultating an artery). Use a high-quality, properly fitting stethoscope, provide a quiet environment, and make sure the body area to be auscultated is sufficiently exposed. Remember that a gown or bed linens can interfere with sound transmission.

Instruct the patient to remain quiet and still. Before starting, warm the stethoscope head (diaphragm and bell) in your hand; otherwise, the cold metal may cause the patient to shiver, possibly causing unwanted sounds. Next, place the diaphragm or bell over the appropriate area. Closing your eyes to help focus your attention, listen intently to individual sounds, and try to identify their characteristics. Determine the intensity, pitch, and duration of each sound, and check the frequency of recurring sounds. To prevent the spread of infection among patients, clean the heads and end pieces with alcohol or a disinfectant. (See *Using a stethoscope.*)

Recording your findings

Begin your documentation with general information, including the patient's age, race, gender, general appearance, height, weight, body mass, vital signs, communication skills, behavior, awareness, orientation, and level of cooperation. Next, precisely record all information you obtained using the four physical assessment techniques.

Just as you followed an organized sequence in your physical examination, you also should follow an organized pattern for recording your findings. Document all information about one body system, for example, before proceeding to another.

Use anatomic landmarks in your descriptions so that other health care providers can compare their findings with yours. For instance, you might describe a wound as "3.8 × 6.4 cm, located 2½″ below the umbilicus at the midclavicular line."

With some body structures, such as the tympanic membrane or breast, you can pinpoint a finding by its position on a clock. For instance, you might write "breast mass at 3 o'clock." If you use this method, however, make sure others recognize the same landmark for the 12 o'clock reference point.

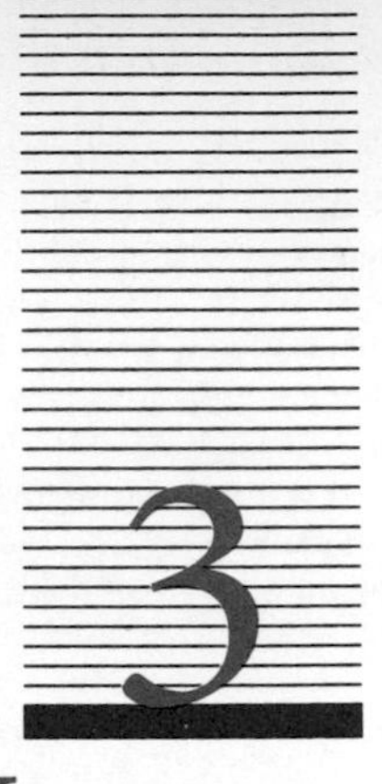

Mental health assessment

Looking at mental health assessment

Effective patient care requires consideration of both psychological and physiologic aspects of health. A patient who seeks medical help for chest pain, for example, may also need to be assessed for anxiety or depression. Knowing the basic function and structures of the brain will help you perform a comprehensive mental health assessment and recognize abnormalities.

The mental health assessment refers to the scientific process of identifying a patient's psychosocial problems, strengths, and possible concerns. Besides serving as the basis for treating psychiatric patients, the mental health assessment has broad clinical applications. Recognizing psychosocial problems and how they affect a person's health is important in any clinical setting. In a medical-surgical unit, for example, you may encounter a patient who experiences depression, has a thought disorder, or has attempted suicide — recognizing these psychosocial problems is key to providing effective treatment.

Obtaining a health history

Begin your assessment by obtaining a health history. For this assessment to be effective, you need to establish a therapeutic relationship with the patient that's built on trust. You must communicate to him that his thoughts and behaviors are important. Effective communication involves both sending and receiving messages, in the form of words and in the form of nonverbal communication — such as eye contact, posture, facial expressions, gestures, clothing, affect, and even silence, all of which can convey a powerful message. (See *Therapeutic communication techniques,* page 38.)

A systematic interview helps you acquire broad information about the patient. The interview should include a description of the patient's behavioral disturbances, a thorough emotional and social history, and mental status tests.

Using this information, you'll be able to assess the patient's psychological functioning, understand his coping methods and their effect on his psychosocial growth, and build a therapeutic alliance that encourages the patient to talk openly. The information you gather during the health history will enable you to develop an effective care plan.

The success of the health history hinges on your ability to listen objectively and respond with empathy. Keep in mind these guidelines when interviewing patients:

- Have clearly set goals in mind. Remember, the assessment interview isn't a random discussion. Your purpose may be to obtain information from a patient, to screen for abnormalities, or to further investigate an identified psychiatric condition, such as depression, paranoia, or suicidal thoughts.
- Don't let personal values obstruct your professional judgment. For example, when assessing appearance, judge attire on its appropriateness and cleanliness, not on whether it suits your taste.
- Pay attention to unspoken signals. Throughout the interview, listen carefully for indications of possible anxiety or distress. What topics does the patient pass over vaguely? You may find important clues in the patient's method of self-expression and in the subjects he avoids about his mental status.

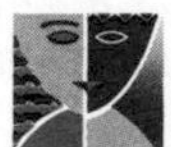

CULTURAL INSIGHT *Keep in mind that a patient's background and values can affect how he responds to illness and adapts to care. Certain questions and behaviors considered acceptable in one culture may be inappropriate in another. For example, a person who blames bad luck on a power called "juju" would be considered delusional in the United States. However, neighbors in Nigeria would consider this quite normal. When dealing with a patient from another culture, consult with an outside resource before drawing conclusions about his mental state.*

- Don't make assumptions about how past events affected the patient emotionally. Try to discover what each event meant to the patient. Don't assume, for example, that the death of a loved one provoked a mood of sadness in a patient. A death by itself doesn't cause sadness, guilt, or anger. What matters is how the patient perceives the loss.
- Monitor your own reactions; the mental health patient may provoke an emotional response strong enough to interfere with your professional judgment. For example, a depressed patient may make you depressed and a hostile patient may provoke your anger. An anxious patient may cause you to develop anxiety after the interview. A violent, psychotic patient who has lost touch with reality may easily induce fear.

In other cases, you may find yourself identifying with a patient. Perhaps the patient has similar interests or experiences or is close to your age. Such feelings pose a real threat to establishing a therapeutic relationship; they may disrupt your objectivity or cause you to avoid or reject the patient. Consult with a psychiatric clinical specialist if you recognize within yourself strong prejudices toward a patient. Develop self-awareness as a tool to monitor patients and to further your own professional growth.

Creating a supportive atmosphere

Choose a quiet, private setting for the mental health assessment interview. Interruptions and distractions threaten confidentiality and interfere with effective listening. If you're meeting the patient for the first time, introduce yourself, address the patient by his surname, and explain the purpose of the interview. Sit a comfortable distance from the patient, and give him your undivided attention.

The patient must feel comfortable enough to discuss his problems. You'll encounter patients who are angry and argumentative. Other patients may be too withdrawn to even say why they're seeking help. You'll also have to deal with diverse cultural norms. Some patients may come from cultural backgrounds that don't discuss intimate details, even with a health care provider. Adolescents may refuse to discuss sexual activity in front of their parents. Lis-

THERAPEUTIC COMMUNICATION TECHNIQUES

Therapeutic communication is the foundation for developing a good relationship with your patient. Here are some techniques that are effective in developing that relationship.

Listening
Listening intently to the patient enables the health care provider to hear and analyze what the patient is saying, alerting the health care provider to the patient's communication patterns.

Rephrasing
Succinct rephrasing of key patient statements helps ensure the health care provider understands and emphasizes important points in the patient's message. For example, the health care provider might say, "You're feeling angry and you say it's because of the way your friend treated you yesterday."

Using broad openings and general statements
Using broad openings and general statements to initiate conversations encourages the patient to talk about any subject that comes to mind. These openings allow the patient to focus the conversation and demonstrate the health care provider's willingness to interact. An example of this technique is: "Is there something you'd like to talk about?"

Clarifying
Asking the patient to clarify a confusing or vague message demonstrates the health care provider's desire to understand what the patient is saying. It can also elicit precise information crucial to the patient's recovery. An example of clarification is: "I'm not sure I understood what you said."

Focusing
Focusing is a technique that assists the patient in redirecting attention toward something specific. It fosters the patient's self-control and helps avoid vague generalizations, thereby enabling the patient to accept responsibility for facing problems. For example, the health care provider might say, "Let's go back to what we were just talking about."

Being silent
Refraining from comment can have several benefits: Silence gives the patient time to talk, think, and gain insight into problems, and it allows the health care provider to gather more information. The health care provider must use this technique judiciously, however, to avoid giving the impression of disinterest or judgment.

Suggesting collaboration
When used correctly, suggesting collaboration gives the patient the opportunity to explore the pros and cons of a suggested approach. It must be used carefully to avoid directing the patient. An example of this technique is: "Perhaps we can meet with your parents to discuss the matter."

Sharing impressions
Sharing impressions gives the health care provider the opportunity to describe the patient's feelings and then seek corrective feedback from the patient. It allows the patient to clarify misperceptions and gives the health care provider a better understanding of the patient's true feelings. For example, the health care provider might say, "Tell me if my perception of what you're telling me agrees with yours."

ten carefully to the patient, and respond with sensitivity. Reassure the patient that you respect his need for privacy. Ask him privately who should be present at the interview. Attempt to make the immediate interview environment calm and quiet, to relax the patient. Reassure him that he's safe, if necessary.

During the interview, adopt a professional but friendly attitude, and maintain eye contact. A calm, nonthreatening tone of voice encourages the patient to talk more openly. Avoid making value judgments about the patient. Don't rush through the interview; building a trusting therapeutic relationship takes time. Remember to allow the patient to carry the conversation, redirecting him as necessary.

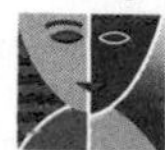

CULTURAL INSIGHT *Communication is the primary component of a mental health assessment. However, communication varies greatly between cultures. Keep in mind that certain qualities that are expected and typically viewed as "normal" (such as maintaining eye contact, a certain degree of openness, insight, and emotional expression) are prevalent in our Western culture but not in others. For instance:*

- *Direct eye contact is considered inappropriate and disrespectful to some Asian, Black, Native American, and Appalachian people.*
- *Some Middle Eastern people are oriented to the present; they may speak of the future only as something to be accepted as it occurs, rather than planned.*
- *Because some Asians strongly value harmonious interpersonal relationships, they may nod and smile and provide answers they feel are expected to maintain harmony, therefore, they may not fully express their true feelings and concerns.*

Avoid making assumptions about behaviors or communication styles such as these, and remember that there may be a cultural explanation for what you would otherwise deem "inappropriate" or "abnormal."

Conducting the patient interview

A patient interview establishes a baseline and provides clues to the underlying or precipitating cause of the patient's current problem. Remember the patient may not be a reliable source of information, particularly if he has a mental illness or other mental impairment. If possible, verify his responses with family members, friends, or health care personnel. Also, check the patient's medical records for previous hospital admissions, if possible, and compare his past and present behavior, symptoms, and circumstances.

Use the following guidelines when conducting a patient interview.

Biographic data

Begin the mental status examination by determining the patient's age, ethnic origin, primary language, birthplace, religion, and marital status. Use this information to establish a baseline and validate the patient's medical record.

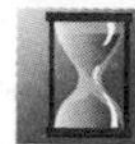

AGE ISSUE *Age-related losses may take a toll on the mental functioning of elderly patients. These may include:*

- *deaths of friends and family*
- *retirement*
- *decrease in income*
- *decreased physical capabilities*
- *impairments in vision and hearing*
- *decreased stimulation*
- *growing isolation.*

Chief complaint

Ask what the patient's chief complaint is and what he expects to accomplish through treatment. In your assessment, include a statement of the chief complaint in the patient's own words. Some patients don't have an overriding concern, whereas others insist that nothing is wrong. Patients enmeshed in a medical problem may fail to recognize their own depression or anxiety. Carefully observe such patients for signs of disturbed mental health.

By asking the patient what he expects to accomplish through treatment you'll learn more about his mental health status. For example, a person with low self-esteem may seek a better self-image. A patient with schizophrenia may want to be rid of his hallucinations. Some patients may not understand the purpose of the interview and subsequent therapy. Help such patients identify the benefits of dealing with problems openly.

The patient may not voice his chief complaint directly. Instead, you or others, such as family members or friends, may note that he's having difficulty coping or that he's exhibiting unusual behavior. If this occurs, determine whether the patient is aware of the problem. When documenting the patient's response, write it down word for word and enclose it in quotation marks. Be sure to note his corresponding physical behavior as well.

When possible, fully discuss the patient's chief complaint with him. Ask about when symptoms began, their severity and persistence, and whether they occurred abruptly or insidiously. If discussing a recurrent problem, ask the patient what prompted him to seek help at this time.

History of psychiatric illnesses
Be sure to discuss past psychiatric disturbances — such as episodes of delusions, violence, attempted suicides, drug or alcohol abuse, or depression. Ask the patient if he has ever undergone psychiatric treatment; if so, did treatment help? Even though the patient may be reluctant to respond, such questions may elicit early warnings of depression, dementia, suicide risk, psychosis, or adverse reactions to drug therapy.

Socioeconomic data
A patient who's suffering personal hardships is more likely to show symptoms of distress during an illness. Information about your patient's educational level, housing conditions, income, employment status, and family situation may provide clues to his current mental health problem.

Family history
Asking questions about family customs, child-rearing practices, and emotional support received during childhood may give important insights into the environmental influences on the patient's development.

How does the patient react while disclosing his family history? For example, when a patient tells you about his parents' divorce, can you detect feelings of jealousy, hostility, or unresolved grief?

Ask about the emotional health of his relatives. Is there a family history of substance abuse, alcoholism, suicide, psychiatric hospitalization, child abuse, or violence? Is there a history of psychological disorders? Ask about physical disorders as well. A family history of diabetes mellitus or thyroid disorders, for instance, can point to the need to investigate whether the patient's problem has an organic basis.

If the patient can't provide answers to important questions or appears unreliable, ask for permission to interview family members or friends.

Medication history
Certain drugs can cause symptoms of mental illness. Review medications the patient is taking, including over-the-counter and herbal preparations, and check for interactions. If he's taking a psychiatric drug, find out how long he has been taking it, if his symptoms have improved, if he's taking the medication as prescribed, and if he has had adverse reactions.

History of physical illnesses
Find out if the patient has a history of medical disorders that may cause distorted thought processes, disorientation, depression, or other symptoms of mental illness. For instance, does he have a history of renal or hepatic failure, infection, thyroid disease, increased intracranial pressure, or a metabolic disorder? (See *Guidelines for an effective mental health interview.*)

Assessing mental status
Most of the mental status assessment can be done during the interview. As you take a health history, you'll quickly learn the patient's level of alertness and orientation, mood, attention, and memory. As his history unfolds, you'll pick up clues regarding his insight, judgment, and recurring or unusual thoughts or perceptions.

The mental status assessment is a tool for assessing psychological dysfunction and for identifying the causes of psychopathology. You should try to integrate certain parts of the mental status assessment with other parts of the examination. This will make the complete assessment more efficient.

Understanding the components of the mental status examination will enable you to plan appropriate interventions. Assess the patient's level of consciousness (LOC), posture and motor behaviors, appearance, behavior, speech, mood and affect, intellectual performance, judgment, insight, perception, coping mechanisms, thought content, sexual drive, competence, and self-destructive behavior.

Level of consciousness
Begin by assessing the patient's LOC, a basic brain function. Identify the intensity of stimulation needed to arouse the patient. When conducting an interview in the office setting, does the patient respond when called in a normal conversational tone or in

a loud voice? If you're conducting the interview in a health care facility, does it take a light touch, vigorous shaking, or painful stimulation to rouse the patient?

Describe the patient's response to stimulation, including the degree of quality of movement, content and coherence of speech, and level of eye opening and eye contact. Finally, describe the patient's actions when the stimulus is removed.

If you discover an alteration in consciousness, refer the patient for a more extensive medical examination.

Posture and motor behavior

Is the patient lying in bed or walking around? Note his posture and ability to relax. Observe the pace, range, and characteristics of his movements. Are they under voluntary control? Are certain body parts immobile? Do his posture and motor behavior change with certain topics of discussion?

Appearance

The patient's appearance helps to indicate his emotional and mental status. Describe the patient's weight, coloring, skin condition, odor, body build, and obvious physical impairments. Note discrepancies between the patient's feelings about his health and your observations. Answer these questions:

- Is the patient's appearance appropriate for his age, gender, and situation?
- Are his skin, hair, nails, and teeth clean?
- Is his manner of dress appropriate?
- If the patient wears cosmetics, are they appropriately applied?
- Does the patient maintain direct eye contact? Does he stare at you for long periods?
- Is the patient's posture erect or slouched? Is his head lowered?
- Observe his gait — is it brisk, slow, shuffling, or unsteady? Does he walk normally?

Behavior

Describe the patient's demeanor and way of relating to others. When entering the room, does the patient appear sad, joyful, or expressionless? Does he use appropriate gestures? Does he acknowledge your initial greeting and introduction? Does he keep an appropriate distance between himself and others? Does he have distinctive mannerisms, such as tics or tremors? Does he gaze directly at you, at the floor, or around the room?

When responding to your questions, is the patient cooperative, mistrustful, embarrassed, hostile, or overly revealing? Describe the patient's activity level during the interview. Is he tense, rigid, restless, or calm? Also, note any extraordinary behavior.

Speech

Observe the content and quality of the patient's speech, noting:

- illogical choice of topics
- irrelevant or illogical replies to questions
- speech defects such as stuttering
- excessively fast or slow speech

GUIDELINES FOR AN EFFECTIVE MENTAL HEALTH INTERVIEW

- Begin the interview with a broad, empathetic statement: "You look distressed; tell me what's bothering you today."
- Explore normal behaviors before discussing abnormal ones: "What do you think has enabled you to cope with the pressures of your job?"
- Phrase inquiries sensitively to lessen the patient's anxiety: "Things were going well at home and then you became depressed. Tell me about that."
- Ask the patient to clarify vague statements: "Explain to me what you mean when you say, 'They're all after me.'"
- Help the patient who rambles to focus on his most pressing problem: "You've talked about several problems. Which one bothers you the most?"
- Interrupt nonstop talkers as tactfully as possible. Use such a statement as: "Thank you for your comments. Now let's move on."
- Express empathy toward tearful, silent, or confused patients who have trouble describing their problem: "I realize that it's difficult for you to talk about this."

- sudden interruptions
- excessive volume
- barely audible speech
- altered voice tone and modulation
- slurred speech
- an excessive number of words (overproductive speech)
- minimal, monosyllabic responses (underproductive speech).

Notice how much time elapses before the patient reacts to your questions. If the patient communicates only with gestures, determine whether this is an isolated behavior or part of a pattern of diminished responsiveness.

Mood and affect

Mood refers to a person's pervading feeling or state of mind. Usually, the patient will project a prevailing mood, although this mood may change in the course of a day. For example, depressed patients may smile occasionally but will revert to their prevailing mood of sadness.

Affect refers to a person's expression of his mood. Variations in affect are referred to as range of emotion.

To assess the patient's mood and affect, begin by asking him about his current feelings. Also, look for indications of mood in facial expression and posture. Does the patient seem able to keep mood changes under control?

Mood swings may indicate a physiologic disorder. Medications, illicit drug or alcohol use, stress, dehydration, electrolyte imbalance, or disease may all induce mood changes. After childbirth and during menopause, many women experience profound depression.

Other indications of a mood disorder include:

- lability of affect — rapid, dramatic fluctuation in the range of emotion
- flat affect — unresponsive range of emotion, possibly an indication of schizophrenia or Parkinson's disease
- inappropriate affect — inconsistency between expression (affect) and mood (for example, a patient who smiles when discussing an anger-provoking situation).

Intellectual performance

An emotionally distressed patient may show an inability to reason abstractly, make judgments, or solve problems. To develop a picture of his intellectual abilities, use the following series of simple tests. Note that these tests screen for organic brain syndrome as well. If organic brain syndrome is suspected, follow up with additional physical, neurobehavioral, and psychological testing.

Orientation. Ask the patient the time, date, place, and circumstance as well as his name. Disorientation occurs when memory or attention is impaired such as in delirium.

Immediate and delayed recall. Assess the patient's ability to recall an incident that just occurred and to remember events after a reasonable amount of time passes.

For example, to test immediate recall say, "I want you to remember three words: apple, house, and umbrella. What are the three words I want you to remember?" Tell the patient to remember these words for future recall. To test delayed recall, ask the patient to repeat the same words in 5 to 10 minutes.

Recent memory. To test the patient about his recent memory, ask him about an event experienced in the past few hours or days. For example, when was he admitted to the health care facility? Make sure you know the correct response or can validate it with a family member. A patient may confabulate plausible answers to mask memory deficits. Impairment of recent memory is seen in the patient with dementia or delirium.

Remote memory. Assess the patient's ability to remember events in the more distant past, such as where he was born or where he attended high school. Remote memory is impaired in the late stage of dementia. Recent memory loss with intact remote memory may indicate an organic disorder.

Attention level. Assess the patient's ability to concentrate on a task for an appropriate length of time. If the patient has a poor attention level, remember to provide simple, written instructions for health care. (See *Testing level of attention.*)

Comprehension. Assess the patient's ability to understand material, retain it, and repeat the content. Ask the patient to read part of a news article and explain it. Evalu-

TESTING LEVEL OF ATTENTION

During your mental status assessment, test the patient for his level of attention. Commonly used tests are digit span, serial 7's, and spelling backward.

Digit span
The digit span test involves reciting a series of numbers and having the patient repeat them back to you. Start with two numbers at a time and increase the number of digits in the series as tolerated. If the patient makes a mistake, try again with another series of the same length. Stop after a second failure.

Next, start again with a series of two digits, and have the patient repeat the numbers backward. Again, increase the number of digits in the series as tolerated.

Normally, the patient can repeat at least five digits forward and at least four digits backward.

Serial 7's
Starting from 100, have the patient subtract 7 and keep subtracting 7. Stop after a third failed attempt by the patient.

Spelling backward
Say a five-letter word to the patient, spell it, and then have the patient spell it backward to you. Repeat the exercise twice, stopping if the patient fails to spell the word backward.

ate his thought processes and cognitive function. (See *Abnormal thought processes*, page 44.)

Concept formation. To test the patient's ability to think abstractly, ask the meaning of common proverbs. If the patient interprets the proverb "People in glass houses shouldn't throw stones" to mean that glass is breakable, he's displaying concrete thinking. If he interprets the proverb as saying "Don't criticize others for what you do yourself" he's showing abstract thinking. You may use other well-known proverbs, such as "A stitch in time saves nine" or "Don't count your chickens before they hatch."

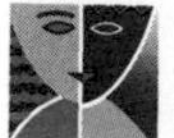

CULTURAL INSIGHT *Keep in mind that some familiar American sayings may confuse your patients from foreign cultures.*

General knowledge. Be sure to determine the patient's store of common knowledge. Do this by asking questions appropriate to his age and level of learning; for example, "Who's the president?" or "Who's the vice president?"

Judgment

Assess the patient's ability to evaluate choices and to draw appropriate conclusions. Ask the patient, "What would you do if you found a stamped, addressed, sealed airmail letter lying on the sidewalk?"

An answer to the above question such as "Track down the recipient" would indicate impaired judgment. Questions that emerge naturally during conversation (for example, "What would you do if you ran out of medication?") may also help to evaluate the patient's judgment.

Defects in judgment also may become apparent while the patient tells his history. Pay attention to how the patient handles his interpersonal relationships as well as his occupational and economic responsibilities.

Insight

Some of your questions at the beginning of the interview will give you valuable information about the patient's own insight. For example, the patient's response to the question "What brings you here today?" can reveal whether he has a mature understanding of his problem.

Can the patient see himself realistically? Is he aware of his illness and its circumstances? To assess insight, ask "What do you

> **ABNORMAL THOUGHT PROCESSES**
>
> During your mental assessment interview, you may identify some of the following abnormalities in the patient's thought processes.
>
> - Derailment — speech vacillation from one subject to another. The subjects are unrelated; ideas slip off track between clauses.
> - Flight of ideas — continuous flow of speech in which the patient jumps abruptly from topic to topic.
> - Neologisms — distorted or invented words.
> - Confabulation — fabrications of facts or events to fill in the gaps where memory loss has occurred.
> - Clanging — words spoken based on sound rather than meaning.
> - Echolalia — repetition of words or phrases that others say.
> - Incoherence — incomprehensible speech.
> - Circumstantiality — indirection and delay in reaching the point due to unnecessary detail.
> - Blocking — sudden interruption of speech.
> - Perseveration — persistent repetition of words or ideas.

think has caused your anxiety?" or "Have you noticed a recent change in yourself?"

Expect patients to show varying degrees of insight. For example, an alcoholic patient may admit to having a drinking problem but blame it on his job. The patient with severe lack of insight may indicate a psychotic state.

Perception

Perception refers to the patient's interpretation of reality as well as use of his senses. Psychologists are placing increasing importance on perception in understanding psychological disorders. For example, psychoanalysts have long said that depression results from internal, unresolved conflicts that became activated after a real or perceived loss. Recently, proponents of the cognitive theory of depression have suggested that depression arises from distorted perception. Depressed patients perceive themselves as worthless, the world as barren, and the future as bleak.

The patient with a sensory perception disorder may experience hallucinations, in which he perceives nonexistent external stimuli, or illusions in which he misinterprets external stimuli. Tactile, olfactory, and gustatory hallucinations usually indicate organic disorders.

However, not all visual and auditory hallucinations are associated with psychological disorders. For example, heat mirages, visions of a recently deceased loved one, and illusions evoked by environmental effects or experienced just before falling asleep don't indicate abnormalities. A patient may also experience mild and transitory hallucinations. Constant visual and auditory hallucinations may, however, give rise to strange or bizarre behavior. Disorders associated with hallucinations include schizophrenia and acute organic brain syndrome after withdrawal from alcohol or barbiturate addiction.

Coping mechanisms

Assess the patient who relies on coping mechanisms. When faced with a stressful situation the patient may adopt coping, or defense, mechanisms — behaviors that operate on an unconscious level to protect the ego. Examples include denial, displacement, fantasy, identification, projection, rationalization, reaction formation, regression, and repression. Look for an excessive reliance on these coping mechanisms during the interview. (See *Exploring coping mechanisms.*)

Thought content

Assess the patient's thought patterns as expressed throughout the examination. Are his thoughts well connected to reality? Are his ideas clear, and do they progress in a logical sequence? Observe the patient for indications of morbid thoughts and preoccupations or abnormal beliefs.

Abnormalities in thought content include delusions and obsessions. Usually associated with schizophrenia, delusions are false beliefs without a firm basis in reality. Grandiose and persecutory delusions are most common. Other types are somatic, nihilistic, and control. Ideas of reference (misinterpreting acts of others in a highly personal way) are closely related to delusions but don't represent the same level of ego disintegration.

Some patients suffer intense preoccupations, also called *obsessions* that interfere with daily living. Patients may constantly think about hygiene, for example. A compulsion is a preoccupation that's acted out such as constantly washing one's hands. Most compulsive patients must exert great effort to control their compulsions.

Also observe the patient for suicidal, self-destructive, violent, or superstitious thoughts; recurring dreams; distorted perceptions of reality; and feelings of worthlessness.

Sexual drive

Changes in sexual drive provide valuable in formation in psychological assessment, but you may have to sharpen your skills in assessing the patient's sexual activity. Prepare yourself for patients who are uncomfortable discussing their sexuality. You should avoid language that assumes a heterosexual orientation. Introduce the subject tactfully but directly. For example, say to the patient, "I'm going to ask you a few questions about your sexual activity because it's an important part of almost everyone's life." Follow-up questions might include:

- Are you sexually active?
- Do you usually have relations with men or women?
- Have you noticed any recent changes in your interest in sexual intercourse?
- Do you have the same pleasure from sexual intercourse now as before?
- What form of protection did you use during your last sexual encounter?

Competence

Assessing your patient's level of competence tells you if he understands reality and the consequences of his actions. Does the patient understand the implications of his illness, its treatment, and the consequences of avoiding treatment? Use extreme caution when assessing changes in competence. Unless behavior strongly indicates otherwise, assume that the patient is competent. Remember that legally, only a judge has the power or right to declare a person incompetent to make decisions regarding personal health and safety or financial matters.

Self-destructive behavior

Assess the patient's self-destructive behavior, keeping in mind that healthy, adventurous people may intentionally take death-defying risks, especially during youth. However, the risks taken by self-destructive patients aren't death-defying but death-seeking.

Suicide — intentional, self-inflicted death — may be carried out with guns, drugs, poisons, rope, automobiles, or razor

EXPLORING COPING MECHANISMS

Coping, or defense, mechanisms help to relieve anxiety. Common coping mechanisms include:

- Denial — refusal to admit truth or reality
- Displacement — transference of emotion from its original object to a substitute
- Fantasy — creation of unrealistic or improbable images to escape from daily pressures and responsibilities
- Identification — unconscious adoption of the personality characteristics, attitudes, values, and behaviors of another person
- Projection — displacement of negative feelings onto another person
- Rationalization — substitution of acceptable reasons for the real or actual reasons motivating behavior
- Reaction formation — behavior in a manner that's opposite from the way the person feels
- Regression — return to behavior of an earlier, more comfortable time
- Repression — exclusion of unacceptable thoughts and feelings from the conscious mind, leaving them to operate in the subconscious.

blades. It also may be carried out through drowning, jumping, or refusing food, fluids, or medications. In a subintentional suicide, a person has no conscious intention of dying but nevertheless engages in self-destructive acts that could easily become fatal.

Risk factors for suicide include:

- history of psychiatric illness
- substance abuse
- personality disorder
- prior suicide attempt
- family history of suicide.

Not all self-destructive behavior is suicidal in intent. Some patients engage in self-destructive behavior because it helps them to feel alive. For example, a patient who has lost touch with reality may cut or mutilate body parts to focus on physical pain, which may be less overwhelming than emotional distress. Such behavior may indicate a borderline personality disorder.

Be sure to assess depressed patients for suicidal tendencies. Not all such patients want to die, but a higher percentage of depressed patients commit suicide than patients with other diagnoses. Chemically dependent and schizophrenic patients also present a high suicide risk as well as people experiencing intolerably high levels of anxiety.

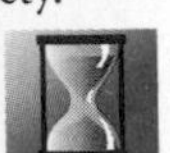

AGE ISSUE *Suicide rates are highest among men older than age 65 but are increasing among teenagers and young adults.*

Suicidal patients with schizophrenia may become agitated instead of depressed. Voices may tell them to kill themselves. Alarmingly, some patients with schizophrenia provide only vague behavioral clues before taking their lives.

If you observe signals of hopelessness, perform a direct suicide assessment. Protect the patient from self-harm during a suicidal crisis. After treatment, the patient should be thinking more clearly and, the hope is that he'll find reasons for living. (See *Recognizing and responding to suicidal patients*.)

Psychological and mental status testing

Although most of your mental status assessment can be done during your interview, you'll also need to evaluate other aspects of your patient's mental status. These aspects can be assessed using the psychological and mental status tests discussed here.

Mini–Mental State Examination

The Mini–Mental State Examination measures orientation, registration, recall, calculation, language, and graphomotor function. This test offers a quick and simple way to quantify cognitive function and screen for cognitive loss. Each section of the test involves a related series of questions or commands. The patient receives one point for each correct answer.

To give the examination, seat the patient in a quiet, well-lit room. Ask him to listen carefully and to answer each question about his cognitive function as accurately as he can.

Don't time the test, but do score it right away. To score, add the number of correct responses. The patient can receive a maximum score of 30 points.

Usually, a score below 24 indicates cognitive impairment, although this may not be an accurate cutoff for highly or poorly educated patients. A score below 20 usually appears in patients with delirium, dementia, schizophrenia, or affective disorder and not in normal elderly people or in patients with neurosis or personality disorder.

Cognitive Capacity Screening Examination

The Cognitive Capacity Screening Examination measures orientation, memory, calculation, and language. It's an interviewer-administered test of 30 questions that's used to assess dementia and delirium.

Cognitive Assessment Scale

The Cognitive Assessment Scale measures orientation, general knowledge, mental ability, and psychomotor function. It's used as a screening tool for the diagnosis of cognitive impairments associated with advancing age.

It takes approximately 45 minutes to administer and is composed of 103 questions grouped into 10 categories, including:

- temporal orientation
- spatial orientation
- attention-concentration and calculation
- immediate recall
- language
- remote memory
- judgment and abstraction

RECOGNIZING AND RESPONDING TO SUICIDAL PATIENTS

Watch for these warning signs of impending suicide:

- Withdrawing from life
- Isolating from any social situation
- Displaying signs of depression, which may include constipation, crying, fatigue, helplessness, hopelessness, poor concentration, reduced interest in sex and other activities, sadness, and weight loss
- Bidding farewell to friends and family
- Putting affairs in order
- Giving away prized possessions
- Expressing covert suicide messages and death wishes
- Voicing of obvious suicide messages such as "I'd be better off dead."

Answering a suicidal threat

If a patient shows signs of impending suicide, assess the seriousness of the intent and the immediacy of the risk. Consider a patient with a chosen method who plans to commit suicide in the next 48 to 72 hours a high risk.

Tell the patient that you're concerned. Then urge him to avoid self-destructive behavior until the staff has an opportunity to help him. You may specify a time for the patient to seek help.

Next, consult with the health care treatment team about arranging for psychiatric hospitalization or a safe equivalent such as having someone watch the patient at home. Initiate safety precautions for those with high suicide risk:

- Provide a safe environment. Check and correct conditions that could be dangerous for the patient. Look for exposed pipes, windows without safety glass, and access to the roof or open balconies.
- Remove dangerous objects, such as belts, razors, suspenders, light cords, glass, knives, nail files, and clippers.
- Make the patient's specific restrictions clear to staff members, plan for observation of the patient, and clarify day- and night-staff responsibilities.

Patients may ask you to keep their suicidal thoughts confidential. Remember, such requests are ambivalent; suicidal patients want to escape the pain of life, but they also want to live. A part of them wants you to tell other staff so they can be kept alive. Tell patients that you can't keep secrets that endanger their lives or conflict with their treatment. You have a duty to keep them safe and to ensure the best care.

Be alert when the patient is shaving, taking medication, or using the bathroom. These normal activities could be dangerous for the suicidal patient. In addition to observing the patient, maintain personal contact with him. Encourage continuity of care and consistency of health care providers. Helping the patient build emotional ties to others is the ultimate technique for preventing suicide.

- agnosia
- apraxia
- recent memory.

Beck Depression Inventory

The Beck Depression Inventory helps diagnose depression, determine its severity, and monitor the patient's response during treatment. This self-administered, self-scored test asks patients to rate how often they experience symptoms of depression, such as poor concentration, suicidal thoughts, guilty feelings, and crying. Questions focus on both cognitive symptoms such as impaired decision making, and on physical symptoms such as loss of appetite. Elderly and physically ill patients commonly score high on questions regarding their physical symptoms; their scores may stem from aging, physical illness, or depression.

The sum of 21 questions gives the total, with a maximum score of 63. A score of 10 to 18 indicates mild depression; 19 to 29, moderate to severe depression; 30 to 63, severe depression.

THE RORSCHACH TEST

The illustration depicts two of ten inkblots shown to patients during a Rorschach test. The patient describes his impressions of each inkblot, and the psychologist analyzes the content of the responses as an aid in personality evaluation.

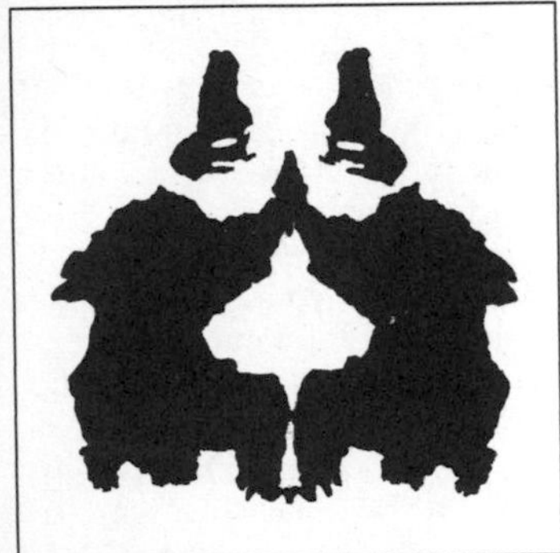

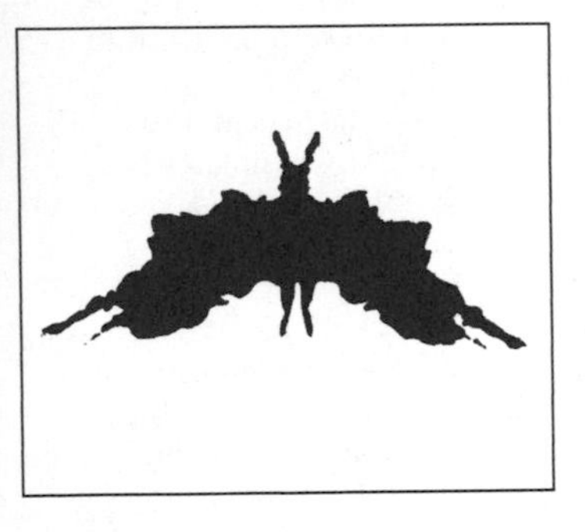

You may help the patient complete the test by reading the questions, but be careful not to influence his answers. Instruct the patient to choose the answer that describes him most accurately.

If you suspect depression, a test score above 17 may provide objective evidence of the need for treatment. To monitor the patient's depression, repeat the test during the course of treatment.

Global Deterioration Scale

The Global Deterioration Scale assesses and stages primary degenerative dementia based on orientation, memory, and neurologic function. It provides caregivers with an overview of the stages of cognitive function for those suffering from a primary degenerative dementia such as Alzheimer's disease. The results are broken down into seven stages:

- Stages 1 to 3 are the predementia stages.
- Stages 4 to 7 are the dementia stages.

Beginning in stage 5, an individual can no longer survive without assistance. Caregivers can get an idea of where an individual is at in the disease process by observing that individual's behavioral characteristics and comparing them with the scale.

Minnesota Multiphasic Personality Inventory

Made up of 566 questions, the Minnesota Multiphasic Personality Inventory test is a structured paper-and-pencil test that provides a practical technique for assessing personality traits and ego function in adolescents and adults. Most patients who read English require little assistance in completing this test.

Psychologists translate a patient's answers into a psychological profile. Use caution in interpreting profiles. Patient answers are compared with diagnostic criteria established and standardized in the 1930s. Critics charge that the personality profile models developed in the 1930s were based on studies of small groups (30 people) and may no longer provide a valid basis for diagnosis.

Test results include information on coping strategies, defenses, strengths, gender identification, and self-esteem. The psychologist combines the patient's profile with data gathered from the interview and explains the test results to the patient.

The test pattern may strongly suggest a diagnostic category. If results indicate a risk of suicide or violence, monitor the patient's behavior. If results show frequent somatic complaints indicating possible hypochondria, evaluate the patient's physical status. If complaints lack medical confirmation, help the patient explore how these symptoms may signal emotional distress.

Draw-a-person test

In the draw-a-person test, the patient draws a human figure of each sex. The psychologist interprets the drawing systematically and correlates his interpretation with diagnosis. This test also provides an estimate of a child's developmental level.

UNDERSTANDING THE DSM-IV-TR

When evaluating a patient with psychiatric problems, considering factors that may have influenced his condition, such as life stresses or physical illness, is an important part in arriving at a diagnosis. To help health care providers accomplish this, the American Psychiatric Association's *Diagnostic and Statistical Manual of Mental Disorders,* Fourth Edition, Text Revision *(DSM-IV-TR)* offers a more flexible approach to diagnosis and a more realistic picture of the patient, which should improve treatment. The key to the *DSM-IV-TR's* effectiveness is its multiaxial evaluation that requires every patient to be assessed on each of five axes.

Axis I
Clinical syndromes; conditions not attributable to a mental disorder that are a focus of attention or treatment; or clinical disorders and other conditions that may be a focus of clinical attention

Axis II
Personality disorders; mental retardation

Axis III
General medical conditions

Axis IV
Psychosocial and environmental problems

Axis V
Global Assessment and Functioning; highest level of adaptive functioning during the past year.

For example, using the above multiaxial evaluation, a patient's diagnosis might read as follows:

Axis I: adjustment disorder with anxious mood

Axis II: obsessive-compulsive personality

Axis III: Crohn's disease, acute bleeding episode

Axis IV: 5 to 6 (moderately severe); recent remarriage, death of father

Axis V: very good; patient has been a successful single parent, new wife, schoolteacher, part-time journalist.

Sentence completion test
In the sentence completion test, the patient completes a series of partial sentences. A sentence might begin, "When I get angry, I...." The response may reveal the patient's fantasies, fears, aspirations, or anxieties.

Thematic apperception test
With the thematic apperception test, the patient views a series of pictures depicting ambiguous situations, he then tells a story describing each picture. The psychologist evaluates these stories systematically to obtain insights into the patient's personality, particularly regarding interpersonal relationships and conflicts.

The Rorschach test
During a Rorschach test, the patient is asked to describe his impressions of 10 inkblots. The psychologist analyzes the content of the responses as an aid in personality evaluation. (See *The Rorschach test.*)

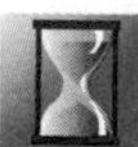

AGE ISSUE *Most elderly patients generally do well on the entire mental health examination, but keep in mind that functional impairments may become evident as they age. Elderly people are slower to retrieve and process data, and they take more time to learn new material. Motor responses may be slow and the ability to perform complex tasks may be impaired. Don't confuse these impairments with mental illness — they may be due to aging.*

Physical assessment
Because mental health problems may stem from organic causes or medical treatment, a physical assessment is also warranted. Observe the patient for key signs and symptoms and examine him by using inspection, palpation, percussion, and auscultation.

Classification of mental disorders
Mental status disorders are classified according to the American Psychiatric Associ-

ation's *Diagnostic and Statistical Manual of Mental Disorders,* Fourth Edition, Text Revision (*DSM-IV-TR*). (See *Understanding the DSM-IV-TR.*)The classification emphasizes observable data and deemphasizes subjective and theoretical impressions. The manual offers a standardized interdisciplinary system for all members of the mental health care team to use. It includes a complete description of psychiatric disorders and other conditions, and describes diagnostic criteria that must be met to support each diagnosis.

Abnormal findings

During a mental health assessment, you may detect abnormalities in thought processes, thought content, and perception because your patient may exhibit vagueness, empty repetition, or obscure phrases. In addition, a patient may seek care for any other of signs and symptoms that may be related to mental health including agitation, anxiety, bizarre gait, depression, fatigue, and psychotic behavior. The following history, physical assessment, and analysis summaries will help you assess each one quickly and accurately. After obtaining further information, begin to interpret the findings. (See *Mental health assessment: Interpreting your findings.*)

Agitation

Agitation refers to a state of hyperarousal, increased tension, and irritability that can lead to confusion, hyperactivity, and overt hostility. It can arise gradually or suddenly and last for minutes or months. Whether it's mild or severe, agitation worsens with increased fever, pain, stress, or external stimuli.

History

Determine the severity of the patient's agitation by examining the number and quality of agitation-induced behaviors, such as emotional lability, confusion, memory loss, hyperactivity, and hostility. Obtain a history from the patient or a family member, including diet, known allergies, and use of herbal medicine.

Ask if the patient is being treated for any illnesses. Find out if he has had any recent infections, trauma, stress, or changes in sleep patterns. Ask him about prescribed or over-the-counter drug use, including supplements and herbal medicines. Ask about alcohol intake.

Physical assessment

Perform a complete physical examination of the patient with special emphasis on mental status. In addition, check for signs of drug abuse, such as needle tracks and dilated pupils. Obtain baseline vital signs and neurologic status for future comparison.

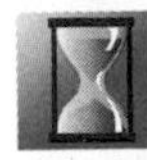

AGE ISSUE *When evaluating an agitated child, remember to use words that he can understand and to look for nonverbal clues. For instance, if you suspect that pain is causing agitation, ask him to tell you where it hurts, watching for other indicators, such as wincing, crying, or moving away.*

Analysis

Agitation alone merely signals a change in the patient's condition. But it's a useful indicator of a developing disorder. Agitation can result from a toxic (poisons), metabolic, or infectious cause; brain injury; or a psychiatric disorder. It can also result from pain, fever, anxiety, drug use and withdrawal, hypersensitivity reactions, and various disorders.

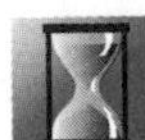

AGE ISSUE *A common sign in children, agitation accompanies the expected childhood diseases as well as more severe disorders that can lead to brain damage, such as hyperbilirubinemia, phenylketonuria, vitamin A deficiency, hepatitis, frontal lobe syndrome, increased intracranial pressure, and lead poisoning. In neonates, agitation can stem from alcohol or drug withdrawal if the mother abused these substances.*

Any deviation from an older person's usual activities or rituals may provoke anxiety or agitation. Any environmental change, such as a transfer to a nursing home or a visit from a stranger in the patient's home, may trigger a need for treatment.

Anxiety

Anxiety is the most common psychiatric symptom and can result in significant impairment. A subjective reaction to a real or imagined threat, anxiety is a nonspecific feeling of uneasiness or dread. It may be mild, moderate, or severe. Mild anxiety may

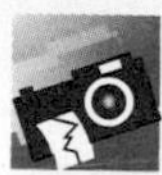

CLINICAL PICTURE

MENTAL HEALTH ASSESSMENT: INTERPRETING YOUR FINDINGS

After you assess the patient, a group of findings may lead you to suspect a particular mental health disorder. The chart below shows you some common groups of findings for major signs and symptoms related to mental health, along with their probable causes.

Sign or symptom and findings	Probable cause
Agitation	
▪ Agitation, mania ▪ Euphoria, irritability ▪ Delusions ▪ Flight of ideas ▪ Extreme talkativeness ▪ Easily distracted ▪ Decreased sleep	Bipolar disorder, manic phase
▪ Varying degrees of agitation ▪ Excessive worry lasting over 6 months disproportionate to situation ▪ Trembling and twitching ▪ Dry mouth ▪ Sweating ▪ Nausea ▪ Urinary frequency or diarrhea	Generalized anxiety disorder
Anxiety	
▪ Chronic anxiety ▪ Recurrent, unshakable thoughts or impulse to perform ritualistic acts ▪ Recognition that acts are irrational with inability to control them ▪ Decreased anxiety after performing ritualistic act	Obsessive-compulsive disorder
Anxiety *(continued)*	
▪ Chronic anxiety ▪ Persistent fear of object, activity, or situation accompanied by intense desire to avoid object, activity, or situation ▪ Inability to suppress fear; recognition that fear is irrational	Phobias
▪ Chronic anxiety of varying severity ▪ Exposure to extreme traumatic event ▪ Intrusive, vivid memories and thoughts of trauma ▪ Reliving of event in nightmares and dreams ▪ Insomnia ▪ Depression ▪ Feelings of numbness and detachment	Posttraumatic stress disorder
Bizarre gait	
▪ Bizarre gait or paralysis developing after severe stress ▪ Unaccompanied by other symptoms ▪ Patient indifference to impairment	Conversion disorder

(continued)

MENTAL HEALTH ASSESSMENT: INTERPRETING YOUR FINDINGS *(continued)*

Sign or symptom and findings	Probable cause
Bizarre gait *(continued)*	
■ Bizarre gait along with any combination of pseudo-neurologic problems ■ Fainting ■ Weakness ■ Memory loss ■ Dysphagia ■ Visual problems ■ Loss of voice ■ Seizures ■ Bladder dysfunction ■ Pain in joints, back, and extremities ■ Complaints in almost any other body system	Somatization disorder
Depression	
■ Depression alternating with mania ■ Low self-esteem ■ Social withdrawal ■ Feelings of hopelessness, apathy, or self-reproach ■ Difficulty concentrating or thinking clearly ■ Sluggish physical movements ■ Slowed speech and responses ■ Sleep disturbances ■ Sexual dysfunction	Bipolar disorders, depressed phase
Depression *(continued)*	
■ Depression accompanied by apathy, decreased interest or pleasure in almost all activities occurring every day ■ Impaired social, occupational, and overall general functioning ■ Severe fatigue ■ Inability to make decisions or concentrate ■ Feelings of worthlessness or extreme guilt ■ Appetite changes ■ Sleep disturbances ■ Decreased libido ■ Suicidal ideation	Major depressive disorder
Fatigue	
■ Persistent fatigue unrelated to exertion ■ Headache ■ Anorexia ■ Constipation ■ Sexual dysfunction ■ Insomnia ■ Slowed speech ■ Bradykinesia or agitation ■ Irritability ■ Loss of concentration ■ Feelings of worthlessness ■ Persistent thoughts of death	Chronic depression

MENTAL HEALTH ASSESSMENT: INTERPRETING YOUR FINDINGS *(continued)*

Sign or symptom and findings	Probable cause
Psychotic behavior	
▪ Psychotic behavior characterized as odd or eccentric behavior ▪ Inaccurate beliefs that others' behaviors or environmental phenomena are meant to have an effect on the patient ▪ Odd beliefs or magical thinking ▪ Unusual perceptual experiences ▪ Vague, circumstantial, metaphorical, overly elaborate, or stereotypical speech ▪ Unfounded suspicion of being followed, talked about, persecuted, or under surveillance ▪ Inappropriate or constricted affect ▪ Social isolation and excessive social anxiety	Schizotypal personality disorder
Psychotic behavior *(continued)*	
▪ Hallucinations ▪ Delusions ▪ Thought blocking, magical thinking ▪ Speech abnormalities, such as clang associations, echolalia, loose association and flight of ideas, word salad, and neologisms ▪ Apathy ▪ Blunted affect ▪ Anhedonia ▪ Asociality ▪ Lack of motivation ▪ Confused thinking and speech ▪ Bizarre behavior	Schizophrenia

cause slight physical or psychological discomfort. Severe anxiety may be incapacitating or even life-threatening.

History

If the patient displays mild or moderate anxiety, ask about its duration. Find out if it's constant or sporadic and if the patient noticed any precipitating factors. Ask him if the anxiety is exacerbated by stress, lack of sleep, or excessive caffeine intake and alleviated by rest, tranquilizers, or exercise. Obtain a complete medical history, especially noting drug use.

CRITICAL POINT *If the patient displays acute, severe anxiety, quickly take his vital signs and determine his chief complaint, which indicates how to proceed. For example, if the patient's anxiety occurs with chest pain and shortness of breath, suspect myocardial infarction and intervene accordingly. While examining the patient, try to keep him calm. Suggest relaxation techniques, and talk to him in a reassuring, soothing voice. Uncontrolled anxiety can alter vital signs and exacerbate the causative disorder.*

Physical assessment

Perform a thorough physical examination, focusing on any complaints that may trigger or be aggravated by anxiety. If significant physical signs don't accompany the patient's anxiety, suspect a psychological basis. Determine the patient's level of consciousness (LOC) and observe his behavior. If appropriate, refer the patient for psychiatric evaluation.

Analysis
Everyone experiences anxiety from time to time — it's a normal response to actual danger, prompting the body (through stimulation of the sympathetic and parasympathetic nervous systems) to purposeful action. It's also a normal response to physical and emotional stress, which can be produced by virtually any illness. In addition, anxiety can be precipitated or exacerbated by many nonpathologic factors, including lack of sleep, poor diet, and excessive intake of caffeine or other stimulants. However, excessive, unwarranted anxiety may indicate an underlying psychological problem.

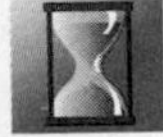

AGE ISSUE *In children, anxiety usually results from painful physical illness or inadequate oxygenation. Its autonomic signs tend to be more common and dramatic than in adults.*

In elderly patients, distractions from their usual activities may provoke anxiety or agitation.

Bizarre gait
A bizarre gait is also called *hysterical gait.* The gait has no consistent pattern.

History
If you suspect that the patient's gait impairment has no organic cause, begin to investigate other possibilities. Ask the patient when he first developed the impairment and whether it coincided with any stressful period or event, such as the death of a loved one or loss of employment. Ask about associated symptoms, and explore any reports of frequent unexplained illnesses and multiple health care provider visits. Subtly try to determine if he'll gain anything from malingering, for instance, added attention or an insurance settlement.

Physical assessment
Begin by testing the patient's reflexes and sensorimotor function, noting any abnormal response patterns. To quickly check his reports of leg weakness or paralysis, perform a test for Hoover's sign: Place the patient in the supine position and stand at his feet. Cradle a heel in each of your palms, and rest your hands on the table. Ask the patient to raise the affected leg. In true motor weakness, the heel of the other leg will press downward; in hysteria, this movement will be absent. As a further check, observe the patient for normal movements when he's unaware of being watched.

Analysis
Bizarre gait is produced unconsciously by a person with a somatoform disorder or consciously by a malingerer, and it has no obvious organic basis. It may mimic an organic impairment but characteristically has a more theatrical or bizarre quality with key elements missing, such as a spastic gait without hip circumduction or leg "paralysis" with normal reflexes and motor strength. Its manifestations may include wild gyrations, exaggerated stepping, leg dragging, or mimicking unusual walks, such as that of a tightrope walker.

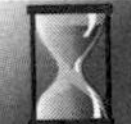

AGE ISSUE *Bizarre gait is rare in patients younger than age 8. More common in prepubescence, it usually results from conversion disorder.*

Depression
Depression is a mood disturbance characterized by feelings of sadness, despair, and loss of interest or pleasure in activities. These feelings may be accompanied by somatic complaints, such as changes in appetite, sleep disturbances, restlessness or lethargy, and decreased concentration. Thoughts of injuring one's self, death, or suicide may also occur.

History
During the examination, determine how the patient feels about himself, his family, and his environment. Explore the nature of his depression, the extent to which other factors affect it, and his coping mechanisms and their effectiveness.

Begin by asking the patient what's bothering him. Find out how his current mood differs from his usual mood. Then ask him to describe the way he feels about himself. Ask about his plans and dreams, determining how realistic they are. Find out if he's generally satisfied with what he has accomplished in his work, relationships, and other interests. Ask about changes in his social interactions, sleep patterns, appetite, normal activities, or ability to make decisions and concentrate. Determine patterns of drug and alcohol use. Listen for clues that may suggest suicidal ideation.

Ask the patient about his family—its patterns of interaction and characteristic responses to success and failure. Ask about what part he feels he plays in his family life. Find out if other family members have been depressed and whether anyone important to the patient recently has been sick or has died. Finally, ask the patient about his environment. Find out if his lifestyle has changed in the past month, 6 months, or year. Find out what he does to feel better when he feels blue. Find out how he feels about his role in the community and the available resources. Determine if he has an adequate support network.

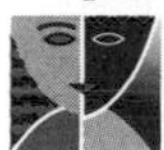

CULTURAL INSIGHT *Patients who don't speak English fluently may have difficulty communicating their feelings and thoughts. Consider using someone outside the family as an interpreter to allow the patient to express his feelings more freely.*

Physical assessment

Complete a thorough physical examination of all body systems to rule out possible medical causes. Pay particular attention to body systems that may be affected due to depression, such as nutritional status, skin, and elimination.

Analysis

Clinical depression must be distinguished from "the blues"—periodic bouts of dysphonia that are less persistent and severe than the clinical disorder. The criterion for major depression is one or more episodes of depressed mood, or decreased interest or the ability to take pleasure in all or most activities, lasting at least 2 weeks.

Major depression strikes 10% to 15% of adults, affecting all racial, ethnic, age, and socioeconomic groups. It's twice as common in women as in men and is especially prevalent among adolescents. Depression has numerous causes, including genetic and family history, medical and psychiatric disorders, and the use of certain drugs. It can also occur in the postpartum period. A complete psychiatric and physical examination should be conducted to exclude possible medical causes.

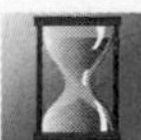

AGE ISSUE *Elderly patients commonly present with physical complaints, somatic complaints, agitation, or changes in intellectual functioning (memory impairment) making the diagnosis of depression difficult. Depressed older adults at highest risk for suicide are those who are over age 85, have low self-esteem, and have a need to be in control.*

Fatigue

Fatigue is a feeling of excessive tiredness, lack of energy, or exhaustion accompanied by a strong desire to rest or sleep. This common symptom is distinct from weakness, which involves the muscles, but may occur with it.

History

Obtain a careful history to identify the patient's fatigue pattern. Ask about related symptoms and any recent viral or bacterial illness or stressful changes in lifestyle. Explore nutritional habits and any appetite or weight changes. Carefully review the patient's medical and psychiatric history for any chronic disorders that commonly produce fatigue. Ask about a family history of such disorders.

Obtain a thorough drug history, noting use of any narcotic or drug with fatigue as an adverse effect. Ask about alcohol and drug use patterns. Determine the patient's risk for carbon monoxide poisoning, and inquire as to whether the patient has a carbon monoxide detector in his home.

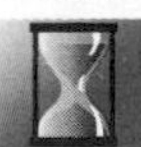

AGE ISSUE *When evaluating a child for fatigue, ask his parents if they've noticed any change in his activity level. Fatigue without an organic cause occurs normally during accelerated growth phases in preschool-age and prepubescent children. However, psychological causes of fatigue must be considered, for example, a depressed child may try to escape problems at home or school by taking refuge in sleep. In the pubescent child, consider the possibility of drug abuse, particularly of hypnotics and tranquilizers.*

Always ask older patients about fatigue because this symptom may be insidious and mask more serious underlying conditions.

Physical assessment

Perform a complete physical examination of all body systems. Observe the patient's general appearance for overt signs of depression or organic illness. Observe if he is unkempt or expressionless and if he appears tired or sickly or has a slumped posture. Evaluate his mental status, noting especially mental clouding, attention deficits, agitation, or psychomotor retardation.

Analysis

Fatigue is a normal and important response to physical overexertion, prolonged emotional stress, and sleep deprivation. However, it can also be a nonspecific symptom of a psychological or physiologic disorder—especially viral or bacterial infection and endocrine, cardiovascular, or neurologic disease.

Fatigue reflects both hypermetabolic and hypometabolic states in which nutrients needed for cellular energy and growth are lacking because of overly rapid depletion, impaired replacement mechanisms, insufficient hormone production, or inadequate nutrient intake or metabolism.

Fatigue that worsens with activity and improves with rest generally indicates a physical disorder; the opposite pattern, a psychological disorder. Fatigue lasting longer than 4 months, constant fatigue that's unrelieved by rest, and transient exhaustion that quickly gives way to bursts of energy are other findings associated with psychological disorders.

Psychotic behavior

Psychotic behavior reflects an inability or unwillingness to recognize and acknowledge reality and to relate with others. It may begin suddenly or insidiously, progressing from vague complaints of fatigue, insomnia, or headache to withdrawal, social isolation, and preoccupation with certain issues resulting in gross impairment in functioning.

History

Because the patient's behavior can make it difficult—or potentially dangerous—to obtain pertinent information via interview and examination, conduct the interview in a calm, safe, and well-lit room. Provide enough personal space to avoid threatening or agitating the patient. The physical assessment may need to be postponed if the patient is agitated or combative.

Physical assessment

Ask the patient to describe his problem and any circumstances that may have precipitated it. Obtain a drug history, noting especially use of an antipsychotic, and explore his use of alcohol and other drugs such as cocaine, indicating duration of use and amount. Ask about any recent illnesses or accidents.

As the patient talks, watch for cognitive, linguistic, or perceptual abnormalities such as delusions. Observe if his thoughts and actions match. Look for unusual gestures, posture, gait, tone of voice, and mannerisms. Observe the patient for his responses to stimuli, for example, if he looks around the room.

Interview the patient's family. Find out which family members he seems closest to. Ask the family how they describe the patient's relationships, communication patterns, and role. Find out if any family member has ever been hospitalized for psychiatric or emotional illness. Ask about the patient's compliance with his drug regimen.

Finally, evaluate the patient's environment, educational and employment history, and socioeconomic status. Find out if community services are available, how he spends his leisure time, if he has friends, and if he has ever had a close emotional relationship.

Analysis

Various behaviors together or separately can constitute psychotic behavior. These include delusions, illusions, hallucinations, bizarre language, and perseveration. Delusions are persistent beliefs that have no basis in reality or in the patient's knowledge or experience, such as delusions of grandeur. Illusions are misinterpretations of external sensory stimuli such as a mirage in the desert. In contrast, hallucinations are sensory perceptions that don't result from external stimuli. Bizarre language reflects a communication disruption. It can range from echolalia (purposeless repetition of a word or phrase) and clang association (repetition of words or phrases that sound similar) to neologisms (creation and use of words whose meaning only the patient knows). Perseveration, a persistent verbal or motor response, may indicate organic brain disease. Motor changes include inactivity, excessive activity, and repetitive movements.

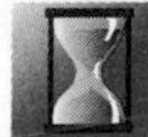

AGE ISSUE *In children, psychotic behavior may result from early infantile autism, symbiotic infantile psychosis, or childhood schizophrenia — any of which can retard development of language, abstract thinking, and socialization. An adolescent patient who exhibits psychotic behavior may have a history of several days' drug use or lack of sleep or food, which must be evaluated and corrected before therapy can begin.*

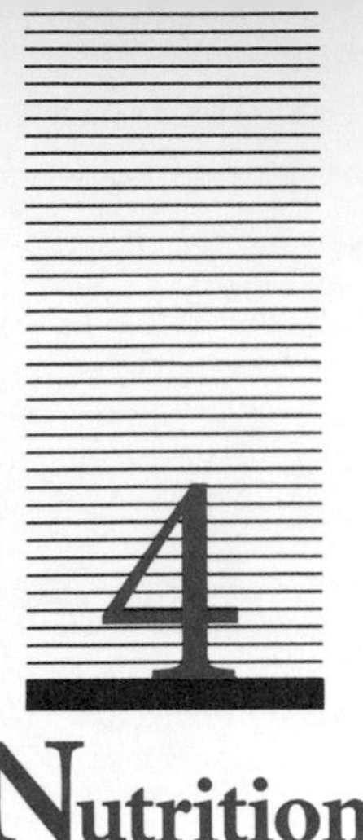

Nutrition

A healthy and balanced nutritional status should be the goal for everyone. This goal is met when nutrient supply, or intake, meets the demand, or requirement. An imbalance occurs when there's overnutrition and supply exceeds demand or undernutrition when demand exceeds supply.

A patient's nutritional status is evaluated by examining information from several sources, including a nutritional screening as well as his medical history, physical assessment findings, and laboratory results, in order to detect potential imbalances. The sources used depend on the patient and setting. A comprehensive nutritional assessment may then be conducted to set goals and determine interventions to correct actual or potential imbalances.

Based on the information gathered in the comprehensive nutritional assessment, the patient may require restrictions in diet, such as a reduction in calories, fat, saturated fat, cholesterol, sodium, or other nutrients. Other diet plans involve therapeutic correction of imbalances, such as by increasing or decreasing certain minerals or vitamins in the patient's diet.

Normal nutrition

Nutrition refers to the sum of the processes by which a living organism ingests, digests, absorbs, transports, uses, and excretes nutrients. For nutrition to be adequate, a person must receive the proper nutrients, including carbohydrates, proteins, lipids, vitamins, minerals, and water. Also, his digestive system must function properly for his body to make use of these nutrients.

The body breaks down nutrients mechanically and chemically into simpler compounds for absorption in the stomach and intestines. The mechanical breakdown of food begins with chewing and then continues in the stomach and intestine as food is churned in the GI tract. The chemical processes start with the salivary enzymes in the mouth and continue with acid and enzyme action throughout the rest of the GI tract.

ANABOLISM AND CATABOLISM

Anabolism is the building up in the body of complex chemical compounds from simpler compounds—for example, proteins from amino acids—to be used for tissue growth, maintenance, and repair.

Catabolism is the breaking down in the body of complex chemical compounds that are then converted into simple compounds and stored or used for energy.

Carbohydrates

Composed of carbon, hydrogen, and oxygen, carbohydrates provide the primary source of energy, yielding 4 kilocalorie (kcal) per gram. Nutritional experts recommend that carbohydrates make up 50% to 60% of an individual's daily dietary intake.

Ingested as complex carbohydrates such as starches and simple carbohydrates such as sugars, carbohydrates are the chief protein-sparing ingredients in a nutritionally sound diet. Carbohydrates are absorbed primarily as glucose; some are absorbed as fructose and galactose and converted to glucose by the liver. A body cell may metabolize glucose to produce the energy needed to maintain cell life or may store it in the muscles and liver as glycogen. It can be converted quickly when the body needs energy fast. If glucose is unavailable, the body breaks down stored fat, a source of energy during periods of starvation. (See *Anabolism and catabolism.*)

Excessive carbohydrate intake— especially of simple carbohydrates—can cause obesity, predisposing the patient to many disorders, including hypertension.

Proteins

Proteins, which consist of amino acids joined by peptide bonds, are complex organic compounds containing carbon, hydrogen, oxygen, and nitrogen atoms. One gram of protein yields 4 kcal. Proteins are necessary for growth, maintenance, and repair of body tissues. The cells of the body can't survive without protein.

Different proteins contain different amino acids; however, not all protein food sources are identical in quality. Complete proteins—such as those found in poultry, fish, meat, eggs, milk, and cheese—can maintain body tissue and promote a normal growth rate; incomplete proteins, such as vegetables and grains, lack essential amino acids. Essential amino acids are organic proteins that the body needs for nitrogen balance but can't produce itself.

The body doesn't store protein because it has a limited life span and constantly undergoes change. The rate of protein turnover varies in different tissues. When the usual sources (carbohydrates and fat) can't meet the body's energy demands, the body uses protein precursors to generate energy.

In a healthy individual with adequate caloric and protein intake, nitrogen intake should equal nitrogen excretion (nitrogen balance). Positive nitrogen balance occurs when nitrogen intake exceeds its output—for example, during pregnancy or growth periods. Negative nitrogen balance occurs when nitrogen output exceeds intake.

CRITICAL POINT *In a patient with inadequate protein intake, negative nitrogen balance occurs, resulting in tissue wasting; insufficient quality of digested dietary protein; or excessive tissue breakdown after stress, injury, immobilization, or disease.*

Lipids

Chemically similar to carbohydrates, lipids consist of carbon, hydrogen, and oxygen.

UNDERSTANDING LIPOPROTEINS

Synthesized primarily in the liver, lipoproteins consist of lipids combined with plasma proteins. The five types of lipoproteins are chylomicrons, very-low-density lipoproteins (VLDLs), low-density lipoproteins (LDLs), intermediate-density lipoproteins (IDLs), and high-density lipoproteins (HDLs).

Chylomicrons
Chylomicrons are the lowest-density lipoproteins, consisting mostly of triglycerides derived from dietary fat, with small amounts of protein and other lipids. In the form of chylomicrons, long-chain fatty acids and cholesterol move from the intestine to the blood and storage areas. Researchers haven't found a connection between an above-normal level of circulating chylomicrons (type I hyperlipoproteinemia) and coronary artery disease (CAD).

VLDLs
VLDLs contain mostly triglycerides with some phospholipids and cholesterol. Produced in the liver and small intestine, VLDLs transport glycerides. Obese patients and those with diabetes and, less commonly, young patients with CAD, may have above normal VLDL levels (type IV hyperlipoproteinemia).

LDLs
LDLs consist mainly of cholesterol, with comparatively few triglycerides. By-products of VLDL breakdown, LDLs have the highest atherogenic potential (conducive to forming plaques containing cholesterol and other lipid material in the arteries). An elevated LDL level (type II hyperlipoproteinemia) commonly accompanies an elevated VLDL level.

IDLs
IDLs are short-lived and contain almost equal amounts of cholesterol and triglycerides and smaller amounts of phospholipids and protein. IDLs are converted to LDLs by lipase.

HDLs
HDLs — which are comprised of 50% protein and 50% phospholipids, cholesterol, and triglycerides — may help remove excess cholesterol. Because patients with high HDL levels have a lower incidence of CAD, many researchers believe HDLs may help protect patients against CAD.

However, they have a smaller proportion of oxygen than carbohydrates, and also differ in their structure and properties.

Lipids and other fats are essential for normal functioning. To be transported throughout the body they must combine with plasma proteins to form lipoproteins. (See *Understanding lipoproteins.*) Likewise, free fatty acids combine with albumin; and cholesterol, triglycerides, and phospholipids bind to globulin.

One gram of fat yields 9 kcal. Fats should make up about 30% of the daily caloric intake — 5% to 10% less than the amount ingested by the average person. Saturated fats should account for only about one-third of total fat consumption, and an individual should consume no more than 300 mg of cholesterol per day.

Vitamins and minerals

Essential for normal metabolism, growth, and development, vitamins and minerals are biologically active organic compounds that contribute to enzyme reactions that facilitate the metabolism of amino acids, fats, and carbohydrates. Although the body requires relatively small amounts of vitamins, inadequate vitamin intake leads to deficiency states and disorders.

Water-soluble vitamins include vitamins C and B complex. Fat-soluble vitamins include vitamins A, D, E, and K. Surgery, disease, medications, metabolic disorders, and trauma affect the activity of vitamins in the body. Because readily observable changes don't occur until the late stages of vitamin deficiency, you must assess the patient's dietary intake and observe for subtle changes that provide an early warning of vitamin depletion.

Minerals are equally essential to good nutrition and participate in various physiologic activities. (See *Role of minerals in metabolism*.)

ROLE OF MINERALS IN METABOLISM

Dietary intake of minerals is essential for these physiologic functions:

- maintenance of acid-base balance and osmotic pressure
- membrane transfer of essential compounds
- metabolism of enzymes
- muscle contractility
- nerve impulse transmission
- growth.

Water

Essential to sustain life, water transports nutrients throughout the body and may contribute minerals when consumed.

Nutritional screening

Nutritional screening looks at certain variables to determine the risk of nutritional problems in certain populations. A screening may target pregnant women, elderly people, or those with particular conditions (such as cardiac disorders) to detect deficiencies or potential imbalances. A dietitian, diet technician, or other qualified health care professional may perform this type of screening. Routine screening takes place during the initial history and physical assessment.

The most commonly examined values include:

- height and weight history
- unintentional weight loss (more than 5% in 30 days)
- laboratory values
- skin integrity
- appetite
- present illness or diagnosis
- medical history
- diet
- functional status
- advanced age (age 80 and older).

Wellness screen

A wellness screen has been developed by the Nutritional Screening Initiative, a project of the American Academy of Family Physicians, the American Dietetic Association, and the National Council on the Aging, Inc. This screening tool also assesses body mass index, which evaluates height in relationship to weight as well as eating habits, living environment, and functional status. (See *Using a wellness screen*, page 62.)

Risk assessment

Once the wellness screening is complete, a level of risk for nutritional problems is assigned. Those individuals at higher risk should be given a comprehensive nutritional assessment, whereas those at lower to moderate risk should be periodically reevaluated. (See *Levels of risk for malnutrition*, page 63.)

USING A WELLNESS SCREEN

A wellness screen is an effective assessment tool for evaluating your patient's nutritional status. It provides useful information about the patient's body mass index (BMI), eating habits, living environment, and functional status. A checkmark next to any statement indicates that the patient is at risk and requires further assessment. If indicated, contact the appropriate resources who can provide additional help.

Patient's name *Robert Harrison* Date *5/30/05*

BMI

BMI measures total body fat based on height and weight. To calculate your patient's BMI, first obtain his height to the nearest inch and his weight to the nearest pound. Calculate his BMI by dividing the body weight in kilograms by height in meters squared or by dividing the weight in pounds by height in inches squared and multiplying that result by 703.

Height (in): *71*
Weight (lb): *220*
BMI: *31*

Check whether:

- ☐ the patient lost or gained 10 lb or more in the past 6 months.
- ☑ BMI is less than 18.5.
- ☐ BMI is greater than 24.9.

Eating habits

Check whether the patient:

- ☐ doesn't have enough food to eat each day.
- ☐ usually eats alone.
- ☐ doesn't eat anything on 1 or more days each month.
- ☑ has a poor appetite.
- ☐ is on a special diet.
- ☑ eats vegetables two or fewer times per day.
- ☐ drinks milk or eats milk products once or less per day.
- ☐ eats fruit or drinks fruit juice once or less daily.
- ☐ eats breads, cereals, pasta, rice, or other grains five or fewer times daily.
- ☑ has difficulty chewing or swallowing.
- ☐ has more than one alcoholic drink per day (if a woman); more than two drinks per day (if a man).
- ☐ has pain in the mouth, teeth, or gums.

Living environment

Check whether the patient:

- ☐ lives on an income of less than $6,000 per year (per individual in the household).
- ☑ lives alone.
- ☐ is housebound.
- ☐ is concerned about home security.
- ☐ lives in a home with inadequate heating or cooling.
- ☐ doesn't have a stove or refrigerator.
- ☐ can't or prefers not to spend money on food (less than $25 per person spent on food each week).

Functional status

- ☐ Check whether the patient needs help with:
- ☐ bathing.
- ☐ dressing.
- ☐ grooming.
- ☐ toileting.
- ☐ eating.
- ☐ walking or moving about.
- ☐ traveling (outside of the home).
- ☑ preparing food.
- ☑ shopping for food or other necessities.

Comprehensive nutritional assessment

When you complete the nutritional screening and have identified a patient at risk, the next step is a comprehensive nutritional assessment that examines additional factors and better determines the degree of malnutrition. Using this assessment, a baseline nutritional status is determined and effective nutritional care can be planned. Because of the extensive training required and the need

LEVELS OF RISK FOR MALNUTRITION

A patient may be assigned a risk level according to protocols established by your facility. An example of such a risk table is shown here. Even if a patient is determined to be at low risk or no risk at all, periodic evaluations should be performed to detect changes in his nutritional status.

Risk factor	Low	Mild	Moderate	High
Weight (% ideal body weight)	>90	80 to 90	70 to 80	<70
Serum albumin (g/dl)	>3.4	3.0 to 3.3	2.5 to 2.9	<2.5
Intake	Adequate	Fair to good	Poor to fair	Poor to fair
Skin (pressure ulcers)	Intact	Stage I or stage II	Stage III or stage IV	Stage III or stage IV
Diet	Solid	Solid, stable enteral nutrition	Nothing by mouth (NPO), clear liquid, unstable enteral nutrition, parenteral nutrition	NPO, clear liquid, unstable enteral nutrition, parenteral nutrition
Action	Monitor; provide basic nutrition care	Provide supplements; assist with food choices; teach and counsel	Refer to dietitian	Refer to dietitian

for accuracy, a registered dietitian is usually responsible for conducting this assessment.

The comprehensive assessment is commonly performed on moderate- to high-risk patients with some degree of protein-calorie malnutrition. Major parameters examined include medical history, physical examination findings, and laboratory test results.

Multiple criteria must be examined to provide an accurate evaluation of the patient's nutritional status. No single criterion can be used to evaluate a patient and it may not be necessary to gather all possible information for every patient. The decision to consider what information to evaluate is left to the dietitian's discretion.

Health history

The first step in a nutritional assessment is the health history. A patient may come to you with various nutrition-related complaints, such as weight gain or loss; changes in energy level, appetite, or taste; dysphagia; GI tract problems, such as nausea and diarrhea; or other body system changes, such as skin and nail abnormalities. A current and past health history is usually gathered from the patient's medical record or through an interview with the patient.

Current health history

In the current health history, it's relevant to obtain information about the patient's current nutritional status. Ask the patient if he has changed his diet recently. If so, ask him to describe specific changes and their dura-

CAFFEINE CONTENT OF COMMON BEVERAGES

To estimate the amount of caffeine your patient consumes daily, use this chart as a guide.

Beverage	Caffeine content
Coffee (brewed), 1 cup	85 mg
Coffee (instant), 1 cup	60 mg
Black tea (brewed), 1 cup	50 mg
Cola, 12 oz	32 to 65 mg
Green tea (brewed), 1 cup	30 mg
Cocoa, 1 cup	8 mg
Decaffeinated coffee, 1 cup	3 mg

tion. Has his caloric intake increased or decreased? A decreased intake contributes to weight loss and may lead to nutritional deficiency. An increased intake may lead to weight gain but doesn't rule out nutritional deficiency.

Find out if the patient experienced any unusual stress or trauma, such as surgery, change in employment, or family illness. Stress and trauma magnify the body's need for essential nutrients.

If the patient has gained or lost a significant amount of weight, ask him if he has undergone a change in appetite, bowel habits, mobility, physical exercise, or lifestyle. Significant changes may indicate underlying disease. For example, weight gain in a patient may indicate an endocrine imbalance, such as Cushing's syndrome or hypothyroidism. Weight loss may result from cancer, GI disorders, diabetes mellitus, or hyperthyroidism.

Ask the patient about prescription or over-the-counter (OTC) drugs, especially vitamin or mineral supplements and appetite suppressants. If he's taking them, find out what the purpose is and the starting date, dose, and frequency of each. Ask if he uses any "natural" or "health" foods. If he does, find out which ones and how much he uses, and why. Also, ask if the patient avoids certain foods such as meat. Answers to this question may reveal a nutritional deficiency requiring supplementation. The patient himself may perceive a nutritional deficiency and self-prescribe a supplement. In other cases, the response may reveal routine drug use that can cause nutritional deficiencies or related problems.

Other questions to ask the patient include those related to alcohol consumption and smoking habits. Find out if he drinks alcohol and if so, how much does he drink per day or week, what type of alcohol does he consume, and what's the duration of his drinking. Alcohol provides calories (7 kcal/g) but no essential nutrients. Chronic alcohol abuse leads to malnutrition. Also, ask about smoking and chewing tobacco or snuff use. Use of tobacco products may affect taste, which in turn affects appetite.

If the patient consumes coffee, tea, cola, and cocoa, find out the quantity and his consumption patterns. These beverages contain caffeine, a habit-forming stimulant that increases heart rate, respiratory rate, blood pressure, and secretion of stress hormones. In moderate amounts of 50 to 200 mg/day, caffeine is relatively harmless. Intake of greater amounts can cause sensations of nervousness and intestinal discomfort. (See *Caffeine content of common beverages.*)

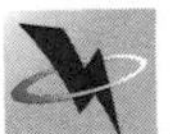

CRITICAL POINT *Patients who drink eight or more cups of coffee per day may complain of insomnia, restlessness, agitation, palpitations, and recurring headaches. Sudden abstinence after long periods of even moderate daily caffeine intake can cause withdrawal symptoms such as headache.*

Past health history

In the past health history, it's also important to identify an existing condition that might affect nutritional status. The condition's impact on nutritional status depends on the severity of the existing condition and how long the patient has been afflicted. (See *Detecting nutritional problems.*)

Ask the patient if he has ever experienced any major illnesses, trauma, extensive dental work, hospitalizations, or chronic medical conditions. Any of these can alter nutritional intake.

Obtain information about food allergies. By causing the patient to eliminate certain foods, allergies increase the risk of nutritional deficiencies. Use information about food allergies to help the patient plan safe, balanced meals and to prevent the hospitalized patient from being served foods that can cause allergic reactions.

Other conditions that compromise nutritional status include eating disorders, such as anorexia nervosa and bulimia, and substance abuse. Ask the patient if he has ever had (or been told he has) any of these conditions. Other problems may also be detected that result in impairment in digestion and absorption, resulting in altered nutritional status. These problems include inflammatory, obstructive, or functional disorders of the GI tract, such as:

- lactose intolerance
- cystic fibrosis
- pancreatic disorders
- inflammatory bowel diseases
- minimal function in the small intestine due to a disorder, such as Crohn's disease or surgical excision (short-gut syndrome)
- radiation enteritis
- liver disorders.

Nutrition may also be affected by conditions known to accelerate metabolism. These conditions include:

- pregnancy
- fever
- sepsis
- thermal injuries
- pressure ulcers
- cancer
- acquired immunodeficiency syndrome
- major surgery
- trauma
- burns.

Some conditions, such as diabetes mellitus, hormonal imbalances, and starvation, alter nutrient metabolism. In addition, diarrhea and malabsorption syndromes, such as celiac disease, cause increased nutrient excretion, whereas other conditions, such as renal insufficiency, impair nutrient excretion.

DETECTING NUTRITIONAL PROBLEMS

Nutritional problems may stem from physical conditions, drugs, diet, or lifestyle factors. The list below will help you find out if your patient is particularly susceptible to nutritional problems.

Physical conditions

- Chronic illnesses, such as diabetes and neurologic, cardiac, or thyroid problems
- Family history of diabetes or heart disease
- Draining wounds or fistulas
- Obesity or a weight gain of 20% above normal body weight
- Unplanned weight loss of 20% below normal body weight
- History of GI disturbances
- Anorexia or bulimia
- Depression or anxiety
- Severe trauma
- Recent chemotherapy or radiation therapy
- Physical limitations, such as paresis or paralysis
- Recent major surgery
- Pregnancy, especially teen or multiple-birth pregnancy
- Mouth, tooth, or denture problems

Drugs and diet

- Fad diets
- Strict vegetarian diet
- Steroid, diuretic, or antacid use
- Liquid diet or nothing by mouth for more than 3 days
- Excessive alcohol intake

Lifestyle factors

- Lack of support from family or friends
- Financial problems

Ask the patient if he has followed a planned weight-loss or weight-gain program within the past 6 months. If so, have him describe the program and determine whether the program is well-balanced.

Family history

Next, explore possible genetic or familial disorders that may affect the patient's nutritional status. Find out if the family history includes such disorders as cardiovascular disease, Crohn's disease, diabetes mellitus, cancer, GI tract disorders, sickle cell anemia, allergies, food intolerance (for example, lactose intolerance), or obesity. These disorders may affect digestion or metabolism of food and alter the patient's nutritional status.

Psychosocial history

The psychosocial history provides valuable information about the patient's current status, beliefs about food, health promotion activities related to nutrition, and possible factors that can interfere with adequate nutrition. This history focuses on areas, such as stress and how the patient copes, including the use of food as a coping mechanism, socioeconomic factors including income and food preparation, self-concept, social support, and typical intake patterns, including factors that may affect these patterns.

In addition, other psychosocial factors could be uncovered during the history that may influence the patient's nutritional habits, including:

- illiteracy
- language barriers
- knowledge of nutrition and food safety
- cultural or religious influences
- social isolation
- limited or low income
- inadequate cooking resources, such as major appliances or kitchen access
- limited access to transportation
- physical inactivity or illness
- use of tobacco or recreational drugs
- limited community resources.

When psychosocial factors have been identified, the patient care plan will need to incorporate these differences as appropriate. For example, if the patient can't read or doesn't read well, using a picture guide on which foods are appropriate to consume and which should be avoided may be more helpful to the patient than written words alone.

Stress and coping mechanisms

First, it's essential to find out how much stress the patient encounters in his daily life and what methods he uses to cope with these stressors. Responses to earlier questions on patterns of activity and nutrition may provide clues to how the patient handles stress.

Ask him if stress, from his job or elsewhere, influences his eating patterns. Daily schedules commonly interfere with mealtimes, predisposing the patient to nutritional deficiencies. Find out if the patient uses food or drink to get through stressful times. Individuals undergoing stress may increase or decrease food intake or change the type of food they eat. Keep in mind that the patient may not be fully aware of his behavior or may be reluctant to discuss it.

Socioeconomic factors

Economic, cultural, and socioeconomic factors can markedly affect a patient's nutritional health. Ask these questions:

- Where and how is your food prepared?
- Do you have access to adequate storage and refrigeration?
- Do you receive welfare payments, Social Security payments, Supplemental Security Income, food stamps, or assistance from Special Supplemental Food Program for Women, Infants, and Children?

If the patient doesn't cook his own food, his nutritional health depends on whether others are available to help him. Inadequate food storage and refrigeration can lead to nutritional problems. A change in economic status or the loss of a food program may also disrupt the patient's nutritional well-being.

Self-concept

Ask the patient if he likes the way he looks and if he's content with his present weight. Today's society places great focus on thinness and physical prowess, causing children to become overweight and adults to feel uncomfortable. Many weight-reduction plans guarantee success; if the patient fails to lose weight or maintain weight loss, he may perceive himself as a failure. Poor self-image may cause these patients to avoid settings that require vigorous exercise or body exposure. To make matters worse, advertisements

UNDERSTANDING DIFFERENCES IN FOOD INTAKE

Your patient's diet may be influenced by various cultural and economic factors. Understanding these factors can give you more insight into your patient's nutritional status:

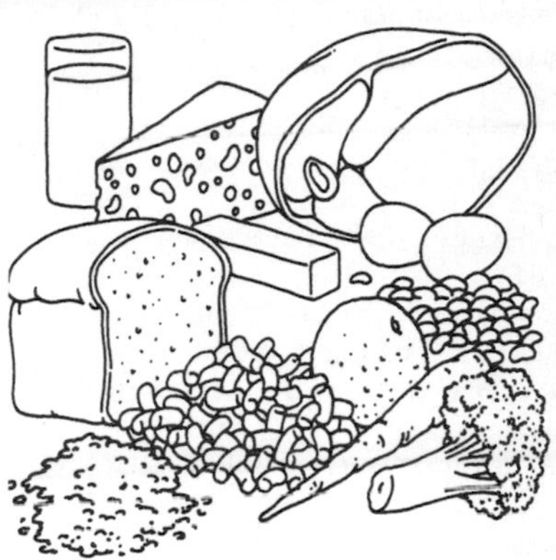

- Socioeconomic status may affect a patient's ability to afford healthful foods in the quantities needed to maintain proper health. Lower socioeconomic status can lead to nutritional problems, especially for younger children, and also pregnant women, who may give birth to neonates with low birth weight or may experience complications during labor.
- Work schedules can affect the amount and type of food a patient eats, especially if the patient works full-time at night.
- Religion can restrict food choices. For example, some Jews and Muslims don't eat pork products, and many Roman Catholics avoid meat on Ash Wednesday and Fridays during Lent.
- Ethnic background influences food choices. For example, fish and rice are staple foods for many Asians.

constantly remind these individuals of the pleasures of food and drink.

Misconception about ideal weight and poor self-image can also lead to eating disorders, such as anorexia nervosa or bulimia.

Social support

Find out if the patient eats alone or with others. Single adults and isolated elderly patients may neglect their nutrition. A person grieving over the recent loss of a loved one may also lose interest in food.

Ask the patient to rate the importance of mealtimes on a scale of 1 to 10, with 10 being the most important. This rating will help determine if meals are enjoyed or endured. The patient who endures meals may develop an eating disorder.

Intake patterns

Asking the patient to describe his typical day will give you important information about his routine activity level and eating habits. Information about intake patterns helps assess what and how much the patient eats. This information can help identify problems in nutritional status and behaviors that need improvement.

Ask him to recount what and how much he ate the day before, how the food was cooked, and who cooked it. The patient's answers will not only tell you about his usual intake but also gives clues about food preferences, eating patterns, and even the patient's memory and mental status.

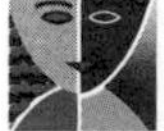

CULTURAL INSIGHT *What the patient eats depends on various cultural and economic influences. Understanding these influences can give you more insight into the patient's nutritional status. (See* Understanding differences in food intake.*)*

Directly observing what the patient eats provides an objective measurement of the kinds and amount of foods consumed. Of course, close observation of a patient is rarely possible. A questionnaire geared to nutritional problems can help provide more specific details about the patient's intake patterns. Open-ended questions are more useful than closed, "yes-or-no" questions for obtaining accurate information. Important areas for questioning include:

- number of meals and snacks eaten in a 24-hour period
- unusual food habits
- time of day most of the calories are consumed
- skipped meals
- meals eaten away from home
- number of fruits and vegetables eaten daily
- number of servings (and types) of grains eaten daily
- how often red meat, poultry, and fish are eaten, including type and amount
- how often meatless meals are consumed
- number of hours of television watched daily while eating snacks or meals
- types and amount of dairy products consumed daily
- how often desserts and sweets are eaten
- types and amount of beverages (including alcohol) consumed
- food allergies or intolerances
- dietary supplements and why they are taken
- medications, including OTC products and herbal supplements.

Dietary history

A patient's dietary history can be obtained using various tools that specify what, how much, and how often a patient typically eats to determine his nutritional status. Two commonly used tools are the 24-hour food recall and the food frequency record.

The 24-hour food recall

A quick and easy method of evaluating a patient's dietary intake is through the 24-hour food recall. To complete this recall, the patient must be able to recount all the types and amounts of foods and beverages he has consumed during a 24-hour period.

The time period may be the past 24 hours or a typical 24-hour period. To help the patient identify portion sizes, food models or pictures of typical portions can be used. Specific details may be necessary in some recall situations such as food preparation (for example, frying versus dry roasting meat). Open-ended questions also reveal more information than typical "yes-or-no" questions. When the information is obtained, recall data is evaluated to see if the patient's nutritional needs are being met.

Food frequency record

The food frequency record is a checklist of particular foods that helps to determine what the patient is specifically consuming and how often. The checklist may list the foods in one column, and the patient checks off how often they're eaten in another column. The choices may include time periods, how often the food is consumed (such as per day, per week, or per month), or if the food is eaten frequently, seldom, or never. The data doesn't typically include the serving size, and it may only include specific foods or nutrients suspected of being deficient or excessive in the patient's diet.

Another method of gathering information for the food frequency record is to use a questionnaire that lists food items organized by food groups. Using this document, the patient records the type of food consumed and how often.

Either checklist provides a more complete dietary picture when used in conjunction with the 24-hour food recall. When deficiencies or excesses are identified, goals may be developed to address nutritional and educational needs.

Physical assessment

Physical assessment helps determine the patient's health status and identifies any illnesses. Physical factors discovered during the comprehensive nutritional assessment may be related to an alteration in nutritional status and malnutrition. However, such findings as height and weight reflect chronic changes in nutritional status rather than acute processes.

After completing the health history, perform a two-part nutritional physical assessment. In part one, assess key body systems. In part two, take anthropometric measurements. Also evaluate the patient's laboratory studies. Remember that nutritional problems may be associated with various disorders or factors.

Body system examination

Before starting your physical assessment, quickly observe the patient's general appearance. Does he look rested? Is his posture good? Are his height and weight proportional to his body build? Are his physical movements smooth with no apparent weaknesses? Is he free from skeletal deformities?

Next, complete a head-to-toe assessment of the patient's major body systems. When performing this head-to-toe assessment, remember that clinical signs are seen late. Nutritional deficiencies are most readily detected in the area of rapid turnover of the epithelial tissues.

Integumentary system

When assessing the integumentary system, which includes the skin, hair, and nails, ask yourself these questions:

- Is his hair shiny and full?
- Is his skin free from blemishes and rashes?
- Is his skin warm and dry, with normal color for that particular patient?
- Are his nails firm with pink nail beds?

Eyes, nose, throat, and neck

When assessing the patient's eyes, nose, throat, and neck, reflect on the following:

- Are the patient's eyes clear and shiny?
- Are the mucous membranes in his nose moist and pink? Is his tongue pink with papillae present?
- Are his gums moist and pink?
- Is his mouth free from ulcers or lesions?
- Is his neck free from masses that would impede swallowing?

Cardiovascular system

Evaluate the following areas:

- Is the patient's heart rhythm regular?
- Are his heart rate and blood pressure normal for his age?
- Are his extremities free from swelling?

Pulmonary system

Investigate the following:

- Are the patient's lungs clear to auscultation?
- Can he clear his own secretions?
- Is lung excursion normal?

GI system

Determine these factors:

- Is the patient's appetite satisfactory, with no reported GI problems?
- Are his elimination patterns regular?
- Is his abdomen free from abnormal masses on palpation?

Neuromuscular system

Assess the following:

- Is the patient alert and responsive?
- Are his reflexes normal?
- Is his behavior appropriate?
- Are his legs and feet free from paresthesia?
- Is there any evidence of muscle wasting?
- Does the patient experience calf pain?

Anthropometric measurements

The second part of the physical assessment is taking anthropometric measurements. These measurements can help identify nutritional problems, especially in patients who are seriously overweight or underweight. All measurements need not be completed each time. However, height and weight are usually necessary. Let the results of the patient's health history be the guide.

Height

Height should be measured with the patient standing as straight as possible, without shoes, against a wall using a fixed measuring stick.

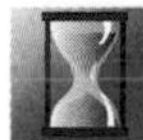

AGE ISSUE *When measuring the height of a child younger than age 2, measure the length of the child in a supine position, while holding the head in the midline position and gently holding the legs in full extension. Be sure to note the growth of children as well as diminishing height in older adults. Growth of children may be noted on standardized charts, such as those developed by the American Academy of Pediatrics, to assess growth patterns for possible abnormalities. Diminishing height in older adults may be related to osteoporotic changes and should be investigated.*

Adaptations may be needed if the patient can't stand or cooperate. (See *Overcoming problems in measuring height,* page 70.)

Weight

Weight may be measured on a beam-balance scale, or a bed scale if the patient is bedridden. The information gathered is more helpful if the weight is measured on the same scale at the same time of day (typically before breakfast and after voiding), in the same amount of clothing, and without shoes.

EXPERT TECHNIQUE

OVERCOMING PROBLEMS IN MEASURING HEIGHT

Wingspan technique
Is your patient confined to a wheelchair? Is he unable to stand straight because of scoliosis? Despite such problems, you can still get an approximate measurement of his height using the "wingspan" technique.

Have the patient hold his arms straight out from the sides of his body. Tell children to hold their arms out "like bird wings." Then measure from the tip of one middle finger to the tip of the other. That distance is the patient's approximate height.

Paper and pencil technique
If the patient is younger than age 2 and a measuring board isn't available, place the child on an examination table that's covered with examining paper. Mark the paper at the top of the child's head and at the bottom of the heels as he's lying in a supine position with his legs fully extended. Measure the distance between the two points to obtain the length.

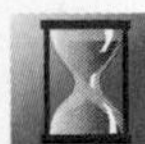

AGE ISSUE *When weighing an infant, use an appropriately sized scale that measures weight to the nearest 0.5 oz or 10 g. Also, be sure to weigh the infant without clothes.*

Ideal body weight. Ideal body weight (IBW), also helpful in assessing nutritional status, is a reference standard for clinical use. For men, this measurement is 106 lb (48.1 kg) for a height of 5′ (1.5 m), plus an additional 6 lb (2.7 kg) for each inch over 5′. For women, IBW is 100 lb (45.4 kg) for a height of 5′, plus 5 lb (2.3 kg) for each inch over 5′. (See *Height and weight table.*)

IBW range can be 10% higher or lower depending on body size. The percentage of IBW is obtained by dividing the patient's true weight by the IBW and then multiplying that number by 100. This percentage can be used to determine the patient's weight status and accompanying health risk:

- An obese person is greater than 120% of IBW.
- An overweight person is 110% to 120% of IBW.
- A person whose weight is normal is 90% to 110% of IBW.
- A mildly underweight person is 80% to 90% of IBW.
- A moderately underweight person is 70% to 79% of IBW.
- A severely underweight person is less than 70% of IBW.

Body mass index

A useful measurement for assessing nutritional status is the body mass index (BMI), which uses a patient's weight and height to help classify him as underweight, normal, or obese. The BMI is calculated by dividing the body weight in kilograms by height in meters squared, or by dividing the weight in pounds by height in inches squared, and multiplying that result by 703. (See *Interpreting BMI,* page 72.)

Body composition measurements

Measurements of body composition include the triceps skinfold measurement, the midarm circumference, and the midarm muscle circumference (MAMC). These measurements provide quantitative information about body composition made up of fat or muscle tissue. Measurements may be compared with reference standards or may be used to evaluate changes. If measurements are less than 90% of the reference value, nutritional intervention is indicated. Keep in mind that the patient and technical variations may limit the use of anthropometric measurements.

Triceps skinfold measurements. Triceps skinfold measures subcutaneous fat stores and is an index of total body fat. To measure the skinfold, the patient's arm hangs freely and a fold of skin located slightly above midpoint is grasped between the thumb and

HEIGHT AND WEIGHT TABLE

Ongoing research suggests that people can carry more weight as they age, without added health risk. Because people of the same height may differ in muscle and bone makeup, a range of weights is shown for each height in this table. The higher weights in each category apply to men, who typically have more muscle and bone than women. Height measurements are without shoes; weight measurements are without clothes.

Height	**Weight**	
	Ages 19 to 34	*Ages 35 and older*
5′0″	97 to 128	108 to 138
5′1″	101 to 132	111 to 143
5′2″	104 to 137	115 to 148
5′3″	107 to 141	119 to 152
5′4″	111 to 146	122 to 157
5′5″	114 to 150	126 to 162
5′6″	118 to 155	130 to 167
5′7″	121 to 160	134 to 172
5′8″	125 to 164	138 to 178
5′9″	129 to 169	142 to 183
5′10″	132 to 174	146 to 188
5′11″	136 to 179	151 to 194
6′0″	140 to 184	155 to 199
6′1″	144 to 189	159 to 205
6′2″	148 to 195	164 to 210
6′3″	152 to 200	168 to 216
6′4″	156 to 205	172 to 222
6′5″	160 to 211	177 to 228
6′6″	164 to 216	182 to 234

forefinger. As the skin is pulled away from underlying muscle, calipers are applied and the measurement is read to the nearest millimeter. (See *Taking anthropometric arm measurements*, page 73.)

Three readings are taken. These readings may be from the same site or other appropriate sites (biceps, thigh, calf, subscapular, or suprailiac skinfolds). The readings are then added together and divided by three to record the average. For men, 11.3 mm is 90% of standard, for women, 14.9 mm.

Midarm circumference. Midarm circumference (MAC) measures muscle mass and subcutaneous fat. This value is taken from

INTERPRETING BMI

Currently, the most widely accepted classification of weight status is the body mass index (BMI). The BMI can be used as a measure of obesity, protein-calorie malnutrition, as well as an indicator of health risk. All measures other than normal place the patient at a higher health risk, and nutritional needs should be assessed accordingly.

Classification	BMI
Underweight	≤ 18.5
Normal	18.5 to 24.9
Overweight	25 to 29.9
Obesity class 1	30 to 34.9
Obesity class 2	35 to 39.9
Obesity class 3	≥ 40

the midpoint of the individual's nondominant arm using a measuring tape. The forearm is flexed at 90 degrees and placed in a dependent position while a tape measure is placed around the mid-upper arm between the top of the acromion process of the scapula and olecranon process of the ulna. Readings are taken while the tape is held firmly—but not too tightly—and recorded to the nearest millimeter.

Midarm muscle circumference. MAMC provides an index of muscle mass and is an indication of somatic protein stores. The value is calculated by multiplying the triceps skin fold measurement by 3.14, then multiplying that value by the MAC measurement. The value is recorded in centimeters. This value is minimally affected by edema and provides a quick estimation.

CRITICAL POINT *The physical examination, which includes observing the patient's general appearance, may reveal signs of malnutrition that are related to a nutritional deficiency. However, signs may also be due to other conditions or disorders and can't be considered indicative of, but only suggestive of, a nutritional deficiency. In addition, remember that physical signs and symptoms may vary among populations because of genetic and environmental differences. (See* Evaluating nutritional assessment findings, *page 74.)*

Laboratory data

Laboratory test results can detect nutritional problems in early stages before physical signs and symptoms appear. Most of the routine tests assess protein-calorie information, with serum albumin used most commonly to screen for nutritional problems. Tests are done to help determine adequacy of protein stores. Some tests measure byproducts of protein catabolism (such as creatinine) and others measure products of protein anabolism (such as albumin level, transferrin level, hemoglobin [Hb] level, hematocrit [HCT], prealbumin, retinol binding protein, and total lymphocyte count).

Albumin

The serum albumin level test assesses protein levels in the body. Albumin makes up more than 50% of total proteins in blood and affects the cardiovascular system because it helps to maintain osmotic pressure. Keep in mind that albumin production requires functioning liver cells and an adequate supply of amino acids, the building blocks of proteins. When a patient's serum albumin level decreases this can be due to serious protein deficiency and loss of blood protein caused by burns, malnutrition, liver or renal disease, heart failure, major surgery, infections, or cancer.

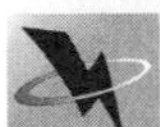

CRITICAL POINT *Decreased albumin levels correlate with poor clinical outcomes, increased length of hospitalization, and increased morbidity and mortality.*

Creatinine height index

The creatinine height index involves a 24-hour urine collection to measure urinary excretion of creatinine. It helps define body protein mass and evaluate protein depletion. Test results are interpreted using a formula that compares results with ideal height standards. The test is of limited value because results are greatly altered by age,

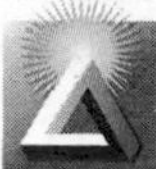

EXPERT TECHNIQUE

TAKING ANTHROPOMETRIC ARM MEASUREMENTS

Follow these steps to determine triceps skinfold thickness, midarm circumference, and midarm muscle circumference.

Triceps skinfold thickness

1. Find the midpoint circumference of the arm by placing the tape measure halfway between the axilla and the elbow. Grasp the patient's skin with your thumb and forefinger, about 3/8" (1 cm) above the midpoint, as shown below.
2. Place the calipers at the midpoint and squeeze for 3 seconds.
3. Record the measurement to the nearest millimeter.
4. Take two more readings and use the average.

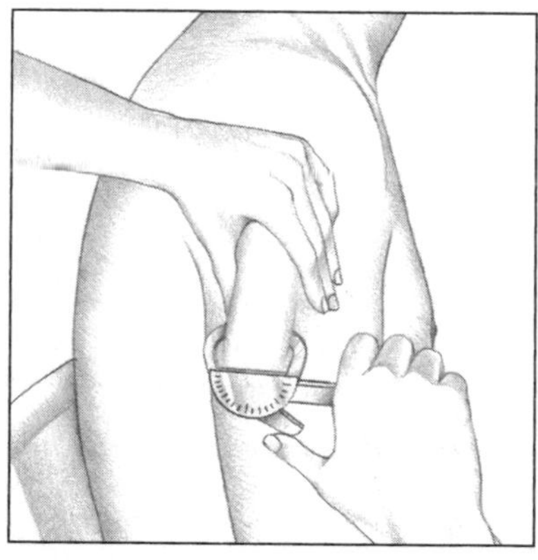

Midarm circumference and midarm muscle circumference

1. At the midpoint, measure the midarm circumference, as shown below. Record the measurement in centimeters.
2. Calculate the midarm muscle circumference by multiplying the triceps skinfold thickness — measured in millimeters — by 3.14.
3. Subtract this number from the midarm circumference.

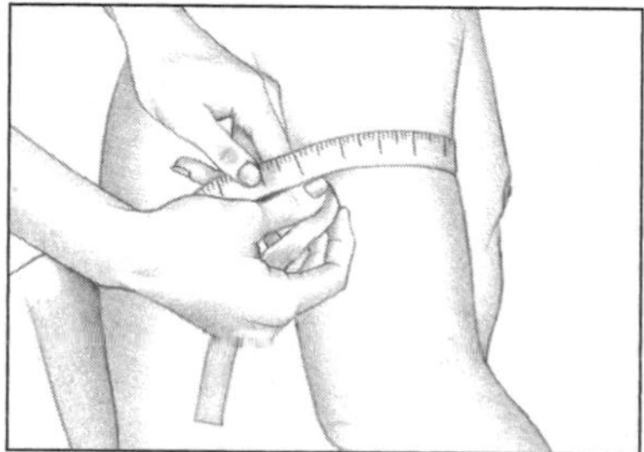

Recording the measurements

Record all three measurements as a percentage of the standard measurements (see chart below) using this formula:

$$\frac{\text{Actual measurement}}{\text{Standard measurement}} \times 100\%$$

After taking and recording the measurements above, consult the chart here to determine your patient's caloric status. Remember a measurement of less than 90% of the standard indicates caloric deprivation. A measurement over 90% indicates adequate or more than adequate energy reserves.

Measurement	Standard	90%
Triceps skinfold thickness	Men: 12.5 mm Women: 16.5 mm	Men: 11.3 mm Women: 14.9 mm
Midarm circumference	Men: 29.3 cm Women: 28.5 cm	Men: 26.4 cm Women: 25.7 cm
Midarm muscle circumference	Men: 25.3 cm Women: 23.3 cm	Men: 22. 8 cm Women: 20.9 cm

EVALUATING NUTRITIONAL ASSESSMENT FINDINGS

Use this chart to determine the implications of the signs and symptoms revealed in the patient's nutritional assessment.

Body system or region	Sign or symptom	Implications
General	▪ Weakness and fatigue ▪ Weight loss	▪ Anemia or electrolyte imbalance ▪ Decreased calorie intake or increased calorie use or inadequate nutrient intake or absorption
Skin, hair, and nails	▪ Dry, flaky skin ▪ Dry skin with poor turgor ▪ Rough, scaly skin with bumps ▪ Petechiae or ecchymoses ▪ Non-healing sore ▪ Thinning, dry hair ▪ Spoon-shaped, brittle, or ridged nails	▪ Vitamin A, vitamin B-complex, or linoleic acid deficiency ▪ Dehydration ▪ Vitamin A deficiency or essential fatty acid deficiency ▪ Vitamin C or K deficiency ▪ Protein, vitamin C, or zinc deficiency ▪ Protein deficiency ▪ Iron deficiency
Eyes	▪ Night blindness; corneal swelling, softening, or dryness; Bitot's spots (gray triangular patches on the conjunctiva) ▪ Red conjunctiva	▪ Vitamin A deficiency ▪ Riboflavin deficiency
Throat and mouth	▪ Cracks at the corner of mouth ▪ Magenta-colored tongue ▪ Beefy, red tongue ▪ Soft, spongy, bleeding gums ▪ Swollen neck (goiter)	▪ Riboflavin or niacin deficiency ▪ Riboflavin deficiency ▪ Vitamin B_{12} deficiency ▪ Vitamin C deficiency ▪ Iodine deficiency
Cardiovascular	▪ Edema ▪ Tachycardia, hypotension	▪ Protein deficiency and zinc deficiency ▪ Fluid volume deficit
GI	▪ Ascites	▪ Protein deficiency
Musculoskeletal	▪ Bone pain and bow leg ▪ Muscle wasting ▪ Pain in calves and thighs	▪ Vitamin D or calcium deficiency ▪ Protein, carbohydrate, and fat deficiency ▪ Thiamine deficiency
Neurologic	▪ Altered mental status ▪ Paresthesia	▪ Dehydration and thiamine or vitamin B_{12} deficiency ▪ Vitamin B_{12}, pyridoxine, or thiamine deficiency

amount of exercise, stress, menstruation, and the presence of severe illness. Increased values may indicate decreased protein stores.

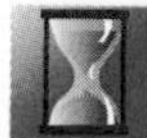

AGE ISSUE *Creatinine values decrease with age because of a normal decrease in lean muscle mass.*

Transferrin

Transferrin is a "carrier" protein that transports iron. The molecule is synthesized mainly in the liver. Transferrin levels decrease along with protein levels and indicate depletion of protein stores. Serum transferrin levels reflect the patient's current protein status more accurately than albumin levels because of their shorter half-life. A normal transferrin value is greater than 200 mg/dl. Decreased transferrin values may indicate inadequate protein production due to liver damage, protein loss from renal disease, acute or chronic infection, or cancer. Elevated levels may indicate severe iron deficiency.

Hemoglobin

Hb is the main component of red blood cells (RBCs), which transport oxygen. Its formation requires an adequate supply of protein in the form of amino acids. Hb levels help to assess the blood's oxygen-carrying capacity and are useful in diagnosing anemia, protein deficiency, and hydration status. Decreased Hb levels suggest iron deficiency anemia, protein deficiency, excessive blood loss, or overhydration. Increased Hb levels suggest dehydration or polycythemia.

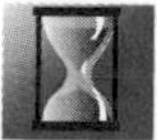

AGE ISSUE *Normal Hb levels vary with the patient's age and type of blood sample tested. These values reflect normal Hb concentrations (in grams per deciliter):*

- *neonates—17 to 22 g/dl (SI, 170 to 220 g/L)*
- *1 week—15 to 20 g/dl (SI, 150 to 200 g/L)*
- *1 month—11 to 15 g/dl (SI, 110 to 150 g/L)*
- *children—11 to 13 g/dl (SI, 110 to 130 g/L)*
- *adult males—14 to 17.4 g/dl (SI, 140 to 174 g/L)*
- *males after middle age—12.4 to 14.9 g/dl (SI, 124 to 149/L)*
- *adult females—12 to 16 g/dl (SI, 120 to 160 g/L)*
- *females after middle age—11.7 to 13.8 g/dl (SI, 117 to 138 g/L).*

Hematocrit

HCT reflects the proportion of blood occupied by the RBCs. This test helps diagnose anemia and dehydration. Decreased HCT suggests iron deficiency anemia or excessive fluid intake or blood loss. Increased HCT suggests severe dehydration or polycythemia.

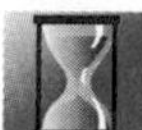

AGE ISSUE *Normal HCT reflect age, gender, sample type, and the laboratory performing the test. These ranges represent normal HCT for different age-groups:*

- *neonates—55% to 68% (SI, 0.55 to 0.68)*
- *1 week—47% to 65% (SI, 0.47 to 0.65)*
- *1 month—37% to 49% (SI, 0.37 to 0.49)*
- *3 months—30% to 36% (SI, 0.30 to 0.36)*
- *1 year—29% to 41% (SI, 0.29 to 0.41)*
- *10 years—36% to 40% (SI, 0.36 to 0.40)*
- *adult males—42% to 52% (SI, 0.42 to 0.52)*
- *adult females—36% to 48% (SI, 0.36 to 0.48).*

Prealbumin

The prealbumin test is also more sensitive than albumin because of its short half-life (2 days). It isn't as affected by liver disease and hydration status as the albumin test; however, it's more expensive to perform. A normal prealbumin value is 16 to 30 mg/dl.

Retinol binding protein

Retinol binding protein is a reliable measurement during acute response. It responds quickly to nutritional repletion due to a small body pool and short half-life (10 to 12 hours). A normal retinol binding protein value is 2.6 to 7.7 mg/dl.

Total lymphocyte count

A leukocyte is a white blood cell (WBC), which is the main cell responsible for fighting infection. Leukocytes are responsible for destroying organisms as well as for phagocytosis, which promotes cellular repair. Normal WBC counts range from 4,000 to 10,000/µl. This test is useful for diagnosing severity of a disease.

There are five different types of leukocytes:

- neutrophils, which fight pyogenic infections
- eosinophils, which fight allergic disorders and parasitic infections
- basophils, which fight parasitic infections
- lymphocytes, which fight viral infections
- monocytes, which fight severe infections.

The WBC differential will provide specific information about which type of WBC is being affected and is a diagnostically useful test.

Malnutrition decreases the total number of lymphocytes, impairing the body's ability to fight infection. The total lymphocyte count is used in evaluating the health of the immune system and assists in evaluation of protein stores. The total lymphocyte count may also be affected by many medical conditions, so the value of this test is limited.

CRITICAL POINT *Decreased total lymphocyte count may indicate malnutrition when no other cause is apparent. It may also point to infection, leukemia, or tissue necrosis.*

Nitrogen balance

A nitrogen balance test involves collecting all urine during a 24-hour period to determine how well the body is using protein. Proteins contain nitrogen. When proteins are broken down into amino acids, nitrogen is excreted in the urine as urea.

Nitrogen intake and excretion should be equal. The nitrogen balance is the difference between nitrogen intake and excretion. It's calculated using a formula, and the results are interpreted to determine whether the patient is receiving the appropriate amount of protein. Results may vary in patients with such conditions as burns and infection.

Triglycerides

Triglycerides are the main storage form of lipids. Measuring triglyceride levels can help identify hyperlipidemia early. However, increased levels alone aren't diagnostic; further studies such as cholesterol measurement are required. Decreased triglyceride levels are common in those who are malnourished.

Cholesterol

A total cholesterol test measures circulating levels of free cholesterol and cholesterol esters. A diet high in saturated fats raises cholesterol levels by stimulating lipid absorption. Increased levels indicate an increased risk of coronary artery disease. Decreased levels are commonly associated with malnutrition.

Additional diagnostic data

In addition to the patient's health history, physical findings, and laboratory data, use additional diagnostic criteria to measure poor nutrition.

Cutaneous hypersensitivity reactions

Immunocompetence may be evaluated by placing small quantities of recall antigens (*Candida*, mumps, or purified protein derivative of tuberculin) under the skin. Normally a positive reaction occurs in 24 to 48 hours with a red area of 5 mm or more. However, in the patient with malnutrition, a delayed reaction, reaction to only one antigen, or no reaction at all (anergy) may occur.

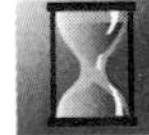

AGE ISSUE *A patient's age can cause delayed cutaneous hypersensitivity reactions, making the cutaneous hypersensitivity test less helpful for determining protein status. Elderly patients may have alterations due to several common factors, including hydration status, chronic diseases, organ function changes, and medications.*

X-rays

X-rays may be used to determine bone integrity, especially in older women, to detect possible osteoporosis. A bone mineral density test is a specialized X-ray that detects the amount of change in a bone. The beam detects the intensity and shows the physician how dense the bones are. A bone scan, another type of X-ray, takes a picture of the bone and identifies fractures, tumors, or inflammation. It's also sensitive enough to recognize structural changes. X-rays may also be used to evaluate the GI tract for integrity and diagnose disorders that may cause malnutrition. The specific X-rays performed will be influenced by the patient's symptoms and diagnosis. Multiple tests may be necessary before a definitive diagnosis is made.

Abnormal findings

If a patient exhibits signs and symptoms related to nutrition, be prepared to complete a thorough assessment of other body systems, such as the integumentary, GI, or musculoskeletal system, and the eyes. In addition, a patient may seek care for any number of signs and symptoms related to nutrition. Some common disorders include anorexia, dyspepsia, dysphagia, and weight loss or weight gain. After obtaining further information, begin to interpret the findings. (See *Nutrition: Interpreting your findings,* pages 78 to 81.)

Anorexia

Anorexia, a lack of appetite in the presence of a physiologic need for food, is a common symptom of GI and endocrine disorders. It's also characteristic of certain severe psychological disturbances.

History

Take the patient's vital signs and weight. Find out previous minimum and maximum weights. Explore dietary habits, such as when and what the patient eats. Ask what foods he likes and dislikes, and why. The patient may identify tastes and smells that nauseate him and cause loss of appetite. Ask about dental problems that interfere with chewing, including poor-fitting dentures. Ask if he has difficulty or pain when swallowing or if he vomits or has diarrhea after meals. Check for a history of stomach or bowel disorders, which can interfere with the ability to digest, absorb, or metabolize nutrients. Find out about changes in bowel habits. Ask about alcohol use and drug use and dosage. Ask the patient how frequently and intensely he exercises.

If the medical history doesn't reveal an organic basis for anorexia, consider psychological factors. Ask the patient if he knows what's causing his decreased appetite. Situational factors, such as a death in the family or problems at school or on the job, can lead to depression and subsequent loss of appetite.

Obtain a 24-hour diet history daily. The patient may consistently exaggerate his food intake (a common occurrence in anorexia nervosa). Determine calorie and nutrient counts for the patient's meals.

Physical assessment

Assess the patient's body systems for changes, being alert for signs of malnutrition. Obtain a baseline anthropometric measurement and compare to standards.

Analysis

The causes of anorexia are diverse and may include acquired immunodeficiency syndrome, Crohn's disease, hypothyroidism, pernicious anemia, anorexia nervosa, or depression. Anorexia can also result from such factors as anxiety, chronic pain, poor oral hygiene, increased blood temperature due to hot weather or fever, and changes in taste or smell that normally accompany aging. Drug therapy or abuse can also cause anorexia. Short-term anorexia rarely jeopardizes health, but chronic anorexia can lead to life-threatening malnutrition.

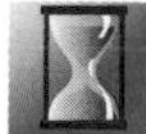

AGE ISSUE *In children, anorexia commonly accompanies many illnesses, but usually resolves promptly. However, in preadolescent and adolescent girls, be alert for the often subtle signs of anorexia nervosa.*

Due to the wide ranging possible causes, diagnostic procedures are necessary and may include thyroid function studies, endoscopy, upper GI series, gallbladder series, barium enema, liver and kidney function tests, hormone assays, computed tomography scans, ultrasonography, and blood studies to assess nutritional status.

Dyspepsia

Dyspepsia refers to an uncomfortable fullness after meals that is associated with nausea, belching, heartburn, and possibly cramping and abdominal distention. Frequently aggravated by spicy, fatty, or high-fiber foods and by excess caffeine intake, dyspepsia without other pathology indicates impaired digestive function. Dyspepsia apparently results when altered gastric secretions lead to excess stomach acidity. Subsequently, dyspepsia can interfere with a patient's nutritional intake.

History

If the patient complains of dyspepsia, begin by asking him to describe it fully. How often and when does it occur, specifically its relation to meals. Question the patient about how this complaint affects his meal patterns

(Text continues on page 81.)

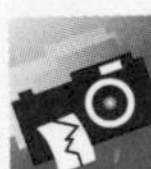

CLINICAL PICTURE

NUTRITION: INTERPRETING YOUR FINDINGS

After you assess the patient, a group of findings may lead you to suspect a particular nutritional disorder. The chart below shows you some common groups of findings for major signs and symptoms related to nutrition, along with their probable causes.

Sign or symptom and findings	Probable cause
Anorexia	
■ Fatigue ■ Afternoon fevers ■ Night sweats ■ Diarrhea ■ Cough ■ Bleeding ■ Lymphadenopathy ■ Opportunistic infection	AIDS
■ Marked weight loss ■ Diarrhea ■ Abdominal pain (right lower quadrant pain) ■ Cramping ■ Fever ■ Weakness ■ Bloody stools ■ Finger clubbing (rare)	Crohn's disease
■ Fatigue ■ Forgetfulness ■ Cold intolerance ■ Unexplained weight gain ■ Constipation ■ Dry flaky skin ■ Facial and hand edema ■ Thick brittle nails ■ Coarse broken hair	Hypothyroidism
Anorexia (continued)	
■ Considerable weight loss ■ Burning tongue ■ Generalized weakness ■ Numbness and tingling of extremities ■ Alternating episodes of constipation and diarrhea ■ Nausea and vomiting ■ Blurred vision ■ Irritability ■ Malaise ■ Fatigue	Pernicious anemia
■ Skeletal muscle atrophy ■ Loss of fatty tissue ■ Constipation ■ Amenorrhea ■ Alopecia ■ Sleep disturbances ■ Distorted self-image ■ Anhedonia ■ Decreased libido ■ Extreme restlessness ■ Avid exercising	Anorexia nervosa
■ Anhedonia ■ Poor concentration ■ Indecisiveness ■ Delusions ■ Menstrual irregularities ■ Decreased libido ■ Sleep disturbances ■ Mood swings ■ Gradual social withdrawal	Depression

NUTRITION: INTERPRETING YOUR FINDINGS *(continued)*

Sign or symptom and findings	Probable cause
Dyspepsia	
■ Biliary colic, radiating to back, shoulders, and chest ■ Diaphoresis ■ Chills ■ Low-grade fever ■ Abdominal pain ■ Jaundice with pruritus ■ Dark urine ■ Clay-colored stools ■ Nausea and vomiting	Cholelithiasis
■ Aggravation by spicy foods or caffeine ■ Relief with antacids ■ Anorexia ■ Vague epigastric pain ■ Belching ■ Nausea and vomiting	Gastritis (chronic)
■ Vague fullness, ranging to pressure or a boring or aching sensation in right or middle epigastrium occurring 1½ to 3 hours after eating and relieved by food or antacids ■ Abdominal tenderness ■ Weight gain ■ Rarely, vomiting	Duodenal ulcer
■ Oppressive, severe, substernal discomfort ■ Tachycardia ■ Tachypnea ■ Dyspnea ■ Pleuritic chest pain ■ Hemoptysis ■ Syncope ■ Hypotension	Pulmonary embolism
Dysphagia	
■ Food regurgitation ■ Chronic cough ■ Hoarseness ■ Halitosis	Esophageal diverticulum
■ Marked salivation ■ Hematemesis ■ Tachypnea ■ Fever ■ Intense pain in mouth and anterior chest aggravated by swallowing	Esophagitis (corrosive)
■ Heartburn exaggerated by strenuous exercise, bending over, or lying down and relieved by sitting up or taking antacids ■ Regurgitation ■ Frequent effortless vomiting ■ Dry nocturnal cough ■ Substernal chest pain	Esophagitis (reflux)
■ Rapid weight loss ■ Painful swallowing ■ Steady chest pain ■ Cough with hemoptysis ■ Hoarseness ■ Sore throat	Esophageal cancer
■ Precipitation or exacerbation by stress ■ Regurgitation of undigested food, especially at night ■ Weight loss ■ Cachexia ■ Hematemesis ■ Heartburn	Achalasia

(continued)

NUTRITION: INTERPRETING YOUR FINDINGS *(continued)*

Sign or symptom and findings	Probable cause
Weight gain, excessive	
▪ Anorexia ▪ Fatigue ▪ Cold intolerance ▪ Constipation ▪ Menorrhagia ▪ Dry, pale, cool skin ▪ Thick, brittle nails	Hypothyroidism
▪ Possible weight loss ▪ Fatigue ▪ Polydipsia ▪ Polyuria ▪ Nocturia ▪ Weakness ▪ Polyphagia ▪ Somnolence	Diabetes mellitus
▪ Edema ▪ Paroxysmal nocturnal dyspnea ▪ Orthopnea ▪ Fatigue	Heart failure
▪ Buffalo hump ▪ Slender extremities ▪ Moon face ▪ Weakness ▪ Purple striae ▪ Emotional lability ▪ Increased susceptibility to infection ▪ Gynecomastia (men) ▪ Hirsutism, acne, and menstrual irregularities (women)	Hypercortisolism
Weight loss, excessive	
▪ Skeletal muscle atrophy ▪ Loss of fatty tissue ▪ Constipation ▪ Dental caries ▪ Cold intolerance ▪ Dryness of scalp hair ▪ Amenorrhea	Anorexia nervosa

Sign or symptom and findings	Probable cause
Weight loss, excessive *(continued)*	
▪ Possible weight gain ▪ Fatigue ▪ Polydipsia ▪ Polyuria ▪ Nocturia ▪ Weakness ▪ Polyphagia ▪ Somnolence	Diabetes mellitus
▪ Nervousness ▪ Heat intolerance ▪ Diarrhea ▪ Increased appetite ▪ Palpitations ▪ Tachycardia ▪ Diaphoresis ▪ Fine tremor ▪ Enlarged thyroid gland (possible) ▪ Exophthalmos	Thyrotoxicosis
▪ Anorexia ▪ Weakness ▪ Fatigue ▪ Irritability ▪ Syncope ▪ Nausea and vomiting ▪ Abdominal pain ▪ Hyperpigmentation	Adrenal insufficiency
▪ Chronic cramping ▪ Abdominal pain ▪ Anorexia ▪ Bloody stools ▪ Nausea ▪ Fever ▪ Abdominal tenderness ▪ Hyperactive bowel sounds ▪ Abdominal distention	Crohn's disease

NUTRITION: INTERPRETING YOUR FINDINGS *(continued)*

Sign or symptom and findings	Probable cause
Weight loss, excessive (continued)	
▪ Intense pain in mouth and anterior chest ▪ Hypersalivation ▪ Dysphagia ▪ Hematemesis	Esophagitis
▪ Emaciated appearance ▪ Muscle wasting ▪ Loss of subcutaneous fat ▪ Subnormal body temperature ▪ Decreased resistance to infection ▪ Hair loss ▪ Dry, atrophic loose skin ▪ Mental and physical growth retardation ▪ Failure to thrive	Marasmus
▪ Generalized illness ▪ Muscle wasting, possibly masked by facial edema or edema in the lower body ▪ Sparse, thin, soft hair ▪ Changes in mucous membranes, such as cracks in the corners of the mouth, mouth ulcers and lesions, and tongue atrophy ▪ Scaly skin ▪ Enlarged liver ▪ Apathy, irritability ▪ Anorexia ▪ Diarrhea ▪ Poor wound healing	Kwashiorkor

and foods eaten. In addition, ask the patient about any drugs or activities that relieve or aggravate the condition Has he had nausea, vomiting, melena, hematemesis, cough, or chest pain? Ask what drugs he's currently taking. Also find out about any recent surgery. Does he have a history of renal, cardiovascular, or pulmonary disease? Has he noticed any change in the amount or color of his urine?

Physical assessment

Focus the physical assessment on the patient's eating habits, especially dietary intake and foods that exacerbate or alleviate the symptoms. Also focus the examination on the abdomen. Inspect for distention, ascites, scars, jaundice, uremic frost, or bruising. Then auscultate for bowel sounds and characterize their motility. Palpate and percuss the abdomen, noting any tenderness, pain, organ enlargement, or tympany.

Last, examine other body systems. Ask about behavior changes and evaluate the patient's level of consciousness. Auscultate for gallops and crackles. Percuss the lungs to detect consolidation. Note peripheral edema and any swelling of lymph nodes.

Analysis

Dyspepsia typically results from GI disorders, such as cholelithiasis, gastritis, ulcer disease, hepatitis and, to a lesser extent, from cardiac, pulmonary, and renal disorders and the effects of drugs. For example, nonsteroidal anti-inflammatory drugs, especially aspirin, commonly cause dyspepsia. Diuretics, antibiotics, antihypertensives, and many other drugs can cause dyspepsia, depending on the patient's tolerance of the dosage. This symptom may also result from emotional upset and overly rapid eating or improper chewing. Usually, it occurs a few hours after eating and lasts for a variable period of time. Its severity depends on the amount and type of food eaten and on GI motility. Additional food or antacids may relieve the discomfort.

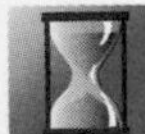

AGE ISSUE *Dyspepsia may occur in an adolescent with peptic ulcer disease, but not due to food; in patients with congenital pyloric stenosis, but projectile vomiting after meals is a more characteristic sign; or in patients who are lactose intolerant.*

Dysphagia

Dysphagia — swallowing difficulty — is a common symptom that's usually easy to localize. It may be constant or intermittent and is classified by the phase of swallowing it affects Among the factors that interfere with swallowing are severe pain, obstruction, abnormal peristalsis, impaired gag reflex, and excessive, scanty, or thick oral secretions.

History

If the patient's dysphagia doesn't suggest airway obstruction, begin a health history. Ask the patient if it's painful to swallow. If so, is the pain constant or intermittent? Have the patient point to where dysphagia feels most intense. Does eating alleviate or aggravate the symptom? Is it more difficult for him to swallow solids than to swallow liquids? If the patient has dysphagia for liquids, ask if hot, cold, and lukewarm fluids affect him differently. Does the symptom disappear after he tries to swallow a few times? Is swallowing easier if he changes position? Ask if he has experienced vomiting, regurgitation, weight loss, anorexia, hoarseness, dyspnea, or cough.

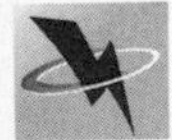

CRITICAL POINT *If the patient suddenly complains of dysphagia and displays signs of respiratory distress, such as dyspnea and stridor, suspect an airway obstruction, and quickly perform abdominal thrusts. Prepare to administer oxygen by mask or nasal cannula, or to assist with endotracheal intubation.*

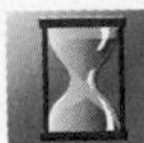

AGE ISSUE *With dysphagia in infants or younger children, pay close attention to their sucking and swallowing ability. Coughing, choking, or regurgitation during feeding suggest dysphagia. Ask the child's parents about the child's feeding patterns and any problems noted.*

Physical assessment

To evaluate the patient's swallowing reflex, place your finger along his thyroid notch and instruct him to swallow. If you feel his larynx rise, this reflex is intact. Next, have him cough to assess his cough reflex. Check his gag reflex if you're sure he has a good swallow or cough reflex. Listen closely to his speech for signs of muscle weakness. Does he have aphasia or dysarthria? Is his voice nasal, hoarse, or breathy? Assess the patient's mouth carefully. Check for dry mucous membranes and thick, sticky secretions. Observe for tongue and facial weakness. Assess for disorientation, which may make him neglect to swallow.

Analysis

Dysphagia is the most common — and sometimes the only — symptom of esophageal disorders, such as esophageal diverticula, esophagitis, narrowing of the esophagus or cancer. However, it may also result from oropharyngeal, respiratory, neurologic, and collagen disorders and the effects of toxins and treatments. Dysphagia increases the risk of choking and aspiration and may lead to malnutrition and dehydration.

Dysphagia may suggest achalasia, most common in patients ages 20 to 40. Here the disorder involves difficulty with solids and liquids. The dysphagia develops gradually and may be precipitated or exacerbated by stress. Occasionally, it's preceded by esophageal colic. Regurgitation of undigested food, especially at night, may cause wheezing, coughing, or choking as well as halitosis. Weight loss, cachexia, hematemesis and, possibly, heartburn are late findings. Additionally, radiation therapy, when directed against oral cancer, may cause scant salivation and temporary dysphagia.

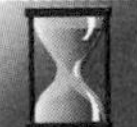

AGE ISSUE *Corrosive esophagitis and esophageal obstruction by a foreign body are more common causes of dysphagia in children than in adults. However, dysphagia may also result from congenital anomalies, such as annular stenosis and esophageal atresia.*

Weight gain, excessive

Weight gain occurs when ingested calories exceed body requirements for energy, causing increased adipose tissue storage.

History

Determine your patient's previous patterns of weight gain and loss. Does he have a family history of obesity, thyroid disease, or diabetes mellitus? Assess his eating and activity patterns. Has his appetite increased? Does he exercise regularly or at all? Next, ask about associated symptoms. Has he experienced visual disturbances, hoarseness, paresthesias, or increased urination and thirst? If the patient is male, has he become impotent? If the patient is female, has she had menstrual irregularities or experienced weight gain during menstruation?

Form an impression of the patient's mental status. Is he anxious or depressed? Does he respond slowly? Is his memory poor? What medications is he currently using?

Physical assessment

During your physical examination, measure height and weight and compare to standards. Also obtain skinfold thickness measurements to estimate fat reserves. Note fat distribution and the presence of localized or generalized edema. Inspect for other abnormalities, such as abnormal body hair distribution or hair loss and dry skin. Take and record the patient's vital signs.

Analysis

Weight gain can occur when fluid retention causes edema. When weight gain results from overeating, emotional factors — most commonly anxiety, guilt, and depression — and social factors may be the primary causes.

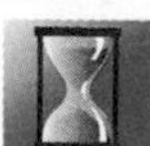

AGE ISSUE *Among elderly patients, weight gain often reflects a sustained food intake in the presence of the normal, progressive fall in basal metabolic rate. Among women, a progressive weight gain occurs with pregnancy, whereas a periodic weight gain usually occurs with menstruation. Weight gain in children can result from endocrine disorders such as hypercortisolism. Other causes include inactivity caused by such disorders as Down syndrome, late stages of muscular dystrophy, and severe cerebral palsy. Nonpathologic causes include poor eating habits, sedentary recreations, and emotional problems, especially among adolescents.*

Weight gain, a primary symptom of many endocrine disorders, also occurs with conditions that limit activity, especially cardiovascular and pulmonary disorders. It can also result from drug therapy that increases appetite, such as with corticosteroids, phenothiazines, tricyclic antidepressants, oral contraceptives (which cause fluid retention), or lithium (which can induce hypothyroidism) or causes fluid retention and from cardiovascular, hepatic, and renal disorders that cause edema.

Weight loss, excessive

Excessive weight loss can reflect decreased food intake, decreased food absorption, increased metabolic requirements, or a combination of the three.

History

Begin with a thorough diet history because weight loss almost always is caused by inadequate caloric intake. If the patient hasn't been eating properly, try to determine why. Ask about his previous weight and if the recent loss was intentional. Be alert to lifestyle or occupational changes that may be a source of anxiety or depression. For example, has he gotten separated or divorced? Has he recently changed jobs?

Inquire about recent changes in bowel habits, such as diarrhea or bulky, floating stools. Has the patient had nausea, vomiting, or abdominal pain, which may indicate a GI disorder? Has he had excessive thirst, excessive urination, or heat intolerance, which may signal an endocrine disorder? Take a careful drug history, noting especially any use of diet pills and laxatives.

Physical assessment

Carefully check the patient's height and weight, and ask about his previous weight. Take his vital signs and note his general appearance: is he well nourished? Do his clothes fit? Is muscle wasting evident?

Examine the patient's skin for turgor and abnormal pigmentation, especially around the joints. Does he have pallor or jaundice? Examine his mouth, including the condition of his teeth or dentures. Look for signs of infection or irritation on the roof of the mouth, and note any hyperpigmentation of the buccal mucosa. Also check the patient's eyes for exophthalmos and his neck for swelling, and evaluate his lungs for adventitious sounds. Inspect his abdomen for signs of wasting, and palpate for masses, tenderness, and an enlarged liver.

Analysis

Excessive weight loss can be caused by endocrine (diabetes or thyrotoxicosis), neoplastic, GI (Crohn's disease, esophagitis or gastroenteritis), and psychiatric disorders; nutritional deficiencies (protein-calorie malnutrition such as marasmus or kwashiorkor); infections; and neurologic lesions that cause paralysis and dysphagia. However, weight loss may accompany conditions that prevent sufficient food intake, such as painful oral lesions, ill-fitting dentures, and loss of teeth. It may be the metabolic sequela of poverty, fad diets, excessive exercise, and certain drugs.

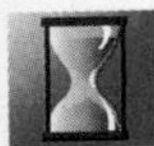

AGE ISSUE *In infants, excessive weight loss may be caused by failure-to-thrive syndrome. In children, severe weight loss may be the first indication of diabetes mellitus. Chronic, gradual weight loss occurs in children with marasmus—nonedematous protein-calorie malnutrition. Weight loss may also occur as result of child abuse or neglect, infections causing high fevers, GI disorders causing vomiting and diarrhea, or celiac disease.*

Excessive weight loss may occur as a late sign in such chronic diseases as heart failure and renal disease. In these diseases, however, it's the result of anorexia.

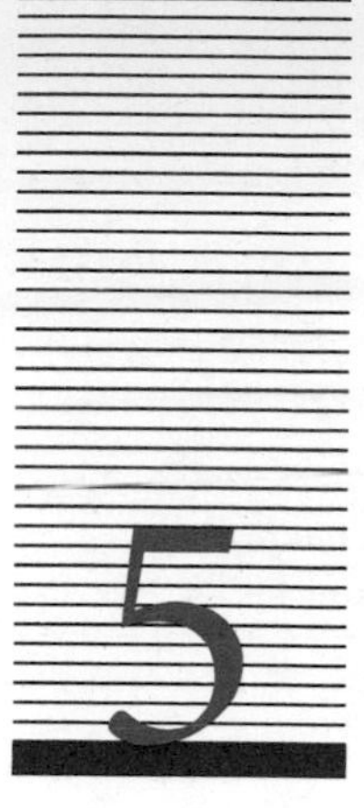

5 Integumentary system

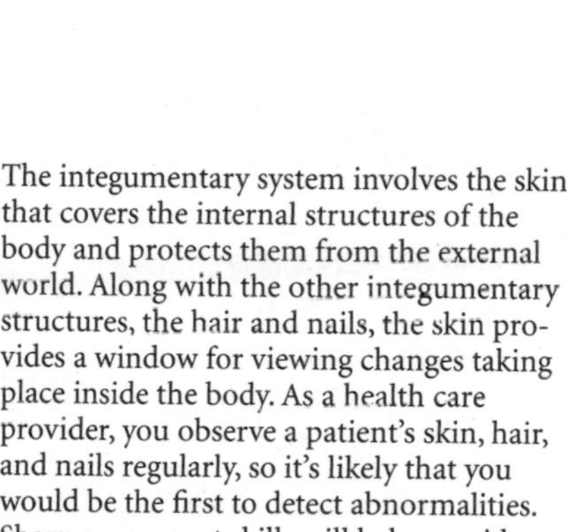

The integumentary system involves the skin that covers the internal structures of the body and protects them from the external world. Along with the other integumentary structures, the hair and nails, the skin provides a window for viewing changes taking place inside the body. As a health care provider, you observe a patient's skin, hair, and nails regularly, so it's likely that you would be the first to detect abnormalities. Sharp assessment skills will help provide a reliable picture of the patient's overall health.

Anatomy and physiology

To perform an accurate physical assessment of the integumentary system, you'll need to understand the anatomy and physiology of the skin, hair, and nails, as well as related structures that include several glands.

Skin

The skin is the body's largest organ. It is the membranous protective covering of the body, consisting of the epidermis and dermis.

Skin functions

The skin performs many functions. These include protection, sensory perception, temperature and blood pressure regulation, vitamin synthesis, and excretion.

Protection. The epidermis protects against trauma, noxious chemicals, and invasion by microorganisms. Langerhans' cells enhance the immune response by helping lymphocytes process antigens entering the epidermis. Melanocytes protect the skin by producing melanin to help filter ultraviolet

SKIN CHANGES WITH AGE

As people age, their skin changes. Listed here are the changes that normally occur with aging.

Change	Findings
Pigmentation	▪ Pale color
Thickness	▪ Wrinkling, especially on the face, arms, and legs ▪ Parchmentlike appearance, especially over bony prominences and on the dorsal surfaces of the hands, feet, arms, and legs
Moisture	▪ Dry, flaky, and rough
Turgor	▪ "Tents" and stands alone (especially in the presence of dehydration)
Texture	▪ Numerous creases and lines

light (irradiation). The intact skin also protects the body by limiting excretion of water and electrolytes.

Sensory perception. Sensory nerve fibers carry impulses to the central nervous system. Autonomic nerve fibers carry impulses to smooth muscles in the walls of the dermal blood vessels, to the muscles around the hair roots, and to the sweat glands. Sensory nerve fibers originate in dorsal nerve roots and supply specific areas of the skin known as *dermatomes*. Through these fibers, the skin can transmit various sensations, including temperature, touch, pressure, pain, and itching.

Temperature and blood pressure regulation. Abundant nerves, blood vessels, and eccrine glands within the dermis help with thermoregulation. When the skin is exposed to cold or when internal body temperature falls, the blood vessels constrict in response to stimuli from the autonomic nervous system. This decreases blood flow through the skin and conserves body heat. When the skin is too hot or internal body temperature rises, the small arteries in the dermis dilate. Increased blood flow through these vessels reduces body heat. If this doesn't adequately lower temperature, the eccrine glands act to increase sweat production; subsequent evaporation cools the skin.

Dermal blood vessels also help with the regulation of systemic blood pressure by vasoconstriction.

Vitamin synthesis. The skin synthesizes vitamin D, or cholecalciferol, when stimulated by ultraviolet light.

Excretion. The skin is also an excretory organ, containing sweat glands that excrete sweat, which contains water, electrolytes, urea, and lactic acid. The skin maintains body surface integrity by migration and shedding. It can repair surface wounds by intensifying normal cell replacement mechanisms. However, regeneration won't occur if the dermal layer is destroyed. The sebaceous glands produce sebum—a mixture of keratin, fat, and cellulose debris. Combined with sweat, sebum forms a moist, oily, acidic film that's mildly antibacterial and antifungal and that protects the skin surface.

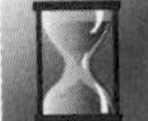

AGE ISSUE *As people age, skin functions decline and normal changes occur. As a result, elderly patients are more prone to skin disease, infection, problems in wound healing, and tissue atrophy.* *(See* Skin changes with age.*)*

Layers of the skin

The skin consists of two distinct layers: the epidermis and the dermis. Subcutaneous

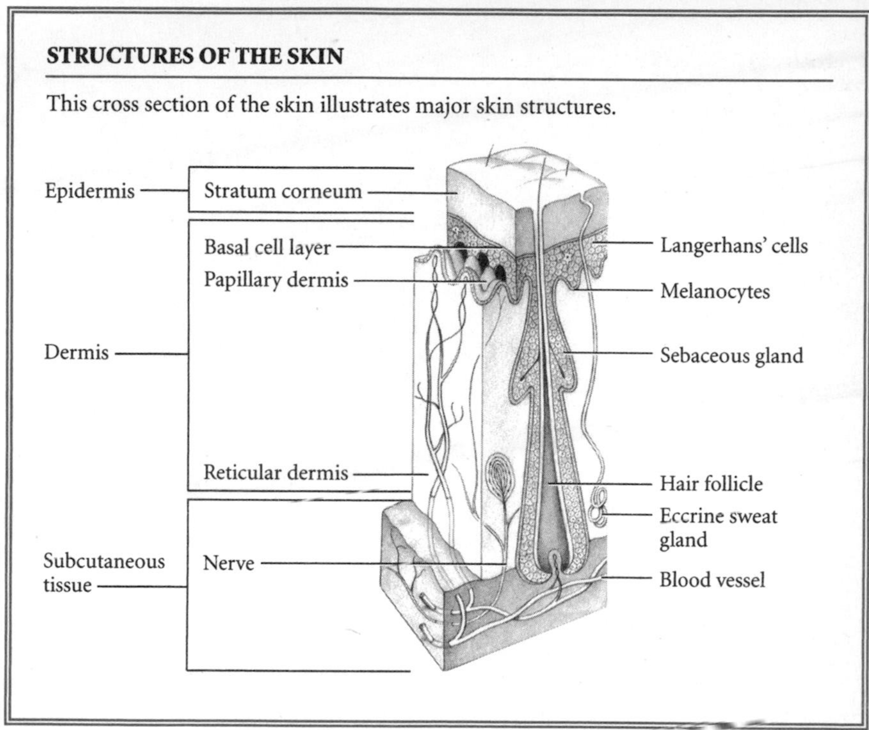

STRUCTURES OF THE SKIN

This cross section of the skin illustrates major skin structures.

tissue lies beneath these layers. (See *Structures of the skin.*)

Epidermis. The epidermis — the outer layer — is made of squamous epithelial tissue. The epidermis is thin and contains no blood vessels. The two major layers of the epidermis are the stratum corneum — the most superficial layer — and the deeper basal cell layer, or stratum germinativum.

Stratum corneum. After mitosis occurs in the germinal layer, epithelial cells undergo a series of changes as they migrate to the outermost part of the epidermis called the *stratum corneum,* which is made up of tightly arranged layers of cellular membranes and keratin.

Langerhans' cells are specialized cells interspersed among the keratinized cells below the stratum corneum. Langerhans' cells have an immunologic function and assist in the initial processing of antigens that enter the epidermis. Epidermal cells are usually shed from the surface as epidermal dust. Differentiation of cells from the basal layer to the stratum corneum takes up to 28 days.

Basal layer. The basal layer produces new cells to replace the superficial keratinized cells that are continuously shed or worn away.

The basal layer also contains specialized cells known as *melanocytes,* which produce the brown pigment melanin and disperse it to the surrounding epithelial cells. Melanin primarily serves to filter ultraviolet radiation (light). Exposure to ultraviolet light can stimulate melanin production. Hormones, the environment, and heredity influence melanocyte production. Because melanocyte production is greater in some people than others, skin color varies considerably.

Dermis. Also called the corium, the dermis is an elastic system that contains and supports the body's blood vessels, lymphatic vessels, nerves, and epidermal appendages, such as the hair, nails, and glands — eccrine and apocrine. The dermis is made up of two

HAIR STRUCTURE

This illustration shows a hair shaft and its associated glands.

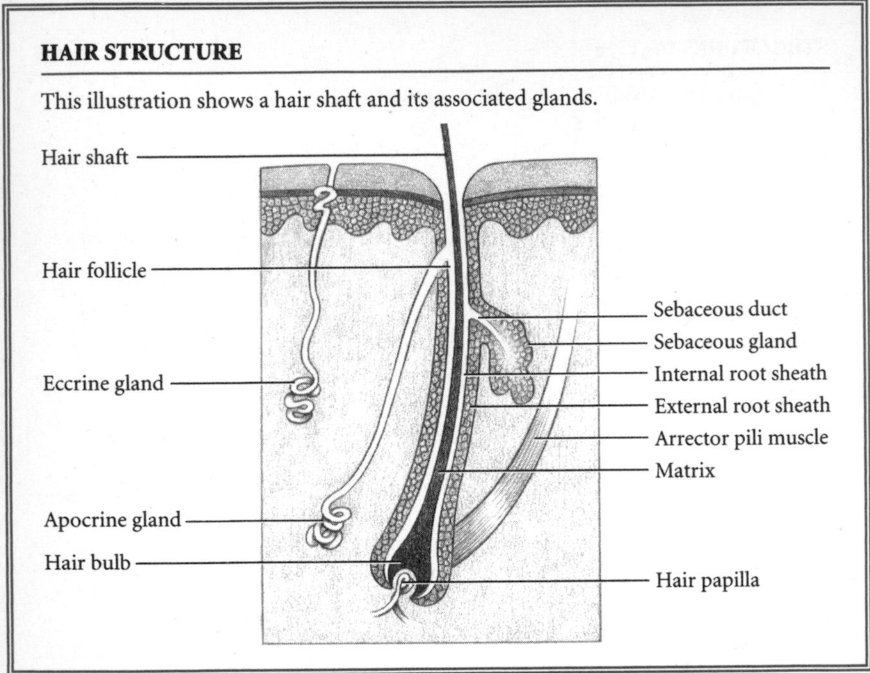

layers, the superficial papillary dermis and the reticular dermis.

The papillary dermis is studded with fingerlike projections, called papillae, that nourish the epidermal cells. The epidermis lies over these papillae and bulges downward to fill the spaces. A collagenous membrane known as the *basement membrane* lies between the epidermis and dermis, holding them together.

The reticular dermis covers a layer of subcutaneous tissue, known as the adipose layer, which is a specialized layer primarily made up of fat cells. It insulates the body to conserve heat, acts as a mechanical shock absorber, and provides energy.

Extracellular material, called matrix, makes up most of the dermis; matrix contains connective tissue fibers called *collagen,* elastin, and reticular fibers. Collagen, a protein, gives strength to the dermis; elastin makes the skin pliable; and reticular fibers bind the collagen and elastin fibers together.

The matrix and connective tissue fibers are produced by spindle-shaped connective tissue cells called dermal fibroblasts, which become part of the matrix as it forms. Fibers are loosely arranged in the papillary dermis, but more tightly packed in the deeper reticular dermis.

Epidermal appendages. The sebaceous, eccrine, and apocrine glands are all epidermal appendages.

SEBACEOUS GLANDS. Sebaceous glands occur on all parts of the skin except for the palms and soles. They're most prominent on the scalp, face, upper body, and genital region and are part of the same structure that contains hair follicles. Their main function is to produce sebum, a lipid substance, which is produced within the lobule and secreted into the hair follicle via the sebaceous duct. Sebum then exits through the hair follicle opening to reach the skin surface. It may help waterproof the hair and skin and promotes the absorption of fat-soluble substances into the dermis. It may also be involved in the production of vitamin D and have some antibacterial function.

ECCRINE GLANDS. Eccrine glands, one type of sweat gland, are widely distributed, coiled glands that produce an odorless, watery

NAIL ANATOMY

The illustration below shows the anatomic components of a fingernail.

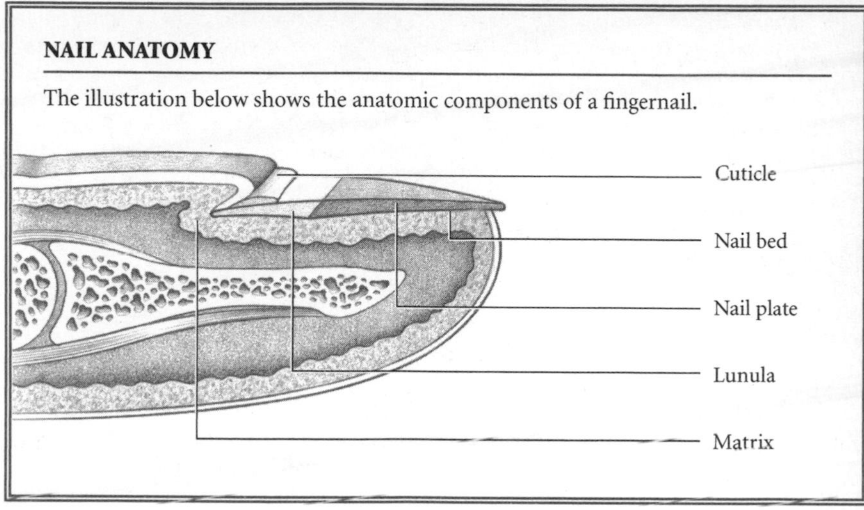

fluid with a sodium concentration equal to that of plasma. A duct from the secretory coils passes through the dermis and epidermis and opens onto the skin surface. Eccrine glands in the palms and soles secrete fluid primarily in response to emotional stress, such as that from taking a test. The remaining 3 million eccrine glands respond primarily to thermal stress, effectively regulating temperature.

Apocrine glands. The second type of sweat gland, located primarily in the axillae and genital areas, are apocrine glands, which have a coiled secretory portion that lies deeper in the dermis than the eccrine glands. A duct connects the apocrine glands to the upper portion of the hair follicle. Apocrine glands, which begin to function at puberty, have no known biological function. Bacterial decomposition of the fluid produced by these glands causes body odor.

Hair

Hair is formed from keratin and produced by matrix cells in the dermal layer. Each hair lies in a hair follicle and receives nourishment from the papilla, a loop of capillaries at the base of the follicle. At the lower end of the hair shaft is the hair bulb that contains melanocytes, which determine hair color. (See *Hair structure.*)

Each hair is attached at the base to a smooth muscle called the arrector pili. This muscle contracts during emotional stress or exposure to cold and elevates the hair, causing goose bumps.

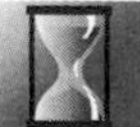

AGE ISSUE *In neonates, the skin is covered with lanugo and hair on the scalp may be lost several weeks after birth, especially at the temple and occiput, but it slowly grows back. As people age, melanocyte function declines, producing light or gray hair, and the hair follicle itself becomes drier as sebaceous gland function decreases. Hair growth also declines with age, decreasing the amount of body hair. In addition, balding, genetically determined in younger people, occurs as a normal result of aging.*

Nails

Nails are formed when the epidermal cells are converted into hard plates of keratin. The nails are made up of the nail root (or nail matrix), nail plate, nail bed, lunula, nail folds, and cuticle. (See *Nail anatomy.*)

The nail plate is the visible, hardened layer that covers the fingertip. The plate is clear with fine longitudinal ridges. Its pink color results from blood vessels underlying vascular epithelial cells. The nail matrix is the site of nail growth and is protected by the cuticle. At the end of the matrix is the white, crescent-shaped area, the lunula, which extends beyond the cuticle.

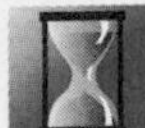

AGE ISSUE *With age, nail growth slows and the nails become brittle and thin. Longitudinal ridges in the nail plate become much more pronounced, making the nails prone to splitting. Also, the nails lose their luster and become yellow in color.*

Health history

When assessing a problem related to the integumentary system, thoroughly explore the patient's chief complaint, current and past health history, family history, psychosocial history, and activities of daily living. Keep in mind that skin, hair, and nail abnormalities may result from a medical problem related to the patient's chief complaint, but they may be overlooked or minimized by the patient.

Skin

Most complaints about the skin involve itching, rashes, lesions, pigmentation abnormalities, or changes in existing lesions.

Begin by asking about changes in the patient's skin and continue with questions about his current and past health history, family history, psychosocial history, and patterns of daily living. Typical questions to ask include:

- How and when did the skin changes occur?
- Are the changes in the form of a skin rash or lesion?
- Is the change confined to one area, or has the condition spread?
- Does the area bleed or have drainage?
- Does the area itch?
- How much time do you spend in the sun, and how do you protect your skin from ultraviolet rays?
- Do you have allergies?
- Do you have a family history of skin cancer or other significant diseases?
- Do you have a fever or joint pain, or have you lost weight?
- Have you had a recent insect bite?
- Do you take any medications or herbal preparations? If yes, which ones?
- What changes in your skin have you observed in the past few years?

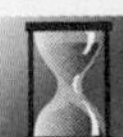

AGE ISSUE *If the patient is an infant or child, ask the parents these questions:*

- *Does the child have any birthmarks?*
- *As a neonate, did he experience any change in skin color—for example, cyanosis or jaundice?*
- *Have you noted any rashes, burns, or bruises? If yes, where and when, and what was the cause?*
- *Has the child been exposed to any contagious skin conditions—such as scabies, lice, or impetigo—or to any communicable diseases?*

Hair

Most concerns about the hair refer either to hair loss or hirsutism, or an increased growth and distribution of body hair. Either of these problems can be caused by such factors as skin infections, ovarian or adrenal tumors, increased stress, or systemic diseases, such as hypothyroidism and malignancies.

Begin by asking about changes in the patient's hair and continue with questions about his current and past health history, family history, psychosocial history, and patterns of daily living. To identify the cause of your patient's hair problem, ask:

- When did you first notice the loss or gain of hair? Was it sudden or gradual?
- Did the change occur in just a few spots or all over your body?
- What was happening in your life when the problem started?
- Are you taking any medications or herbal preparations?
- Are you experiencing itching, pain, discharge, fever, or weight loss?
- What serious illnesses, if any, have you had?

Nails

Most complaints about the nails concern changes in growth or color. Either of these problems may result from infection, nutritional deficiencies, systemic illnesses, or stress.

Begin by asking about changes in a patient's nails and continue with questions about his current and past history, family history, psychosocial history, and patterns of daily living. Typical questions to ask about changes in a patient's nails include:

- When did you first notice the changes in your nails?
- What types of changes have you noticed, for example, in nail shape, color, or brittleness?
- Were the changes sudden or gradual?
- Do you have other signs or symptoms, such as bleeding, pain, itching, or discharge?
- What is the normal condition of your nails?
- Do you have a history of serious illness?
- Do you have a history of nail problems?
- Do you bite your nails?
- Have you had artificial nail tips attached?

Physical assessment

To assess skin, hair, and nails, use the techniques of inspection and palpation. Before beginning the examination, make sure the room is well lit and comfortably warm. Wear gloves during the examination.

Skin inspection

Before beginning the skin examination, gather the following equipment: a clear ruler with centimeter and millimeter markings, a tongue blade, a penlight or flashlight, a Wood's lamp, and a magnifying glass. This equipment will enable you to measure and closely inspect skin lesions and other abnormalities.

Start by observing the overall appearance of the skin. Such observation will help identify areas that need further assessment. Inspect and palpate the skin area by area, focusing on color, texture, turgor, moisture, and temperature.

Skin color

Look for localized areas of bruising, cyanosis, pallor, and erythema. Check for uniformity of color and hypopigmented or hyperpigmented areas. (See *Assessing skin color variations,* page 92.)

Parts of the body that are exposed to the sun may show a darker pigmentation than other areas.

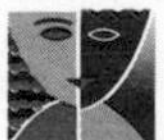

CULTURAL INSIGHT *Depending on the patient's skin pigmentation, skin color changes may vary. However, some local skin color changes are normal variations that appear in certain cultures. For example, Mongolian spots are bluish black areas of pigmentation more commonly noted on the back and buttocks of dark-skinned neonates.* *(See* Detecting color variations in dark-skinned people, *page 92.)*

Skin texture and turgor

Inspect and palpate the patient's skin texture, noting its thickness and mobility. It should look smooth and be intact. Rough, dry skin is common in patients with hypothyroidism, psoriasis, and excessive keratinization. Skin that isn't intact may indicate local irritation or trauma.

Palpation will also help you evaluate the patient's hydration status. Dehydration and edema cause poor skin turgor. Because poor skin turgor may also be caused by aging, it may not be a reliable indicator of the hydration status of elderly patients. Overhydration causes the skin to appear edematous and spongy. Localized edema also can result from trauma or systemic disease. (See *Evaluating skin turgor,* page 93.)

Skin moisture

Observe the skin's moisture content. The skin should be relatively dry with a minimal amount of perspiration. Skin-fold areas should also be fairly dry. Overly dry skin will look red and flaky.

Overly moist skin can be caused by anxiety, obesity, or an environment that's too warm. Heavy sweating, or diaphoresis, usually accompanies fever; strenuous activity; cardiac, pulmonary, and other diseases; and any activity or illness that elevates the metabolic rate.

Skin temperature

Palpate the skin bilaterally for temperature, which can range from cool to warm. Warm skin suggests normal circulation; cool skin, a possible underlying disorder. Distinguish between generalized and localized coolness and warmth. Localized skin coolness can result from vasoconstriction associated with cold environments or impaired arterial circulation to a limb. General coolness can result from such conditions as shock or hypothyroidism. (See *Assessing skin temperature,* page 93.)

Localized warmth occurs in areas that are infected, inflamed, or burned. Generalized warmth occurs with fever or systemic dis-

ASSESSING SKIN COLOR VARIATIONS

When assessing your patient's skin color, note its variations. To interpret your findings more quickly, refer to this chart.

Color	Distribution	Possible cause
Absent	▪ Small circumscribed areas ▪ Generalized	▪ Vitiligo ▪ Albinism
Blue	▪ Around lips or generalized	▪ Cyanosis (*Note:* In blacks, blue gingivae are normal.)
Deep red	▪ Generalized	▪ Polycythemia vera (increased red blood cell count)
Pink	▪ Local or generalized	▪ Erythema (superficial capillary dilation and congestion)
Tan to brown	▪ Facial patches	▪ Chloasma of pregnancy; butterfly rash of lupus erythematosus
Tan to brown-bronze	▪ Generalized (not related to sun exposure)	▪ Addison's disease
Yellow to yellowish brown	▪ Sclera or generalized	▪ Jaundice from liver dysfunction (*Note:* In blacks, yellowish brown pigmentation of sclera is normal.)
Yellow-orange	▪ Palms, soles, and face; not sclera	▪ Carotenemia (carotene in the blood)

EXPERT TECHNIQUE

DETECTING COLOR VARIATIONS IN DARK-SKINNED PEOPLE

Cyanosis
Examine the conjunctivae, palms, soles, buccal mucosa, and tongue. Look for dull, dark color.

Edema
Examine the area for decreased color and palpate for tightness.

Erythema
Palpate the area for warmth.

Jaundice
Examine the sclerae and hard palate in natural, not fluorescent, light if possible. Look for a yellow color.

Pallor
Examine the sclerae, conjunctivae, buccal mucosa, tongue, lips, nail beds, palms, and soles. Look for an ashen color.

Petechiae
Examine areas of lighter pigmentation such as the abdomen. Look for tiny, purplish red dots.

Rashes
Palpate the area for skin texture changes.

EXPERT TECHNIQUE

EVALUATING SKIN TURGOR

To assess skin turgor in an adult, gently squeeze the skin on the forearm or sternal area between your thumb and forefinger, as shown. In an infant, roll a fold of loosely adherent abdominal skin between your thumb and forefinger. Then release the skin.

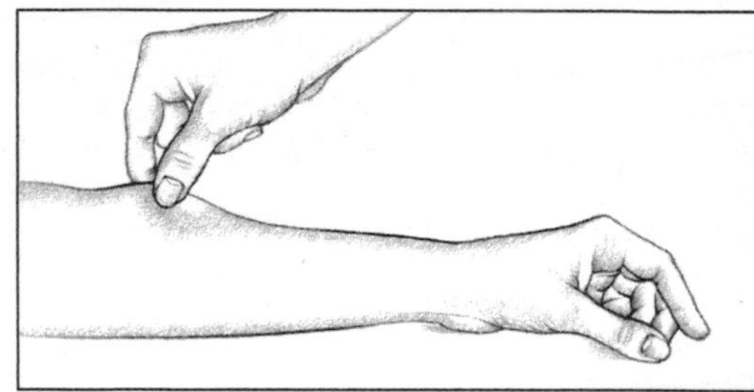

If the skin quickly returns to its original shape, the patient has normal turgor. If it returns to its original shape slowly, over 30 seconds, or maintains a tented position as shown, the skin has poor turgor.

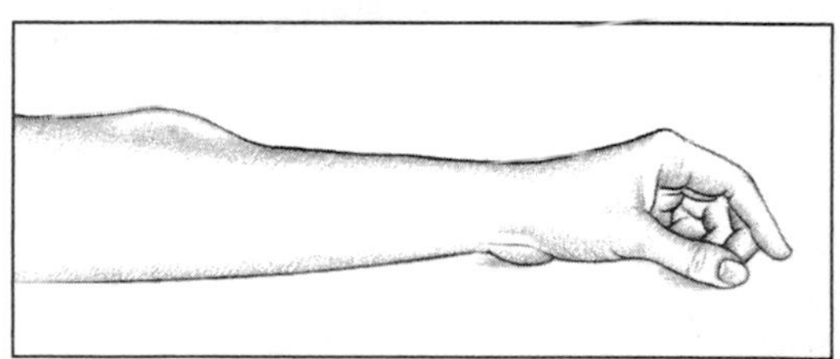

EXPERT TECHNIQUE

ASSESSING SKIN TEMPERATURE

When trying to compare subtle temperature differences in one area of the body to another, use the dorsal surface of your hands and fingers. They're the most sensitive to changes in temperature.

eases such as hyperthyroidism. Be sure to check skin temperature bilaterally.

Skin lesions

During inspection, you may see normal variations in the patient's skin texture and pigmentation. Red lesions caused by vascular changes include hemangiomas, telangiectases, petechiae, purpura, and ecchymoses and may indicate disease.

Other normal variations include birthmarks, freckles, and nevi, or moles. Birthmarks are generally flat and range in color from tan to red or brown. They can be found on all areas of the body. Freckles are small, flat macules located primarily on the face, arms, and back. They're usually red brown to brown. Nevi are either flat or raised, and may be pink, tan, or dark brown. Like birthmarks, they can be found on all areas of the body.

Whenever a lesion is noted, evaluate it to determine its origin. Start by classifying it as primary or secondary. A primary lesion is new and changes in a primary lesion constitute a secondary lesion. Examples of secondary lesions include fissures, scales, crusts, scars, and excoriations. (See *Recognizing skin lesions,* pages 94 and 95.)

Determine if the lesion is solid or fluid-filled. Macules, papules, nodules, wheals, and hives are solid lesions. Vesicles, bullae,

RECOGNIZING SKIN LESIONS

These illustrations depict the most common primary and secondary lesions.

Primary lesions

Bulla

Fluid-filled lesion that's more than 2 cm in diameter (also called a *blister*) — for example, severe poison oak or ivy dermatitis, bullous pemphigoid, second-degree burn

Comedo

Plugged pilosebaceous duct, exfoliative, formed from sebum and keratin — for example, blackhead (open comedo), whitehead (closed comedo)

Cyst

Semisolid or fluid-filled encapsulated mass extending deep into dermis — for example, acne

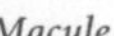

Macule

Flat, pigmented, circumscribed area that's less than 1 cm in diameter — for example, freckle, rubella

Nodule

Firm, raised lesion that's deeper than a papule, that extends into the dermal layer, and that's 0.5 to 2 cm in diameter — for example, dermatofibroma

Papule

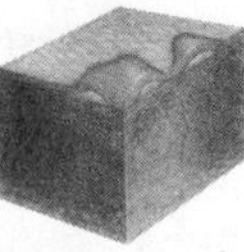

Firm, inflammatory, raised lesion that's up to 0.5 cm in diameter and that may be the same color as skin or pigmented — for example, acne papule, lichen planus

Patch

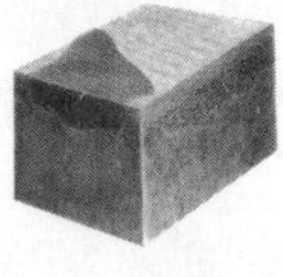

Flat, pigmented, circumscribed area that's more than 2 cm in diameter — for example, herald patch (pityriasis rosea)

Plaque

Circumscribed, solid, elevated lesion that's more than 1 cm in diameter — for example, psoriasis (Elevation above skin surface occupies larger surface area in comparison with height.)

Pustule

Raised, circumscribed lesion that's usually less than 1 cm in diameter and contains purulent material, making it a yellow-white color — for example, acne pustule, impetigo, furuncle

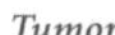

Tumor

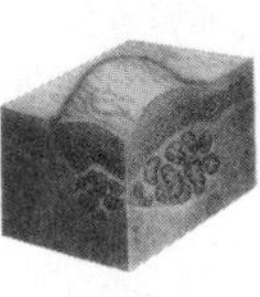

Elevated solid lesion that's more than 2 cm in diameter, extending into dermal and subcutaneous layers — for example, carcinoma

Vesicle

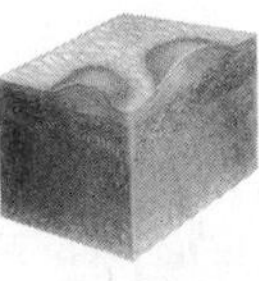

Raised, circumscribed, fluid-filled lesion that's less than 0.5 cm in diameter — for example, chickenpox, herpes simplex

Wheal

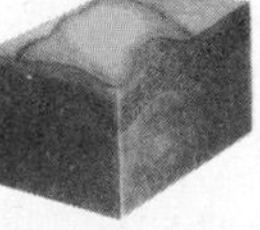

Raised, firm lesion (with intense localized skin edema) that varies in size, shape, and color (from pale pink to red) and disappears within hours — for example, hive (urticaria), insect bite

RECOGNIZING SKIN LESIONS *(continued)*

Secondary lesions

Atrophy
Thinning of skin surface at the site of the disorder — for example, striae, aging skin

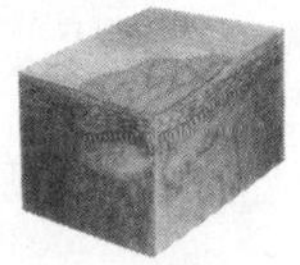

Crust
Dried sebum, serous, sanguineous, or purulent exudate, overlying an erosion or weeping vesicle, bulla, or pustule — for example, impetigo

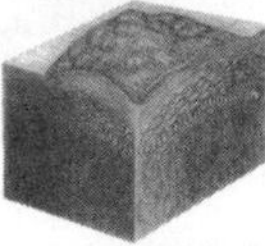

Erosion
Circumscribed lesion involving loss of superficial epidermis — for example, rug burn, abrasion

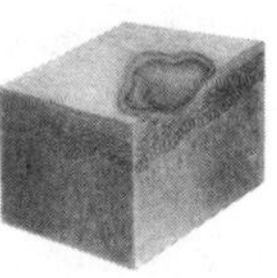

Excoriation
Linear scratched or abraded areas, commonly self induced — for example, abraded acne lesions, eczema

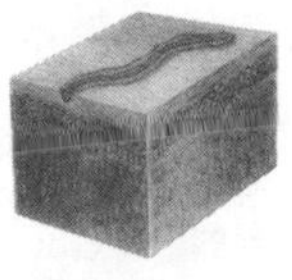

Fissure
Linear cracking of the skin extending into the dermal layer — for example, hand dermatitis (chapped skin)

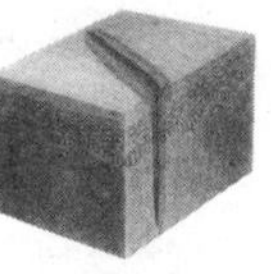

Lichenification
Thickened, prominent skin markings caused by constant rubbing — for example, chronic atopic dermatitis

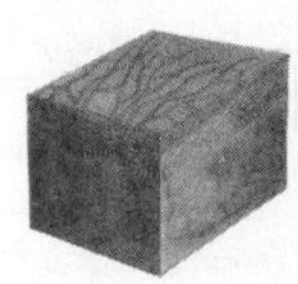

Scale
Thin, dry flakes of shedding skin — for example, psoriasis, dry skin, neonate desquamation

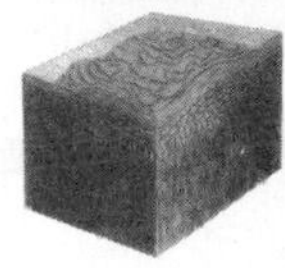

Scar
Fibrous tissue (caused by trauma, deep inflammation, or surgical incision) that's red and raised when it's new, pink and flat for up to 6 weeks, and pale and depressed when it's old — for example, a healed surgical incision

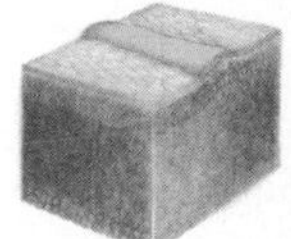

Ulcer
Epidermal and dermal destruction that may extend into subcutaneous tissue and that usually heals with scarring — for example, pressure or stasis ulcer

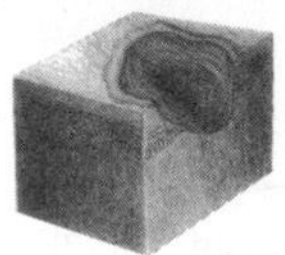

pustules, and cysts are fluid-filled lesions. Using a flashlight or penlight will help you determine whether a lesion is solid or fluid-filled. (See *Illuminating lesions,* page 96.)

To identify lesions that fluoresce, use a Wood's lamp, which gives out specially filtered ultraviolet light. Darken the room and shine the light on the lesion. If the lesion looks bluish green, the patient has a fungal infection.

After identifying the type of lesion, describe its characteristics, pattern, location, and distribution. A detailed description will help you determine whether the lesion is a normal or pathologic skin change.

Symmetry and border. Examine the lesion to see if it looks the same on both sides. Also, check the borders to see if they're regular or irregular. An asymmetrical lesion with an irregular border may indicate malignancy.

Color. Lesions occur in a variety of colors and can change color over time. Therefore, watch for such changes in your patient. For example, if a lesion such as a mole (nevus)

EXPERT TECHNIQUE

ILLUMINATING LESIONS

Illuminating a lesion will help you see it better and learn more about its characteristics. Here are two techniques worth perfecting.

Macule or papule
To determine whether a lesion is a macule or a papule, use this technique: Reduce the direct lighting and shine a penlight or flashlight at a right angle to the lesion. If the light casts a shadow, the lesion is a papule. Macules are flat and don't produce shadows.

Solid or fluid-filled
To determine whether a lesion is solid or fluid-filled, use this technique: Place the tip of a flashlight or penlight against the side of the lesion. Solid lesions don't transmit light. Fluid-filled lesions will transilluminate with a red glow.

has changed from tan or brown to multiple shades of tan, dark brown, black, or a mixture of red, white, and blue, the lesion might be malignant.

Configuration and distribution. Pay close attention as well to the configuration and distribution of the lesion. Many skin diseases have typical configuration patterns. Identifying those patterns will help you determine the cause of the problem. (See *Recognizing common lesion configurations.*)

Diameter. Measure the diameter of the lesion using a millimeter/centimeter ruler. If you estimate the diameter, you may not be able to determine subtle changes in size. An increase in the size or elevation of a mole over a period of many years is common and probably normal. Still, be sure to take note of moles that rapidly change size, especially moles that are 6 mm or larger.

Drainage. If you note drainage, document the type, color, and amount. Also note if the lesion has a foul odor, which can indicate a superimposed infection.

Hair inspection

Start by inspecting and palpating the hair over the patient's entire body, not just on his head. Note the distribution, quantity, texture, and color. The quantity and distribution of head and body hair varies between patients. However, hair should be evenly distributed over the entire body.

Check for patterns of hair loss and growth. If you notice patchy hair loss, look for regrowth. Also, examine the scalp for erythema, scaling, and encrustation. Excessive hair loss with scalp crusting may indicate ringworm infestation. The only way to detect scalp crusting is by using a Wood's lamp. Also, note areas of excessive hair growth, which may indicate a hormone imbalance or be a sign of a systemic disorder such as Cushing's syndrome.

The texture of scalp hair also varies between patients. As a rule, hair should be shiny and smooth, not dry or brittle. Differences in grooming and hairstyling may affect the texture and quality of the hair. Dryness or brittleness can result from the use of harsh hair treatments or hair care products or can be due to a systemic illness. Extreme oiliness is usually related to an excessive production of sebum or to poor grooming habits.

Nail inspection

Inspecting and palpating the nails is vital for two reasons: The appearance of the nails can be a critical indicator of systemic illness, and their overall condition reveals much about the patient's grooming habits and ability to care for himself. Examine the nails for color, shape, thickness, consistency, and contour.

First, look at the color of the nails. Light-skinned people generally have pinkish nails. Dark-skinned people generally have brown nails. Brown-pigmented bands in the nail

RECOGNIZING COMMON LESION CONFIGURATIONS

Identify the configuration of the patient's skin lesion by matching it to one of these illustrations.

Discrete
Individual lesions are separate and distinct.

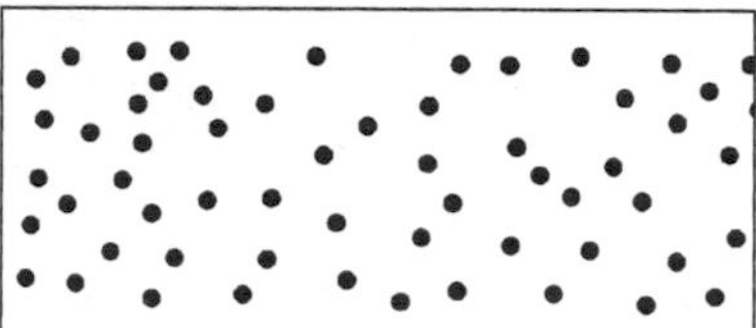

Annular
Lesions are arranged in a single ring or circle.

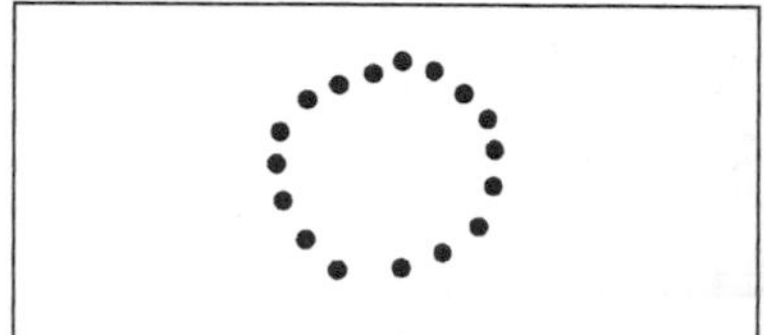

Grouped
Lesions are clustered together.

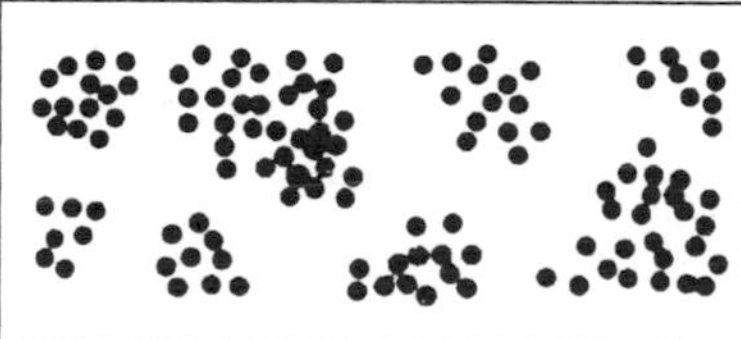

Polycyclic
Lesions are arranged in multiple circles.

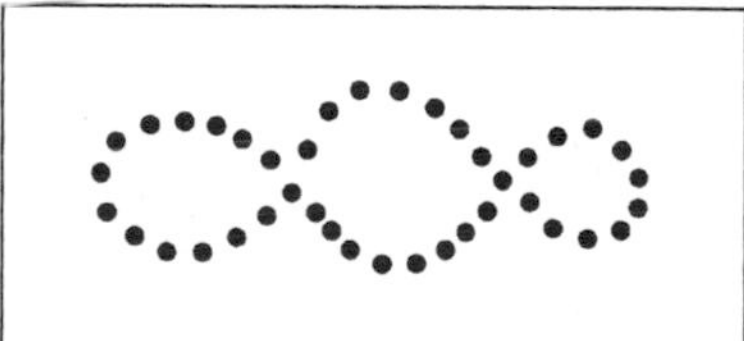

Confluent
Lesions merge so that individual lesions aren't visible or palpable.

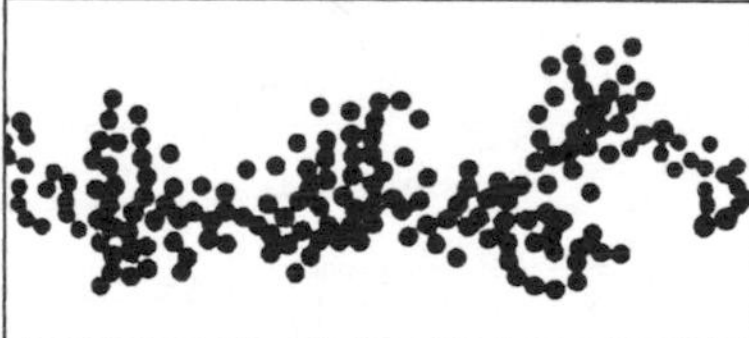

Arciform
Lesions form arcs or curves.

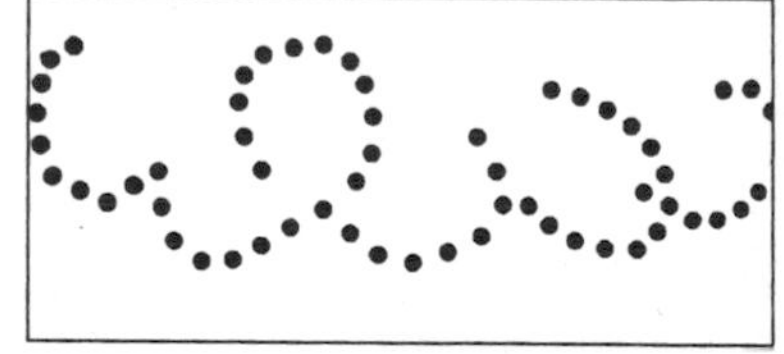

Linear
Lesions form a line.

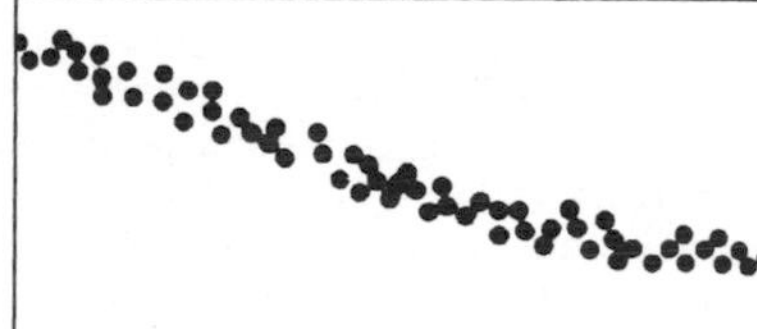

Reticular
Lesions form a meshlike network.

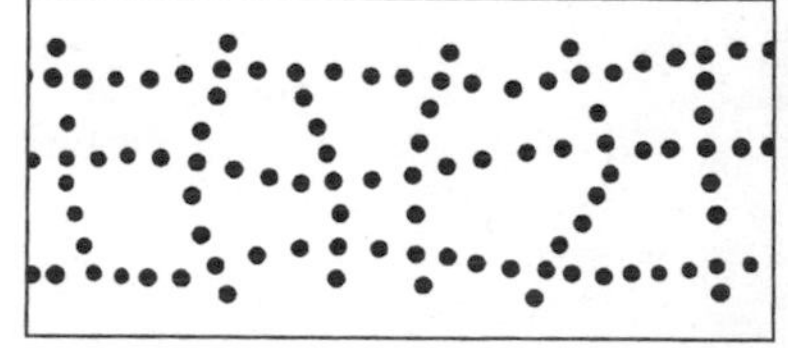

beds are normal in dark-skinned people and abnormal in light-skinned people. Yellow nails may occur in smokers as a result of nicotine stains.

Nail beds can be used to assess a patient's peripheral circulation. Press on the nail bed and then release, noting how long the color

EXPERT TECHNIQUE

EVALUATING CLUBBED FINGERS

In a patient whose fingers are clubbed, suspect hypoxia. When examining a patient's fingers for early clubbing, gently palpate the bases of the nails. Normally they'll feel firm, but in early clubbing they'll feel springy.

To evaluate late clubbing, have the patient place the first phalanges of the forefingers together, as shown in the first illustration. Normal nail bases are concave and create a small, diamond-shaped space when the first phalanges are opposed, as shown.

NORMAL FINGERS

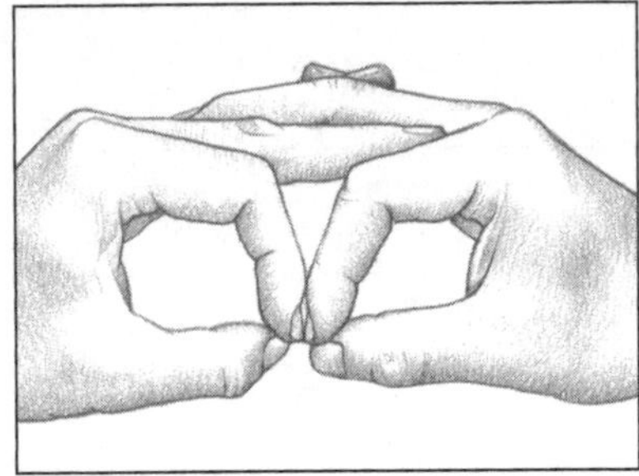

Late clubbing

In late clubbing, however, the now convex nail bases can touch without leaving a space, as shown. This condition is associated with pulmonary or cardiovascular disease. When you spot clubbed fingers, think about the possible causes, such as emphysema, chronic bronchitis, lung cancer, or congestive heart failure.

CLUBBED FINGERS

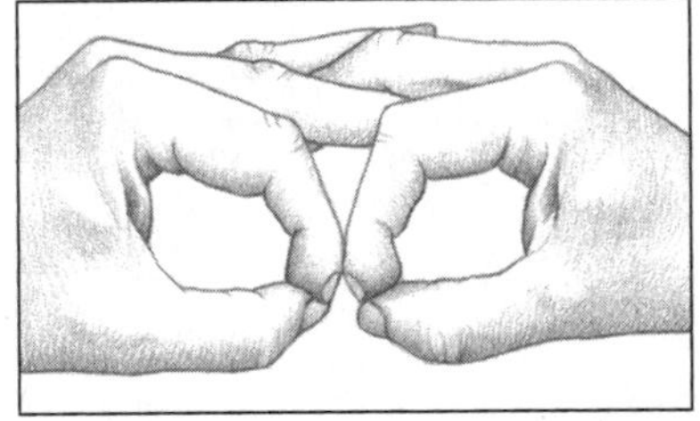

takes to return. It should return immediately, or at least within 3 seconds.

Next, inspect the shape and contour of the nails. The surface of the nail bed should be either slightly curved or flat. The edges of the nail should be smooth, rounded, and clean. The normal angle of the nail base is usually 160 degrees. An increase in the nail angle suggests clubbing. (See *Evaluating clubbed fingers.*) Curved nails are a normal variation. They may appear to be clubbed until you notice that the nail angle is still less than 180 degrees.

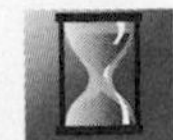

AGE ISSUE *In children, clubbing is most common in those with cyanotic congenital heart disease and cystic fibrosis. Surgical correction of heart defects may reverse clubbing. In elderly patients, arthritic deformities of the fingers or toes may disguise the presence of clubbing.*

Finally, palpate the nail bed to check the thickness of the nail and the strength of its attachment to the bed.

Abnormal findings

A patient's chief complaint may stem from any of the number of signs and symptoms related to the integumentary system. Some common conditions include anhidrosis, alopecia, butterfly rash, clubbing, cyanosis, diaphoresis, erythema, hyperpigmentation, hypopigmentation, jaundice, rashes of various types, pruritus, purpura, and urticaria. The following history, physical assessment, and analysis summaries will help you assess each one quickly and accurately. After obtaining further information, begin to interpret the findings. (See *Integumentary system: Interpreting your findings.*)

Anhidrosis

Anhidrosis refers to an abnormal deficiency of sweat. This abnormality can be generalized (complete) or localized (partial). Generalized anhidrosis can lead to life-threatening impairment of thermoregula-

(Text continues on page 107.)

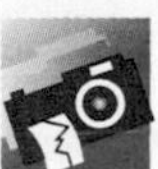

CLINICAL PICTURE

INTEGUMENTARY SYSTEM: INTERPRETING YOUR FINDINGS

After you assess the patient, a group of findings may lead you to suspect a particular integumentary disorder. The chart below shows you some common groups of findings for major signs and symptoms related to the integumentary system, along with their probable causes.

Sign or symptom and finding	Probable cause
Alopecia	
▪ Patchy alopecia, typically on the lower extremities ▪ Thin, shiny atrophic skin ▪ Thickened nails ▪ Weak or absent peripheral pulses ▪ Cool extremities ▪ Paresthesia	Arterial insufficiency
▪ Translucent, charred, or ulcerated skin ▪ Pain	Burns
▪ Loss of the outer third of the eyebrows ▪ Thin, dull, coarse, brittle hair on the face, scalp, and genitals ▪ Fatigue ▪ Constipation ▪ Cold intolerance ▪ Weight gain ▪ Puffy face, hands, and feet	Hypothyroidism
Anhidrosis	
▪ Located on palms and soles of feet ▪ Motor disturbances ▪ Sensory disturbances specific to site of lesion	Cerebral lesion
***Anhidrosis** (continued)*	
▪ Symmetrical distribution below the level of the lesion ▪ Compensatory hyperhidrosis in adjacent areas ▪ Partial or total loss of motor or sensory function depending on site of lesion	Spinal lesion
▪ Localized finding ▪ Small erythematous papules with centrally placed blisters on trunk and neck ▪ Possible pustules in extensive cases ▪ Paroxysmal itching ▪ Paresthesias	Miliaria rubra
▪ Acute onset and generalized finding ▪ Rectal temperature greater than 102.2° F (39° C) ▪ Severe headache ▪ Muscle cramps ▪ Fatigue ▪ Nausea and vomiting ▪ Dizziness ▪ Palpitations ▪ Substernal tightness ▪ Elevated blood pressure followed by hypotension	Anhidrotic asthenia (heatstroke)

(continued)

INTEGUMENTARY SYSTEM: INTERPRETING YOUR FINDINGS *(continued)*

Sign or symptom and finding	Probable cause
Butterfly rash	
■ Alopecia ■ Erythema ■ Mucous membrane lesions ■ Photosensitivity ■ Plaques ■ Scaling ■ Telangiectases	Discoid lupus erythematosus
■ Red, often scaly, sharply demarcated, macular eruption ■ Possibly transient and progressing to include forehead, chin, and area around ears ■ Photosensitivity ■ Scaling ■ Patchy alopecia ■ Mottled erythema of palms and fingers ■ Periungual erythema with edema ■ Macular, reddish purple lesions on volar surfaces of fingers ■ Telangiectasia of base of nails or eyelids ■ Petechiae ■ Joint pain, stiffness, and deformities	Systemic lupus erythematosus
■ Initially appearing as prominent, nonscaling intermittent erythema limited to lower half of nose, eventually increasing ■ Oily skin with papules, pustules, nodules, and telangiectases restricted to the central oval of the face	Rosacea
Butterfly rash *(continued)*	
■ Greasy, scaling, slightly yellow macules and papules of varying sizes ■ Crusts and fissures ■ Pruritus ■ Redness ■ Blepharitis ■ Stye ■ Severe acne and oily skin	Seborrheic dermatitis
Clubbing	
■ Anorexia ■ Malaise ■ Dyspnea ■ Tachypnea ■ Diminished breath sounds ■ Pursed-lip breathing ■ Barrel chest ■ Peripheral cyanosis	Emphysema
■ Wheezing ■ Dyspnea ■ Fatigue ■ Neck vein distention ■ Palpitations ■ Unexplained weight gain ■ Dependent edema ■ Crackles on auscultation	Heart failure
■ Hemoptysis ■ Dyspnea ■ Wheezing ■ Chest pain ■ Fatigue ■ Weight loss ■ Fever	Lung and pleural cancer

INTEGUMENTARY SYSTEM: INTERPRETING YOUR FINDINGS *(continued)*

Sign or symptom and finding	Probable cause
Cyanosis	
■ Occurrence in legs when in dependent position ■ Intermittent claudication ■ Pain at rest ■ Paresthesia ■ Pallor ■ Muscle atrophy ■ Weak leg pulses ■ Leg ulcers and possible gangrene	Arteriosclerotic occlusive disease (chronic)
■ Centrally occurring, usually aggravated by exertion ■ Exertional dyspnea ■ Productive cough with thick sputum ■ Anorexia ■ Weight loss ■ Purse lipped breathing ■ Tachypnea ■ Accessory muscle use ■ Barrel chest ■ Clubbing	Chronic obstructive pulmonary disease
■ Often occurring as a late sign, central, peripheral or both ■ Tachycardia ■ Fatigue ■ Dyspnea ■ Cold intolerance ■ Orthopnea ■ Cough ■ Ventricular or atrial gallop ■ Crackles	Left-sided heart failure
Cyanosis *(continued)*	
■ Resultant from exposure to stress or cold ■ Blanching of fingers and hands first then turning cold then cyanotic ■ Eventually to red with return of normal temperature ■ Numbness and tingling	Raynaud's disease
Diaphoresis	
■ Primarily on palms, soles, and forehead ■ Palpitations ■ Tachycardia ■ Tachypnea ■ Tremor ■ GI distress ■ Fear ■ Difficulty concentrating ■ Behavior changes	Anxiety disorder
■ Fatigue ■ Weakness ■ Anxiety ■ Possibly progressing to confusion thready pulse, hypotension, tachycardia, and cold clammy skin ■ Ashen grey appearance ■ Dilated pupils ■ Normal or subnormal temperature	Heat exhaustion

(continued)

INTEGUMENTARY SYSTEM: INTERPRETING YOUR FINDINGS *(continued)*

Sign or symptom and finding	Probable cause
Diaphoresis *(continued)*	
▪ Irritability ▪ Tremors ▪ Hypotension ▪ Blurred vision ▪ Tachycardia ▪ Hunger ▪ Loss of consciousness	Hypoglycemia
▪ Severe vertigo ▪ Tinnitus ▪ Hearing loss ▪ Nausea ad vomiting ▪ Nystagmus	Meniere's disease
Erythema	
▪ Urticaria ▪ Flushing ▪ Facial edema ▪ Diaphoresis ▪ Weakness ▪ Sneezing ▪ Possible airway edema with hoarseness and laryngospasm ▪ Shock	Anaphylaxis
Erythema *(continued)*	
▪ Sudden and hive-like in appearance with blisters, and petechial lesions, usually appearing symmetrically and bilaterally on face, hands, and feet ▪ Blisters on lips, tongue and buccal mucosa prior to erythema ▪ Thick gray film over mucous membranes ▪ Increased salivation ▪ Cough ▪ Vomiting ▪ Diarrhea ▪ Corneal ulcers ▪ Conjunctival injection with copious purulent discharge ▪ Coryza ▪ Epistaxis ▪ Fever ▪ Tachypnea ▪ Weak rapid pulse ▪ Muscle and joint pain	Erythema multiforme (major)
▪ Silvery white scales over erythematous base ▪ Thick pitted fingernails	Psoriasis

INTEGUMENTARY SYSTEM: INTERPRETING YOUR FINDINGS *(continued)*

Sign or symptom and finding	Probable cause
Hyperpigmentation	
▪ Diffuse brown, tan or bronze to black of exposed and unexposed areas ▪ Loss of axillary and pubic hair ▪ Possible vitiligo ▪ Progressive fatigue ▪ Weakness ▪ Anorexia ▪ Nausea and vomiting ▪ Weight loss ▪ Orthostatic hypotension ▪ Abdominal pain ▪ Irritability ▪ Weak irregular pulse ▪ Diarrhea or constipation ▪ Decreased libido ▪ Amenorrhea ▪ Syncope ▪ Possible enhanced sense of taste, smell, and hearing	Adrenocortical insufficiency
▪ Common sites of deep pigmentation on head, neck, and back ▪ Skin lesion that changes color, becomes inflamed, itches, ulcerates, bleeds, changes texture, or develops associated halo nevus or vitiligo	Malignant melanoma
▪ Raised or macular scaly lesions usually on upper trunk, neck and arms (hyperpigmented in fair-skinned individuals)	Tinea versicolor

Sign or symptom and finding	Probable cause
Hypopigmentation	
▪ Inflammatory skin eruptions sharply defined, separate or fused macules, papules, or plaques varying in color from pink to purple, with a yellowish or brown crust ▪ Scaly enlarged hair follicles ▪ Telangiectasia ▪ Noncontractile scaring and atrophy	Discoid lupus erythematosus
▪ Sharply defined flat white macules and patches; bilaterally symmetrical appearing on sun-exposed areas, body folds, around eyes, nose, mouth and rectum, and over bony prominences ▪ Possible pruritus ▪ Hypopigmented patches surrounding pigmented moles	Vitiligo
Jaundice	
▪ Biliary colic with pain localizing in right upper quadrant ▪ Nausea and vomiting ▪ Fever ▪ Profuse diaphoresis ▪ Chills ▪ Tenderness on palpation ▪ Possible abdominal distention and rigidity	Cholecystitis

(continued)

INTEGUMENTARY SYSTEM: INTERPRETING YOUR FINDINGS *(continued)*

Sign or symptom and finding	Probable cause
Jaundice *(continued)*	
▪ Pruritus ▪ Ascites ▪ Weakness ▪ Leg edema ▪ Nausea and vomiting ▪ Diarrhea or constipation ▪ Anorexia ▪ Weight loss ▪ Right upper quadrant pain ▪ Hematemesis ▪ Bleeding tendencies	Cirrhosis
▪ Epigastric pain often radiating to the back; relieved by sitting up or knees flexed on chest ▪ Nausea ▪ Persistent vomiting ▪ Abdominal distention ▪ Fever ▪ Tachycardia ▪ Abdominal rigidity ▪ Hypoactive bowel sounds	Pancreatitis (acute)
▪ Impaired growth and development ▪ Increased susceptibility to infection ▪ Leg ulcers ▪ Painful swollen joints with fever ▪ Chills ▪ Hematuria ▪ Pallor ▪ Chronic fatigue ▪ Tachycardia	Sickle cell anemia
Papular rash	
▪ Maculopapular rash similar to rubella ▪ Headache ▪ Malaise ▪ Fatigue ▪ Sore throat ▪ Fever ▪ Cervical lymphadenopathy ▪ Splenomegaly and hepatomegaly ▪ Cervical lymphadenopathy ▪ Splenomegaly and hepatomegaly	Infectious mononucleosis
▪ Purple or blue papule or macules on extremities, nose, and ears ▪ Lesions decreasing in size on firm pressure ▪ Scales and ulcerations with bleeding	Kaposi's sarcoma
▪ Slightly raised oval lesion, 2 to 6 cm in diameter initially ▪ Yellow to tan or erythematous patches with scaly edges on trunk, arms, legs, in a characteristic pine tree pattern	Pityriasis rosea
▪ Small yellow brown papules on chest, back or abdomen ▪ Eventually enlarging, becoming deeply pigmented	Seborrheic keratosis

INTEGUMENTARY SYSTEM: INTERPRETING YOUR FINDINGS *(continued)*

Sign or symptom and finding	Probable cause
Pruritus	
■ Intense, severe pruritus ■ Erythematous rash on dry skin at flexion points ■ Possible edema, scaling, and pustules	Atopic dermatitis
■ Scalp excoriation from scratching ■ Matted, foul-smelling, lusterless hair ■ Occipital and cervical lymphadenopathy ■ Oval, gray-white nits on hair shafts	Pediculosis capitis (head lice)
■ Gradual or sudden pruritus ■ Ammonia breath odor ■ Oliguria or anuria ■ Fatigue ■ Irritability ■ Muscle cramps	Chronic renal failure
Purpura	
■ Scattered petechiae most common on the distal arms and legs ■ Epistaxis ■ Easy bruising ■ Hematuria ■ Hematemesis ■ Menorrhagia	Idiopathic thrombocytopenia purpura
■ Petechiae on skin, mucous membranes, retina and serosal surfaces ■ Swollen bleeding gums ■ Epistaxis ■ Lymphadenopathy and splenomegaly	Leukemia
Purpura *(continued)*	
■ Perifollicular petechiae, coalescing to form ecchymoses in saddle areas of thighs and buttocks ■ Scaly dermatitis ■ Pallor ■ Tender, swollen, bleeding gums and loosened teeth ■ Dry mouth ■ Poor wound healing ■ Weakness ■ Lethargy ■ Anorexia ■ Irritability ■ Depression ■ Insomnia	Vitamin C deficiency
■ Scaling dermatitis ■ Pruritus ■ Pink to brown nodules and diffuse pigmentation ■ Painless peripheral lymphadenopathy usually of cervical nodes ■ Fever ■ Fatigue ■ Malaise ■ Weight loss ■ Hepatosplenomegaly	B-cell lymphoma
Pustular rash	
■ Small painless nonpruritic macules or papules enlarging to well circumscribed verrucous crusted or ulcerated lesions ■ Pleuritic chest pain ■ Dry hacking or productive cough ■ Occasional hemoptysis	Blastomycosis

(continued)

INTEGUMENTARY SYSTEM: INTERPRETING YOUR FINDINGS *(continued)*

Sign or symptom and finding	Probable cause
Pustular rash *(continued)*	
■ Purulent skin lesions affecting hair follicles and sebaceous glands ■ Local pain, swelling, and redness ■ Rupture of pustule leading to reduction in pain	Furunculosis
■ Vesicles form and break with crust formation from exudates ■ Thick yellow crust ■ Painless itching	Impetigo
■ Threadlike burrows or channels under the skin ■ Crusted lesions ■ Pruritus, increasing with inactivity and warmth	Scabies
Urticaria	
■ Rapid eruption of diffuse urticaria and angioedema with wheals ranging from pinpoint to palm-size or larger ■ Pruritic, stinging lesions ■ Profound anxiety ■ Weakness ■ Shortness of breath ■ Nasal congestion ■ Dysphagia ■ Warm, moist skin	Anaphylaxis
■ Nonpitting, nonpruritic edema of an extremity or the face ■ Possibly acute laryngeal edema.	Hereditary angioedema
Urticaria *(continued)*	
■ Erythema chronicum migrans that results in urticaria ■ Constant malaise and fatigue ■ Fever ■ Chills ■ Lymphadenopathy ■ Neurologic and cardiac abnormalities ■ Arthritis	Lyme disease
Vesicular rash	
■ Vesicles on an inflamed base, usually on the lips and lower face; possibly in genital region ■ Itching, tingling, burning or pain preceding vesicles ■ Single or appearing in groups	Herpes simplex
■ Erythema and possible nodular skin eruption preceding vesicles ■ Unilateral sharp shooing chest pain mimicking myocardial infarction ■ Burning pain ■ Fever ■ Malaise ■ Pruritus ■ Paresthesia or hyperesthesia of involved area	Herpes zoster

INTEGUMENTARY SYSTEM: INTERPRETING YOUR FINDINGS *(continued)*

Sign or symptom and finding	Probable cause
Vesicular rash *(continued)*	
▪ Vesicles and scaling between toes or entire sole ▪ Inflammation ▪ Pruritus ▪ Difficulty walking	Tinea pedis

Sign or symptom and finding	Probable cause
Vesicular rash *(continued))*	
▪ Vesicles and bullae preceded by diffuse, erythematous rash ▪ Large scale epidermal necrolysis and desquamation ▪ Large flaccid bullae development after mucous membrane inflammation ▪ Burning sensation in conjunctiva ▪ Malaise ▪ Fever ▪ Generalized skin tenderness	Toxic epidermal necrolysis

tion. Localized anhidrosis rarely interferes with thermoregulation, because it affects only a small percentage of the body's eccrine glands.

History
If anhidrosis is localized or the patient reports local hyperhidrosis or unexplained fever, take a brief health history. Ask the patient to characterize his sweating during heat spells or strenuous activity.

Does he usually sweat slightly or profusely? Ask about recent prolonged or extreme exposure to heat and about the onset of anhidrosis or hyperhidrosis. Obtain a complete medical history, focusing on neurologic disorders; skin disorders, such as psoriasis and scleroderma; systemic diseases that can cause peripheral neuropathies, such as diabetes mellitus; and drug use.

Physical assessment
Inspect the patient's skin color, texture, and turgor. If you detect any skin lesions, document their location, size, color, texture, and pattern.

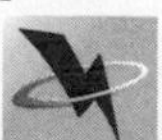

CRITICAL POINT *If you detect anhidrosis in a patient whose skin feels hot and appears flushed, ask if he's also experiencing nausea, dizziness, palpitations, or substernal tightness. If so, quickly take a rectal temperature, assess other vital signs, and evaluate the patient's level of consciousness (LOC). If rectal temperature exceeding 102.2° F (39° C) occurs with tachycardia, tachypnea, altered blood pressure, and a decreased LOC, suspect life-threatening anhidrotic asthenia (heatstroke). Start rapid cooling measures, such as immersing the patient in ice or cold water and giving I.V. fluid replacements. Continue these measures, and frequently check vital signs and neurologic status until the patient's temperature drops below 102.2° F, and then place him in an air-conditioned room.*

Analysis
Anhidrosis results from neurologic (cerebral and spinal cord lesions) and skin disorders; congenital, atrophic, or traumatic changes to sweat glands; and use of certain drugs such as anticholinergics. Neurologic disorders disturb central or peripheral nervous pathways that normally activate sweating, causing retention of excess body heat and perspiration. The absence, obstruction, atrophy, or degeneration of sweat glands can

produce anhidrosis at the skin surface, even if neurologic stimulation is normal.

Anhidrosis may go unrecognized until significant heat or exertion fails to raise sweat. However, localized anhidrosis often provokes compensatory hyperhidrosis in the remaining functional sweat glands. Often the patient's chief complaint, this compensatory hyperhidrosis should lead to the suspicion of anhidrosis.

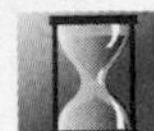

AGE ISSUE *Neonates — especially premature ones — may be anhidrotic for several weeks after birth due to delayed development of the thermoregulatory center. In infants and children, miliaria rubra (prickly heat) and congenital skin disorders, such as ichthyosis and anhidrotic ectodermal dysplasia, are the most common causes of anhidrosis.*

Alopecia

Alopecia usually affects the scalp and develops gradually. It can be classified as diffuse or patchy, and scarring or nonscarring. Scarring alopecia, or permanent hair loss, results from hair follicle destruction, which smoothes the skin surface, erasing follicular openings. Nonscarring alopecia, or temporary hair loss, results from hair follicle damage that spares follicular openings, allowing future hair growth.

History

If the patient isn't receiving chemotherapeutic drugs or radiation therapy, begin by asking when he first noticed the hair loss or thinning. Does it affect the scalp alone or occur elsewhere on the body? Is it accompanied by itching or rashes? Then carefully explore other signs and symptoms to help distinguish between normal and pathologic hair loss. Ask about recent weight change, anorexia, nausea, vomiting, and altered bowel habits. Also ask about urine changes, such as hematuria or oliguria. Has the patient been especially tired or irritable? Does he have a cough or difficulty breathing? Ask about joint pain or stiffness and about heat or cold in tolerance. Inquire about exposure to insecticides.

For a female patient, find out if she has had menstrual irregularities, and note her pregnancy history. For a male patient, ask about sexual dysfunction, such as decreased libido or impotence.

Next, ask about hair care. Does the patient frequently use a hot blow dryer or electric curlers? Does he periodically dye, bleach, or perm his hair? Ask the black patient if he uses a hot comb to straighten his hair or a long-toothed comb to achieve an Afro look. Does he ever braid the hair in cornrows?

Check for a family history of alopecia, and ask what age relatives were when they started experiencing hair loss. Also ask about nervous habits, such as pulling the hair or twirling it around a finger.

Physical assessment

Begin the physical examination by assessing the extent and pattern of scalp hair loss. Is it patchy or symmetrical? Is the hair surrounding a bald area brittle or lusterless? Is it a different color from other scalp hair? Does it fall out easily? Inspect the underlying skin for follicular openings, erythema, loss of pigment, scaling, induration, broken hair shafts, and hair regrowth.

Then examine the rest of the skin. Note the size, color, texture, and location of any lesions. Check for jaundice, edema, hyperpigmentation, pallor, or duskiness. Examine the patient's nails for vertical or horizontal pitting, thickening, brittleness, or whitening. As you do so, watch for fine tremors in the hands. Observe the patient for muscle weakness and ptosis. Palpate for lymphadenopathy, enlarged thyroid or salivary glands, and masses in the abdomen or chest.

Analysis

One of the most common causes of alopecia is the use of certain chemotherapeutic drugs. Alopecia may also result from the use of other drugs; radiation therapy; a skin, connective tissue, endocrine, nutritional, or psychological disorder; a neoplasm; an infection; a burn; or exposure to toxins.

Normally, everyone loses about 50 hairs per day, and these hairs are replaced by new ones. However, aging, genetic predisposition, and hormonal changes may contribute to gradual hair thinning and hairline recession. This type of alopecia occurs in about 40% of adult men and may also occur in postmenopausal women.

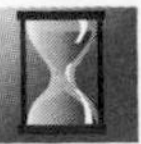

AGE ISSUE *Alopecia normally occurs during the first 6 months of life, as either a sudden, diffuse hair*

loss or a gradual thinning that's hardly noticeable. In addition, bald areas can result if infants are left in one position for too long.

In men, hair loss commonly affects the temporal areas, producing an M-shaped hairline. In women, diffuse thinning marks the centrofrontal area. In both sexes, hair loss also occurs on the trunk, pubic area, axillae, arms, and legs. Another normal pattern of alopecia occurs 2 to 4 months postpartum. This temporary, diffuse hair loss on the scalp may be scant or dramatic and possibly accentuated at the frontal areas. Anxiety, high fever, and even certain hair styles or grooming methods may also cause alopecia.

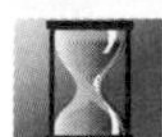

AGE ISSUE *In children, common causes of alopecia include chemotherapy or radiation therapy, seborrheic dermatitis (known as "cradle cap" in infancy), alopecia mucinosa, tinea capitis, and hypopituitarism. Tinea capitis may produce a kerion lesion — a boggy, raised, tender, and hairless lesion. Trichotillomania, a psychological disorder more common in children than adults, may produce patchy baldness with stubby hair growth due to habitual hair pulling. Other causes of alopecia include progeria and congenital hair shaft defects such as trichorrhexis nodosa.*

Butterfly rash

A butterfly rash appears in a malar distribution across the nose and cheeks. Similar rashes may appear on the neck, scalp, and other areas. Butterfly rash is sometimes mistaken for sunburn, because it can be provoked or aggravated by ultraviolet rays.

History

Ask the patient when he first noticed the butterfly rash and if he has been recently exposed to sun. Next, ask about recent weight or hair loss and about the presence of rashes elsewhere on his body. Does he have a family history of lupus erythematosus? Is he taking hydralazine or procainamide, which are common causes of drug-induced lupus erythematosus?

Physical assessment

Inspect the butterfly rash, noting any macules, papules, pustules, and scaling. Is the rash edematous? Are areas of hypopigmentation or hyperpigmentation present? Look for blisters or ulcers in the mouth, and note any inflamed lesions. Check for rashes elsewhere on the body.

Analysis

The presence of a butterfly rash is a sign of systemic lupus erythematosus. However, it can also signal dermatologic disorders, such as rosacea or seborrheic dermatitis.

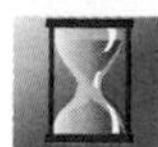

AGE ISSUE *In children, a butterfly rash may occur as part of an infectious disease such as erythema infectiosum, or "slapped cheek syndrome."*

Clubbing

A nonspecific sign of pulmonary and cyanotic cardiovascular disorders, clubbing is the painless, usually bilateral increase in soft tissue around the terminal phalanges of the fingers or toes. It doesn't involve changes in the underlying bone. In early clubbing, the normal 160-degree angle between the nail and the nail base approximates 180 degrees. As clubbing progresses, this angle widens and the base of the nail be comes visibly swollen. In late clubbing, the angle where the nail meets the now convex nail base extends more than halfway up the nail.

History

Because clubbing is usually detected while other symptoms of pulmonary or cardiovascular disease are being evaluated, review the patient's current treatment plan; clubbing may resolve with correction of the underlying disorder.

Physical assessment

Evaluate the extent of clubbing in fingers and toes. Don't mistake curved nails, a normal variation, for clubbing. To quickly examine a patient's fingers for early clubbing, gently palpate the nail bases. Normally, they feel firm, but in early clubbing, nail bases feel springy when palpated. To evaluate late clubbing, have the patient place the first phalanges of the forefingers together, gently pressing the fingernails together. Normal nail bases are concave and create a small, diamond-shaped space when the first phalanges are opposed. In late clubbing, however, the now convex nail bases can touch without leaving a space.

Analysis

Clubbing is typically a sign of pulmonary or cardiovascular disease, such as emphysema, chronic bronchitis, lung cancer, or heart failure. Although clubbing may also result from such hepatic and GI disorders as cirrhosis, Crohn's disease, and ulcerative colitis, it occurs only rarely in these disorders. So first check for more common signs and symptoms.

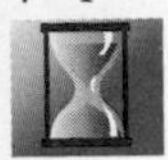

AGE ISSUE *In older adults, arthritic deformities of the fingers or toes may disguise the presence of clubbing. In children, clubbing is most common in those with congenital heart disease and cystic fibrosis.*

Cyanosis

Cyanosis—a bluish or bluish black discoloration of the skin and mucous membranes —results from excessive concentration of unoxygenated hemoglobin in the blood. This common sign may develop abruptly or gradually. It can be classified as central or peripheral, although the two types may exist together.

History

If cyanosis accompanies less acute conditions, perform a thorough examination. Begin with a history, focusing on cardiac, pulmonary, and hematologic disorders. Ask about previous surgery.

CRITICAL POINT *If the patient displays sudden, localized cyanosis and other signs of arterial occlusion, protect the affected limb from injury; however, don't massage the limb. If you observe central cyanosis that stems from a pulmonary disorder or shock, perform a rapid evaluation. Take immediate steps to maintain the patient's airway, assist his breathing, and monitor his circulation.*

Physical assessment

Begin the physical assessment by taking vital signs. Inspect the skin and mucous membranes to determine the extent of cyanosis. Ask the patient when he first noticed the cyanosis. Does it subside and recur? Is it aggravated by cold, smoking, or stress? Alleviated by massage or rewarming? Check for cool, pallid skin, redness, and ulceration. Also note clubbing.

Next, evaluate the patient's LOC. Ask about headache, dizziness, or blurred vision. Test his motor strength. Ask about pain in the arms and legs, especially with walking, and about abnormal sensations, such as numbness, tingling, or coldness.

Ask about chest pain and its severity. Can the patient identify any aggravating and alleviating factors? Palpate peripheral pulses and test capillary refill time. Note edema. Auscultate heart rate and rhythm, noting gallops and murmurs. Auscultate the abdominal aorta and femoral arteries to detect any bruits.

Ask about a cough. Is it productive? If so, have the patient describe the sputum. Evaluate respiratory rate and rhythm. Check for nasal flaring and use of accessory muscles. Ask about sleep apnea. Does he sleep with his head propped up on pillows? Inspect for asymmetrical chest expansion or barrel chest. Percuss the lungs for dullness or hyperresonance, and auscultate for decreased or adventitious breath sounds.

Analysis

Central cyanosis reflects inadequate oxygenation of systemic arterial blood caused by right-to-left cardiac shunting or pulmonary disease, or by hematologic disorders. It may occur in any location on the skin and also on the mucous membranes of the mouth, lips, and conjunctiva.

Peripheral cyanosis reflects sluggish peripheral circulation caused by vasoconstriction, reduced cardiac output, or vascular occlusion. It may be widespread or it may occur locally in one extremity; however, it doesn't affect mucous membranes. Typically, peripheral cyanosis appears on exposed areas, such as the fingers, nail beds, feet, nose, and ears.

Although cyanosis is an important sign of cardiovascular and pulmonary disorders, it isn't always an accurate gauge of oxygenation. Several factors contribute to its development: hemoglobin concentration and oxygen saturation, cardiac output, and partial pressure of oxygen (PO_2). Cyanosis is usually undetectable until the oxygen saturation of hemoglobin falls below 80%. Severe cyanosis is quite obvious, whereas mild cyanosis is more difficult to detect—even in natural, bright light. In dark-skinned patients, cyanosis is most apparent in the mucous membranes and nail beds. A transient, nonpathologic cyanosis may result from environmental factors. For example, peripheral cyanosis may result from cutaneous vasoconstriction following brief exposure to cold air or water. Central cyanosis may result from reduced Po_2 at high altitudes.

AGE ISSUE *In children, circumoral cyanosis may precede generalized cyanosis. Acrocyanosis (also called "glove and bootee" cyanosis) may occur in infants due to excessive crying or exposure to cold. Exercise and agitation enhance cyanosis. Many pulmonary disorders responsible for cyanosis in adults also cause cyanosis in children. In addition, central cyanosis may result from cystic fibrosis, asthma, airway obstruction by a foreign body, acute laryngotracheobronchitis, and epiglottiditis. It may also result from congenital heart defects such as transposition of the great vessels that cause right-to-left intracardiac shunting.*

Diaphoresis

Diaphoresis is profuse sweating—at times, amounting to more than 1 liter of sweat per hour. Usually diaphoresis begins abruptly and may be accompanied by other autonomic system signs, such as tachycardia and increased blood pressure.

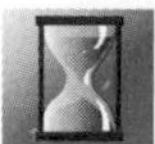

AGE ISSUE *Diaphoresis varies with age because sweat glands function immaturely in infants and are less active in elderly adults. As a result, these age-groups may fail to display diaphoresis associated with its common causes.*

History

If the patient is diaphoretic, quickly rule out the possibility of a life-threatening cause.

CRITICAL POINT *If the patient with diaphoresis complains of blurred vision, ask him about increased irritability and anxiety. Has he been unusually hungry lately? Does he have tremors? Note hypotension and tachycardia. Then ask about a history of insulin-dependent diabetes as the patient may be experiencing hypoglycemia. If profuse diaphoresis is noted in a weak, tired and apprehensive patient, suspect heatstroke. Suspect autonomic hyperreflexia in a patient with diaphoresis with a spinal cord lesion above T6 or T7. If the complains of chest pain and dyspnea, suspect myocardial infarction or heart failure.*

Begin the health history by having the patient describe his chief complaint. Then explore associated signs and symptoms. Note general fatigue and weakness. Does the patient have insomnia, headache, and changes in vision or hearing? Is the patient often dizzy? Does he have palpitations? Ask about pleuritic pain, cough, sputum, and difficulty breathing; nausea, vomiting, altered bowel or bladder habits; and abdominal pain. Ask the female patient about amenorrhea. Is she menopausal? Note weight loss or gain. Ask about paresthesia, muscle cramps or stiffness and joint pain.

Complete the history by asking about travel to tropical countries. Note recent exposure to high environmental temperatures or to pesticides. Does the patient have a recent bug bite? Check for a history of partial gastrectomy or of drug or alcohol abuse. Finally, obtain a thorough drug history.

Physical assessment

First, determine the extent of diaphoresis by inspecting the trunk and extremities as well as the palms, soles, and forehead. Also, check the patient's clothing and, if accessible, his bedding for dampness. Note whether diaphoresis occurs during the day or at night. Observe for flushing, abnormal skin texture or lesions, and increased coarse body hair. Note poor skin turgor and dry mucous membranes. Check for splinter hemorrhages and Plummer's nails. Evaluate the patient's mental status and take his vital signs. Observe for fasciculations and flaccid paralysis. Be alert for seizures. Note the patient's facial expression and examine the eyes for pupillary dilation or constriction, exophthalmos, and excessive tearing. Test visual fields. Also check for hearing loss and for tooth or gum disease. Percuss the lungs for dullness and auscultate for crackles, diminished or bronchial breath sounds, and increased vocal fremitus. Look for decreased respiratory excursion. Palpate for lymphadenopathy and hepatosplenomegaly.

Analysis

Diaphoresis represents an autonomic nervous system response to physical or psychogenic stress, or to fever or high environmental temperature. When caused by stress, diaphoresis may be generalized or limited to the palms of the hands, soles of the feet, and the forehead. When caused by fever or high environmental temperature, it's usually generalized.

Intermittent diaphoresis may accompany chronic disorders characterized by recurrent fever; isolated diaphoresis may mark an episode of acute pain or fever. Night sweats may characterize intermittent fever because body temperature tends to return to normal between 2 a.m. and 4 a.m. before rising again.

When caused by excessive external temperature, diaphoresis is a normal response. Acclimatization usually requires several days of exposure to high temperatures; during this process, diaphoresis helps maintain normal body temperature. Diaphoresis also commonly occurs during menopause. It's preceded by a sensation of intense heat known as a hot flash. Other causes include exercise or exertion that accelerates metabolism, creating internal heat, and mild-to-moderate anxiety that helps initiate the fight-or-flight response.

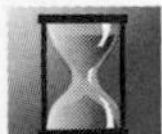

AGE ISSUE *In infants and children, diaphoresis often results from environmental heat or overdressing. Typically, it's most apparent around the head. Other causes include drug withdrawal associated with maternal addiction, heart failure, thyrotoxicosis, and the effects of drugs such as antihistamines, haloperidol, and thyroid hormone.*

Erythema

Dilated or congested blood vessels produce red skin, or erythema, the most common sign of skin inflammation or irritation. Erythema may be localized or generalized and may occur suddenly or gradually. Skin color can range from bright red in acute conditions to pale violet or brown in chronic problems. Erythema must be differentiated from purpura, which causes redness from bleeding into the skin. When pressure is applied directly to the skin, erythema blanches momentarily, but purpura doesn't.

History

If the patient's erythema isn't associated with anaphylaxis, obtain a detailed health history. Find out how long he has had the erythema and where it first began. Ask if he has had any associated pain or itching. Has he recently had a fever, upper respiratory infection, or joint pain? Does he have a history of skin disease or other illness? Does he or anyone in his family have allergies, asthma, or eczema? Has he been exposed to someone who has had a similar rash or is now ill?

Obtain a complete drug history, including recent immunizations. Ask about the patient's food intake and any exposure to chemicals.

Physical assessment

Begin the physical examination by assessing the extent, distribution, and intensity of erythema. Look for edema and other skin lesions, such as hives, scales, papules, and purpura. Examine the affected area for warmth, and gently palpate it to check for tenderness or crepitus.

Analysis

Usually, erythema results from changes in the arteries, veins, and small vessels, which lead to increased small-vessel perfusion. Drugs and neurogenic mechanisms may also allow extra blood to enter the small vessels. In addition, erythema can result from trauma and tissue damage as well as from changes in supporting tissues, which increase vessel visibility.

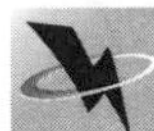

CRITICAL POINT *If your patient has sudden progressive erythema with a rapid pulse, dyspnea, hoarseness, and agitation, quickly take his vital signs. He may be suffering from anaphylactic shock.*

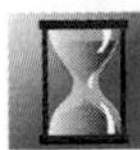

AGE ISSUE *Normally, erythema toxicum neonatorum — a pink papular rash — develops in the first 4 days after birth and spontaneously disappears by day 10. Neonates and infants can also develop erythema from infections and other disorders. For instance, candidiasis can produce thick white lesions over an erythematous base on the oral mucosa, as well as diaper rash with beef red erythema.*

Hyperpigmentation

Hyperpigmentation, or excessive skin coloring, usually reflects overproduction, abnormal location, or maldistribution of melanin — the dominant brown or black pigment found in skin, hair, mucous membranes, nails, brain tissue, cardiac muscle, and parts of the eye. This sign can also reflect abnormalities of other skin pigments: carotenoids (yellow), oxyhemoglobin (red), and hemoglobin (blue).

History

Hyperpigmentation isn't an acute process, but an end result of another process — the main target of the examination. Begin with a detailed patient history. Do any other family members have the same problem? Was the patient's hyperpigmentation present at birth? Did other signs or symptoms, such as skin rash, accompany or precede it? Obtain a history of medical disorders (especially endocrine), as well as contact with or ingestion of chemicals, metals, plants, vegetables, citrus fruits, or perfumes. Was the hyperpigmentation related to exposure to sunlight or a change of season? Is the patient pregnant or taking prescription or over-the-counter drugs?

In addition, explore any other signs and symptoms. Ask about fatigue, weakness, muscle aches, chills, irritability, fainting, and itching. Does the patient have any cardiopulmonary signs or symptoms, such as cough, shortness of breath, or swelling of the ankles, hands, or other areas? Does he have any GI complaints, such as anorexia, nausea, vomiting, weight loss, abdominal pain, diarrhea, constipation, or epigastric fullness? Also ask about genitourinary signs and symptoms, such as dark or pink urine, increased or decreased urination, menstrual irregularities, and loss of libido.

Physical assessment

Examine the patient's skin and note the color of hyperpigmented areas: brown suggests excess melanin in the epidermis; slate gray or a bluish tone suggests excess pigment in the dermis. Inspect for other changes, too — thickening and leatherlike texture and changes in hair distribution. Check the patient's skin and sclera for jaundice, and note any spider angiomas, palmar erythema, or purpura.

Take the patient's vital signs, noting any fever, hypotension, or pulse irregularities. Evaluate the patient's general appearance. Do you note exophthalmos or an enlarged jaw, nose, or hands? Palpate for an enlarged thyroid and auscultate for a bruit over the gland. Palpate muscles for atrophy and joints for swelling and tenderness. Assess the abdomen for ascites and edema, and palpate and percuss the liver and spleen to evaluate their size and position. Check the male patient for testicular atrophy and gynecomastia.

Analysis

Hyperpigmentation most commonly results from exposure to sunlight. However, it can also result from metabolic, endocrine, neoplastic, and inflammatory disorders; chemical poisoning; drugs; genetic defects; thermal burns; ionizing radiation; and localized activation by sunlight of certain photosensitizing chemicals on the skin.

Many types of benign hyperpigmented lesions occur normally. Some — such as acanthosis nigricans and carotenemia — may also accompany certain disorders, but their significance is unproven. Chronic nutritional insufficiency may lead to dyspigmentation — increased pigmentation in some areas and decreased pigmentation in others.

Typically asymptomatic and chronic, hyperpigmentation is a common problem that can have distressing psychological and social implications. It varies in location and intensity and may fade over time.

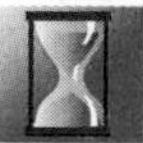

AGE ISSUE *In children, most moles are junctional nevi — flat, well demarcated, brown-to-black, and appearing anywhere on the skin. Although they're considered benign, recent evidence suggests that some of these may become malignant in later life.*

Hypopigmentation

Hypopigmentation is a decrease in normal skin, hair, mucous membrane, or nail color. It typically results from a deficiency, absence, or abnormal degradation of the pigment melanin.

History

Ask the patient if any other family member has hypopigmentation and if it was present from birth or followed skin lesions or a rash. Were the lesions painful? Does the patient have any medical problems or a history of burns, physical injury, or physical contact with chemicals? Is he taking prescription or over-the-counter drugs. Find out if he has noticed other skin changes — such as erythema, scaling, ulceration, or hyperpigmentation — or if sun exposure causes unusually severe burning.

Physical assessment

Examine the patient's skin, noting any erythema, scaling, ulceration, areas of hyperpigmentation, and other findings.

Analysis

This sign may be congenital or acquired, asymptomatic or associated with other findings. Its causes include genetic disorders, nutritional deficiency, chemicals and drugs, inflammation, infection, and physical trauma. Typically chronic, hypopigmentation can be difficult to identify if the patient is light-skinned or has only slightly decreased coloring.

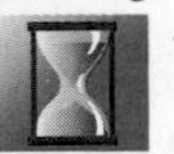

AGE ISSUE *In children, hypopigmentation results from genetic or acquired disorders, including albinism, phenylketonuria, and tuberous sclerosis. In neonates, it may indicate a metabolic or nervous system disorder.*

Jaundice

Jaundice is the yellow discoloration of the skin or mucous membranes, indicating excessive levels of conjugated or unconjugated bilirubin in the blood. In fair-skinned patients, it's most notice able on the face, trunk, and sclera. In dark-skinned patients, it's most noticeable on the hard palate, sclera, and conjunctiva.

Jaundice is most apparent in natural sunlight. In fact, it may be undetectable in artificial or poor light. It's commonly accompanied by pruritus (because bile pigment damages sensory nerves), dark urine, and clay-colored stools.

History

A history of the patient's jaundice is critical in determining its cause. Begin the history by asking the patient when he first noted the jaundice. Does he also have pruritus? Clay-colored stools or dark urine? Ask about past episodes or a family history of jaundice. Does he have any nonspecific signs or symptoms, such as fatigue, fever, or chills; GI signs or symptoms, such as anorexia, abdominal pain, nausea, or vomiting; or cardiopulmonary symptoms, such as shortness of breath or palpitations? Ask about alcohol use and any history of cancer, or liver or gall bladder disease. Has the patient lost weight? Obtain a medication history.

Physical assessment

Perform the physical examination in a room with natural light. Inspect the skin for texture and dryness and for hyperpigmentation and xanthomas. Look for spider angiomas or petechiae, clubbed fingers, or gynecomastia. If the patient has heart failure, auscultate for arrhythmias, murmurs, and gallops. For all patients, auscultate for crackles and abnormal bowel sounds. Palpate the lymph nodes for swelling and the abdomen for tenderness, pain, or swelling. Palpate and percuss the liver and spleen for enlargement, and test for ascites with the shifting dullness and fluid wave techniques. Obtain baseline data on the patient's mental status: slight changes in sensorium may be early signs of deteriorating hepatic function.

Analysis

Jaundice may result from any of three pathophysiologic processes: massive hemolysis leading to large amounts of unconjugated bilirubin passing into the blood causing increased intestinal conversion of this bilirubin to water soluble urobilinogen for excretion; inability of the liver to conjugate or excrete bilirubin leading to increased blood levels of conjugated and unconjugated bilirubin; normal formation rate for bilirubin whose flow into the intestine is blocked causing an accumulation of conjugated bilirubin in the blood. Jaundice may be the only warning sign of certain disorders such as pancreatic carcinoma.

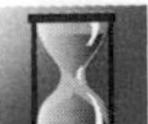

AGE ISSUE *In the neonate, physiologic jaundice is common, developing between 3 to 5 days after birth. In infants, obstructive jaundice usually results from congenital biliary atresia. Choledochal cyst — a congenital cystic dilatation of the common bile duct — may also cause jaundice in children, particularly of Japanese descent.*

Papular rash

Papular rash consists of small, raised, circumscribed — and perhaps discolored — lesions known as papules. It may erupt anywhere on the body in various configurations and may be acute or chronic.

History

Find out when the rash first erupted. Has the patient noticed any changes in the rash since then? Is it itchy or burning? Painful or tender? Have him describe associated signs and symptoms, such as fever, headache, and GI distress.

Next, obtain a medical history, including allergies, previous rashes or skin disorders, infections, childhood diseases, sexually transmitted diseases, and neoplasms. Has the patient recently been bitten by an insect or rodent, or been exposed to anyone with an infectious disease? Finally, obtain a complete drug history.

Physical assessment

Evaluate the papular rash fully. Note its color, configuration, and location on the patient's body.

Analysis

Papular rashes characterize many cutaneous disorders; they may also result from allergic, infectious, neoplastic, and systemic disorders. Transient maculopapular rashes, usually on the trunk, may accompany reactions to many drugs, including antibiotics, such as tetracycline, ampicillin, cephalosporins, and sulfonamides; benzodiazepines such as diazepam; lithium; gold salts; allopurinol; isoniazid; and salicylates.

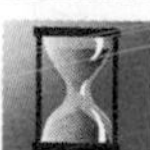

AGE ISSUE *In children, common causes of papular rashes include infectious diseases, such as molluscum contagiosum, and scarlet fever; scabies; insect bites; allergies or drug reactions; and miliaria, which occurs in three forms, depending on the depth of sweat gland involvement.*

Pruritus

Pruritis is an unpleasant itching sensation that usually provokes scratching as the patient tries to gain relief. It affects the skin, certain mucous membranes, and the eyes. Most severe at night, pruritus may be exacerbated by increased skin temperature, poor skin turgor, local vasodilation, dermatoses, and stress.

History

If the patient reports pruritus, have him describe its onset, frequency, and intensity. If pruritus occurs at night, ask him whether it prevents him from falling asleep or awakens him after he falls asleep. Generally, pruritus related to dermatoses prevents—but doesn't disturb—sleep. Is the itching localized or generalized? When is it most severe? How long does it last? Is there a relationship to such activities as physical exertion, bathing, makeup application, or use of perfume?

Ask the patient how he cleans his skin. In particular, look for excessive bathing, harsh soaps, contact allergy, and excessively hot water. Does he have occupational exposure to known skin irritants, such as glass fiber insulation or chemicals? Ask about the patient's general health and the medications he takes; new medications are suspect. Has he recently traveled abroad? Does he have pets? Has anyone else in the house reported itching? Ask about contact with skin irritants, previous skin disorders, and related symptoms. Then obtain a complete drug history.

Physical assessment

Examine the patient for signs of scratching, such as excoriation, purpura, scabs, scars, or lichenification. Look for primary lesions to help confirm dermatoses.

Analysis

The most common symptom of dermatologic disorders, pruritus may also result from a local or systemic disorder or from use of certain drugs. Physiologic pruritus, such as pruritic urticarial papules and plaques of pregnancy, may occur in primigravidas late in the third trimester. Pruritus can also stem from emotional upset or contact with skin irritants.

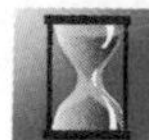

AGE ISSUE *In children, pruritis may be caused by certain adult disorders, but they may affect different parts of the body. For instance, scabies may affect the head in infants, but not in adults. Pityriasis rosea may affect the face, hands, and feet of adolescents. Some childhood diseases, such as measles and chickenpox, can also cause pruritus. Hepatic diseases can also produce pruritus in children as bile salts accumulate on the skin.*

Purpura

Purpura is the extravasation of red blood cells from the blood vessels into the skin, subcutaneous tissue, or mucous membranes. It's characterized by discoloration—

usually purplish or brownish red—that's easily visible through the epidermis. Purpuric lesions include petechiae, ecchymoses, and hematomas. Purpura differs from erythema in that it doesn't blanch with pressure because it involves blood in the tissues, not just dilated vessels.

History
After you detect purpura, ask the patient when he first noticed the lesion and if he has also noticed other lesions on his body. Does he or his family have a history of bleeding disorders or easy bruising? Find out what medications the patient is taking, if any, and ask him to describe his diet. Ask about recent trauma or transfusions and the development of associated signs, such as epistaxis, bleeding gums, hematuria, and hematochezia. Also, ask about systemic complaints such as fever, which may suggest infection. If the patient is female, ask about heavy menstrual flow.

Physical assessment
Inspect the patient's entire skin surface to determine the type, size, location, distribution, and severity of purpuric lesions. Also inspect the mucous membranes. Remember that the same mechanisms that cause purpura can also cause internal hemorrhage, although purpura isn't a cardinal indicator of this condition.

Analysis
Purpura results from damage to the endothelium of small blood vessels, coagulation defects, ineffective perivascular support, capillary fragility and permeability, or a combination of these factors. In turn, these faulty hemostatic factors can result from thrombocytopenia or other hematologic disorders, invasive procedures and, of course, anticoagulant drugs. Additional causes are nonpathologic.

AGE ISSUE *Purpura can be a consequence of aging because loss of collagen decreases connective tissue support of upper skin blood vessels. In the elderly or cachectic patient, skin atrophy and inelasticity and loss of subcutaneous fat increase susceptibility to minor trauma, causing purpura to appear along the veins of the forearms, hands, legs, and feet.*

Prolonged coughing or vomiting can produce crops of petechiae in loose face and neck tissue. Violent muscle contraction, as occurs in seizures or weight lifting, sometimes results in localized ecchymoses from increased intraluminal pressure and rupture. High fever, which increases capillary fragility, can also produce purpura.

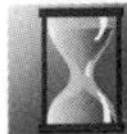

AGE ISSUE *Neonates commonly have petechiae, particularly on the head, neck, and shoulders, after vertex deliveries. Perhaps a result from the trauma of birth, these petechiae disappear within a few days. Other causes in infants include thrombocytopenia, vitamin K deficiency, and infantile scurvy. The most common type of purpura in children is allergic purpura.*

Pustular rash
A pustular rash is made up of crops of pustules—vesicles and bullae that fill with purulent exudate. These lesions vary greatly in size and shape and can be generalized or localized to the halt follicles or sweat glands.

History
Have the patient describe the appearance, location, and onset of the first pustular lesion. Did another type of skin lesion precede the pustule? Find out how the lesions spread. Ask what medications the patient takes and if he has applied any topical medication to his rash. If so, what type and when was it last applied? Find out if he has a family history of skin disorders.

Physical assessment
Examine the entire skin surface, noting if it's dry, oily, moist, or greasy. Record the exact location and distribution of the skin lesions and their color, shape, and size.

Analysis
Pustules appear in skin and systemic disorders; with use of certain drugs, and with exposure to skin irritants. For example, people who have been swimming in salt water commonly develop a papulopustular rash under the bathing suit or elsewhere on the body from irritation by sea organisms. Although many pustular lesions are sterile, pustular rash usually indicates infection. Any vesicular eruption, or even acute contact dermatitis, can become pustular if secondary infection occurs.

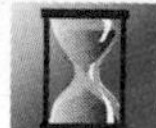

AGE ISSUE *In children, the various disorders that produce pustular rash are varicella, erythema toxicum neonatorum, candidiasis, and impetigo.*

Urticaria

Also known as *hives*, urticaria is a vascular skin reaction characterized by the eruption of transient pruritic wheals — smooth, slightly elevated patches with well-defined erythematous margins and pale centers. It's produced by the local release of histamine or other vasoactive substances as part of a hypersensitivity reaction.

History

If the patient isn't in distress, obtain a complete health history. Does the urticaria follow a seasonal pattern? Do certain foods or drugs seem to aggravate it? Is there any relationship to physical exertion? Is the patient routinely exposed to chemicals on the job or at home? Obtain a detailed drug history, including use of prescription and over-the-counter drugs. Note any history of chronic or parasitic infections, skin disease, or GI disorders.

Physical assessment

Fully evaluate the lesions — note their color, configuration, and location on the patient's body.

Analysis

Acute urticaria evolves rapidly and usually has a detectable cause, such as hypersensitivity to a certain drug, food, insect bite, inhalant, or contactant; emotional stress; or an environmental factor. Although individual lesions usually subside within 12 to 24 hours, new crops of lesions may erupt continuously, thus prolonging the attack.

Urticaria lasting longer than 6 weeks is classified as chronic. The lesions may recur for months or years, and the underlying cause is usually unknown. Occasionally, a diagnosis of psychogenic urticaria is made.

Angioedema, or giant urticaria, is characterized by the acute eruption of wheals involving the mucous membranes and, occasionally, the arms, legs, or genitals.

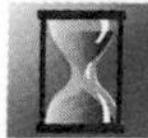

AGE ISSUE *Pediatric forms of urticaria include acute papular urticaria, which usually occurs after an insect bite and urticaria pigmentosa, which is rare. Hereditary angioedema may also cause urticaria.*

Vesicular rash

A vesicular rash is a scattered or linear distribution of vesicles — sharply circumscribed lesions filled with clear, cloudy, or bloody fluid. The lesions, which are usually less than 0.5 cm in diameter, may occur singly or in groups. They sometimes occur with bullae — fluid filled lesions larger than 0.5 cm in diameter.

History

Ask your patient when the rash began, how it spread, and whether it has appeared before. Did other skin lesions precede eruption of the vesicles? Obtain a thorough drug history. If the patient has used any topical medication, what type did he use and when was it last applied? Also ask about associated signs and symptoms. Find out if he has a family history of skin disorders, and ask about allergies, recent infections, insect bites, and exposure to allergens.

Physical assessment

Examine the patient's skin, noting if it's dry, oily, or moist. Observe the general distribution of the lesions and record their exact location. Note the color, shape, and size of the lesions, and check for crusts, scales, scars, macules, papules, or wheals. Palpate the vesicles or bullae to determine if they're flaccid or tense. Slide your finger across the skin to see if the outer layer of epidermis separates easily from the basal layer.

Analysis

A vesicular rash may be mild or severe and temporary or permanent. It can result from infection, inflammation, or allergic reactions.

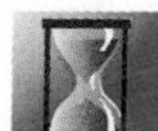

AGE ISSUE *In children, vesicular rashes are caused by staphylococcal infections (staphylococcal scalded skin syndrome is a life-threatening infection occurring in infants), varicella, hand-foot-and-mouth disease, and miliaria rubra.*

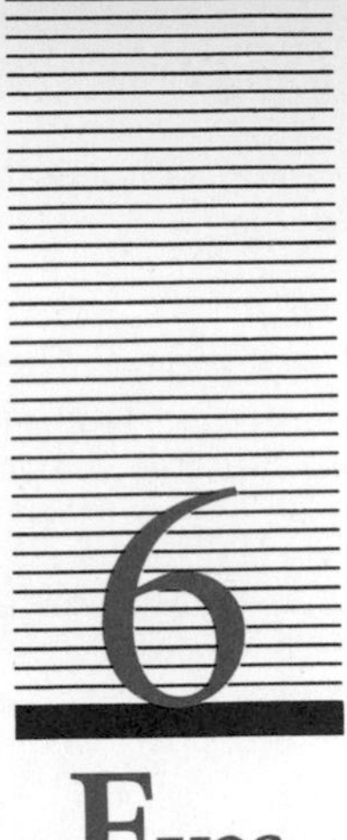

6 Eyes

About 70% of all sensory information reaches the brain through the eyes. Disorders in vision can interfere with a patient's ability to function independently, perceive the world, and enjoy beauty.

A thorough assessment of the patient's eyes and vision can help to identify problems that can affect the patient's health and quality of life. In many cases, early detection can lead to successful, sight-saving treatment.

Today, fewer people lose their sight from infections or injuries than in the past. Still, the overall incidence of blindness is rising as the population ages. Primary causes of vision loss include diabetic retinopathy, glaucoma, cataracts, and macular degeneration — conditions more common in elderly patients than in younger ones. Young people can lose their sight due to opportunistic infections associated with human immunodeficiency virus and acquired immunodeficiency syndrome. The opportunistic infections toxoplasmosis and cytomegalovirus retinitis typically cause blindness. Other vision disorders that may limit a person's ability to function include strabismus, amblyopia, and refractory errors.

Anatomy and physiology

To perform an accurate assessment of the eyes, you need to understand the anatomy and physiology of the eye and its structures. Extraocular (external) and intraocular (internal) structures form the eye, and extraocular muscles and cranial nerves (CNs) control it. (See *Structures of the eye.*)

The sensory organ of sight, the eye transmits visual images to the brain for interpre-

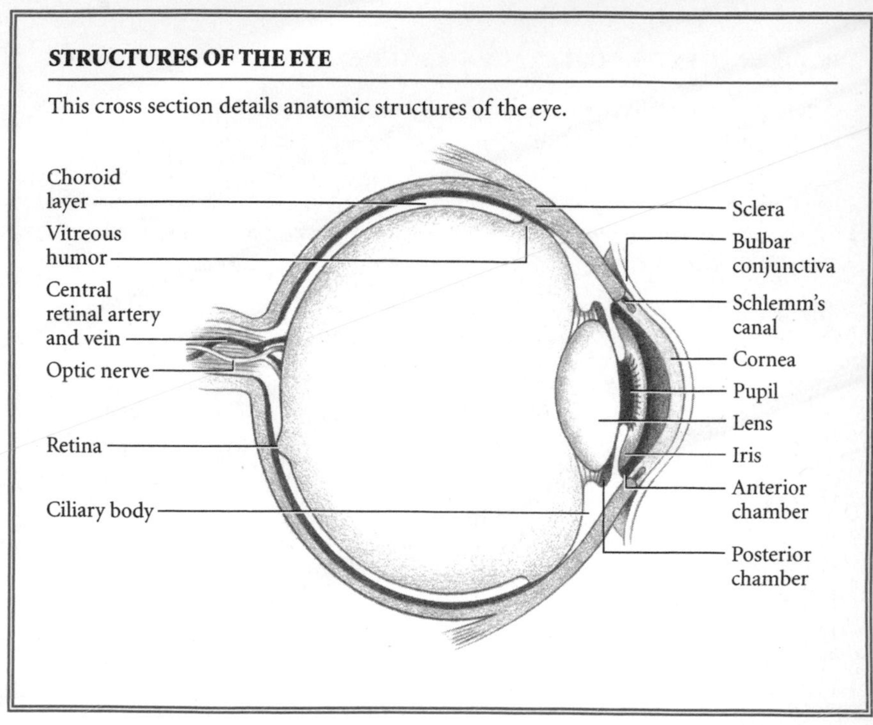

STRUCTURES OF THE EYE

This cross section details anatomic structures of the eye.

tation. The eyeball is about 1″ (2.5 cm) in diameter and occupies the bony orbit, a skull cavity formed anteriorly by the frontal, maxillary, zygomatic, acromial, sphenoid, ethmoid, and palatine bones. Nerves, adipose tissue, and blood vessels cushion and nourish the eye posteriorly.

Extraocular structures

The eyelids, conjunctivae, and lacrimal apparatus form the eye's extraocular structures.

Eyelids

Also called palpebrae, the eyelids are loose folds of skin covering the anterior eye. The eyelids protect the eye from foreign bodies, regulate the entrance of light, and distribute tears over the eye by blinking. The lid margins contain hair follicles, which contain eyelashes and sebaceous glands. When closed, the upper and lower eyelids cover the eye completely. When open, the upper eyelid extends beyond the limbus (the junction of the cornea and the sclera) and covers a small portion of the iris. The lower lid margin lies even with, or just below, the limbus. The palpebral fissure, which is the distance between the lid margins, should be equal in both eyes.

Conjunctivae

Serving to protect the eye from foreign bodies, the conjunctivae are transparent mucous membranes extending from the lid margins. The palpebral conjunctiva lines the highly vascular eyelids and therefore appears shiny pink or red. The bulbar conjunctiva, which contains many small, normally visible blood vessels, joins the palpebral portion and covers the sclera up to the limbus.

A small, fleshy elevation called the caruncle sits at the nasal aspect of the conjunctivae. The tarsal plates are lined posteriorly by conjunctivae and contain meibomian glands in vertical columns, which create the appearance of light yellow streaks. These glands secrete sebum, which is made up of keratin, fat, and cellular debris, onto the posterior lid margins to retain tears and keep the eye lubricated.

REVIEWING EXTRAOCULAR MUSCLES AND STRUCTURES

In this illustration the extraocular muscles and structures are shown. Each work together to support and protect the eyes.

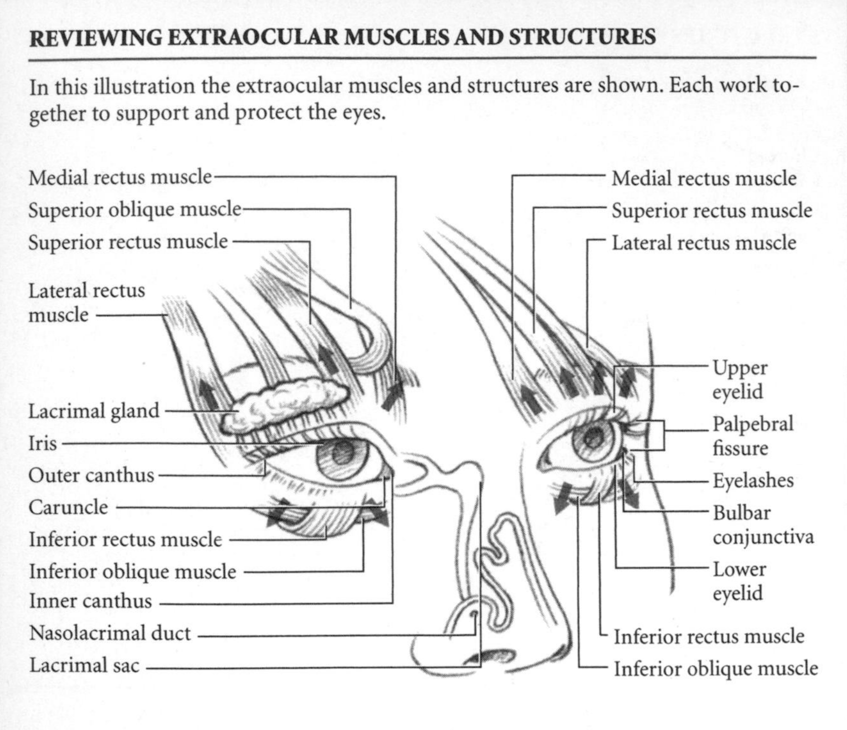

Lacrimal apparatus

The lacrimal apparatus — consisting of the lacrimal glands, the punctum, the lacrimal sac, and the nasolacrimal duct — lubricates and protects the cornea and the conjunctivae by producing and absorbing tears.

After washing across the eyeball, the tears drain through the punctum. The punctum, which is the only visible portion of the lacrimal apparatus, is a tiny opening at the medial junction of the upper and lower eyelids. From there, the tears flow through the lacrimal canals into the lacrimal sac. They then drain through the nasolacrimal duct and into the nose.

Extraocular muscles and cranial nerves

The coordinated action of six eye muscles — the superior, inferior, medial, and lateral rectus muscles, and the superior and inferior oblique muscles — controls eye movement. By functioning together, the extraocular muscles hold both eyes parallel and create binocular vision. The superior and inferior rectus muscles move the eye up and down on a transverse axis; the medial and lateral rectus muscles move the eye toward the nose and toward the temple on an anteroposterior axis; and the superior and inferior oblique muscles move the eye to the right and left on a vertical axis.

Six CNs — the optic (II), oculomotor (III), trochlear (IV), trigeminal (V), abducens (VI), and facial (VII) — innervate the eye, ocular muscles, and lacrimal apparatus. (See *Reviewing extraocular muscles and structures.*)

Intraocular structures

Easily visible anterior intraocular structures include the sclera, cornea, anterior chamber, iris, and pupil. Other intraocular structures are visible only with the use of an ophthalmoscope or other instrument. These include the aqueous humor, lens, ciliary body vitreous humor, retina, and choroid. The eye must be surgically rotated in order to see the posterior sclera.

With ophthalmoscopic (funduscopic) examination of the posterior portion of the eye (the fundus), the retinal blood vessels, optic disk, physiologic cup of the optic disk, macula, and fovea centralis can be seen.

Sclera, choroid, and vitreous humor

The white coating on the outside of the eyeball, the sclera, maintains the eye's size and shape. The choroid, which lines the recessed portion of the eyeball beneath the sclera, contains a network of arteries and veins that maintain blood supply to the eye. The vitreous humor is a thick, gelatinous material that fills the space directly behind the lens and maintains the retina's placement and the eyeball's spherical shape.

Bulbar conjunctiva and cornea

A thin, transparent membrane, the bulbar conjunctiva lines the eyelids and covers and protects the anterior portion of the white sclera. The cornea is a smooth, avascular, transparent tissue that merges with the sclera at the limbus. It refracts, or bends, light rays entering the eye.

The cornea, which is located in front of the pupil and iris, is fed by the ophthalmic branch of CN V (the trigeminal nerve). Stimulation of this nerve initiates a protective blink, the corneal reflex.

Iris

The iris is a circular, contractile diaphragm that contains smooth and radial muscles and is perforated in the center by the pupil. Varying amounts of pigment granules within the smooth muscle fibers give it color. Its posterior portion contains involuntary muscles that control pupil size and regulate the amount of light entering the eye.

Pupil

The iris's central opening, the pupil is normally round and equal in size to the opposite pupil. The pupil permits light to enter the eyes.

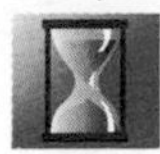

AGE ISSUE *Depending on the patient's age, pupil diameter can range from 0.3 to 0.5 cm. At birth, the pupil is small and unresponsive to light. It enlarges during childhood, and then progressively decreases in size throughout adulthood.*

Anterior and posterior chambers

The posterior chamber, located directly behind the lens, is filled with a watery fluid called aqueous humor. This fluid bathes the lens capsule as it flows through the pupil into the anterior chamber.

The anterior chamber is filled with the clear, aqueous humor. The amount of fluid in the chamber varies in an effort to maintain pressure in the eye. Fluid drains from the anterior chamber through collecting channels into Schlemm's canal.

Ciliary body and choroids

The iris, ciliary body, and choroid make up the eyeball's middle layer. Suspensory ligaments attached to the ciliary body control the lens's shape for close and distant vision. The pigmented, vascular choroid supplies the outer retina's blood supply and then drains blood through its remaining vasculature.

Lens

Located directly behind the iris at the pupillary opening, the lens consists of avascular transparent fibrils in an elastic membrane called the lens capsule. The lens refracts and focuses light onto the retina.

Vitreous chamber

The vitreous chamber, located behind the lens, occupies four-fifths of the eyeball. This chamber is filled with vitreous humor, an avascular gelatinous substance that maintains the shape of the eyeball.

Retina

The innermost region of the eyeball, the retina receives visual stimuli and transmits images to the brain for processing. Four sets of retinal blood vessels—the superonasal, inferonasal, superotemporal, and inferotemporal—are visible through an ophthalmoscope.

Each set of vessels contains a transparent arteriole and vein. As these vessels leave the optic disc, they become progressively thinner, intertwining as they extend to the periphery of the retina.

Optic disc and physiologic cup. A well-defined, round or oval area measuring less than ⅛″ (0.3 cm) within the retina's nasal portion, the optic disc is the opening through which the ganglion nerve axons (fibers) exit the retina to form the optic nerve. This area is called the blind spot because no light-sensitive cells, or photoreceptors, are located there.

The physiologic cup is a light-colored depression within the temporal side of the optic disc where blood vessels enter the retina. It covers one-fourth to one-third of the disc but doesn't extend completely to the margin.

Photoreceptor neurons. Photoreceptor neurons make up the retina's visual receptors. Not visible through the ophthalmoscope, these receptors — some shaped like rods and some like cones — are responsible for vision. Rods respond to low-intensity light, but they don't provide sharp images or color vision. Cones respond to bright light and provide high-acuity color vision.

Macula and fovea centralis. Located laterally from the optic disc, the macula is slightly darker than the rest of the retina and contains no visible retinal vessels. Because its borders are poorly defined, the macula is difficult to see on an ophthalmologic examination. It's best identified by having the patient look straight at the ophthalmoscope's light.

The fovea centralis, a slight depression in the macula, appears as a bright reflection when examined with an ophthalmoscope. Because the fovea contains the heaviest concentration of cones, it acts as the eye's clearest vision and color receptor.

Physiology of vision

Every object reflects light. For an individual to perceive an object clearly, this reflected light must be intercepted by the eye and pass through numerous intraocular structures, including the cornea, anterior chamber, pupil, lens, and vitreous humor. The lens focuses the light into an upside-down and reversed image on the retina. Reacting to the light, specialized photoreceptor cells, known as rods and cones, in the retina send nerve impulses via the optic nerve and optic tract to the visual cortex of the occipital lobe, which then interprets the image.

Health history

The most common eye-related complaints related to the eyes include double vision (diplopia), visual floaters, photophobia (light sensitivity), vision loss, and eye pain. Other complaints include decreased visual acuity or clarity, defects in color vision, and difficulty seeing at night. Even if a patient's chief complaint or previous diagnosis isn't eye-related, question him about his eyes and vision. Keep in mind that poor vision can affect the patient's ability to comply with treatment. (See *Common eye complaints.*)

To obtain an accurate and complete patient history, adjust questions to the patient's specific complaint and compare the answers with the results of the physical assessment.

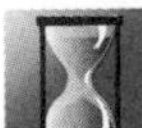

AGE ISSUE *Further modify questions according to the patient's age; for example, ask a child if the writing on the school chalkboard is readable or ask an elderly patient about peripheral vision, visual acuity, glaucoma testing, problems with glare, and abnormal tearing. (See* Assessing the eyes of children and older adults, *page 124.)*

Current health history

Begin by asking about the patient's current eye health status. Carefully document the patient's chief complaint using his own words. Ask for a complete description of this problem and any others. During the interview, observe the patient's eye movements and focusing ability for clues to visual acuity and eye muscle coordination. To investigate further, ask the following questions about eye function:

- Do you have problems with your eyes? Besides indicating visual disturbances, problems with the eyes can result from other conditions, such as diabetes, hypertension, or neurologic disorders.
- Do you wear or have you ever worn corrective lenses? If so, for how long? This establishes how long the patient has had a vision disorder and informs the health care provider of the patient's need to wear corrective lenses during the visual acuity check.
- If you wear corrective lenses, are they glasses or hard or soft contact lenses? Improperly fitted contact lenses or prolonged wearing of contact lenses can cause eye in-

COMMON EYE COMPLAINTS

If the patient is seeking medical attention for a vision problem, his chief complaint will probably be one of these disorders.

Decreased visual acuity
Lack of visual acuity—the ability to see clearly—is commonly associated with refractive errors. In nearsightedness or myopia, the eye focuses the visual image in front of the retina, causing objects in close view to be seen clearly and those at a distance to be blurry. In farsightedness, or hyperopia, the eye focuses the visual image behind the retina, causing objects in close view to be blurry and those at a distance to be clear. Both problems are caused by a difference in the shape of the eyeball from normal.

Diplopia
Also called double vision, diplopia is caused by extraocular muscle misalignment. It occurs when the visual axes aren't directed at the object of sight at the same time.

Eye pain
A complaint of eye pain needs immediate attention because it may signal an emergency. Ask the patient about the intensity, duration, frequency, and onset of the pain; what causes it (for example, bright light); whether headaches accompany it; and what he does to relieve it.

Diseases that can cause eye pain include acute angle-closure glaucoma and conjunctivitis. Corneal damage caused by a foreign body or abrasions and trauma to the eye can also cause eye pain.

Visual halos or bright light rings
Increased intraocular pressure, as occurs in glaucoma, causes the patient to see halos and rainbows around bright lights. It can be caused by corneal edema, as a result of prolonged contact lens wear, or fluctuation in blood glucose levels.

Night blindness
The patient may complain of poor vision once darkness descends. Night blindness, or the inability to adapt to dim light or darkness, is caused by retinal degeneration, such as retinitis pigmentosa, optic nerve disease, glaucoma, or vitamin A deficiency related to malnutrition or chronic alcoholism.

Vision loss
Your patient may complain of central or peripheral vision loss, or he may report a scotoma—a blind spot in the visual field that is surrounded by an area of normal vision. A disorder in any structure of the eye can result in vision loss. The degree and location of blindness depend on the disease causing the problem and the location of the lesion. The major causes of blindness in the United States are glaucoma, untreated cataracts, retinal disease, and macular degeneration.

Visual floaters
Visual floaters are specks of varying shape and size that float through the visual field and disappear when the patient tries to look at them. They're caused by small cells floating in the vitreous humor. Visual floaters require further investigation because they may indicate vitreous hemorrhage and retinal separation. A large, black floater that appears suddenly may indicate vitreous detachment.

flammation and corneal abrasions. Wearers of soft lenses are especially vulnerable to conjunctival inflammation and infection because the lenses, worn for long periods, can irritate the eye.

- For what eye condition do you wear corrective lenses? Besides providing information about an existing eye condition, the answer allows adjustment of the diopters for ophthalmoscopic examination of nearsightedness or farsightedness.

> **ASSESSING THE EYES OF CHILDREN AND OLDER ADULTS**
>
> If your patient is a child, ask a parent or guardian these additional questions:
>
> - Was the child delivered vaginally or by cesarean delivery? If he was delivered vaginally, did his mother have a vaginal infection at the time? (Inform the parents that infections — chlamydia, gonorrhea, genital herpes, or candidiasis — can cause eye problems in neonates.)
> - Did he have erythromycin ointment instilled in his eyes at birth?
> - Has he had an eye examination before? If so, when was the most recent examination?
> - Has he passed the normal developmental milestones?
> - Has he ever had an eye injury?
> - Does he know how to hold and handle sharp objects such as scissors?
> - Does he complain of eye pain or headaches?
> - Does he squint to see objects at a distance?
> - Does he hold objects close to his eyes to see them?
>
> If your patient is an aging adult, ask him these additional questions:
>
> - Have you had any difficulty climbing stairs or driving?
> - Have you ever been tested for glaucoma? If so, when and what was the result?
> - If you have glaucoma, has your health care provider prescribed eyedrops for you? If so, what kind?
> - How well are you able to instill your eyedrops?
> - Do your eyes ever feel dry? Do they burn? If so, how do you treat the problem?

- If you wear corrective lenses, do you wear them all the time or just for certain activities, such as reading or driving? The answers provide information about the severity and type of vision disturbance.
- If you once wore corrective lenses and have stopped wearing them, why and when did you stop? Eyestrain or excessive tearing may occur if the patient isn't wearing necessary lenses.

Past health history

During the next part of the health history, ask the following questions to gather additional information about the patient's eyes:

- When did you last have your corrective lenses changed? A recent lens change with continued visual disturbances could indicate an underlying health problem, such as a brain tumor.
- Have you ever had blurred vision? Blurred vision can indicate a need for corrective lenses or suggest a neurologic disorder such as a brain tumor, or an endocrine disorder such as diabetic retinopathy. If the patient isn't in distress, ask him how long he has had the visual blurring. Does it occur only at certain times? Ask about associated symptoms, such as pain or discharge. If visual blurring followed injury, obtain details of the accident and ask if vision was impaired immediately after the injury. Obtain a medical and medication history.
- Have you ever seen spots, floaters, or halos around lights? If yes, is this a sudden change or has it occurred for a while?

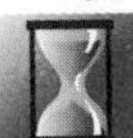

AGE ISSUE *In elderly patients with myopia, the chronic appearance of spots or floaters is a normal occurrence.*

- Do you suffer from frequent eye infections or inflammation? Frequent infections or inflammation of the eye can indicate low resistance to infection, eyestrain, allergies, or occupational or environmental exposure to an irritant.
- Have you ever had eye surgery? A history of eye surgery may indicate glaucoma, cataracts, or injuries such as detached retina, which may appear as abnormalities on ophthalmoscopic examination.
- Have you ever had an eye injury? Injuries, such as those from a penetrating foreign body, can distort the ophthalmoscopic examination.

- Do you often have sties? Sties, infected meibomian glands, or glands of Zeis, tend to recur.
- Do you have a history of high blood pressure?

CRITICAL POINT *Patients with high blood pressure are at risk for arteriosclerosis of the retinal blood vessels and vision disturbances.*

- Do you have a history of diabetes?
- Are you taking prescription medications for your eyes? If so, which medications and how often? Ask the patient to describe how he administers his medications, eyedrops, ointments, or gel. Review with the patient how to take his medication. Prescription eye medications should alert you to an eye disorder. For example, a patient who's taking pilocarpine probably has glaucoma.
- What other medications are you taking, including prescription drugs, over-the-counter medications, and home remedies? Certain medications can cause vision disturbances. For example, digoxin overdose can cause a patient to see yellow halos around bright lights. In addition, also remember to ask about herbal preparations, eyedrops, and eyewashes.

Family history

Next, investigate for familial eye disorders. Ask if any member of the patient's family has ever been treated for myopia, cataracts, glaucoma, or loss of vision.

Psychosocial history

Explore the patient's daily habits that affect the eyes by asking these questions:

- Does your occupation require close use of your eyes, such as long-term reading or prolonged use of a computer display terminal? These activities can cause eyestrain or dryness when the person forgets to blink.
- Does the air where you work or live contain anything that causes you eye problems? Cigarette smoke, formaldehyde insulation, or occupational materials such as glues or chemicals can cause eye irritation.
- Do you wear goggles when working with power tools, chain saws, or table saws, or when engaging in sports that might irritate or endanger the eye, such as swimming, fencing, or playing racquetball? Serious eye irritation or injury can occur with these activities.
- Do you smoke or are you exposed regularly to secondhand smoke? Warn him that smoking increases the risk of vascular disease, which can damage vision and lead to blindness.

If your patient is visually impaired, ask him how well he can manage activities of daily living. Assess whether he and his family need assistance in learning to use adaptive devices or a referral to an agency that helps visually impaired people.

Physical assessment

A complete physical assessment of the eye involves inspecting the external eye and lids, testing visual acuity, assessing eye muscle function, palpating the nasolacrimal sac, and examining intraocular structures with an ophthalmoscope.

Before starting the examination, gather the necessary equipment, including a good light source, one or two opaque cards, an ophthalmoscope, vision-test cards, gloves, tissues, and cotton-tipped applicators. Make sure the patient is seated comfortably and that you're seated at eye level with him.

Eye inspection

Start the inspection by observing the patient's face. With the scalp line as the starting point, check that his eyes are in a normal position. They should be about one-third of the way down the face and about one eye's width apart from each other. Next assess the conjunctiva, cornea, anterior chamber, iris, pupil, and eyelid.

Eyelids

Each upper eyelid should cover the top quarter of the iris so the eyes look alike. Check for an excessive amount of visible sclera above the limbus (corneoscleral junction). Ask the patient to open and close his eyes to see if they close completely. If the downward movement of the patient's upper eyelid in a down gaze is delayed, then the patient has lid lag, which is a common sign of hyperthyroidism. Protrusion of the eyeball, called exophthalmos or proptosis, is common in patients with hyperthyroidism.

Assess the lids for redness, edema, inflammation, or lesions. Also, inspect the eyes for excessive tearing or dryness. The eyelid mar-

EXPERT TECHNIQUE

ASSESSING CORNEAL SENSITIVITY

To test corneal sensitivity, touch a wisp of cotton from a cotton ball to the cornea, as shown. Remember, a wisp of cotton is the only safe object to use for this test. Even though 4″ × 4″ gauze pads and tissues are soft, they can cause corneal abrasions and irritation.

The patient should blink. If he doesn't, he may have suffered damage to the sensory fibers of cranial nerve V or to the motor fibers controlled by cranial nerve VI. Keep in mind that people who wear contact lenses may have reduced sensitivity because they're accustomed to having foreign objects in their eyes.

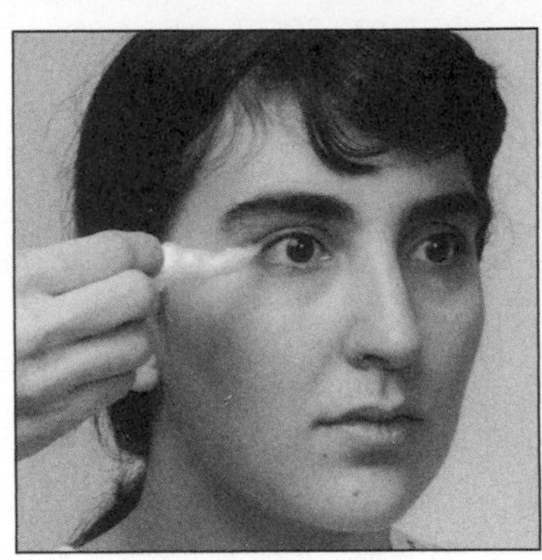

gins should be pink, and the eyelashes should turn outward. Observe whether the lower eyelids turn inward toward the eyeball, called *entropion,* or outward, called *ectropion.* Examine the eyelids for lumps. Swelling around the patient's eyes, or periorbital edema, may result from allergies, local inflammation, fluid-retaining disorders, or crying. In a patient with ptosis, or a drooping upper eyelid, there may be an interruption in sympathetic innervation to the eyelid, muscle weakness, or damage to the oculomotor nerve. A patient with acute hordeolum, also called a stye, has a bacterial infection in a sweat or sebaceous gland on the eyelid. The affected area becomes red and painful, and you may observe a green-yellow discharge.

Before palpating the nasolacrimal sac, explain the procedure to the patient. Then put on examination gloves. With the patient's eyes closed, gently palpate the area below the inner canthus, noting tenderness, swelling, or discharge through the lacrimal point. If tenderness, swelling, or discharge through the lacrimal point occurs upon palpation, these findings could indicate blockage of the nasolacrimal duct.

Conjunctiva

Next, have your patient look up. Gently pull the lower eyelid down to inspect the bulbar conjunctiva, which is the delicate mucous membrane that covers the exposed surface of the sclera. It should be clear and shiny. Note excessive redness or exudate. The palpebral conjunctiva, the membrane that lines the eyelids, in patients with a history of allergies may have a cobblestone appearance.

To examine the palpebral conjunctiva, have the patient look down. Then lift the upper lid, holding the upper lashes against the eyebrow with your finger. The palpebral conjunctiva should be uniformly pink.

With the lid still secured, inspect the bulbar conjunctiva for color changes, foreign bodies, and edema. Also, observe the sclera's color, which should be white to buff. A bluish discoloration may indicate scleral thinning.

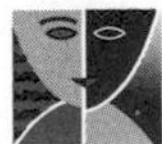

CULTURAL INSIGHT *In black patients, you may see flecks of tan in the conjunctiva.*

Cornea

Examine the cornea by shining a penlight first from both sides and then from straight ahead. The cornea should be clear and without lesions. Test corneal sensitivity by lightly touching the cornea with a wisp of cotton. (See *Assessing corneal sensitivity.*)

Anterior chamber and iris

The anterior chamber of the eye is bordered anteriorly by the cornea and posteriorly by the iris. The iris should appear flat, and the cornea should appear convex. Excess pressure in the eye—such as that caused by acute angle-closure glaucoma—may push the iris forward, making the anterior chamber appear very small. The irises should be the same size, color, and shape.

Pupil

Each pupil should be equal in size, round, and about one-fourth the size of the irises in normal room light. Approximately one person in four has asymmetrical pupils without disease.

CRITICAL POINT *Unequal pupils generally indicate neurologic damage, iritis, glaucoma, or therapy with certain medications. A fixed pupil that doesn't react to light can be an ominous neurologic sign.*

Test the pupils for direct and consensual response. In a slightly darkened room, hold a penlight about 20″ (50 cm) from the patient's eyes, and direct the light at the eye from the side. Note the reaction of the pupil you're testing (direct response) and the opposite pupil (consensual response). They should both react the same way. Also note sluggishness or inequality in the response. Repeat the test with the other pupil.

CRITICAL POINT *If you shine the light into the eye of a blind patient, neither pupil will respond. If you shine the light into the eye of a seeing patient, both pupils will respond consensually.*

To test the pupils for accommodation, place your finger approximately 4″ (10 cm) from the bridge of the patient's nose. Ask the patient to look at a fixed object in the distance and then to look at your finger. His pupils should constrict and his eyes converge as he focuses on your finger.

To document that the patient's pupils appear normal, use the abbreviation PERRLA (which stands for pupils equal, round, reactive to light, and accommodation) and the terms direct and consensual.

Testing visual acuity

To test your patient's far and near vision, use a Snellen chart and a near-vision chart. To test his peripheral vision, use confrontation. Before each test, ask the patient to remove corrective lenses, if he wears them.

Snellen chart

Have the patient sit or stand 20′ (6 m) from the chart, and cover his left eye with an opaque object. Ask him to read the letters on one line of the chart and then to move downward to increasingly smaller lines until he can no longer discern all of the letters. Have him repeat the test covering his right eye. Finally, have him read the smallest line he can read with both eyes uncovered to test his binocular vision. (See *Visual acuity charts*, page 128.)

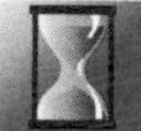

AGE ISSUE *In young children (and patients who can't read), use the Snellen E chart to test visual acuity. Cover the patient's left eye to check the right eye, point to an E on the chart, and ask the patient to point which way the letter faces. Repeat the test with the left eye.*

If the patient wears corrective lenses, have him repeat the test wearing them. If the test values between the two eyes differ by two lines, such as 20/30 in one eye and 20/50 in the other, suspect an abnormality such as amblyopia, especially in children. Record the vision with and without correction.

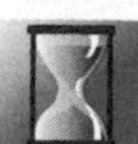

AGE ISSUE *In adults and children ages 6 and older, normal vision is measured as 20/20. For children younger than age 6, normal vision varies. For children ages 3 and younger, normal vision is 20/50; for children age 4, 20/40; and for children age 5, 20/30.*

Near-vision chart

To test near vision, cover one of the patient's eyes with an opaque object and hold a Rosenbaum near-vision card 14″ (35 cm) from his eyes. Have him read the line with the smallest letters he's able to distinguish. Repeat the test with the other eye. If the patient wears corrective lenses, have him repeat the test while wearing them. Record the visual accommodation with and without lenses.

Any patient who complains of blurring with the card at 14″ or who can't read it accurately needs retesting and then referral to an ophthalmologist if necessary. Keep in mind that a patient who's illiterate may be too embarrassed to say so. If a patient seems to be struggling to read the type, or stares at

VISUAL ACUITY CHARTS

The most commonly used charts for testing visual acuity are the Snellen alphabet chart (as shown) and the Snellen E chart (as shown), the latter of which is used for young children and adults who can't read. Both charts are used to test distance vision and measure visual acuity. The patient reads each chart at a distance of 20′(6 m).

Recording results
Visual acuity is recorded as a fraction. The top number (20) is the distance between the patient and the chart. The bottom number is the distance from which a person with normal vision could read the line. The larger the bottom number, the poorer the patient's vision.

SNELLEN ALPHABET CHART

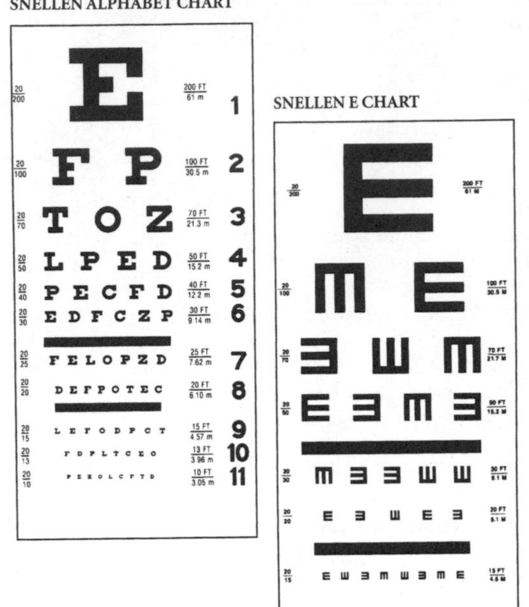

it without attempting to read, change to the E chart.

Testing color perception

Congenital color blindness is usually a sex-linked recessive trait passed from mothers to male offspring. Acquired color deficit is pathologic. People with color blindness can't distinguish among red, green, and blue.

Of the many tests to detect color blindness, the most common involves asking a patient to identify patterns of colored dots on colored plates. The patient who can't discern colors will miss the patterns.

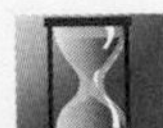

AGE ISSUE *In a child, early detection of color blindness allows him to learn to compensate for the deficit and also alerts teachers to the student's special needs.*

Assessing eye muscle function

A thorough assessment of the eyes includes an evaluation of the extraocular muscles. To evaluate these muscles, assessment involves testing the corneal light reflex and the cardinal positions of gaze and the cover-uncover test.

Corneal light reflex

To assess the corneal light reflex, ask the patient to look straight ahead; shine a penlight on the bridge of his nose from about 12″ to 15″ (30 cm to 38 cm) away. The light should fall at the same spot on each cornea. If it doesn't, the eyes aren't being held in the same plane by the extraocular muscles. This reaction typically occurs in patients who lack muscle coordination, a condition called *strabismus*.

Cardinal positions of gaze

Cardinal positions of gaze evaluates the oculomotor, trigeminal, and abducent nerves as well as the extraocular muscles. To perform this test, ask the patient to remain still while you hold a pencil or other small object directly in front of his nose at a distance of about 18″ (45 cm).

Ask him to follow the object with his eyes without moving his head. Then move the object to each of the six cardinal positions,

TESTING EXTRAOCULAR MUSCLES

The coordinated action of six muscles controls eyeball movements. To test the function of each muscle and the cranial nerve (CN) that innervates it, ask the patient to look in the direction controlled by that muscle. The six directions you can test make up the *cardinal fields of* gaze. The patient's inability to turn the eye in the designated direction indicates muscle weakness or paralysis.

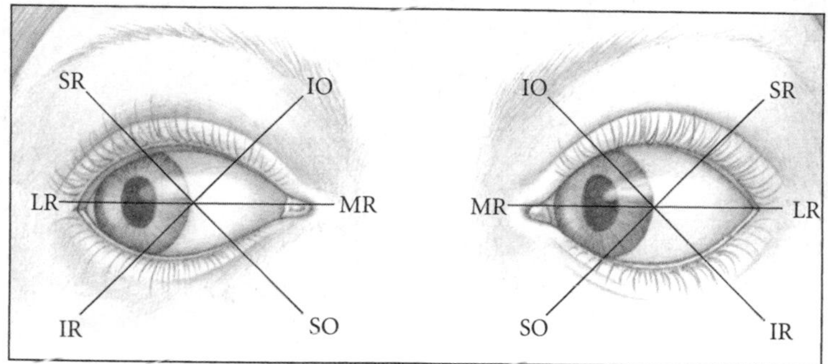

SR — superior rectus (CN III)
IR — inferior rectus (CN III)
MR — medial rectus (CN III)
LR — lateral rectus (CN VI)
IO — inferior oblique (CN III)
SO — superior oblique (CN IV)

returning to the midpoint after each movement. The patient's eyes should remain parallel as they move. Note abnormal findings such as nystagmus and amblyopia, the failure of one eye to follow an object. (See *Testing extraocular muscles.*)

Cover-uncover test

Another test to assess extraocular muscles is the cover-uncover test. This test usually isn't done unless you detect an abnormality during one of the two previous tests. To perform a cover-uncover test, have the patient stare at a wall on the other side of the room. Cover one eye and watch for movement in the uncovered eye. Remove the eye cover and watch for movement again. Repeat the test with the other eye. When you cover and uncover the patient's eye, his eye should remain still.

Eye movement, while covering or uncovering the eye is considered abnormal. It may result from weak or paralyzed extraocular muscles, which may be caused by cranial nerves (CN) impairment.

Testing peripheral vision

Assessment of peripheral vision tests the optic nerve (CN II) and measures the retina's ability to receive stimuli from the periphery of its field. You can grossly evaluate peripheral vision by assessing visual fields, which compares the patient's peripheral vision with your own. However, because this assumes you have normal vision, the test can be subjective and inaccurate.

To test peripheral visual fields, follow this procedure. Sit facing the patient, about 2′ (61 cm) away, with your eyes at the same level as his. Have him stare straight ahead. Cover one of your eyes with an opaque cover or your hand, and ask him to cover the eye directly opposite your covered eye. Next, bring an object, such as a penlight, from the periphery of the superior field toward the center of the field of vision. The object should be equidistant between you and the patient. Ask him to tell you the moment the object appears. If your peripheral vision is intact, you and the patient should see the object at the same time.

Repeat the procedure clockwise at 45-degree angles, checking the superior, inferior, temporal, and nasal visual fields. When testing the temporal field, you'll have difficulty moving the penlight far enough out so that neither person can see it, so test the temporal field by placing the penlight somewhat behind the patient and out of his

EXPERT TECHNIQUE

EXAMINING THE EYE

This illustration shows the correct position for the health care provider and the patient when an ophthalmoscope is used to examine the internal structures of the eye.

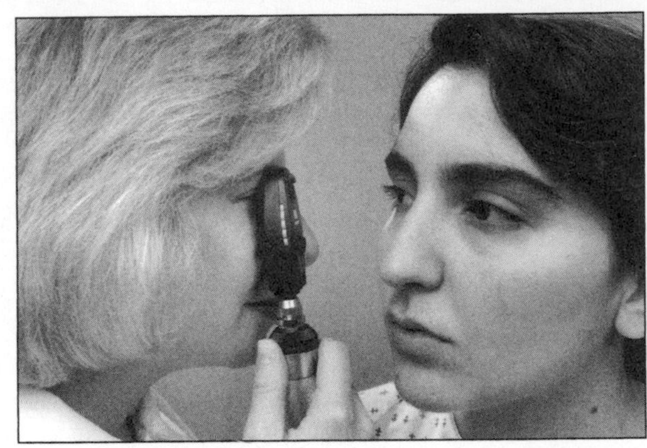

visual field. Slowly bring the penlight around until the patient can see it.

Examining intraocular structure

The ophthalmoscope allows direct observation of internal structures of the eye. To see those structures properly, you'll need to adjust the lens dial. Use the black, positive numbers on the dial to focus on near objects such as the patient's cornea and lens. Use the green, minus numbers to focus on distant objects such as the retina.

Before the examination, have the patient remove his contact lenses (if they're tinted) or eyeglasses, and darken the room to dilate his pupils and make the examination easier. Ask the patient to focus on a point behind you. Tell him that you'll be moving into his visual field and blocking his view. Also, explain that you'll be shining a bright light into his eye, which may be uncomfortable but not harmful. (See *Examining the eye.*)

Set the lens dial at zero, hold the ophthalmoscope about 4″ (10 cm) from the patient's eye, and direct the light through the pupil to elicit the red reflex, a reflection of light off the choroid. Check the red reflex for depth of color. Now, move the ophthalmoscope closer to the eye. Adjust the lens dial so you can focus on the anterior chamber and lens. Look for clouding, foreign matter, or opacities. If the lens is opaque, indicating cataracts, you may not be able to complete the examination.

To examine the retina, start with the dial turned to zero. Rotate the lens-power dial to adjust for your refractive correction and the patient's refractive error. Observe the vitreous body for clarity. The first retinal structures you'll see are the blood vessels. Rotating the dial into the negative numbers will bring the blood vessels into focus. The arteries will look thinner and brighter than the veins. Follow one of the vessels along its path toward the nose until you reach the optic disk, where all vessels in the eye originate. Examine arteriovenous crossings for arteriovenous nicking, which are localized constrictions in the retinal vessels that might be a sign of hypertension.

The optic disk is a creamy pink to yellow-orange structure with clear borders and a round-to-oval shape. With practice, you'll be able to identify the physiologic cup, a small depression that occupies about one-third of the disk's diameter. The disk may fill or exceed your field of vision. If you don't see it, follow a blood vessel toward the center until you do. The nasal border of the disk may be somewhat blurred. Completely scan the retina by following four blood vessels from the optic disk to different peripheral areas. The retina should have a uniform color and be free from scars and pigmenta-

LOOKING AT THE RETINA

This illustration shows the complex anatomy of the retina and its structures.

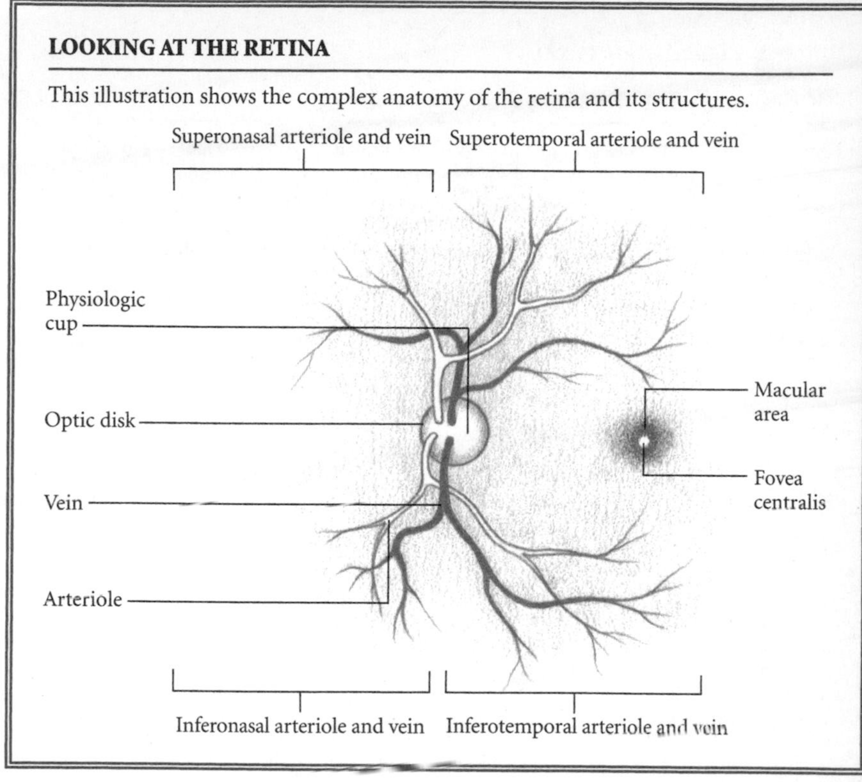

tion. As you scan, note lesions or hemorrhages. (See *Looking at the retina.*)

Finally, move the light laterally from the optic disk to locate the macula, the part of the eye most sensitive to light. It appears as a darker structure, free from blood vessels. Your view may be fleeting because most patients can't tolerate having a beam of light fall on the macula. If you locate it, ask the patient to shift his gaze into the light.

Abnormal findings

A patient's chief complaint may be caused by any number of signs and symptoms related to the eyes. Some common conditions include diplopia, eye discharge, eye pain, miosis, mydriasis, ocular deviation, photophobia, nonreactive or sluggish pupils, tunnel vision, vision loss, visual blurring, and visual floaters. The following history, physical assessment, and analysis summaries will help you assess each one quickly and accurately. After obtaining further information, begin to interpret the findings. (See *Eyes: Interpreting your findings,* pages 132 to 136).

Diplopia

Diplopia is double vision — seeing one object as two. This symptom results when extraocular muscles fail to work together, causing images to fall on noncorresponding parts of the retinas.

History

Find out when the patient first noticed diplopia. Are the images side-by-side (horizontal), one above the other (vertical), or a combination? Does diplopia affect near or far vision? Does it affect certain directions of gaze? Ask if diplopia has worsened, remained the same, or subsided. Does its severity change throughout the day? Worsening of diplopia or its appearance by evening may indicate myasthenia gravis. Find out if the patient can correct diplopia by tilting his head.

(Text continues on page 136.)

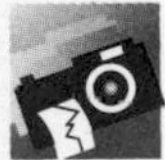

CLINICAL PICTURE

EYES: INTERPRETING YOUR FINDINGS

After you assess the patient, a group of findings may lead you to suspect a particular eye disorder. The chart below shows some common groups of findings for the signs and symptoms of the eyes, along with their probable causes.

Sign or symptom and findings	Probable cause
Diplopia	
▪ Confusion ▪ Slurred speech ▪ Halitosis ▪ Staggering gait ▪ Behavior changes ▪ Nausea and vomiting ▪ Conjunctival injection (possible)	Alcohol intoxication
▪ Blurred vision ▪ Paresthesia ▪ Nystagmus ▪ Constipation ▪ Muscle weakness ▪ Paralysis ▪ Spasticity ▪ Hyperreflexia ▪ Gait ataxia ▪ Dysphagia ▪ Emotional lability ▪ Urinary dysfunction	Multiple sclerosis
▪ Sudden onset ▪ Eye deviation ▪ Pain ▪ Purulent drainage ▪ Lid edema ▪ Chemosis ▪ Redness ▪ Proptosis ▪ Nausea ▪ Fever	Orbital cellulitis
Eye discharge	
▪ Purulent or mucopurulent, greenish-white discharge that occurs unilaterally ▪ Sticky crusts that form on the eyelids during sleep ▪ Itching and burning ▪ Excessive burning ▪ Sensation of a foreign body in the eye	Bacterial conjunctivitis
▪ Scant but continuous purulent discharge that's easily expressed from the tear sac ▪ Excessive tearing ▪ Pain and tenderness near the tear sac ▪ Eyelid inflammation and edema noticeable around the lacrimal punctum	Dacryocystitis
▪ Continuous frothy discharge ▪ Chronically red eyes with inflamed lid margins ▪ Soft, foul-smelling, cheesy yellow discharge elicited by pressure on the meibomian glands	Meibomianitis

EYES: INTERPRETING YOUR FINDINGS *(continued)*

Sign or symptom and findings	Probable cause
Eye pain	
▪ Sudden blurred vision with excruciating pain ▪ Nausea and vomiting ▪ Halo vision ▪ Fixed nonreactive moderately dilated pupil ▪ Rapidly decreasing visual acuity	Acute angle-closure glaucoma
▪ Burning in both eyelids ▪ Itching ▪ Sticky discharge ▪ Foreign body sensation ▪ Lid ulcerations ▪ Loss of eyelashes	Blepharitis
▪ Purulent eye discharge ▪ Sticky eyelids ▪ Photophobia ▪ Impaired visual acuity	Corneal ulcer
▪ Severe tenderness ▪ Conjunctival injection ▪ Bluish purple sclera ▪ Photophobia ▪ Excessive tearing	Scleritis
Miosis	
▪ Ipsilateral location ▪ Conjunctival injection ▪ Ptosis ▪ Facial flushing ▪ Sweating ▪ Bradycardia ▪ Restlessness ▪ Nasal stuffiness or rhinorrhea	Cluster headache

Sign or symptom and findings	Probable cause
Miosis *(continued)*	
▪ Ipsilaterally located to the lesion ▪ Sluggish papillary reflex ▪ Slight enophthalmos ▪ Moderate ptosis ▪ Facial anhidrosis ▪ Vascular headache	Horner's syndrome
▪ Moderate to severe eye pain ▪ Severe conjunctival injection ▪ Photophobia	Anterior uveitis
Mydriasis	
▪ Unilaterally located ▪ Ptosis ▪ Diplopia ▪ Decreased papillary reflexes ▪ Exotropia ▪ Complete loss of accommodation ▪ Focal neurologic signs	Oculomotor nerve palsy
▪ Loss of papillary reflex in affected eye ▪ Abrupt onset of excruciating pain ▪ Decreased visual acuity ▪ Visual blurring ▪ Halo vision ▪ Conjunctival injection ▪ Cloudy cornea	Acute angle-closure glaucoma

(continued)

EYES: INTERPRETING YOUR FINDINGS *(continued)*

Sign or symptom and findings	Probable cause
Ocular deviation	
▪ Diplopia ▪ Blurred vision ▪ Sensory dysfunction such as paresthesia ▪ Nystagmus ▪ Constipation ▪ Muscle weakness ▪ Paralysis ▪ Spasticity ▪ Hyperreflexia ▪ Gait ataxia ▪ Dysphagia ▪ Emotional lability ▪ Urinary dysfunction	Multiple sclerosis
▪ Diplopia ▪ Abrupt onset of fever, headache, and vomiting ▪ Nuchal rigidity ▪ Seizures ▪ Aphasia ▪ Ataxia ▪ Hemiparesis ▪ Cranial nerve palsies ▪ Photophobia ▪ Changes in level of consciousness	Encephalitis
▪ Diplopia ▪ Unilateral eyelid edema ▪ Erythema ▪ Hyperemia ▪ Chemosis ▪ Extreme orbital pain ▪ Purulent discharge	Orbital cellulitis
Photophobia	
▪ Nuchal rigidity ▪ Hyperreflexia ▪ Opisthotonos ▪ Fever and chills ▪ Headache ▪ Vomiting ▪ Seizures ▪ Changes in level of consciousness	Bacterial meningitis
▪ Conjunctival injection ▪ Increased tearing ▪ Foreign body sensation ▪ Eye pain ▪ Burning ▪ Itching	Conjunctivitis
▪ Noise sensitivity ▪ Aching or throbbing headache ▪ Fatigue ▪ Blurred vision ▪ Nausea and vomiting	Migraine headache
▪ Visible conjunctival follicles ▪ Red and edematous eyelids ▪ Pain ▪ Increased tearing ▪ Discharge ▪ Possibly progressing to yellow or gray inflamed papillae, entropion with corneal scarring	Trachoma

EYES: INTERPRETING YOUR FINDINGS *(continued)*

Sign or symptom and findings	Probable cause
Pupils, nonreactive	
■ Initially sluggish and progressing to nonreactive and dilated ■ Decreased accommodation ■ Dysphagia ■ Decreased level of consciousness occurring within 48 hours	Encephalitis
■ Initially dilated, nonreactive pupils and loss of accommodation, unilaterally or bilaterally ■ Bilateral midposition pupils suggesting central herniation; unilateral dilated nonreactive pupil suggesting uncal herniation	Oculomotor nerve palsy
Pupils, sluggish	
■ Longstanding history of diabetes ■ Orthostatic hypotension ■ Syncope ■ Dysphagia ■ Episodic constipation or diarrhea ■ Painless bladder distention with overflow incontinence	Diabetic neuropathy
■ Small, irregularly shaped pupils reacting better to accommodation than light ■ Ptosis ■ Nystagmus ■ Diplopia ■ Blurred vision ■ Sensory impairments	Multiple sclerosis
Vision loss	
■ Sudden and unilateral loss, partial or complete ■ Sluggish direct papillary response ■ Normal consensual response ■ Potential for blindness within hours	Central retinal artery occlusion
■ Gradual or sudden with partial or complete loss ■ Visual field deficits ■ Shard or curtain coming over the field ■ Visual floaters ■ Gray, opaque, detached retina with an indefinite margin and black retinal vessels on ophthalmoscopic examination	Retinal detachment
■ Sudden unilateral loss ■ Visual floaters ■ Partial vision with a reddish haze	Vitreous hemorrhage
Visual blurring	
■ Gradual visual blurring ■ Halo vision ■ Visual glare in bright light ■ Progressive vision loss ■ Gray pupil that later turns milky white	Cataract

(continued)

EYES: INTERPRETING YOUR FINDINGS *(continued)*

Sign or symptom and findings	Probable cause	Sign or symptom and findings	Probable cause
Visual blurring		***Visual floaters***	
▪ Constant morning headache that decreases in severity during the day ▪ Possible severe, throbbing headache ▪ Restlessness ▪ Confusion ▪ Nausea and vomiting ▪ Seizures ▪ Decreased level of consciousness	Hypertension	▪ Gradual or sudden, partial or complete vision loss ▪ Flashes of light in visual field ▪ Cloud or shadow falling in front on eye ▪ Gray, opaque, detached retina with an indefinite margin and black retinal vessels on ophthalmoscopic examination	Retinal detachment
▪ Paroxysmal attacks of severe, throbbing, unilateral or bilateral headache ▪ Nausea and vomiting ▪ Sensitivity to light and noise ▪ Sensory or visual auras	Migraine headache	▪ Shower of red or black dots or red haze across visual field ▪ Sudden blurring in affected eye ▪ Greatly reduced visual acuity	Vitreous hemorrhage

If the patient has a fourth nerve lesion, tilting his head toward the opposite shoulder causes compensatory tilting of the unaffected eye. If he has incomplete sixth nerve palsy, tilting of his head toward the side of the paralyzed muscle may relax the affected lateral rectus muscle. Explore associated symptoms such as eye pain. Ask about hypertension, diabetes mellitus, allergies, and thyroid, neurologic, or muscular disorders. Also, note a history of extraocular muscle disorders, trauma, or eye surgery.

Physical assessment

If the patient complains of double vision, first check his neurologic status and find out about associated neurologic symptoms because diplopia can accompany serious disorders. Evaluate his level of consciousness, pupil size and response to light, and motor and sensory functions. Take his vital signs. Briefly ask about associated symptoms, especially severe headache.

Observe the patient for ocular deviation, ptosis, proptosis, lid edema, and conjunctival injection. Distinguish monocular and binocular diplopia by asking the patient to occlude one eye. If he still sees double, he has monocular diplopia. Test visual acuity and extraocular muscles. Check vital signs.

Analysis

The causes of this muscle incoordination include orbital lesions, the effects of surgery, or impaired function of CNs that supply extraocular muscles (oculomotor, CN III; trochlear, CN IV; abducens, CN VI). Diplopia usually begins intermittently or affects near or far vision exclusively. It can be classified as monocular or binocular. More common, binocular diplopia may result from ocular deviation or displacement, extraocular muscle palsies, or psychoneurosis. It may also follow retinal surgery. Monocular diplopia may result from an early cataract, retinal edema, scarring, iridodialysis, subluxated lens, poorly fitting contact lens, or uncorrected refractive error. Diplopia may also occur in hysteria or malingering.

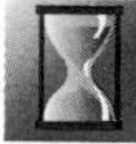

AGE ISSUE *In young children, the congenital disorder strabismus produces diplopia. However, the brain rapidly compensates for double vision by suppressing one image, so diplopia is a rare complaint among young children. School-age children who complain of double vision require careful examination to rule out serious disorders such as brain tumor.*

Eye discharge

Commonly associated with conjunctivitis, eye discharge is the excretion of a substance other than tears. This common sign may occur in one or both eyes, producing scant to copious discharge. The discharge may be purulent, frothy, mucoid, cheesy, serous, clear, or stringy and white. Occasionally the discharge can be expressed by applying pressure to the tear sac, punctum, meibomian glands, or canaliculus.

History

Begin your evaluation by finding out when the discharge began. Does it occur at certain times of day or in connection with certain activities? If the patient complains of pain, ask him to show you its exact location and to describe its character. Is the pain dull, continuous, sharp, or stabbing? Do his eyes itch or burn? Do they tear excessively? Are they sensitive to light? Does he feel like something is in them?

Physical assessment

After checking vital signs, carefully inspect the eye discharge. Note the amount and consistency. Then test visual acuity, with and without correction. Examine external eye structures, beginning with the unaffected eye to prevent cross-contamination. Check for eyelid edema, entropion, crusts, lesions, and trichiasis. Next, ask the patient to blink as you watch for impaired lid movement. If the eyes seem to bulge, measure them with an exophthalmometer. Test the six cardinal fields of gaze. Examine for conjunctival injection and follicles and for corneal cloudiness or white lesions.

Analysis

Eye discharge is common in patients with an inflammatory or infectious eye disorder, but it may also occur in patients with certain systemic disorders. Because this sign may accompany a disorder that threatens vision, it must be assessed and treated immediately.

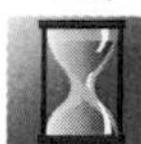

AGE ISSUE *In infants, the prophylactic eye medication silver nitrate commonly causes eye irritation and discharge. However, in children, discharges usually result from eye trauma, eye infection, or upper respiratory tract infection.*

Eye pain

Eye pain may be described as a burning, throbbing, aching, or stabbing sensation in or around the eye. It may also be characterized as a foreign-body sensation. This sign varies from mild to severe; its duration and exact location provide clues to the causative disorder.

History

If the patient's eye pain doesn't result from a chemical burn, take a complete history. Have the patient describe the eye pain fully. Is it an ache or a sharp pain? How long does it last? Is it accompanied by burning or itching? Find out when it began. Is it worse in the morning or late in the evening? Ask about recent trauma or surgery, especially if the patient complains of sudden, severe pain. Does he have headaches? If so, find out how often and at what time of day they occur.

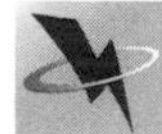

CRITICAL POINT *If the patient's eye pain results from a chemical burn, remove contact lenses, if present, and irrigate the eye with at least 1 liter of normal saline solution over 10 minutes. Evert the lids and wipe the fornices with a cotton-tipped applicator to remove particles or chemicals.*

Physical assessment

During the physical examination, don't manipulate the patient's eye if you suspect trauma. Carefully assess the lids and conjunctiva for redness, inflammation, and swelling. Examine the eyes for ptosis or exophthalmos. Finally, test visual acuity with and without correction, assess extraocular movements, and characterize discharge.

Analysis

Typically, eye pain results from corneal abrasion. It may also result from glaucoma and other eye disorders, trauma, and neurologic and systemic disorders. Any of these may stimulate nerve endings in the cornea or external eye, producing pain.

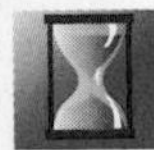

AGE ISSUE *In children, trauma and infection are the most common causes of eye pain. Be alert for nonverbal clues to pain, such as tightly shutting or frequent rubbing of the eyes.*

Miosis

Miosis—pupillary constriction caused by contraction of the sphincter muscle in the iris—occurs normally as a response to fatigue, increased light, and administration of miotic drugs; as part of the eye's accommodation reflex; and as part of the aging process.

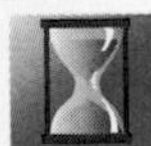

AGE ISSUE *Pupil size steadily decreases from adolescence to about age 60. Miosis occurs frequently in neonates because they sleep or are sleepy most of the time.*

History

Begin by asking the patient if he's experiencing other ocular symptoms, and have him describe their onset, duration, and intensity. Does he wear contact lenses? During the history, be sure to ask about trauma, serious systemic disease, and use of topical and systemic medications.

Physical assessment

Perform a thorough eye examination. Inspect and compare both pupils for size (many people have a normal discrepancy), color, shape, reaction to light, accommodation, and consensual light response. Examine both eyes for additional signs, then evaluate extraocular muscle function by evaluating the six cardinal fields of gaze. Finally, test visual acuity in each eye, with and without correction, paying particular attention to blurred or decreased vision in the miotic eye.

Analysis

Miosis can also stem from ocular and neurologic disorders, trauma, contact lens overuse, and systemic drugs, such as barbiturates, cholinergics, cholinesterase inhibitors, guanethidine, opiates, and reserpine. A rare form of miosis—Robertson's pupils—can stem from tabes dorsalis and diverse neurologic disorders. Occurring bilaterally, these miotic (usually pinpoint), unequal, and irregularly shaped pupils don't dilate properly with mydriatic drug use and fail to react to light, although they do constrict on accommodation.

Mydriasis

Mydriasis—pupillary dilation caused by contraction of the dilator of the iris—is a normal response to decreased light, long emotional stimuli, and topical administration of mydriatic and cycloplegic drugs.

History

Begin by asking the patient about other eye problems, such as pain, blurring, diplopia, or visual field defects. Obtain a health history, focusing on eye or head trauma, glaucoma and other ocular problems, and neurologic and vascular disorders. In addition, obtain a complete medication history.

Physical assessment

Perform a thorough eye and pupil examination. Inspect and compare the pupils' size, color, and shape (many people normally have unequal pupils). Also, test each pupil for light reflex, consensual response, and accommodation. Be sure to check the eyes for ptosis, swelling, and ecchymosis. Test visual acuity in both eyes with and without correction. Evaluate extraocular muscle function by checking the six cardinal fields of gaze.

Analysis

Mydriasis can also result from ocular and neurologic disorders, eye trauma, and disorders that decrease level of consciousness. Mydriasis may be an adverse effect of certain drugs, such as anticholinergics, antihistamines, sympathomimetics, barbiturates (in overdose), estrogens, and tricyclic antidepressants; it also commonly occurs early in anesthesia induction.

Ocular deviation

Ocular deviation refers to abnormal eye movement that may be conjugate, when both eyes move together, or dysconjugate, when one eye moves differently from the other. Normally, eye movement is directly controlled by the extraocular muscles innervated by the oculomotor, trochlear, and abducens nerves (CNs III, IV, and VI). Together, these muscles and nerves direct a visual stimulus to fall on corresponding parts of the retina.

History

If the patient isn't in distress, find out how long he has had the ocular deviation. Is it accompanied by double vision, eye pain, or headache? Also, ask if he has noticed associated motor or sensory changes or fever.

CRITICAL POINT *If the patient displays ocular deviation, quickly take his vital signs and look for altered level of consciousness, pupil changes, motor or sensory dysfunction, and severe headache. If possible, ask the patient's family about behavioral changes. Find out if there's a history of recent head trauma. Respiratory support may be necessary. Also prepare the patient for emergency neurologic tests such as a computed tomography scan.*

Check for a history of hypertension, diabetes, allergies, and thyroid, neurologic, or muscular disorders. Then obtain a thorough ocular history. Ask the patient if he has ever had extraocular muscle imbalance, eye or head trauma, or eye surgery.

Physical assessment

During the physical examination, observe the patient for partial or complete ptosis. Does he spontaneously tilt his head or turn his face to compensate for ocular deviation? Check for eye redness or periorbital edema. Assess visual acuity, then evaluate extraocular muscle function by testing the six cardinal fields of gaze.

Analysis

Ocular deviation may result from ocular, neurologic, endocrine, and systemic disorders that interfere with the muscles, nerves, or brain centers governing eye movement. Occasionally it signals a life-threatening disorder such as ruptured cerebral aneurysm. Dysconjugate ocular deviation may result from unequal muscle tone (nonparalytic strabismus) or from muscle paralysis associated with CN damage (paralytic strabismus). Conjugate ocular deviation may result from disorders that affect the centers in the cerebral cortex and brain stem responsible for conjugate eye movement. Typically, such disorders cause gaze palsy—difficulty moving the eyes in one or more directions.

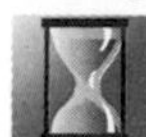

AGE ISSUE *In children, the most common cause of ocular deviation is nonparalytic strabismus. Normally, children achieve binocular vision by age 3 to 4 months. Although severe strabismus is readily apparent, mild strabismus must be confirmed by tests for misalignment, such as the corneal light reflex test and the cover-uncover test. Testing is crucial—early corrective measures help preserve binocular vision and cosmetic appearance.*

Photophobia

A common symptom, photophobia is an abnormal sensitivity to light. It can be benign or can indicate an underlying problem.

History

If your patient reports photophobia, find out when it began and how severe it is. Did it follow eye trauma? A chemical splash or exposure to the rays of a sun lamp? If photophobia results from trauma, avoid eye manipulation. Ask the patient about eye pain and have him describe its location, duration, and intensity. Does he have a sensation of a foreign body in his eye? Does he have other signs and symptoms, such as increased tearing and vision changes?

Physical assessment

Obtain the patient's vital signs and assess his neurologic status. Follow this with a careful eye examination, inspecting the eyes' external structures for abnormalities. Examine the conjunctiva and sclera, noting especially their color. Characterize the amount and consistency of discharge. Then check pupillary reaction to light. Evaluate extraocular muscle function by testing the six cardinal fields of gaze, and test visual acuity in both eyes.

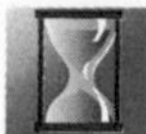

AGE ISSUE *Suspect photophobia in a child who squints, rubs his eyes frequently, or wears sunglasses while indoors and outdoors.*

Analysis
In many patients, photophobia simply indicates increased eye sensitivity without an underlying disease. In some patients, it can indicate excessive wearing of contact lenses or poorly fitted lenses. However, in others, this symptom can indicate systemic disorders, ocular disorders or trauma, or use of certain drugs such as mydriatics.

Pupils, nonreactive
Nonreactive (fixed) pupils fail to constrict in response to light or dilate when the light is removed. The development of a unilateral or bilateral nonreactive response indicates an important change in the patient's condition and could signal a life-threatening emergency and possibly brain death.

History
If the patient is conscious, obtain a brief history. Ask him what type of eye drops he's using, if any, and when they were last instilled. Also, ask if the patient is experiencing pain and, if so, try to determine its location, intensity, and duration.

CRITICAL POINT *If the patient is unconscious and develops unilateral or bilateral nonreactive pupils, quickly take his vital signs. Be alert for decerebrate or decorticate posture, bradycardia, elevated systolic blood pressure, widened pulse pressure, and the development of other untoward changes in the patient's condition. Remember, a unilateral dilated, nonreactive pupil may be an early sign of uncal brain herniation.*

Physical assessment
Evaluate pupillary reaction to light. First test the patient's direct light reflex. Darken the examination room, and cover one of the patient's eyes while you hold open the opposite eyelid. Using a bright penlight, bring the light toward the patient from the side and shine it directly into his opened eye. If normal, the pupil will promptly constrict. Now test the consensual light reflex. Hold the patient's eyelids open and shine the light into one eye while watching the pupil of the opposite eye. If normal, both pupils will promptly constrict. Repeat both procedures in the opposite eye.

Determine the patient's visual acuity in both eyes. Then test the pupillary reaction to accommodation. Normally, both pupils constrict equally as the patient shifts his glance from a distant to a near object. Hold a penlight at the side of each eye, and examine the cornea and iris for abnormalities. Measure intraocular pressure (IOP) with a tonometer, or estimate IOP by placing your second and third fingers over the patient's closed eyelid. If the eyeball feels rock hard, suspect elevated intraocular pressure. If the patient has experienced ocular trauma, don't manipulate the affected eve. After the examination, cover the affected eye with a protective metal shield but don't let the shield rest on the globe.

Analysis
In addition to signaling a possible life-threatening emergency situation, nonreactive pupils occur with use of certain optic drugs, such as mydriatics and cycloplegics. A unilateral or bilateral nonreactive response indicates dysfunction of CNs II and III, which mediate the pupillary light reflex.

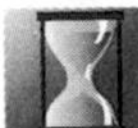

AGE ISSUE *Children have nonreactive pupils for the same reasons as adults. The most common cause is oculomotor nerve palsy from increased intracranial pressure (ICP).*

Pupils, sluggish
Sluggish pupillary reaction is an abnormally slow pupil response to light. It can occur in one pupil or both, unlike the normal reaction, which is always bilateral.

History
Obtain a brief health history. Ask the patient about the use of eye drops and when they were last instilled. Also, ask if he's experiencing pain and, if so, try to determine its location, intensity, and duration.

Physical assessment
To assess pupillary reaction to light, first test the patient's direct light reflex. Darken the room, and cover one of the patient's eyes while you hold open the opposite eyelid. Using a bright penlight, bring the light toward the patient from the side and shine it directly into his opened eye. If normal, the pupil will promptly constrict. Now test the consensual light reflex. Hold both of the patient's eyelids open, and shine the light into one eye while watching the pupil of the op-

posite eye. If normal, both pupils will promptly constrict. Repeat both procedures to test light reflexes in the opposite eye.

Determine the patient's visual function. Test visual acuity in both eyes. Then test the pupillary reaction to accommodation. The pupils should constrict equally as the patient shifts his glance from a distant to a near object. Hold a penlight at the side of each eye and examine the cornea and iris for irregularities, scars, and foreign bodies. Measure IOP with a tonometer. Alternatively, estimate IOP without a tonometer by placing fingers over the patient's closed eyelid. If the eyeball feels rock hard, suspect elevated IOP.

Analysis

A sluggish reaction in one or both pupils indicates dysfunction of CNs II and III, which mediate the pupillary light reflex. A sluggish reaction accompanies degenerative disease of the central nervous system and diabetic neuropathy.

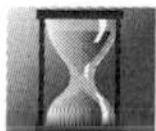

AGE ISSUE *In elderly patients, sluggish pupils occur normally because their pupils become smaller and less responsive with age.*

Vision loss

Vision loss — the inability to perceive visual stimuli — can be sudden or gradual and temporary or permanent. The deficit can range from a slight impairment of vision to total blindness.

History

If the patient's vision loss occurred gradually, ask him if the vision loss affects one eye or both, and all or only part of the visual field. Ask the patient if he has experienced photosensitivity, and ask him about the location, intensity, and duration of eye pain. In addition, you should obtain an ocular history and a family history of eye problems or systemic diseases that may lead to eye problems, such as hypertension; diabetes mellitus; thyroid, rheumatic, or vascular disease; infections; and cancer.

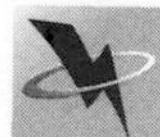

CRITICAL POINT *Sudden vision loss can signal an ocular emergency. Don't touch the eye if the patient has perforating or penetrating ocular trauma.*

Physical assessment

Carefully inspect both eyes, noting edema, foreign bodies, drainage, or conjunctival or scleral redness. Observe whether lid closure is complete or incomplete, and check for ptosis. Using a flashlight, examine the cornea and iris for scars, irregularities, and foreign bodies. Observe the size, shape, and color of the pupils, and test the direct and consensual light reflex and the effect of accommodation. Evaluate extraocular muscle function by testing the six cardinal positions of gaze. Evaluate the extent of vision loss by testing visual acuity in each eye.

Analysis

Vision loss can result from ocular, neurologic, and systemic disorders, as well as from trauma and reactions to certain drugs, such as chloroquine, phenylbutazone, and digoxin.

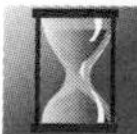

AGE ISSUE *Children who complain of slowly progressive vision loss may have an optic nerve glioma (a slow-growing, usually benign tumor) or retinoblastoma (a malignant tumor of the retina). Congenital rubella and syphilis may cause vision loss in infants.*

Visual blurring

Visual blurring is a common symptom that refers to the loss of visual acuity with indistinct visual details.

History

If the patient isn't in distress, ask him how long he has had the visual blurring. Does it occur only at certain times? Ask about associated symptoms, such as pain or discharge. If visual blurring followed injury, obtain details of the accident, and ask if vision was impaired immediately after the injury. Obtain a medical and drug history.

Physical assessment

Inspect the patient's eye, noting lid edema, drainage, or conjunctival or scleral redness. Also note an irregularly shaped iris, which may indicate previous trauma, and excessive blinking, which may indicate corneal damage. Check for pupillary changes, and test visual acuity in both eyes. If the patient has visual blurring accompanied by sudden, severe eye pain, a history of trauma, or sudden vision loss, perform an ophthalmologic examination. If the patient has a penetrating or perforating eye injury, don't touch the eye.

Analysis

Visual blurring may result from an eye injury, a neurologic or eye disorder or a disorder with vascular complications such as diabetes mellitus. Visual blurring may also result from mucus passing over the cornea, refractive errors, improperly fitted contact lenses, or the use of certain drugs.

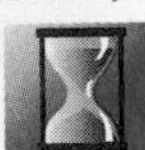

AGE ISSUE *In children, visual blurring may stem from congenital syphilis, congenital cataracts, refractive errors, an eye injury or infection, or increased ICP. Refer the child to an ophthalmologist if appropriate. Test vision in school-age children as you would in adults. Test children ages 3 to 6 with the Snellen symbol chart; test toddlers with Allen cards, each illustrated with a familiar object such as an animal. Ask the child to cover one eye and identify the objects and then ask him to identify them as you gradually back away. Record the maximum distance at which he can identify at least three pictures.*

Visual floaters

Visual floaters are particles of blood or cellular debris that move about in the vitreous. As these enter the visual field, they appear as spots or dots.

History

If the patient's condition permits, obtain a drug and allergy history. Ask about nearsightedness (a predisposing factor), use of corrective lenses, eye trauma, or other eye disorders. Also ask about a history of granulomatous disease, diabetes mellitus, or hypertension, which may have predisposed him to retinal detachment, vitreous hemorrhage, or uveitis.

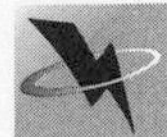

CRITICAL POINT *Sudden onset of visual floaters may signal retinal detachment. Ask the patient if he also sees flashing lights or spots in the affected eye. Also, find out if he's experiencing a curtainlike loss of vision. If so, notify an ophthalmologist immediately. Restrict his eye movements until the proper diagnosis is made.*

Physical assessment

If appropriate, inspect the patient's eyes for signs of injury. Note bruising or edema. Test his visual acuity and papillary reaction to light and accommodation.

Analysis

The sudden onset of visual floaters commonly signals retinal detachment, an ocular emergency.

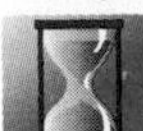

AGE ISSUE *In elderly or myopic patients, chronic floaters may occur normally. Visual floaters in children usually follow trauma that causes retinal detachment or vitreous hemorrhage. However, they may also result from vitreous debris, a benign congenital condition with no other signs or symptoms.*

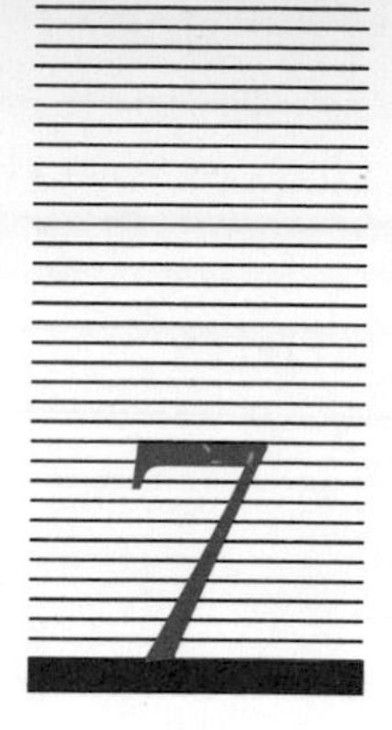

Ears, nose, and throat

The ability to hear, smell, and taste allows individuals to communicate with others, connect with the world, and take pleasure in life. Because these senses play such vital roles in daily life, a thorough assessment of a patient's ears, nose, and throat, and their related structures, is necessary.

Besides revealing impairments in hearing, smell, and taste, the assessment can also uncover important clues to physical problems in the patient's integumentary, musculoskeletal, cardiovascular, respiratory, immune, and neurologic systems.

To perform an accurate physical assessment, an understanding of the anatomy and physiology of the ears, nose, and throat, and their related structures, is crucial.

Anatomy and physiology

The ear is divided into three parts: external, middle, and inner. The anatomy and physiology of each part play separate but important roles in hearing.

Structures of the ear

The ear can be divided into three main parts—the external ear, the middle ear, and the inner ear. (See *Structures of the ear,* page 144.)

External ear

The flexible external ear consists mainly of elastic cartilage. This part of the ear contains the ear flap, also known as the *auricle* or *pinna,* and the auditory canal. The outer third of this canal has a bony framework. Although not part of the external ear, the mastoid process is an important bony landmark behind the lower part of the auricle.

STRUCTURES OF THE EAR

This illustration presents the structures of the ear including the external, middle, and inner ear.

EXTERNAL EAR
External auditory canal (meatus)
Auricle (pinna)
Helix
Anthelix
Concha
Antitragus
Tragus
Lobule

MIDDLE EAR
Incus
Malleus
Tympanic membrane
Footplate of stapes

INNER EAR
Semicircular canals
Acoustic nerve branches
Cochlea
Round window
Oval window
Eustachian tube
Vestibule

Bone covered by thin skin forms the inner two-thirds. The adult's external canal leads inward, downward, and forward to the middle ear. It's lined with glands that secrete cerumen, which lubricates and protects the ear. The external ear functions to collect sounds and transmit them to the middle ear.

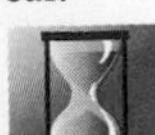

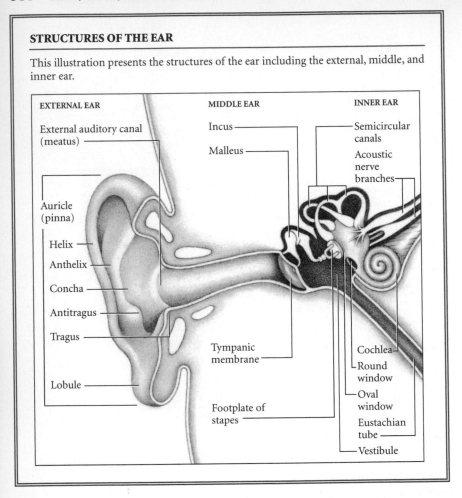

AGE ISSUE *In elderly male patients you will observe coarse hair in the ear canal.*

Middle ear

The tympanic membrane separates the external and middle ear. This pearl gray structure consists of three layers that include skin, fibrous tissue, and a mucous membrane. Its upper portion, the pars flaccida, has little support; its lower portion, the pars tensa, is held taut. The center, or umbo, is attached to the tip of the long process of the malleus on the other side of the tympanic membrane.

A small, air-filled structure, the middle ear performs three vital functions:

- It transmits sound vibrations across the bony ossicle chain to the inner ear.
- It protects the auditory apparatus from intense vibrations.
- It equalizes the air pressure on both sides of the tympanic membrane to prevent it from rupturing.

The middle ear contains three small bones of the auditory ossicles: the malleus, or hammer; the incus, or anvil; and the stapes, or stirrup. These bones are linked like a chain and vibrate in place. The long process of the malleus fits into the incus, forming a true joint, and allows the two structures to move as a single unit. The proximal end of the stapes fits into the oval window, an opening that joins the middle and inner ear.

The eustachian tube connects the middle ear with the nasopharynx, equalizing air pressure on either side of the tympanic membrane. This tube also connects the ear's sterile area to the nasopharynx. The tube is opened during yawning or swallowing. A normally functioning eustachian tube keeps the middle ear free from contaminants from the nasopharynx. Upper respiratory tract infections and allergies can block the tube, obstructing middle ear drainage, which may cause otitis media or effusion.

Inner ear

The inner ear consists of closed, fluid-filled spaces within the temporal bone. It contains the bony labyrinth, which includes three connected structures — the vestibule, the semicircular canals, and the cochlea. These structures are lined with the membranous labyrinth. A fluid called perilymph fills the space between the bony labyrinth and the membranous labyrinth, cushioning these sensitive organs.

The vestibule and semicircular canals help maintain equilibrium. The cochlea, a spiral chamber that resembles a snail shell, is the organ of hearing. The organ of Corti, part of the membranous labyrinth, contains hair cells that receive auditory sensations. The vestibular branch of the acoustic nerve contains peripheral nerve fibers that terminate in the epithelium of the semicircular canals, and the central branch terminates in the medulla at the vestibular nucleus.

Functions of the ear

The ear, a sensory organ, enables hearing and helps maintains equilibrium.

Hearing

When sound waves reach the external ear, structures there transmit the waves through the auditory canal to the tympanic membrane, causing it to vibrate and sending it to the stapes, through the oval window, producing sound waves of the perilymph. Finally, the cochlear branch of the acoustic nerve (cranial nerve VIII) transmits the vibrations to the temporal lobe of the cerebral cortex, where the brain interprets the sound.

Sound waves travel through the ear by two pathways — air conduction and bone conduction. Air conduction occurs when sound waves travel in the air through the external and middle ear to the inner ear. Bone conduction occurs when sound waves travel through the bone to the inner ear.

Equilibrium

Besides controlling hearing, structures in the middle and inner ear control equilibrium, or balance. The semicircular canals of the inner ear contain cristae — hairlike structures that respond to body movements. Endolymph fluid bathes the cristae.

When a person moves, the cristae bend, releasing impulses through the vestibular portion of the acoustic nerve to the brain, which controls equilibrium. When a person is stationary, nerve impulses to the brain orient him to this position, and the pressure of gravity on the inner ear helps him maintain equilibrium.

Nose

The nose is more than the sensory organ of smell. It also plays a key role in the respiratory system by filtering, warming, and humidifying inhaled air. When assessing the nose, be sure to also assess the paranasal sinuses. (See *Anatomic structure of the nose, mouth, and oropharynx,* page 146.)

External and internal nose

The lower two-thirds of the external nose consists of flexible cartilage; the upper one-third is rigid bone. Posteriorly, the internal nose merges with the pharynx. Anteriorly, it merges with the external nose.

Nasal septum

The internal and external nose are divided vertically by the nasal septum, which is straight at birth and in early life but becomes slightly deviated or deformed in almost every adult. Only the posterior end, which separates the posterior nares, remains constantly in the midline.

ANATOMIC STRUCTURE OF THE NOSE, MOUTH, AND OROPHARYNX

These illustrations show the anatomic structure of the nose, mouth, and oropharynx.

NOSE AND MOUTH

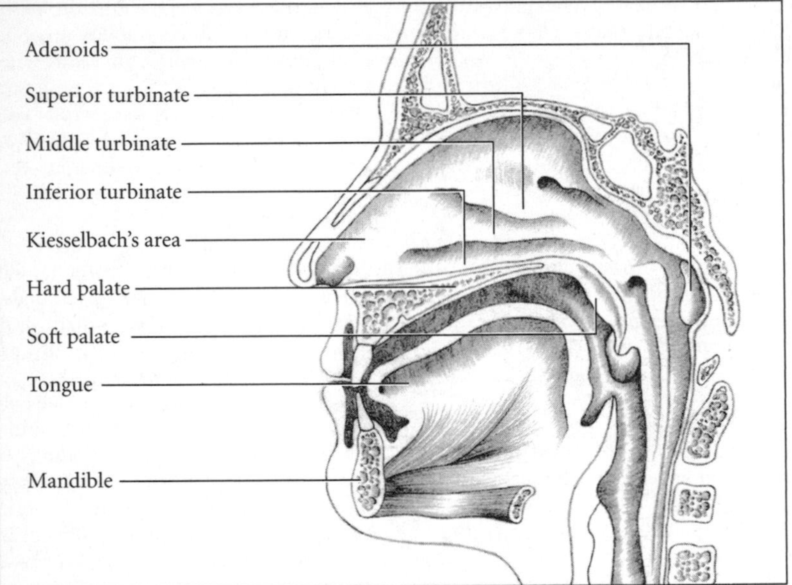

MOUTH AND OROPHARYNX

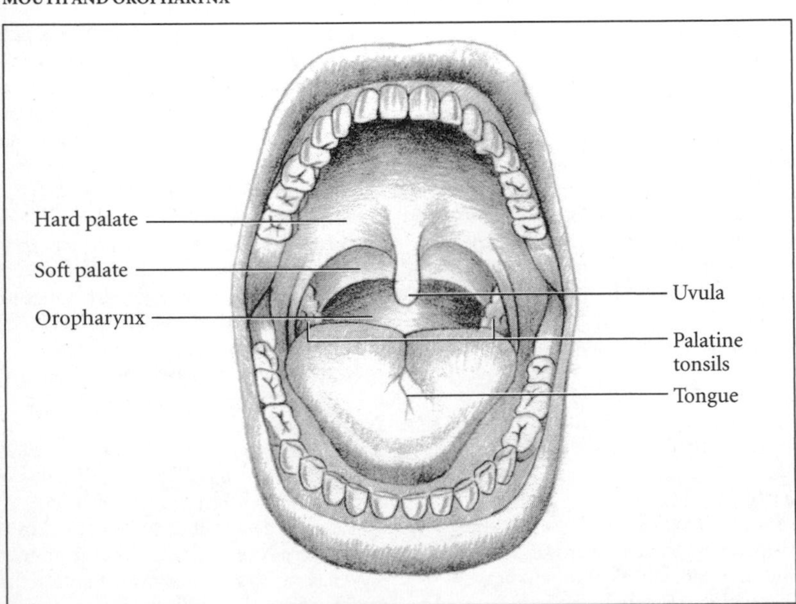

Vestibule

Air entering the nose passes through the vestibule, which is lined with coarse hair that helps filter out dust. Olfactory receptors lie above the vestibule in the roof of the nasal cavity and the upper one-third of the septum. Known as the olfactory region, this area is rich in capillaries and mucus-producing goblet cells that help warm, moisten, and clean inhaled air. Kiesselbach's area, the most common site of nosebleeds, is located in the anterior portion of the septum. Because of its rich blood supply, the nasal mucosa is redder than the oral mucosa.

Turbinates

Further along the nasal passage are the superior, middle, and inferior turbinates. Separated by grooves called meatuses, the curved bony turbinates and their mucosal covering ease breathing by warming, filtering, and humidifying inhaled air.

Paranasal sinuses

Four pairs of paranasal sinuses open into the internal nose, including:

- maxillary sinuses, located on the cheeks below the eyes
- frontal sinuses, located above the eyebrows
- ethmoidal and sphenoidal sinuses, located behind the eyes and nose in the head.

The sinuses serve as resonators for sound production and provide mucus. You'll be able to assess the maxillary and frontal sinuses, but the ethmoidal and sphenoidal sinuses aren't readily accessible.

CRITICAL POINT *The small openings between the sinuses and the nasal cavity are easily obstructed because they're lined with mucous membranes that can become inflamed and swollen.*

Throat and neck

The throat, or pharynx, is divided into the nasopharynx, the oropharynx, and the laryngopharynx. Located within the throat are the hard and soft palates, the uvula, and the tonsils. The mucous membrane lining the throat normally is smooth and bright pink to light red.

Food travels through the pharynx to the esophagus. Air travels through it to the larynx. The epiglottis diverts material away from the glottis during swallowing and helps prevent aspiration. By vibrating expired air through the vocal cords, the larynx produces sound. Changes in vocal cord length and air pressure affect the voice's pitch and intensity. The larynx also stimulates the vital cough reflex when a foreign body touches its sensitive mucosa. The most important function of the larynx is to act as a passage for air between the pharynx and the trachea.

The neck is formed by the cervical vertebrae and the major neck and shoulder muscles, together with their ligaments. Other important structures of the neck include the trachea, thyroid gland, and chains of lymph nodes.

The thyroid gland lies in the anterior neck, just below the larynx. Its two cone-shaped lobes are located on either side of the trachea and are connected by the isthmus below the cricoid cartilage, which gives the gland its butterfly shape. The largest endocrine gland, the thyroid produces the hormones triiodothyronine (T_3) and thyroxine (T_4), which affect the metabolic reactions of every cell in the body.

Health history

To investigate a patient's chief complaint about the ears, nose, and throat, and their related structures, ask about the onset, location, duration, and characteristics of the symptom as well as what aggravates and relieves it.

Ear assessment

The most common ear complaints are hearing loss, tinnitus, pain, discharge, and dizziness. Hearing loss and tinnitus usually are due to long-term problems. Pain, discharge, and dizziness usually result from short-term conditions.

If the patient reports hearing loss, ask him to describe it fully. Find out if it's unilateral or bilateral, and continuous or intermittent. Ask the patient about a family history of hearing loss. Obtain the patient's medical history, noting chronic ear infections, ear surgery, and ear or head trauma. Also find out if the patient recently had an upper respiratory infection. After taking a drug history, have the patient describe his occupation and work environment.

CRITICAL POINT *Patients taking certain antibiotics and other medications may experience hearing loss.*

Ask the patient to be more specific about complaints of pain, such as onset, location, intensity, and associated symptoms. The patient may describe such signs and symptoms as:

- pain caused by touching or pulling the ear, which usual indicates an external ear infection
- deep, throbbing pain, which indicates a middle ear disorder
- severely inflamed outer ear, which results from a swollen or completely blocked ear canal
- feeling of pressure or blockage, which may stem from a eustachian tube dysfunction that creates negative pressure in the middle ear or from muscle spasm or temporomandibular joint arthralgia.

Earaches in patients usually result from disorders of the external and middle ear associated with infection, obstruction, or trauma. Their severity ranges from a feeling of fullness or blockage to deep, boring pain; at times, earaches may be difficult to localize precisely. Signs and symptoms may be intermittent or continuous and may develop suddenly or gradually.

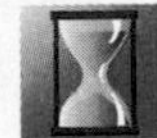

AGE ISSUE *In children, common causes of earache are acute otitis media and insertion of foreign bodies that become lodged or infected. Be alert for crying or ear tugging in a young child—nonverbal clues that signal earache.*

Investigate complaints of ear discharge. Ask about color and consistency, onset, and any history of head injury. Ask if the patient has feelings of abnormal movement or vertigo (spinning). Determine when episodes occur, how often, any recurrence, or if nausea, vomiting, or tinnitus occur with it. Also evaluate the patient if he has allergies.

CRITICAL POINT *Patients with environmental or seasonal allergies may experience serous otitis media, or inflammation of the middle ear. Otitis externa, or inflammation of the external ear, can be caused by allergic reactions to hair dyes, cosmetics, perfumes, and other personal care products.*

Nose assessment

The most common complaints about the nose include nasal stuffiness, nasal discharge, and epistaxis (nosebleed). Ask if the patient has had any of these problems. Ask about the color and consistency of any discharge. Also ask about frequent colds, hay fever, headaches, and sinus trouble. Ask whether certain conditions or environments seem to cause or aggravate the patient's problem.

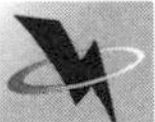

CRITICAL POINT *Environmental allergies can cause nasal stuffiness and discharge, and stagnant nasal discharge can act as a culture medium and lead to sinusitis and other nasal infections.*

Ask if he has ever had nose or head trauma. Also ask about insertion of a foreign body.

If the patient's chief complaint is epistaxis and he isn't in any distress, ask these questions:

- Is there a history of recent trauma?
- How often have nosebleeds occurred in the past?
- Have the nosebleeds been long or unusually severe?
- Has the patient recently had surgery in the sinus area?

Also ask about a family history of hypertension, bleeding, or liver disorders and other illnesses. Ask whether the patient bruises easily. Find out what drugs he uses, especially anti-inflammatories such as aspirin and anticoagulants such as warfarin.

If the patient complains of nasal obstruction, ask him about the duration and frequency of the obstruction. Find out if it began suddenly or gradually, and if it's intermittent or persistent, or unilateral or bilateral. Inquire about the presence and character of drainage, such as watery, purulent, or bloody. Nasal obstruction in a patient may result from an inflammatory, neoplastic, endocrine, or metabolic disorder; a structural abnormality; or a traumatic injury. It may cause discomfort, alter a patient's sense of taste and smell, and cause voice changes.

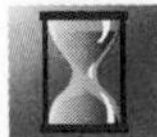

AGE ISSUE *In children, acute nasal obstruction usually results from the common cold. In infants and children, especially between ages 3 and 6, chronic nasal obstruction typically results from large adenoids. In neonates, choanal*

atresia is the most common congenital cause of nasal obstruction and can be unilateral or bilateral. Cystic fibrosis may cause nasal polyps in children, resulting in nasal obstruction. However, if the child has unilateral nasal obstruction and rhinorrhea, assume that there's a foreign body in the nose until proven otherwise.

Investigate if the patient has any nasal or sinus pain or headaches. Ask about recent travel, the use of drugs or alcohol, and previous trauma or surgery.

CRITICAL POINT *Although a frequent and typically benign symptom, nasal obstruction may herald certain life-threatening disorders, such as a basilar skull fracture or a malignant tumor.*

Throat and neck assessment

Ask the patient if he has bleeding or sore gums, mouth or tongue ulcers, a bad taste in his mouth, bad breath, toothaches, loose teeth, frequent sore throats, hoarseness, or facial swelling. Also ask whether he smokes or uses other types of tobacco.

If the patient is having neck problems, ask if he has neck pain or tenderness, neck swelling, or trouble moving his neck.

Further assess throat pain by asking the patient when he first noticed the pain, and have him describe it. Find out if he has had throat pain before and whether it's accompanied by fever, ear pain, or dysphagia. Review the patient's medical history for throat problems, allergies, and systemic disorders. If a patient experiences throat pain — commonly known as a sore throat — he has discomfort in any part of the pharynx that includes the nasopharynx, the oropharynx, or the hypopharynx. This common symptom ranges from a sensation of scratchiness to severe pain. It's typically accompanied by ear pain because cranial nerves IX and X innervate the pharynx as well as the middle and external ear.

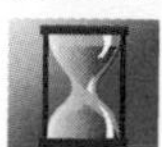

AGE ISSUE *In children, sore throat is a common complaint and may result from many of the same disorders that affect adults. Acute epiglottiditis, herpangina, scarlet fever, acute follicular tonsillitis, and retropharyngeal abscess are other common causes of sore throat in children.*

If the patient complains of dysphagia or difficulty swallowing, ask him these questions:

- Is swallowing painful? If so, is the pain constant or intermittent? (Have the patient point to where dysphagia feels most intense.)
- Does eating alleviate or aggravate the symptom?
- Are solids or liquids more difficult to swallow? If the answer is liquids, do hot, cold, or lukewarm fluids affect him differently?
- Does the symptom disappear after he tries to swallow a few times?
- Is swallowing easier if he changes position?
- Has he has recently experienced vomiting, regurgitation, weight loss, anorexia, hoarseness, dyspnea, or a cough?

In patients with esophageal disorders, dysphagia is the most common — and sometimes only — symptom. However, it may also result from an oropharyngeal, respiratory, neurologic, or collagen disorder or from the effects of toxins and treatments. (See *Classifying dysphagia,* page 150.)

CRITICAL POINT *Dysphagia increases the risk of choking and aspiration and may lead to malnutrition and dehydration.*

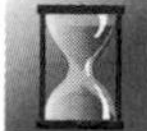

AGE ISSUE *In infants and young children, be sure to pay close attention to sucking and swallowing ability. Coughing, choking, or regurgitation during feeding suggests dysphagia. More common in children than adults, corrosive esophagitis and esophageal obstruction by a foreign body are causes of dysphagia. However, dysphagia may also result from congenital anomalies, such as annular stenosis, dysphagia lusoria, and esophageal atresia. In patients over age 50 with head or neck cancer, dysphagia is usually the first symptom that causes them to seek care.*

General health history

After asking specific questions about the ears, nose, and throat, and their related structures, ask questions about the patient's general health.

Ask the patient these questions pertaining to signs and symptoms:

- Have you noticed changes in the way you tolerate hot and cold weather?
- Has your weight changed recently?
- Do you have breathing problems or feel as if your heart is skipping beats?

CLASSIFYING DYSPHAGIA

Dysphagia is classified by the phase of swallowing it affects.

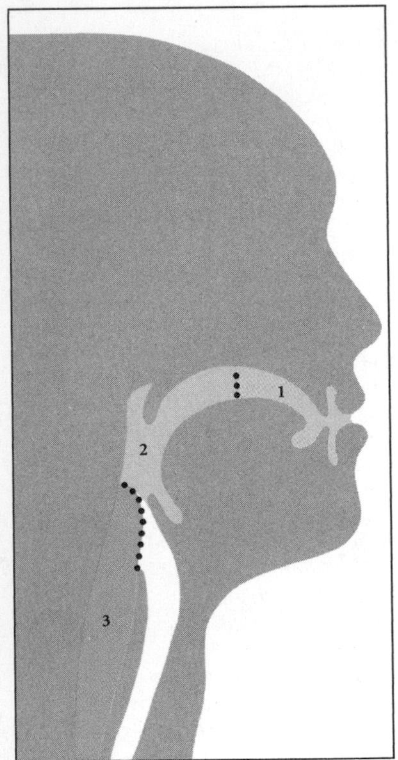

Phase 1
Dysphagia in phase 1, or the transfer phase, occurs when the tongue presses against the hard palate to transfer the chewed food to the back of the throat. Cranial nerve V then stimulates the swallowing reflex. This phase usually results from a neuromuscular disorder.

Phase 2
Dysphagia in phase 2, or the transport phase, occurs when the soft palate closes against the pharyngeal wall to prevent nasal regurgitation. At the same time, the larynx rises and the vocal chords close to keep food out of the lungs. Breathing stops momentarily as the throat muscles constrict to move food into the esophagus. This phase usually indicates spasm or cancer.

Phase 3
Dysphagia in phase 3, or the entrance phase, occurs as food moves through the esophageal sphincter and into the stomach. This phase results from lower esophageal narrowing by diverticula, esophagitis, and other disorders.

- Have you noticed a change in your menstrual pattern?
- Do you have a family history of Graves' disease?
- Have you noticed any tremors, agitation, difficulty concentrating, or sleeping?

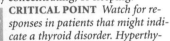

CRITICAL POINT *Watch for responses in patients that might indicate a thyroid disorder. Hyperthyroidism can cause heat intolerance, weight loss, and a short menstrual pattern with scant flow. Hypothyroidism can cause cold intolerance, weight gain, an increase in menstrual pattern and flow and, in extreme cases, bradycardia and dyspnea from low cardiac output.*

Physical assessment

Examining the ears, nose, and throat, and their related structures, mainly involves using the techniques of inspection, palpation, and auscultation. An ear assessment also requires the use of an otoscope and the administration of hearing acuity tests.

Ear examination

To assess your patient's ears, inspect and palpate the external structures, perform an otoscopic examination of the ear canal and test his hearing acuity.

Inspection and palpation

Begin by observing the patient's ears for position and symmetry. The top of the ear

RECOGNIZING COMMON ABNORMAL SKIN FINDINGS

On this page and the pages that follow, you'll find photos of common abnormal skin findings along with brief descriptions of each. Use the photos to guide your assessment.

Basal cell carcinoma

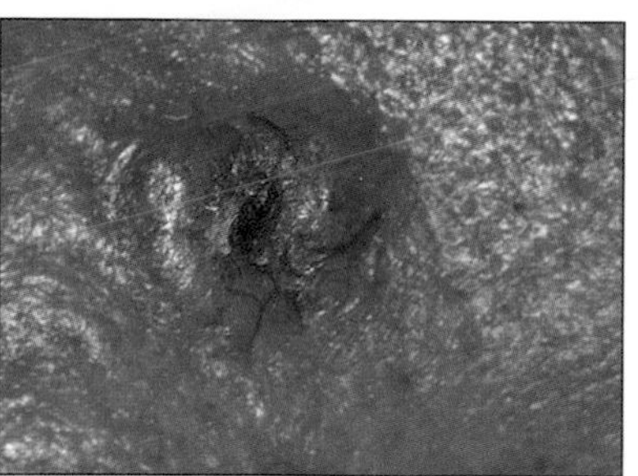

The most common type of skin cancer, basal cell carcinoma results from sun exposure. It usually appears as a small waxy-looking nodule that ulcerates and forms a central depression. Basal cell carcinoma typically starts as a skin-colored papule (may be deeply pigmented) with a translucent top and overlying telangiectases. It rarely metastasizes and commonly appears on the head and neck.

Malignant melanoma

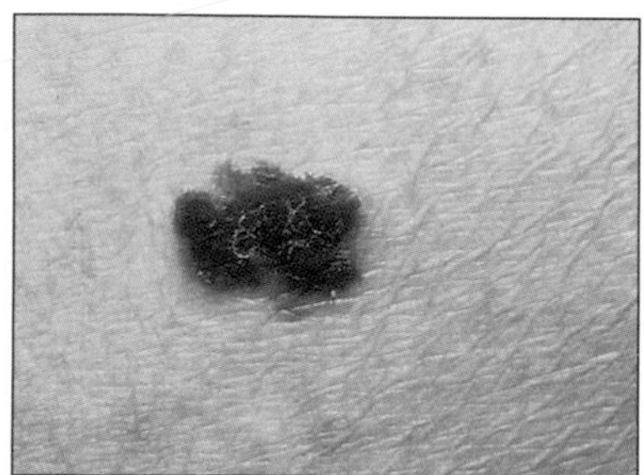

Malignant melanoma can occur anywhere on the body and can arise from a preexisting mole. Its border, color, and surface are usually irregular. The lesion is usually black or purple (although some may be pink, red, or whitish-blue) and may be accompanied by scaling, flaking, or oozing. Melanoma spreads through the lymphatic and vascular systems and can metastasize to the regional lymph nodes liver, lungs, and central nervous system.

Squamous cell carcinoma

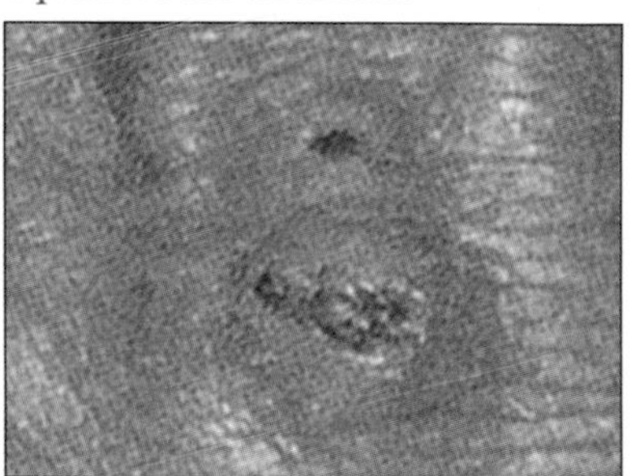

Squamous cell carcinoma results from sun exposure and can metastasize. It appears as a raised border with a central ulcer and may be rough, thickened, or scaly. It most commonly appears on the face and neck as an erythematous scaly patch with sharp edges.

Kaposi's sarcoma

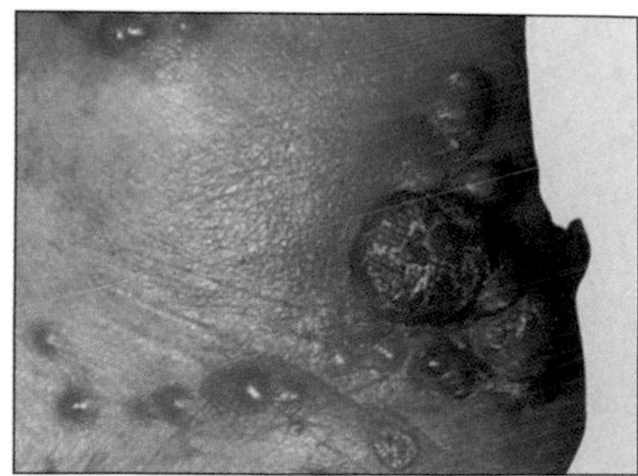

Kaposi's sarcoma commonly appears first on the lower legs; however, the lesions may develop anywhere. Initially, you'll note multiple brown or bluish red nodules of varying shapes and sizes. These nodules develop into larger plaques that may open and drain or cause edema of the legs.

(continued)

RECOGNIZING COMMON ABNORMAL SKIN FINDINGS *(continued)*

Lupus erythematosus (discoid or systemic)

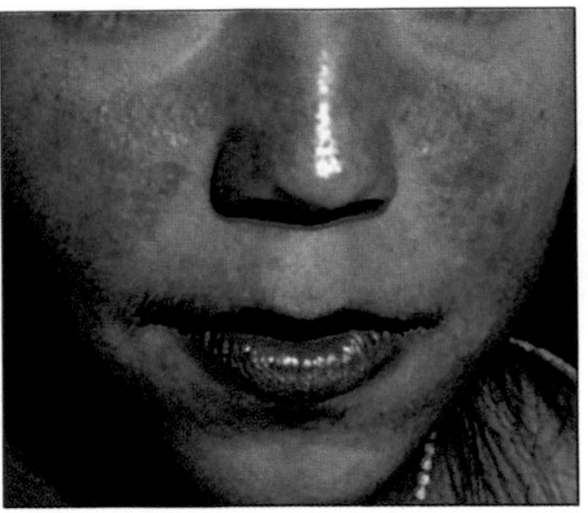

The typical sign of lupus erythematosus, a butterfly-shaped rash, appears as a red, scaly, sharply demarcated rash over the cheeks and nose. The rash may extend to other areas of the face or to other exposed areas, such as the ears and neck.

Scabies

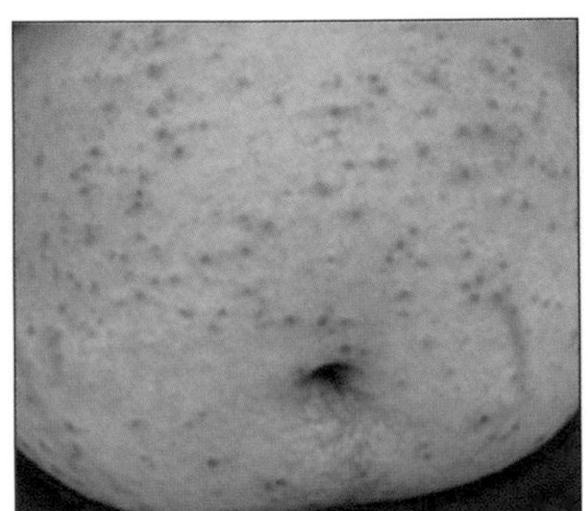

Mites, which can be picked up from an infested person, burrow under the skin and cause scabies lesions. The lesions appear in a straight or zigzagging line about 1 cm long with a black dot at the end. Commonly seen between the fingers, at the bend of the elbow and knee, and around the groin or perineal area, scabies lesions itch and may cause a rash.

Telangiectasia

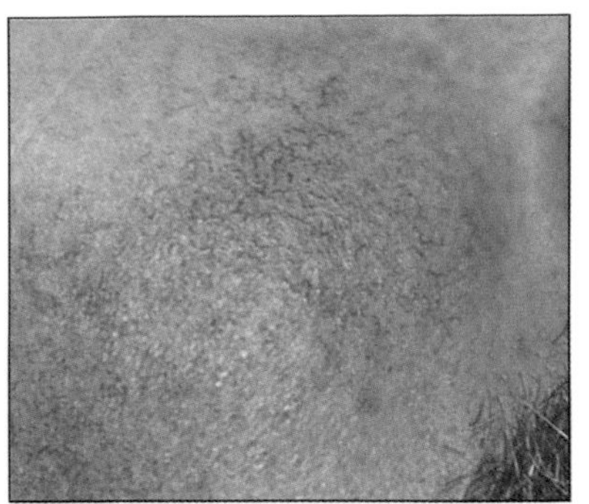

Formed by dilation of small blood vessels, telangiectasia blanches when pressure is applied. This type of lesion may be a normal finding in an elderly person or may be associated with cirrhosis or lupus erythematosus.

Vitiligo

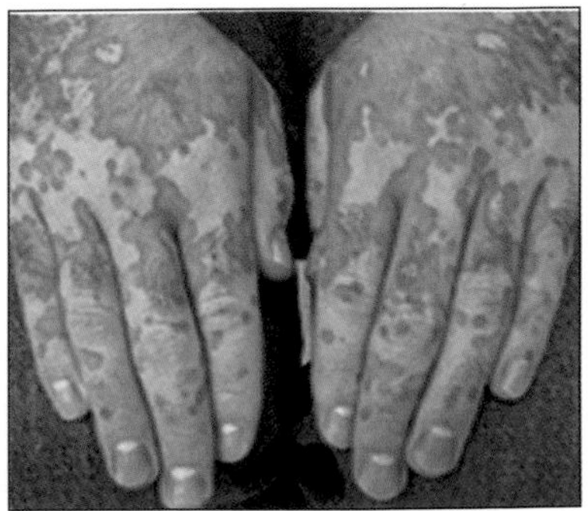

Vitiligo is a slowly progressive disease of hypopigmentation that causes irregular areas of pigmented skin around milk-colored patches. These areas commonly appear on the face, hands, and feet.

Psoriasis

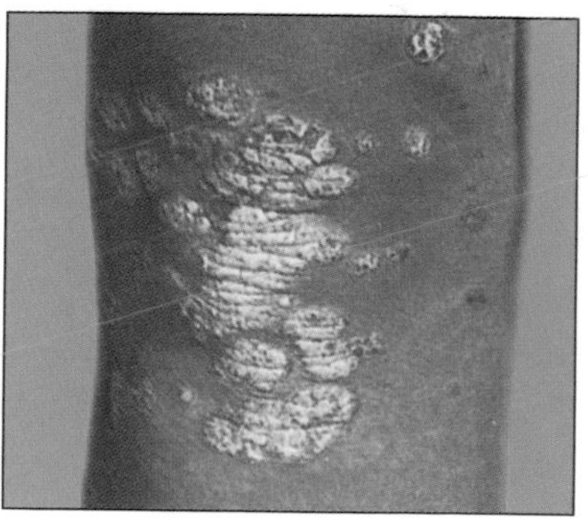

Psoriasis is a chronic disease of marked epidermal thickening and plaques that are symmetrical and that generally appear as red bases topped with silvery scales. The lesions, which may connect with one another, occur most commonly on the scalp, elbows, and knees.

Contact dermatitis

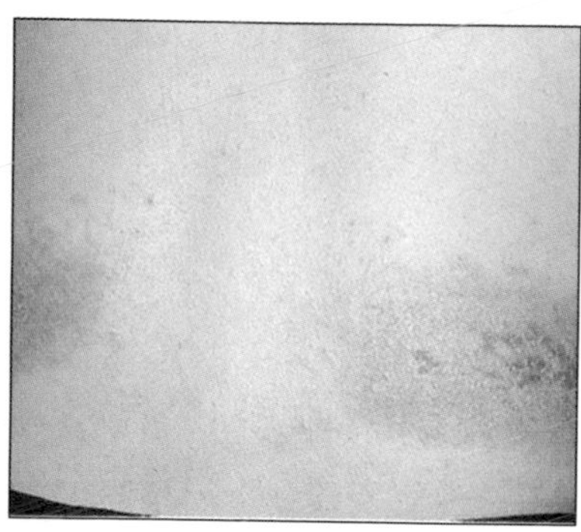

Contact dermatitis is an inflammatory disorder that results from contact with an irritant. Primary lesions, including vesicles, large oozing bullae, and red macules that appear at localized areas of redness, may itch and burn.

Urticaria (hives)

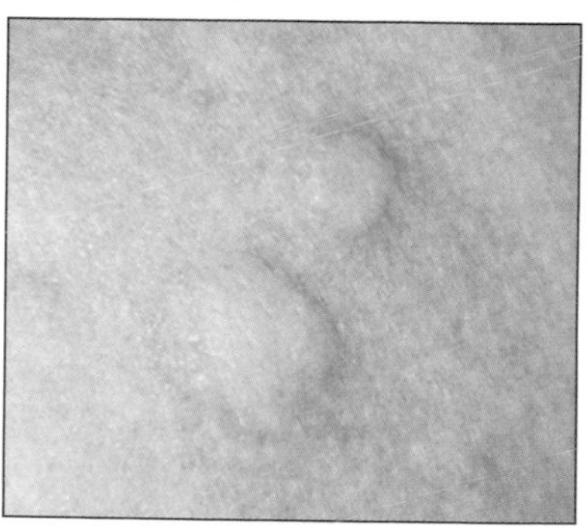

Occurring as an allergic reaction, urticaria appears suddenly as pink, edematous papules or wheals (round elevations of the skin) that cause intense itching. The lesions may become large and contain vesicles.

Eczema

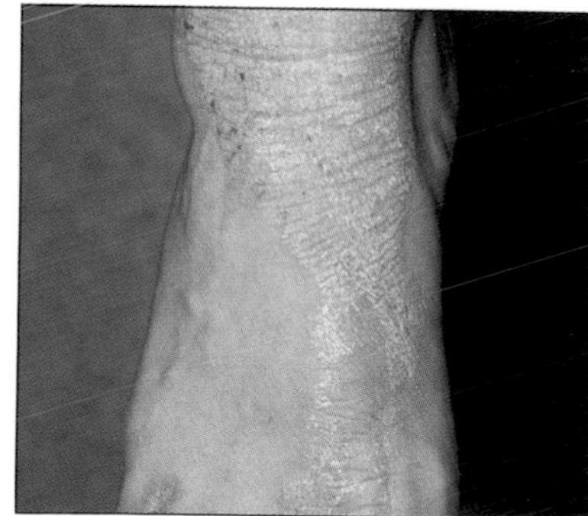

Eczema may be acute or chronic and may be accompanied by severe itching. It appears as reddened papules, vesicles, or pustular lesions and typically affects the antecubital and popliteal areas. Blisters, oozing, and crusting may occur. Thickening, excoriation, and extreme dryness of the skin can also occur.

(continued)

RECOGNIZING COMMON ABNORMAL SKIN FINDINGS *(continued)*

Herpes zoster

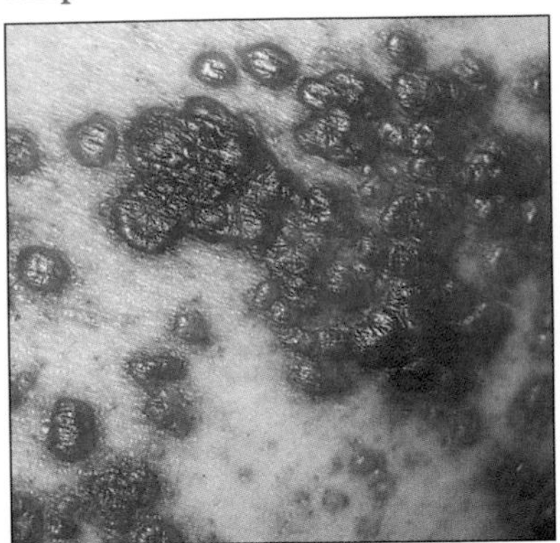

Herpes zoster appears as a group of vesicles or crusted lesions along a nerve root. The vesicles are usually unilateral and typically appear on the face, hands, and neck. These lesions cause pain but not itching or rash.

Candidiasis

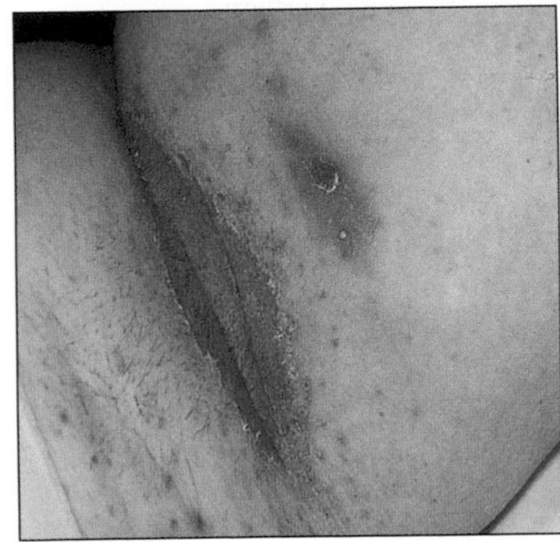

Candidiasis is a fungal infection that produces erythema and a scaly, papular rash. Because the fungus thrives in moist environments, it usually occurs under the breasts and in the axillae.

Tinea corporis (ringworm)

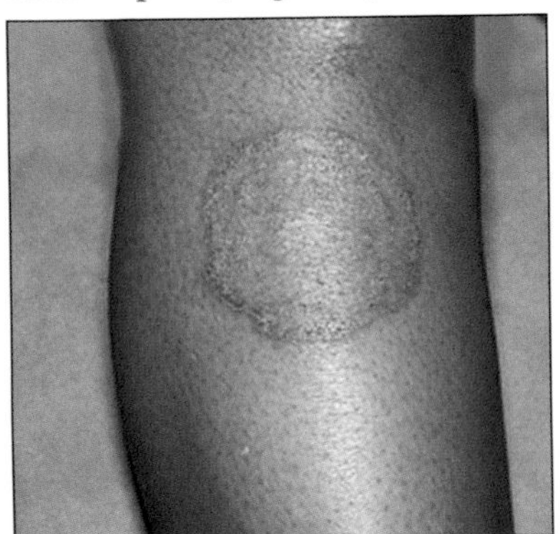

Tinea corporis are round, red, scaly lesions that are accompanied by intense itching. These lesions have slightly raised, red borders consisting of tiny vesicles. Individual rings may connect to form patches with scalloped edges. They usually appear on exposed areas of the body.

Impetigo

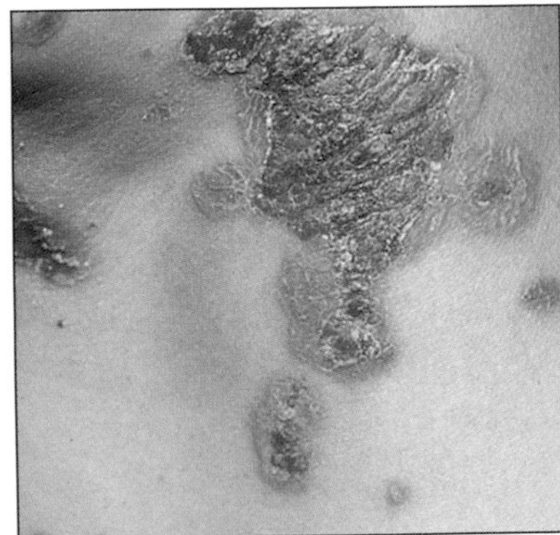

Impetigo is a rash that usually appears on the face. It's caused by a bacterial infection. When ruptured, fragile vesicles in the rash ooze a honey-colored fluid and crusts may form.

ABNORMAL FINDINGS OF THE EAR

Otitis media

Otitis media is an inflammation of the middle ear. It can be caused by bacteria, viruses, allergies, or malfunctions of the eustachian tubes.

Inflammation may be accompanied by an accumulation of fluid in the middle ear that may restrict the movement of the eardrum and may result in hearing loss. Pain may occur if there's pressure from the fluid against the eardrum.

NORMAL RIGHT EARDRUM

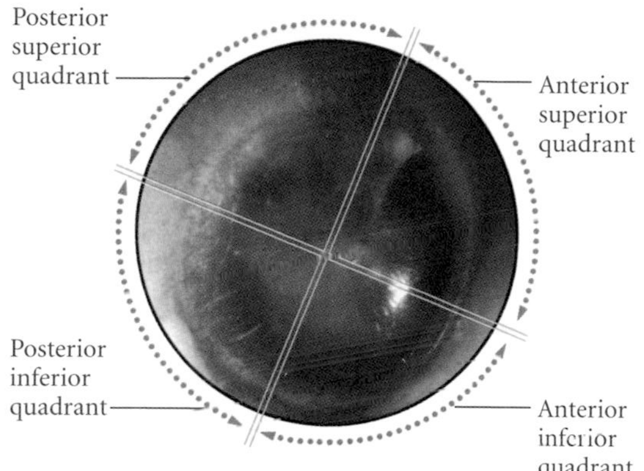

Classification and common complications of otitis media

The illustrations below show three of the classifications along with common complications of otitis media.

ACUTE OTITIS MEDIA

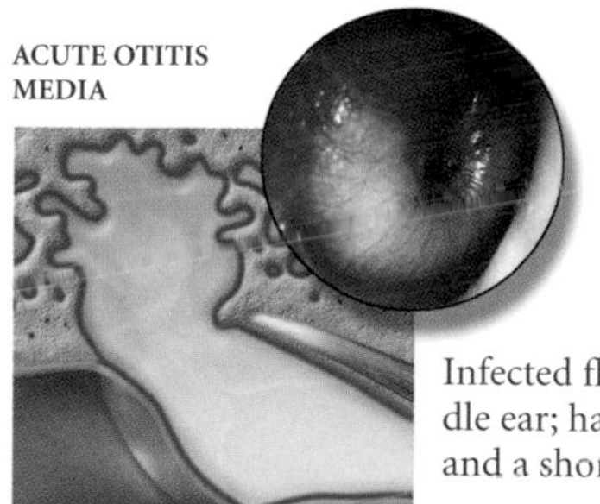

Infected fluid in the middle ear; has a rapid onset and a short duration

OTITIS MEDIA WITH EFFUSION

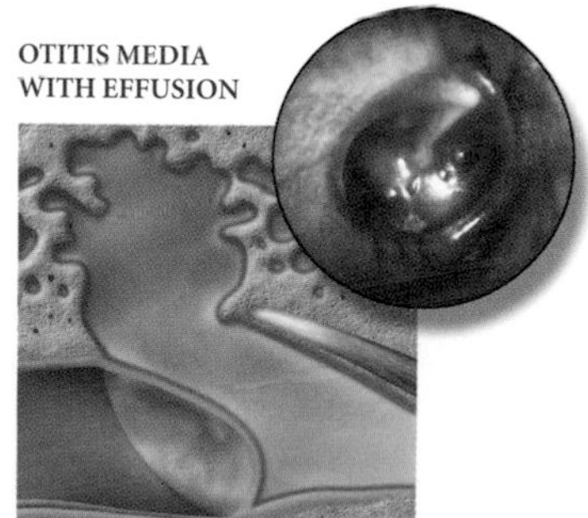

Fluid in the middle ear that may be acute, subacute, or chronic; produces relatively few symptoms

PERFORATION

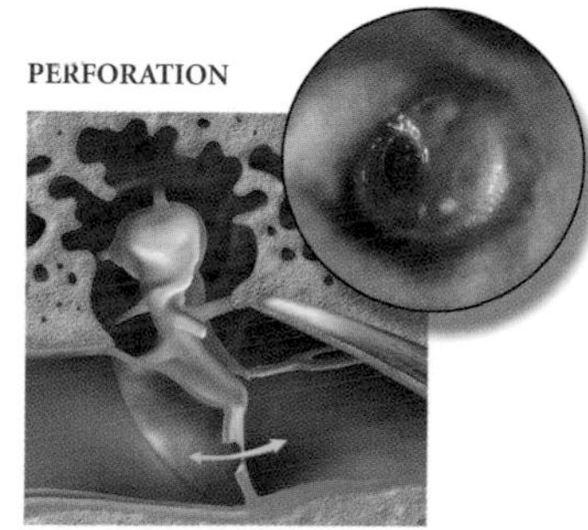

A hole in the tympanic membrane caused by chronic negative middle ear pressure, inflammation, or trauma

ABNORMAL FINDINGS OF THE EYE

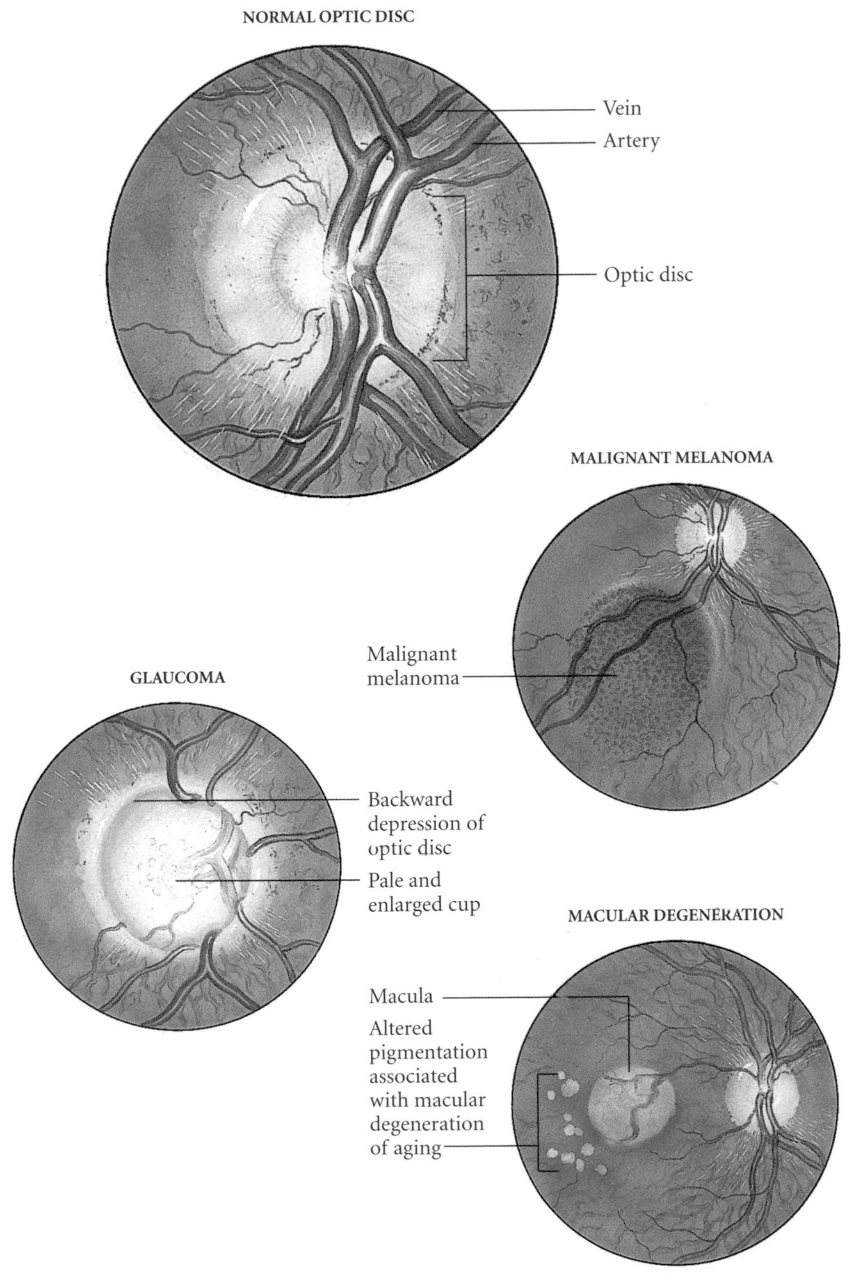

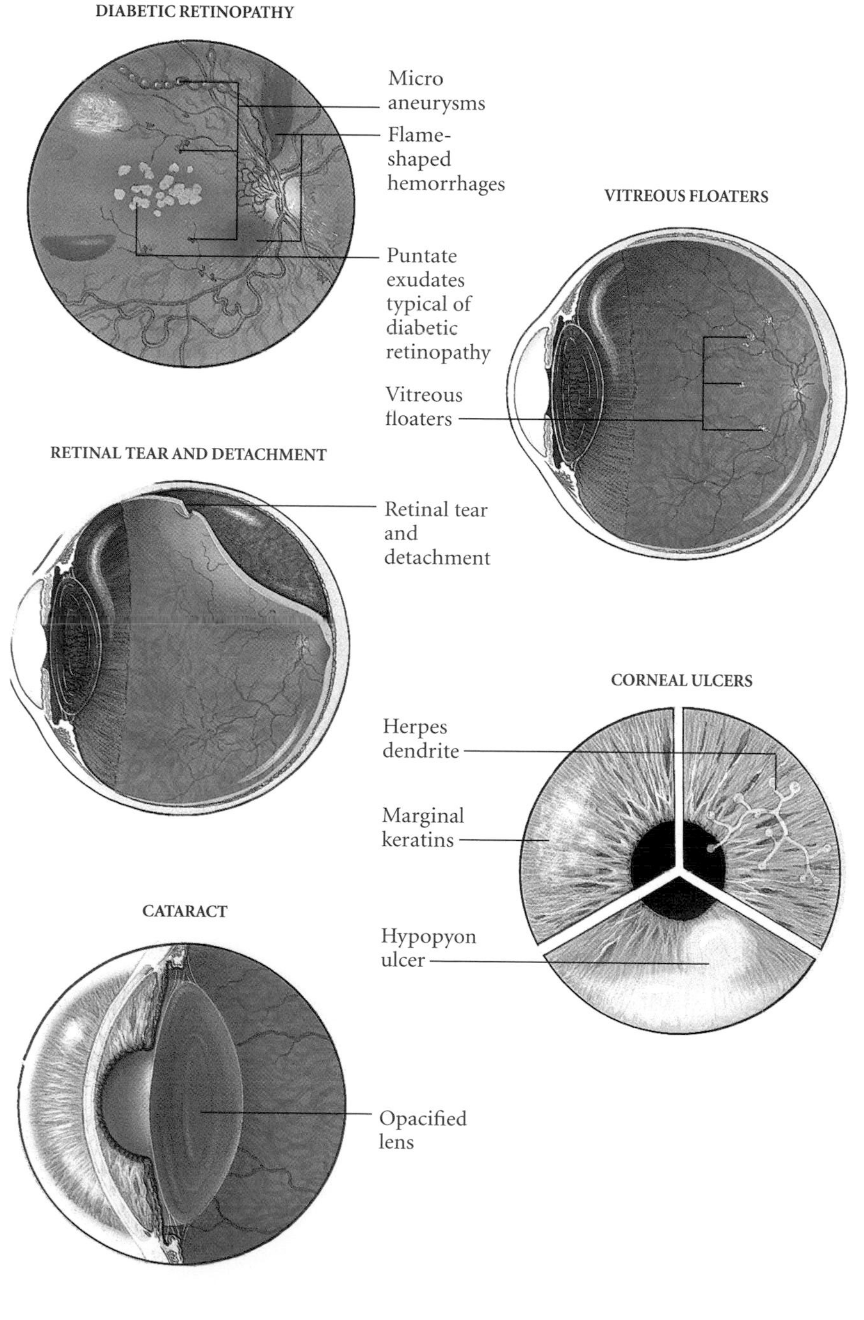
DIABETIC RETINOPATHY
Micro aneurysms
Flame-shaped hemorrhages
Puntate exudates typical of diabetic retinopathy
VITREOUS FLOATERS
Vitreous floaters
RETINAL TEAR AND DETACHMENT
Retinal tear and detachment
CORNEAL ULCERS
Herpes dendrite
Marginal keratins
Hypopyon ulcer
CATARACT
Opacified lens

ABNORMAL FINDINGS OF THE NOSE AND MOUTH

Abnormal findings of the nose and mouth can result from the common cold, an upper respiratory tract infection, or acute rhinitis. Look for swelling and increased discharge from the mucous membranes lining the nose as well as inflammation of the mucous membranes of the head and throat.

Paranasal sinuses
Within the bones surrounding the nose are many air-filled sacs called *sinuses.* The mucous membranes lining these sinuses are continuous with the nasal lining, and infections may easily spread through the openings in the nose. If bacteria invade the sinuses *(sinusitis)*, look for gray, yellow, or green nasal discharge.

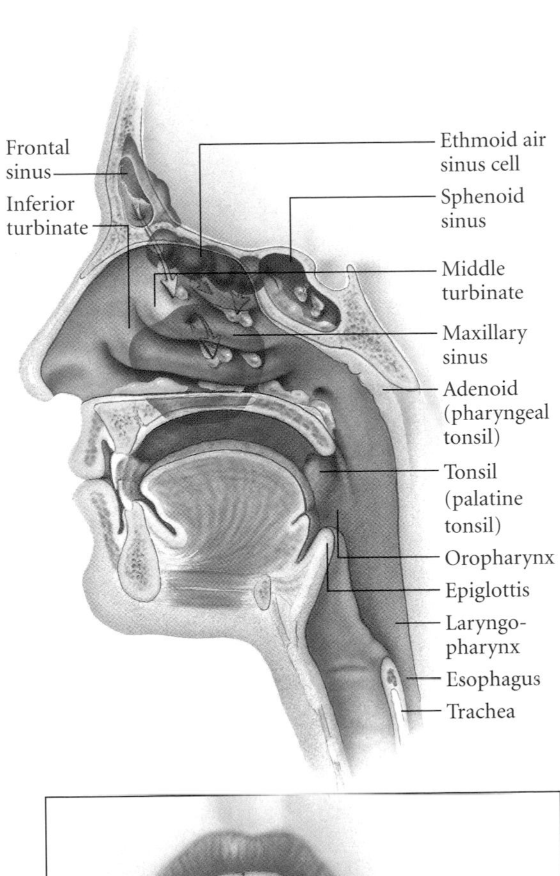

The throat and tonsils
Airborne particles, viruses, and bacteria that aren't trapped in the nose or in the mouth may land on the pharynx. As shown in the illustration at right, a circle of lymphatic tissue surrounds the pharynx and serves as a first line of defense. Inflammation affecting the throat and tonsils causes swelling, redness, and pain with swallowing and is commonly called a *sore throat.* Bacteria (most frequently *Streptococcus*) may cause a more severe infection called *strep throat*. An infection of the palatine tonsils is called *tonsillitis* and their enlargement may cause discomfort.

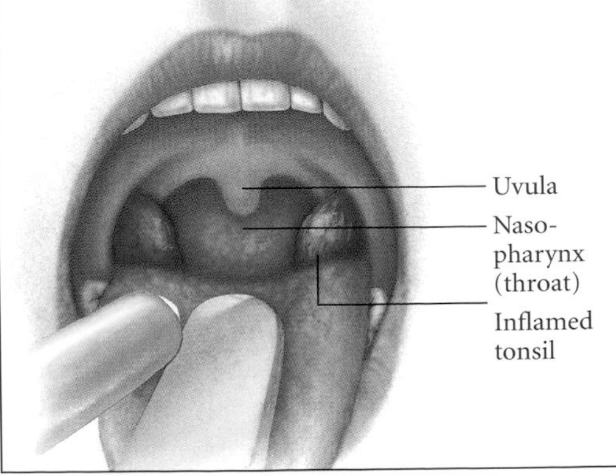

should line up with the outer corner of the eye, and the ears should look symmetrical, with an angle of attachment no more than 10 degrees. The face and ears should be the same shade and color.

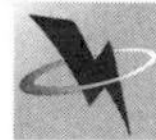

CRITICAL POINT *Low-set ears commonly accompany congenital disorders, including kidney problems.*

Auricles that protrude from the head, or "lop" ears, are fairly common and don't affect hearing ability.

Inspect the auricle for lesions, drainage, nodules, or redness. Pull the helix back, and note if it's tender. If the patient feels pain when you pull the ear back, he may have otitis externa. If the patient has crusted, indurated, or ulcerated lesions that fail to heal, they should be excised and examined. These lesions may indicate a fairly common disorder known as carcinoma of the auricle, which may be either basal cell or squamous cell. Advanced lesions are easy to diagnose, but small growths are commonly overlooked.

Next, inspect and palpate the mastoid area behind each auricle. Assess for tenderness, redness, or warmth. Tenderness behind the ear may be present in otitis media. Redness or warmth could signal a local infection.

Finally, inspect the opening of the ear canal. Patients normally have varying amounts of hair and cerumen, or earwax, in the ear canal. Cerumen may be flaky and vary in color.

CRITICAL POINT *Be alert for ear discharge, redness, or odor. Also look for nodules or cysts. In acute otitis externa, the ear canal is often swollen, narrowed, moist, pale, tender, and sometimes, reddened. In chronic otitis externa, the ear canal is usually thickened, red, and itchy. Cerumen shouldn't be impacted in a normal ear canal.*

Temporomandibular joints

Inspect and palpate the temporomandibular joints, which are located anterior to and slightly below the auricle. To palpate these joints, place the middle three fingers of each hand bilaterally over each joint. Then gently press on the joints as the patient opens and closes his mouth. Evaluate the joints for movability, approximation (drawing of bones together), and discomfort. Normally, this process should be smooth and painless for the patient. The patient shouldn't experience neck pain, vertigo, otalgia, or stuffiness in the ear. Dislocation of the temporomandibular joints may be related to trauma. Arthritis may cause swelling, tenderness, and decreased range of motion. Crepitus or clicking may occur with poor occlusion, meniscus injury, or swelling caused by trauma.

Otoscopic examination

The next part of the ear assessment involves examining the patient's auditory canal, tympanic membrane, and malleus with the otoscope. (See *Using an otoscope,* page 152.)

Before inserting the speculum into the patient's ear canal, check the canal for foreign particles or discharge.

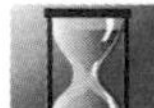

AGE ISSUE *In younger children, obstruction of the ear canal by a foreign body commonly occurs. Inanimate objects and vegetables are the most common objects found in a child's ear canal; cotton is the most common object found in an adult's ear canal. Pain and drainage may signal a foreign body, but sometimes no signs or symptoms occur, and the object may be found during a routine examination.*

Next, palpate the tragus — the cartilaginous projection anterior to the external opening of the ear — and pull the auricle up.

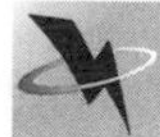

CRITICAL POINT *If the patient's tragus is tender, don't insert the speculum. He could have otitis externa, and inserting the speculum could cause pain.*

To insert the speculum of the otoscope, tilt the patient's head away from you. Grasp the superior posterior auricle with your thumb and index finger and pull it up and back to straighten the canal. Keep your hand along the patient's face to steady the otoscope. As everyone's ear canal is shaped differently, vary the angle of the speculum until you can see the tympanic membrane.

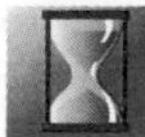

AGE ISSUE *Because an ear examination may upset the child with an earache, perform this part at the end of your physical examination. To examine the child's ears, place him in a supine position with his arms extended and held securely by his parent. Hold the otoscope with*

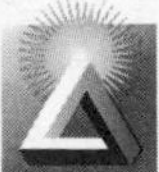

EXPERT TECHNIQUE

USING AN OTOSCOPE

The instructions below describe how to use an otoscope to examine the patient's ears.

Inserting the speculum
Before inserting the speculum into the patient's ear, straighten the ear canal by grasping the auricle and pulling it up and back, as shown.

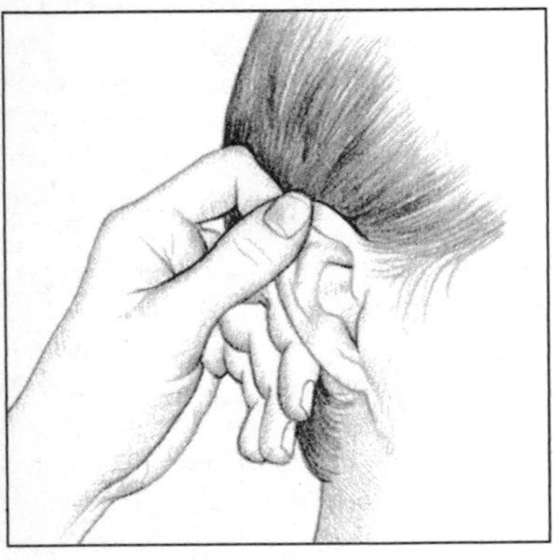

Positioning the scope
To examine the ear's external canal, hold the otoscope with the handle parallel to the patient's head, as shown. Bracing your hand firmly against his head prevents you from hitting the ear canal with the speculum.

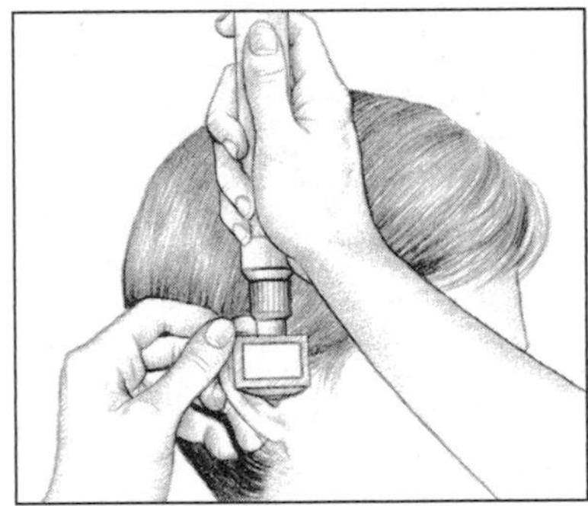

Viewing the structures
When the otoscope is positioned properly, you should see the tympanic membrane structures shown here.

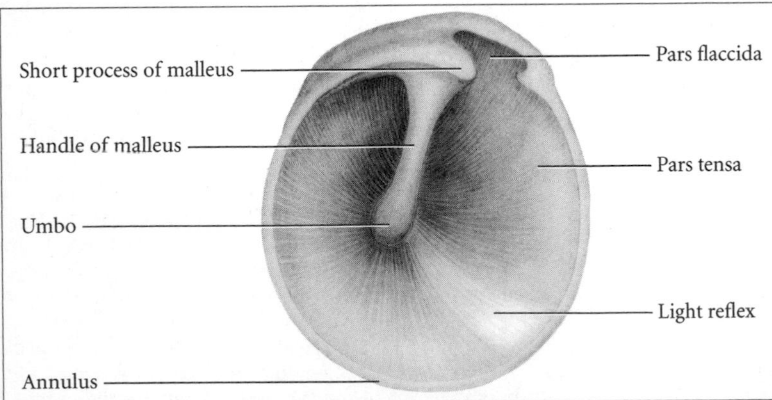

the handle pointing toward the top of the child's head and brace it against him using one or two fingers. If your patient is younger than age 3, pull the auricle down to get a better view of the tympanic membrane.

Insert the speculum to about one-third its length when inspecting the ear canal. Make sure you insert it gently because the inner two-thirds of the canal is sensitive to pressure. Note the color of the cerumen.

Cerumen that's grayish brown and dry-looking is old. The external canal should be free from inflammation and scaling.

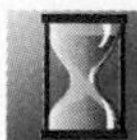

AGE ISSUE *The elderly patient may have harder, drier cerumen because of rigid cilia in the ear canal. A cloudy appearing eardrum is a normal finding related to aging.*

Examine the tympanic membrane for the light reflex. The light reflex in the right ear should be between 4 and 6 o'clock; in the left ear, it should be between 6 and 8 o'clock. If the light reflex in a patient's ear is displaced or absent, the tympanic membrane may be bulging, inflamed, or retracted.

If necessary, carefully rotate the speculum for a complete view of the tympanic membrane. The membrane should be pearl gray, glistening, and transparent. The annulus should be white and denser than the rest of the membrane.

If excessive cerumen obstructs the view of the tympanic membrane, don't try to remove it with an instrument or you could cause the patient excessive pain. Instead, use ceruminolytic drops and warm water irrigation as ordered.

Check the patient's tympanic membrane carefully for bulging, retraction, bleeding, lesions, or perforations, especially at the periphery. A perforated tympanic membrane appears as a hole surrounded by reddened tissue. You may see discharge draining through the perforated area.

Finally, look for the bony landmarks. The malleus will appear as a dense, white streak at the 12 o'clock position. At the top of the light reflex, find the umbo, the inferior point of the malleus.

Hearing acuity testing

The last part of an ear assessment is testing the patient's hearing acuity. Begin by estimating hearing by performing the whispered voice test and the ticking watch test. For the whispered voice test, ask the patient to occlude one ear, or occlude it for him. Move your finger quickly, but gently, in the ear canal. Then stand 1′ to 2′ (30.5 to 61 cm) from the patient, exhale fully, and whisper softly toward the unoccluded ear. Choose numbers or words that have two syllables that are equally accented such as "nine-four" or "baseball." To perform the ticking watch test, hold a ticking watch close to the patient's ear. Then move it away from his ear until he can't hear the ticking. Note the distance.

If hearing is diminished, use the Weber's and Rinne tests to assess conductive hearing loss, which is impaired sound transmission to the inner ear, and sensorineural hearing loss, which is impaired auditory nerve conduction or inner ear function. (See *Performing the Weber's and Rinne tests,* page 154.)

Weber's test

Weber's test is performed when the patient reports diminished or lost hearing in one ear. This test involves using a tuning fork to evaluate bone conduction. The tuning fork should be tuned to the frequency of normal human speech, 512 cycles per second.

To perform Weber's test, strike the tuning fork lightly against your hand and place the fork on the patient's forehead at the midline or on the top of his head. If he hears the tone equally well in both ears, record this as a normal Weber's test. If he hears the tone better in one ear, record the result as right or left lateralization.

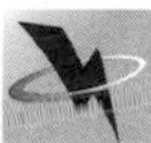

CRITICAL POINT *In a patient with conductive hearing loss, during lateralization the tone will sound louder in the ear with hearing loss because bone conducts the tone to the ear. Because the unaffected ear picks up other sounds, it doesn't hear the tone as clearly. In a patient with sensorineural hearing loss, sound is present in the unaffected ear.*

Rinne test

Perform the Rinne test after completing Weber's test to compare air conduction of sound with bone conduction of sound. To do this test, strike the tuning fork against your hand and place it over the patient's mastoid process. Ask him to tell you when the tone stops and note this time in seconds. Next, move the still-vibrating tuning fork to the opening of the ear without touching the ear. Ask him to tell you when the tone stops and note the time in seconds.

The patient should hear the air-conducted tone twice as long as he hears the bone-conducted tone. During the Rinne test, if the patient doesn't hear the air-conducted tone longer than the bone-conducted tone,

EXPERT TECHNIQUE

PERFORMING THE WEBER'S AND RINNE TESTS

The Weber's and Rinne tests can help determine whether the patient's hearing loss is conductive or sensorineural. The Weber's test evaluates bone conduction; the Rinne test, bone and air conduction. Using a 512-Hz tuning fork, perform these preliminary tests as described here.

Weber's test

Place the base of a vibrating tuning fork firmly against the midline of the patient's skull at the forehead. Ask her if she hears the tone equally well in both ears. If she does, the Weber's test is generally midline — a normal finding. In an abnormal Weber's test (graded right or left), sound is louder in one ear, suggesting a conductive hearing loss in that ear, or a sensorineural loss in the opposite ear.

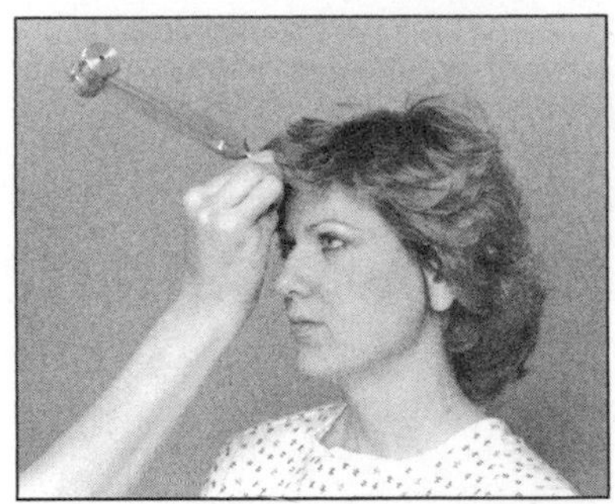

Rinne test

Hold the base of a vibrating tuning fork against the patient's mastoid process to test bone conduction. Then quickly move the vibrating fork in front of her ear canal to test for conduction. Ask her to tell you when a location has the louder or longer sound. Repeat the procedure for the other ear. In a positive Rinne test, air conduction lasts longer or sounds louder than bone conduction — a normal finding. In a negative test, the opposite is true: Bone conduction lasts longer or sounds louder than air conduction.

After performing both tests, correlate the results with other assessment data.

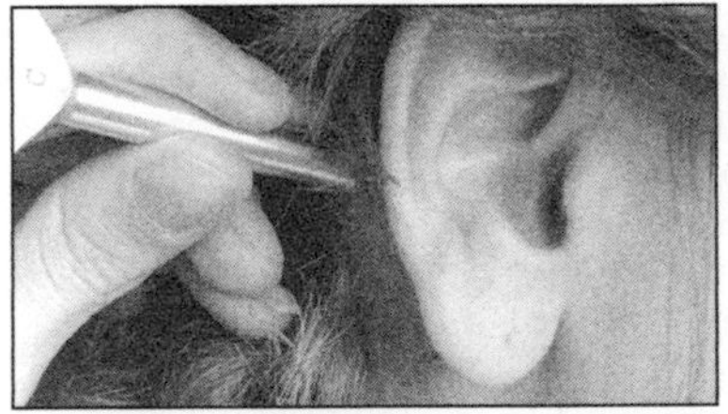

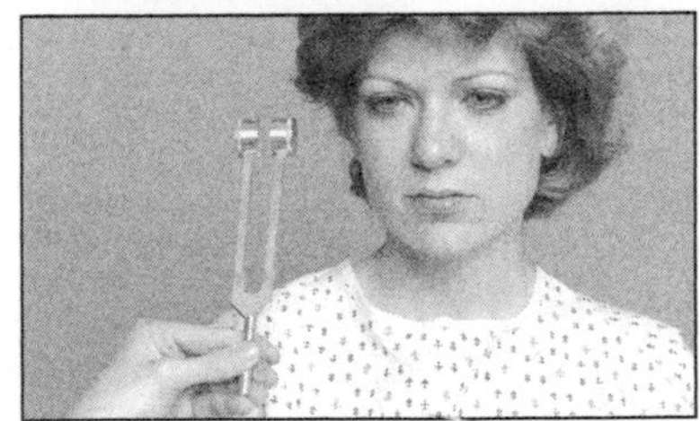

Implications of results

Conductive hearing loss produces:
- abnormal Weber's test results
- negative Rinne test result
- improved hearing in noisy areas
- normal ability to discriminate sounds
- difficulty hearing when chewing
- a quiet speaking voice.

Sensorineural hearing loss produces:
- positive Rinne test
- poor hearing in noisy areas
- difficulty hearing high-frequency sounds
- complaints that people mumble or shout
- tinnitus.

he has a conductive hearing loss in the affected ear.

Nose and sinus examination

A complete examination of the nose also includes assessing the sinuses. To perform this examination, use the techniques of inspection and palpation.

Nose inspection and palpation

Begin by observing the patient's nose for position, symmetry, and color. On inspection and palpation, you may find:

- variations, such as discoloration, swelling, deformity, or skin breakdown (Variations in size and shape are largely due to differences in cartilage and in the amount of fibroadipose tissue.)
- nasal discharge or flaring, which may be normal during quiet breathing in adults and in children

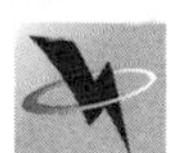

CRITICAL POINT *Marked, regular nasal flaring in an adult signals respiratory distress.*

- obstruction of the nasal mucous membranes along with a discharge of thin mucus, which can signal systemic disorders; nasal or sinus disorders such as a deviated septum; trauma, such as a basilar skull or nasal fracture; excessive use of vasoconstricting nose drops or sprays; and allergies or exposure to irritants, such as dust, tobacco smoke, or fumes
- nasal drainage accompanied by sinus tenderness and fever, which suggests acute sinusitis usually involving the frontal or maxillary sinuses
- bloody discharge, which usually results from the patient blowing his nose, but spontaneous or traumatic epistaxis can also occur
- thick, white, yellow, or greenish drainage, which suggests infection
- clear, thin drainage, which may simply indicate rhinitis, but must be monitored closely as it could be cerebrospinal fluid leaking due to a basilar skull fracture.

To test nasal patency and olfactory nerve (cranial nerve I) function, ask the patient to block one nostril and inhale a familiar aromatic substance through the other nostril. Possible substances include soap, coffee, citrus, tobacco, or nutmeg. Ask him to identify the aroma. Then repeat the process with the other nostril, using a different aroma.

Inspect the nasal cavity. Ask the patient to tilt his head back slightly and push the tip of his nose up. Use the light from the otoscope to illuminate his nasal cavities. Check the patient for severe deviation or perforation of the nasal septum. Examine the vestibule and turbinates for redness, softness, and discharge.

Examine the nostrils by direct inspection, using a nasal speculum and a penlight or small flashlight, or an otoscope with a short, wide-tip attachment. Have the patient sit in front of you with his head tilted back. Put on gloves and insert the tip of the closed nasal speculum into one nostril to the point where the blade widens. Slowly open the speculum as wide as possible without causing discomfort. Shine the flashlight in the nostril to illuminate the area.

Observe the color and patency of the nostril and check for exudate. The mucosa should be moist, pink to light red, and free from lesions and polyps. After inspecting one nostril, close the speculum, remove it, and inspect the other nostril. (See *Inspecting the nostrils,* page 156.)

In patients with viral rhinitis, the mucosa will appear red and swollen. In patients with allergic rhinitis, the mucosa may be pale, bluish, or red.

Finally, palpate the patient's nose with the thumb and forefinger, assessing for pain, tenderness, swelling, and deformity.

Sinus inspection and palpation

When examining the sinuses, remember, only the frontal and maxillary sinuses are accessible; you won't be able to palpate the ethmoidal and sphenoidal sinuses. However, if the frontal and maxillary sinuses are infected, you can assume that the other sinuses are as well.

Begin by checking for swelling around the eyes, especially over the sinus area. Then palpate the sinuses, checking for tenderness. (See *Palpating the sinuses,* page 156.) To palpate the frontal sinuses, place your thumbs above the patient's eyes just under the bony ridges of the upper orbits, and place your fingertips on the patient's forehead. Apply gentle pressure. Next, palpate the maxillary sinuses. If the patient complains of tenderness during palpation of the sinuses, use transillumination to see if the sinuses are filled with fluid or pus. Transillumination

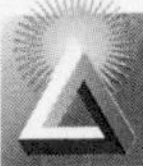

EXPERT TECHNIQUE

INSPECTING THE NOSTRILS

This illustration shows the proper placement of the nasal speculum during direct inspection and the structures you should be able to see during this examination.

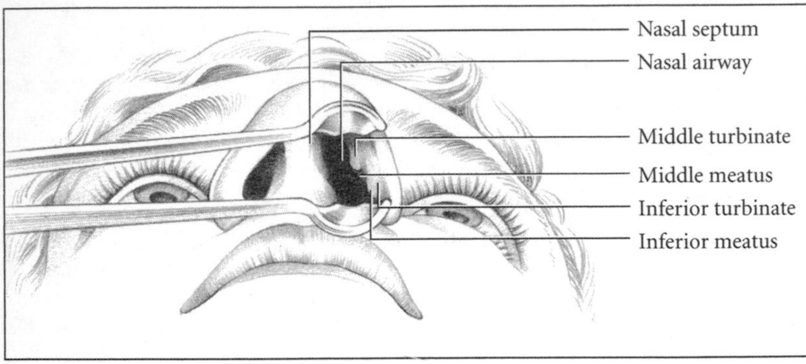

EXPERT TECHNIQUE

PALPATING THE SINUSES

This illustration shows the location of the frontal sinuses located on the forehead and maxillary sinuses located on each side of the nose. To palpate the maxillary sinuses, gently press your thumbs on each side of the nose just below the cheekbones, as shown.

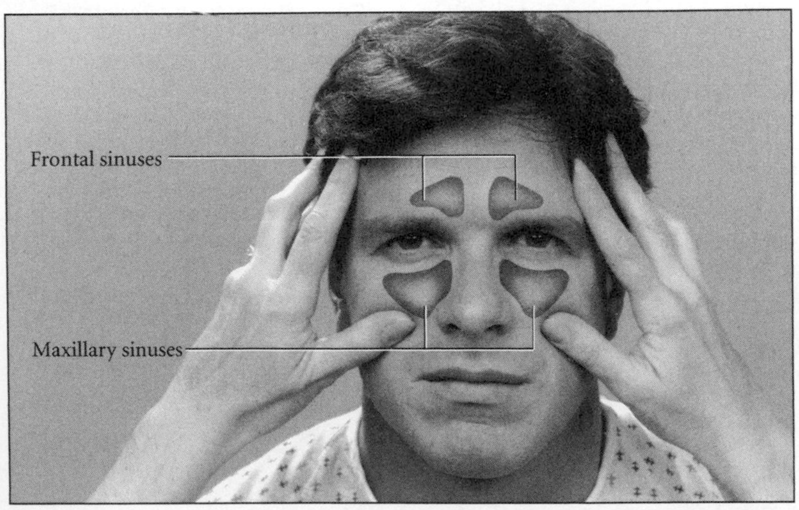

EXPERT TECHNIQUE

TRANSILLUMINATING THE SINUSES

Using a penlight you can transilluminate the sinuses so that you'll be able to detect sinus tumors and obstruction. Before you start, darken the room.

Frontal sinuses
Place the penlight on the supraorbital ring and direct the light upward to illuminate the frontal sinuses just above the eyebrow, as shown.

Maxillary sinuses
Place the penlight on the patient's cheekbone just below the eye and ask her to open her mouth. The light should transilluminate easily and equally.

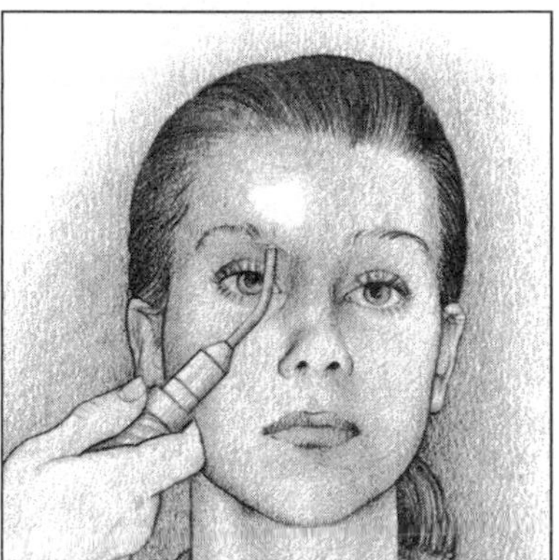

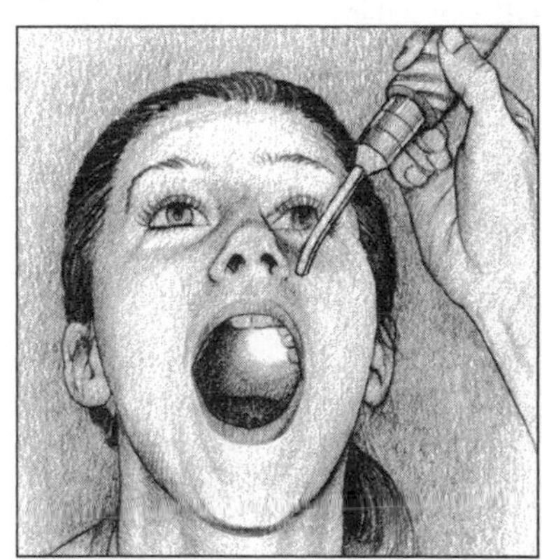

can also help reveal tumors and obstructions. (See *Transilluminating the sinuses.*) If the patient experiences local tenderness and other symptoms such as pain, fever, and nasal discharge, these suggest acute sinusitis.

Mouth, throat, and neck examination

Assessing the mouth and throat requires the techniques of inspection and palpation. Assessing the neck also involves auscultation.

Mouth inspection and palpation

First, inspect the patient's lips. They should be pink, moist, symmetrical, and without lesions. Put on gloves and palpate the lips for lumps or surface abnormalities.

Use a tongue blade and a bright light to inspect the oral mucosa. Have the patient open his mouth and place the tongue blade on top of his tongue. The oral mucosa should be pink, smooth, moist, and free from lesions and unusual odors.

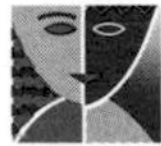

CULTURAL INSIGHT *A bluish hue or flecked pigmentation of the lips is common in dark-skinned patients, as well as increased pigmentation of the oral mucosa.*

Next, observe the gingivae, or gums. They should be pink, moist, have clearly defined margins at each tooth, and not be retracted. Inspect the teeth, noting their number, condition, and whether any are missing or crowded. If a patient is wearing dentures, ask him to remove them and then examine the gums.

Finally, inspect the tongue. It should be midline, symmetrical, moist, pink, and free from lesions. The posterior surface should be smooth and the anterior surface should be slightly rough with small fissures. The tongue should move easily in all directions, and it should lie straight to the front at rest.

CRITICAL POINT *Asymmetric protrusion of the patient's tongue suggests a lesion of cranial nerve XII.*

Ask the patient to raise the tip of his tongue and touch his palate directly behind his front teeth. Inspect the ventral surface of the tongue and the floor of the mouth. The area underneath the tongue is a common site for the development of oral cancers, so be sure to assess it thoroughly.

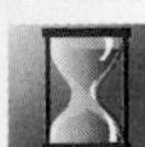

AGE ISSUE *Elderly patients may have varicose veins on the ventral surface of the tongue.*

Next, wrap a piece of gauze around the tip of the patient's tongue and move it first to one side then the other to inspect the lateral borders. They should be smooth and even-textured.

Inspect the patient's oropharynx by asking him to open his mouth while you shine the penlight on the uvula and palate. If necessary, insert a tongue blade into the mouth and depress the tongue. Place the tongue blade slightly off-center to avoid eliciting the gag reflex. The uvula and oropharynx should be pink and moist, without inflammation or exudates. The tonsils should be pink and shouldn't be hypertrophied. Ask the patient to say "ah," and then observe for movement of the soft palate and uvula.

CRITICAL POINT *If your patient has painful swallowing and a displaced, beefy, red uvula, he may have a peritonsillar abscess that's usually caused by acute tonsillitis and can be a potential emergency because it can cause airway obstruction. In this condition, a streptococcal infection spreads from the tonsils to the surrounding soft tissue. If the patient has cranial nerve X paralysis the soft palate fails to rise and the uvula deviates to the opposite side when the patient says "ah."*

Finally, palpate the patient's lips, tongue, and oropharynx. Note lumps, lesions, ulcers, or edema of the lips or tongue. Swelling of the lips and tongue could indicate angioedema, which is usually allergic in nature. Lesions and ulcerations on the lips may be related to herpes simplex infection or syphilis. Carcinoma may appear as a scaly plaque, an ulcer, or a nodular lesion — it usually affects the lower lip.

Assess the patient's gag reflex by gently touching the back of the pharynx with a cotton-tipped applicator or tongue blade. This should produce a bilateral response.

Neck inspection and palpation

First, observe the patient's neck. It should be symmetrical and the skin should be intact. Note any scars. Visible pulsations, masses, swelling, venous distention, or thyroid or lymph node enlargement should be absent. A diffusely enlarged thyroid is commonly related to Graves' disease, Hashimoto's thyroiditis, or endemic goiter. Multiple nodules on the thyroid suggest a metabolic cause; a single nodule may be a benign cyst or a tumor. Lymph node enlargement could indicate infection. Venous distention is seen with heart failure.

Ask the patient to move his neck through the entire range of motion and to shrug his shoulders. Also ask him to swallow. Note rising of the larynx, trachea, or thyroid.

Lymph node palpation. Palpate the patient's neck to gather more data. Using the finger pads of both hands, bilaterally palpate the chain of lymph nodes under the patient's chin in the preauricular area; then proceed to the area under and behind the ears. (See *Locating lymph nodes.*)

Assess the lymph nodes for size, shape, mobility, consistency, and tenderness. Compare nodes on one side with those on the other. When assessing the lymph nodes, your findings may include:

- enlargement of a supraclavicular node, especially on the left, which suggests possible metastasis from a thoracic or abdominal cancer
- tender nodes, which are indicative of inflammation; hard or fixed nodes, which suggest malignancy
- generalized lymphadenopathy, which requires further investigation; human immunodeficiency virus infection or acquired immunodeficiency syndrome may be the cause.

Trachea palpation. Palpate the trachea, normally located midline in the neck. Place your thumbs along each side of the trachea near the lower part of the neck. Note any

LOCATING LYMPH NODES

This illustration shows the location of lymph nodes in the patient's head and neck.

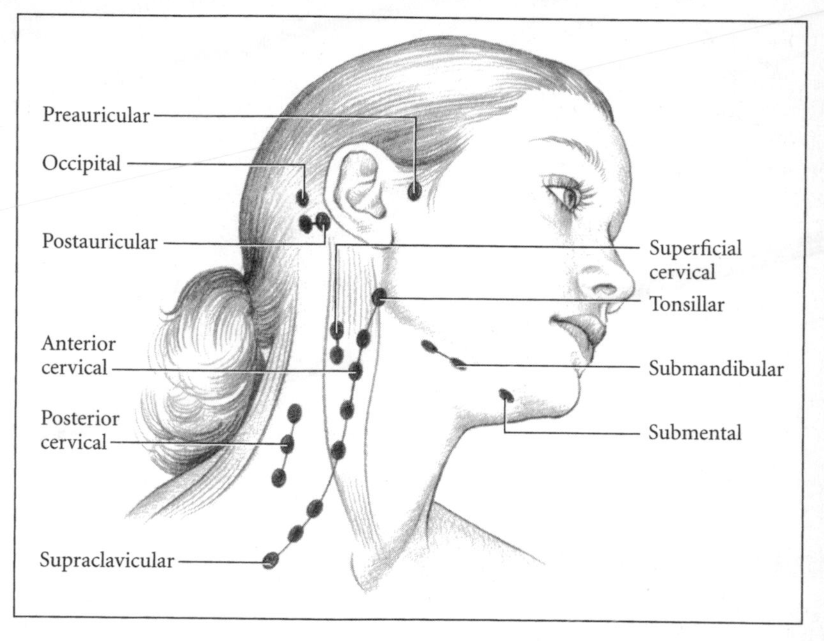

pain or tenderness. Check whether the distance between the trachea's outer edge and the sternocleidomastoid muscle is equal on both sides. Tracheal deviation may result from a mass in the neck, or mediastinal mass, atelectasis, or a pneumothorax.

Thyroid gland palpation. To palpate the thyroid, stand behind the patient and put your hands around his neck, with the fingers of both hands over the lower trachea. Ask him to swallow as you feel the thyroid isthmus. The isthmus should rise with swallowing because it lies across the trachea, just below the cricoid cartilage.

Displace the thyroid to the right and then to the left, palpating both lobes for enlargement (a possible goiter), nodules, tenderness, a gritty sensation, or a pulsation. (See *Structure of the thyroid gland,* page 160.)

Lowering the patient's chin slightly and turning toward the side being palpated helps relax the muscle and facilitate assessment.

Neck auscultation

Finally, auscultate the neck. Using light pressure on the bell of the stethoscope, listen over the carotid arteries. Ask the patient to hold his breath while listening to prevent breath sounds from interfering with the sounds of circulation. When auscultating the neck, listen for bruits, which signal turbulent blood flow.

During the neck auscultation, if you detect an enlarged thyroid gland, also auscultate the thyroid area with the bell. Check for a bruit or a soft rushing sound, which indicates a hypermetabolic state.

STRUCTURE OF THE THYROID GLAND

This illustration shows the structure and location of the thyroid gland.

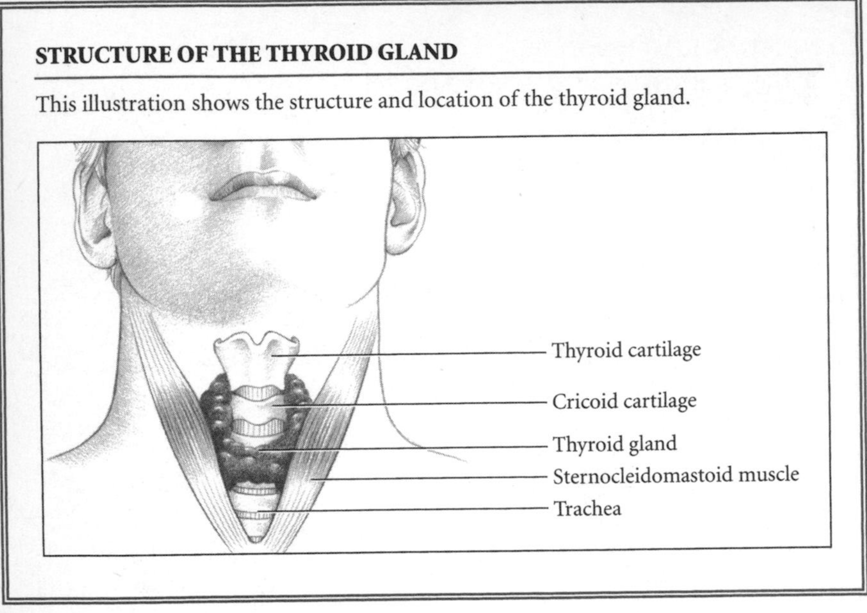

Abnormal findings

A patient's chief complaint may be for any of a number of signs and symptoms related to the ears, nose, and throat, and their related structures. Common findings include dysphagia, earache, epistaxis, hearing loss, lymphadenopathy, nasal flaring, nasal obstruction, rhinorrhea, and throat pain. The following history, physical examination, and analysis summaries will help you assess each one quickly and accurately. After obtaining further information, begin to interpret the findings. (See *Ears, nose, and throat: Interpreting your findings.*)

Dysphagia

Dysphagia, or difficulty swallowing, is a common symptom that's usually easy to localize. It may be constant or intermittent and is classified by the phase of swallowing it affects. Among the factors that interfere with swallowing are severe pain, obstruction, abnormal peristalsis, impaired gag reflex, and excessive, scanty, or thick oral secretions.

History

If the patient with dysphagia doesn't suggest airway obstruction, begin a health history. Ask the patient if swallowing is painful and if the pain is constant or intermittent. Have the patient point to where the dysphagia feels most intense and ask him if eating alleviates or aggravates it. Find out if solids or liquids are more difficult to swallow; if the answer is liquids, ask if hot, cold, or lukewarm fluids affect him differently. Ask the patient if the symptom disappears after he tries to swallow a few times. Find out if swallowing is easier if he changes position. Ask if he has recently experienced vomiting, regurgitation, or weight loss.

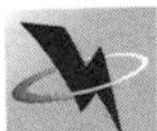

CRITICAL POINT *If the patient suddenly complains of dysphagia and displays signs of respiratory distress, such as dyspnea and stridor, suspect an airway obstruction and quickly perform abdominal thrusts. Prepare to administer oxygen by mask or nasal cannula, or to assist with endotracheal intubation.*

Physical assessment

To evaluate the patient's swallowing reflex, place your finger along his thyroid notch and instruct him to swallow. If you feel his larynx rise, the reflex is intact. Next, have him cough to assess his cough reflex. Check his gag reflex if you're sure he has a good

(Text continues on page 165.)

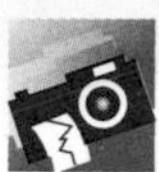

CLINICAL PICTURE

EARS, NOSE, AND THROAT: INTERPRETING YOUR FINDINGS

After you assess the patient, a group of findings may lead you to a particular disorder of the ears, nose, and throat. The chart below shows some common groups of findings for major signs and symptoms related to an assessment of the ears, nose, and throat, along with their probable causes.

Sign or symptom and findings	Probable cause
Dysphagia	
▪ Signs of respiratory distress, such as crowing and stridor ▪ Phase 2 dysphagia with gagging and dysphonia	Airway obstruction
▪ Phase 2 and 3 dysphagia ▪ Rapid weight loss ▪ Steady chest pain ▪ Hoarseness ▪ Sore throat ▪ Hiccups	Esophageal cancer
▪ Painless, progressive dysphagia ▪ Lead line on the gums ▪ Metallic taste ▪ Papilledema ▪ Ocular palsy ▪ Footdrop or wristdrop ▪ Mental impairment or seizures	Lead poisoning
▪ Phase 2 or 3 dysphagia occurring suddenly ▪ Gagging ▪ Coughing ▪ Esophageal pain ▪ Dyspnea, if accompanied by tracheal compression	Esophageal obstruction by foreign body
▪ Phase 2 dysphagia for solids and liquids ▪ Dry sore throat ▪ Cough ▪ Thick mucus in throat	Pharyngitis, chronic

Sign or symptom and findings	Probable cause
Earache	
▪ Sensation of blockage or fullness in the ear ▪ Itching ▪ Partial hearing loss ▪ Possible dizziness	Cerumen impaction
▪ Mild to moderate ear pain that occurs with tragus manipulation ▪ Low-grade fever ▪ Sticky yellow or purulent ear discharge ▪ Partial hearing loss ▪ Feeling of blockage in the ear ▪ Swelling of the tragus, external meatus, and external canal ▪ Lymphadenopathy	Otitis externa, acute
▪ Severe, deep, throbbing ear pain ▪ Hearing loss ▪ High fever ▪ Bulging, fiery red eardrum	Otitis media, acute suppurative

(continued)

EARS, NOSE, AND THROAT: INTERPRETING YOUR FINDINGS *(continued)*

Sign or symptom and findings	Probable cause
Epistaxis	
■ Ecchymoses ■ Petechiae ■ Bleeding from the gums, mouth, and I.V. puncture sites ■ Menorrhagia ■ Signs of GI bleeding, such as melena and hematemesis	Coagulation disorders
■ Unilateral or bilateral epistaxis ■ Nasal swelling ■ Periorbital ecchymoses and edema ■ Pain ■ Nasal deformity ■ Crepitation of the nasal bones	Nasal fracture
■ Oozing epistaxis ■ Dry cough ■ Abrupt onset of chills and high fever ■ "Rose-spot" rash ■ Vomiting ■ Profound fatigue ■ Anorexia	Typhoid fever
■ Extreme bleeding usually from posterior nose ■ Pulsation above middle turbinate ■ Dizziness ■ Throbbing headache ■ Anxiety ■ Peripheral edema ■ Nocturia ■ Nausea and vomiting ■ Drowsiness ■ Mental impairment	Hypertension
Epistaxis *(continued)*	
■ Nasal discharge, bloody or blood-tinged; possibly becoming purulent and copious after 24 to 48 hours ■ Nasal congestion ■ Pain and tenderness ■ Malaise ■ Headache ■ Low-grade fever ■ Red, erythematous nasal mucosa	Sinusitis, acute
■ Direct or indirect blow ■ Abrasions, contusions, lacerations, or avulsions If severe: ■ Severe headache ■ Changes in level of consciousness ■ Hemiparesis ■ Dizziness ■ Seizures ■ Projectile vomiting ■ Decreased pulse and respirations	Skull fracture
Hearing loss	
■ Conductive hearing loss ■ Ear pain or a feeling of fullness ■ Nasal congestion ■ Conjunctivitis	Allergies
■ Sudden or intermittent conductive hearing loss ■ Bony projections visible in the ear canal ■ Normal tympanic membrane	Osteoma

EARS, NOSE, AND THROAT: INTERPRETING YOUR FINDINGS *(continued)*

Sign or symptom and findings	Probable cause
Hearing loss *(continued)*	
▪ Abrupt hearing loss ▪ Ear pain ▪ Tinnitus ▪ Vertigo ▪ Sense of fullness in the ear	Tympanic membrane perforation
Lymphadenopathy	
▪ Single or multiple node involvement ▪ Pruritus ▪ Fatigue ▪ Weakness ▪ Night sweats ▪ Malaise ▪ Weight loss ▪ Unexplained fever	Hodgkin's disease
▪ Painful lymph nodes, primarily axillary, cervical, and inguinal nodes ▪ Prodromal symptoms, including headache, malaise, and fatigue occurring 3 to 5 days before onset of lymphadenopathy ▪ Sore throat ▪ Temperature fluctuations ▪ Stomatitis ▪ Exudative tonsillitis or pharyngitis	Mononucleosis, infectious
▪ Painless enlargement of one or more lymph nodes ▪ Dyspnea ▪ Cough ▪ Hepatosplenomegaly ▪ Fever ▪ Night sweats ▪ Fatigue ▪ Malaise ▪ Weight loss	Non-Hodgkin's lymphoma
Nasal flaring	
▪ Dyspnea ▪ Tachypnea ▪ Prolonged expiratory wheezing ▪ Accessory muscle use ▪ Cyanosis ▪ Dry or productive cough	Asthma, acute
▪ Dyspnea ▪ Tachypnea ▪ High fever ▪ Sudden shaking chills ▪ Hacking cough that becomes productive ▪ Stabbing chest pain worsening with movement and respiration ▪ Decreased or absent breath sounds ▪ Fine crackles ▪ Pleural friction rub	Pneumonia
Nasal obstruction	
▪ Watery nasal discharge ▪ Sneezing ▪ Temporary loss of smell and taste ▪ Sore throat ▪ Malaise ▪ Arthralgia ▪ Mild headache	Common cold
▪ Anosmia ▪ Clear, watery nasal discharge ▪ History of allergies, chronic sinusitis, trauma, cystic fibrosis, or asthma ▪ Translucent, pear-shaped polyps that are unilateral or bilateral	Nasal polyps

(continued)

EARS, NOSE, AND THROAT: INTERPRETING YOUR FINDINGS *(continued)*

Sign or symptom and findings	Probable cause
Nasal obstruction *(continued)*	
▪ Thick, purulent drainage ▪ Severe pain over the sinuses ▪ Fever ▪ Inflamed nasal mucosa with purulent mucus	Sinusitis
Rhinorrhea	
▪ Initially, watery nasal discharge becoming thicker and mucopurulent ▪ Sneezing ▪ Nasal congestion ▪ Dry, hacking cough ▪ Sore throat ▪ Transient loss of smell and taste ▪ Malaise ▪ Myalgia ▪ Dry lips ▪ Red upper lip and nose	Common cold
▪ Usually with severe unilateral headache ▪ Miosis ▪ Ipsilateral tearing ▪ Conjunctival injection ▪ Possible flushing, facial diaphoresis, bradycardia, and restlessness	Headache, cluster
Rhinorrhea *(continued)*	
▪ Episodic, profuse watery discharge ▪ Increased lacrimation ▪ Nasal congestion ▪ Itchy, watery eyes, nose, and throat ▪ Postnasal drip ▪ Frontal or temporal headache	Allergic rhinitis
▪ Thick purulent discharge leading to purulent postnasal drip resulting in throat pain and halitosis ▪ Nasal congestion ▪ Severe pain and tenderness over involved sinuses ▪ Fever ▪ Malaise	Sinusitis
Throat pain	
▪ Seasonal or year-round occurrence ▪ Nasal congestion with a thin nasal discharge and postnasal drip ▪ Paroxysmal sneezing ▪ Decreased sense of smell ▪ Frontal or temporal headache ▪ Pale and glistening nasal mucosa with edematous nasal turbinates ▪ Watery eyes	Allergic rhinitis

EARS, NOSE, AND THROAT: INTERPRETING YOUR FINDINGS *(continued)*

Sign or symptom and findings	Probable cause
Throat pain *(continued)*	
▪ Mild to severe hoarseness ▪ Temporary loss of voice ▪ Malaise ▪ Low-grade fever ▪ Dysphagia ▪ Dry cough ▪ Tender, enlarged cervical lymph nodes	Laryngitis
▪ Mild to severe sore throat ▪ Pain may radiate to the ears ▪ Dysphagia ▪ Headache ▪ Malaise ▪ Fever with chills ▪ Tender cervical lymphadenopathy	Tonsillitis, acute

swallow or cough reflex. Listen closely to his speech for signs of muscle weakness. Does he have aphasia or dysarthria? Is his voice nasal, hoarse, or breathy? Assess the patient's mouth carefully. Check for dry mucous membranes and thick, sticky secretions. Observe for tongue and facial weakness and obvious obstructions, for example, enlarged tonsils. Assess the patient for disorientation, which may make him neglect to swallow.

AGE ISSUE *In infants or small children, look for dysphagia by paying close attention to their sucking and swallowing ability. Coughing, choking, or regurgitation during feeding suggests dysphagia.*

Analysis

Dysphagia is the most common—and sometimes the only—symptom of esophageal disorders. However, it may also result from oropharyngeal, respiratory, neurologic, and collagen disorders, or from the effects of toxins and treatments. Dysphagia increases the risk of choking and aspiration and may lead to malnutrition and dehydration.

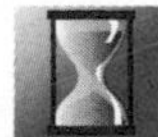

AGE ISSUE *In children, corrosive esophagitis and esophageal obstruction by a foreign body are more common causes of dysphagia. It may also result from congenital defects, such as annular stenosis, dysphagia lusoria, and esophageal atresia. In patients older than age 50, dysphagia is typically the chief complaint in cases of head or neck cancer. The incidence of such cancers increases markedly in this age-group.*

Earache

Earaches usually result from disorders of the external and middle ear associated with infection, obstruction, or trauma. Their severity ranges from a feeling of fullness or blockage to deep, boring pain; at times, they may be difficult to localize precisely. Earaches are a common symptom that may be intermittent or continuous and may develop suddenly or gradually.

History

Ask the patient to characterize the earache. Find out how long he has had it, if it's intermittent or continuous, or painful or slightly annoying. Ask if he can localize the site of the ear pain and if he has pain in other areas such as the jaw.

Ask about recent ear injury or other trauma. Find out if such activities as swimming or showering trigger his ear discomfort and if it's associated with itching. If so, find out where the itching is most intense and when it began. Ask about ear drainage and, if present, have the patient characterize it. Ask if he hears ringing or noise in his ears. Ask about dizziness or vertigo and if it worsens when the patient changes position. Find out if he has difficulty swallowing, hoarseness, neck pain, or pain when he opens his mouth.

Find out if the patient has recently had a head cold or problems with his eyes, mouth, teeth, jaws, sinuses, or throat. Disorders in these areas may refer pain to the ear along the cranial nerves.

Physical assessment

Begin the physical examination by inspecting the external ear for redness, drainage, swelling, or deformity. Then apply pressure to the mastoid process and tragus to elicit any tenderness. Using an otoscope, examine the external auditory canal for lesions, bleeding, discharge, impacted cerumen, foreign bodies, tenderness, or swelling. Examine the tympanic membrane for intactness and a normal pearly gray color. Look for tympanic membrane landmarks including the cone of light, umbo, pars tensa, and the handle and short process of the malleus.

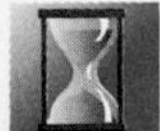

AGE ISSUE *Examine the child's ears by placing him in a supine position with his arms extended and held securely by his parent. Holding the otoscope with the handle pointing toward the top of the child's head, brace it against him using one or two fingers.*

Perform the ticking watch, whispered voice, Rinne, and Weber's tests to assess the patient for hearing loss.

Analysis

The particular symptoms the patient describes and the signs you observe help pinpoint the cause. Pain caused by touching or pulling the ear, for instance, usually indicates an external ear infection; a deep throbbing pain, a middle ear disorder. A severely inflamed outer ear may result from a swollen or completely blocked ear canal. A feeling of pressure or blockage can stem from a eustachian tube dysfunction that creates negative pressure in the middle ear or from muscle spasm or temporomandibular joint arthralgia.

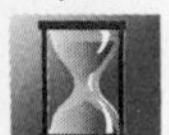

AGE ISSUE *In children, common causes of earache are acute otitis media and insertion of foreign bodies that become lodged or infected. Be alert for crying or ear tugging in a young child — nonverbal clues of an earache.*

Epistaxis

A common sign, epistaxis (nosebleed) can be spontaneous or induced from the front or back of the nose. Most nosebleeds occur in the anterior-inferior nasal septum (Kiesselbach's plexus), but they may also occur at the point where the inferior turbinates meet the nasopharynx. Usually unilateral, they seem bilateral when blood runs from the bleeding side behind the nasal septum and out the opposite side. Epistaxis ranges from mild oozing to severe — possibly life-threatening — blood loss.

History

If your patient isn't in distress, take a health history. Ask him if he has a history of recent trauma and how often he has had nosebleeds in the past. Find out if the nosebleeds were long or unusually severe. Ask about recent surgery in the sinus area, as well as a history of hypertension, bleeding or liver disorders, and other recent illnesses. Ask if the patient bruises easily. Find out what drugs he uses, especially anti-inflammatories, such as aspirin, and anticoagulants such as warfarin.

CRITICAL POINT *If your patient has severe epistaxis, quickly take his vital signs. Be alert for tachypnea, hypotension, and other signs of hypovolemic shock. Insert a large-gauge I.V. line for rapid fluid and blood replacement, and attempt to control bleeding by pinching the nares closed. (However, if you suspect a nasal fracture, don't pinch the nares. Instead, place gauze under the patient's nose to absorb the blood.) Have the patient with hypovolemia lie down and turn his head to the side to prevent blood from draining down the back of his throat, which could cause aspiration or vomiting. If the patient isn't hypovolemic, have him sit upright and tilt his head forward. Constantly check airway patency. If the patient's condition is unstable, begin cardiac monitoring and give supplemental oxygen by mask.*

Physical assessment

Begin the physical examination by inspecting the patient's skin for other signs of bleeding, such as ecchymoses and petechiae, and noting any jaundice, pallor, or other abnormalities. When examining a trauma patient, look for associated injuries, such as eye trauma or facial fractures.

Analysis
A rich supply of fragile blood vessels makes the nose particularly vulnerable to bleeding. Air moving through the nose can dry and irritate the mucous membranes, forming crusts that bleed when they're removed; dry mucous membranes are also more susceptible to infections, which can produce epistaxis as well. Trauma is another common cause of epistaxis. Additional causes include septal deviations; hematologic, coagulation, renal, and GI disorders; and certain drugs, such as anticoagulants, anti-inflammatory agents, cocaine, and treatments.

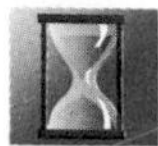

AGE ISSUE *In elderly and young people, vigorous nose blowing may rupture superficial blood vessels causing nosebleeds. Children are more likely to experience anterior nosebleeds, usually the result of nose-picking or allergic rhinitis. Elderly patients are more likely to experience posterior nosebleeds.*

Hearing loss
Affecting nearly 16 million people in the United States, hearing loss may be temporary or permanent, and partial or complete. Hearing loss is a common symptom that may involve reception of low-, middle-, or high-frequency tones. If hearing loss doesn't affect speech frequencies, the patient may be unaware of it.

History
If the patient reports hearing loss, ask him to describe it fully. Find out if it's unilateral or bilateral, and continuous or intermittent. Ask about a family history of hearing loss. Then obtain the patient's medical history, noting chronic ear infections, ear surgery, and ear or head trauma. Find out if the patient recently had an upper respiratory tract infection. After taking a drug history, have the patient describe his occupation and work environment.

Next, explore associated signs and symptoms. If the patient has ear pain, find out if it's unilateral or bilateral, and continuous or intermittent. Ask the patient if he has noticed discharge from one or both ears. If so, have him describe its color and consistency, and note when it began. Find out if he hears ringing, buzzing, hissing, or other noises in one or both ears. If so, ask him if the noises are constant or intermittent. Ask if he experiences dizziness and if so, find out when he first noticed it.

Physical assessment
Begin the physical examination by inspecting the external ear for inflammation, boils, foreign bodies, and discharge. Then apply pressure to the tragus and mastoid to elicit tenderness. If you detect tenderness or external ear abnormalities, notify the health care provider to discuss whether an otoscopic examination should be done. During the otoscopic examination, note color change, perforation, bulging, or retraction of the tympanic membrane, which normally looks like a shiny, pearl gray cone.

Next, evaluate the patient's hearing acuity, using the ticking watch and whispered voice tests. Then perform Weber's and Rinne tests to obtain a preliminary evaluation of the type and degree of hearing loss.

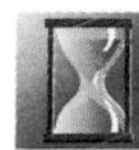

AGE ISSUE *When assessing an infant or a young child for hearing loss, remember that you can't use a tuning fork. Instead, test the startle reflex in infants younger than age 6 months, or have an audiologist test brain stem-evoked response in neonates, infants, and young children. Also obtain a gestational, perinatal, and family history from the parents.*

Analysis
Normally, sound waves enter the external auditory canal, then travel to the middle ear's tympanic membrane and ossicles — that is, the incus, malleus, and stapes — and into the inner ear's cochlea. The cochlear division of the eighth cranial, or auditory, nerve carries the sound impulse to the brain. This type of sound transmission, air conduction, is normally better than bone conduction — sound transmission through bone to the inner ear.

Hearing loss can be classified as conductive, sensorineural, mixed, and functional. Conductive hearing loss results from external or middle ear disorders that block sound transmission. This type of hearing loss usually responds to medical or surgical intervention, or in some cases, both. Sensorineural hearing loss results from disorders of the inner ear or of the eighth cranial nerve. Mixed hearing loss combines aspects of conductive and sensorineural hearing loss. Functional hearing loss results from psychological factors rather than identifiable organic damage.

Hearing loss may also result from trauma, infection, allergy, a tumor, certain systemic and hereditary disorders, or the use of ototoxic drugs and treatments. In most cases, though, it results from presbycusis, a sensorineural hearing loss that usually affects people older than age 50. Other physiologic causes of hearing loss include cerumen impaction; barotitis media, or unequal pressure on the eardrum, associated with descent in an airplane or elevator, diving, or close proximity to an explosion; and chronic exposure to noise over 90 decibels, which can occur in certain occupations, with particular hobbies, or from listening to live or recorded music.

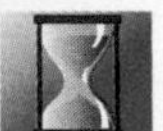
AGE ISSUE *In children, mumps is the most common cause of unilateral sensorineural hearing loss. Other causes are meningitis, measles, influenza, and acute febrile illness. Disorders that may produce congenital conductive hearing loss include atresia, ossicle malformation, and other abnormalities. Serous otitis media commonly causes bilateral conductive hearing loss in children. Conductive hearing loss may also occur in children who put foreign objects in their ears. In older patients, presbycusis may be aggravated by exposure to noise as well as other factors.*

Lymphadenopathy

Lymphadenopathy — enlargement of one or more lymph nodes — may result from increased production of lymphocytes or reticuloendothelial cells, or from infiltration of cells that aren't normally present. This sign may be generalized, involving three or more node groups, or localized.

History

Ask the patient when he first noticed the lymph node swelling, and whether it's located on one side of his body or both. Are the swollen areas sore, hard, or red? Ask the patient if he has recently had an infection or other health problem. Also ask if a biopsy has ever been done on any lymph node because this may indicate a previously diagnosed cancer. Find out if the patient has a family history of cancer.

Physical assessment

Palpate the entire lymph node system to determine the extent of lymphadenopathy and to detect any other areas of local enlargement. Use the pads of your index and middle fingers to move the skin over underlying tissues at the nodal area. If you detect enlarged nodes, note their size in centimeters and whether they're fixed or mobile, tender or nontender, and erythematous or not. Note their texture, for example, if the node is discrete, or if the area is matted. If you detect tender, erythematous lymph nodes, check the area drained by that part of the lymph system for signs of infection, such as erythema and swelling. Also palpate for and percuss the spleen.

Analysis

Normally, lymph nodes are discrete, mobile, soft, nontender and, except in children, nonpalpable; however, palpable nodes may be normal in adults. Nodes that are more than 1 cm in diameter are cause for concern. They may be tender and the skin overlying the lymph node may be erythematous, suggesting a draining lesion. Alternatively, they may be hard and fixed, tender or nontender, suggesting a malignant tumor.

Generalized lymphadenopathy may be caused by an inflammatory process, such as bacterial or viral infection, connective tissue disease, an endocrine disorder, or neoplasm. Localized lymphadenopathy most commonly results from infection or trauma affecting a specific area.

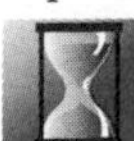
AGE ISSUE *In children, infection is the most common cause of lymphadenopathy. It's commonly associated with otitis media and pharyngitis.*

Nasal flaring

Nasal flaring is the abnormal dilation of the nostrils. Usually occurring during inspiration, nasal flaring may occasionally occur during expiration or throughout the respiratory cycle.

History

Once the patient's condition is stabilized, obtain a pertinent history. Ask about cardiac and pulmonary disorders such as asthma. Find out if the patient has allergies, and if he has experienced a recent illness, such as a respiratory tract infection, or trauma. Ask the patient if he smokes and if he has a history of smoking. Obtain a drug history.

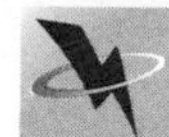

CRITICAL POINT *If you note nasal flaring in the patient, quickly evaluate his respiratory status. Absent breath sounds, cyanosis, diaphoresis, and tachycardia point to complete airway obstruction.*

Physical assessment
If the patient is stabilized, inspect the nose and examine the patient's chest and lungs.

Analysis
Nasal flaring indicates respiratory dysfunction, ranging from mild difficulty to potentially life-threatening respiratory distress. Pulmonary function tests, such as vital capacity testing, can produce nasal flaring with forced inspiration or expiration. Certain respiratory treatments, such as deep breathing, can cause nasal flaring.

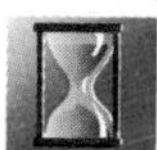

AGE ISSUE *In infants and young children, nasal flaring is an important sign of respiratory distress because they can't verbalize their discomfort. Common causes include airway obstruction, respiratory distress syndrome, croup, and acute epiglottiditis.*

Nasal obstruction
Nasal obstruction, as the name implies, involves a blockage in the nasal passageway. It may cause discomfort, alter a person's sense of taste and smell, and cause voice changes.

History
Begin the health history by asking the patient about the duration and frequency of the obstruction. Find out if it began suddenly or gradually, and if it's intermittent or persistent, and unilateral or bilateral. Inquire about the presence and character of drainage, such as if it's watery, purulent, or bloody. Find out if the patient has nasal or sinus pain or headaches. Ask about recent travel, the use of drugs or alcohol, and previous trauma or surgery.

Physical assessment
Examine the patient's nose; assess air flow and the condition of the turbinates and nasal septum. Evaluate the orbits for any evidence of dystopia, decreased vision, excess tearing, or abnormal appearance of the eye. Palpate over the frontal and maxillary sinuses for tenderness. Examine the ears for signs of middle ear effusions. Inspect the oral cavity, pharynx, nasopharynx, and larynx to detect inflammation, ulceration, excessive mucosal dryness, and neurologic deficits. Lastly, palpate the neck for lymphadenopathy.

Analysis
Nasal obstruction may result from an allergic, inflammatory, neoplastic, endocrine, or metabolic disorder; a structural abnormality; a traumatic injury; or a mechanical obstruction, such as a foreign object. It's frequently and typically a benign symptom, but may signal certain life-threatening disorders, such as a basilar skull fracture or malignant tumor.

Rhinorrhea
Common but rarely serious, rhinorrhea is the free discharge of thin nasal mucus. It can be self-limiting or chronic. Depending on the cause, the discharge may be clear, purulent, bloody, or serosanguineous.

History
Begin the health history by asking the patient if the discharge runs from both nostrils and find out if it's intermittent or persistent, if it began suddenly or gradually, and if the position of his head affects it.

Next, ask the patient to characterize the discharge, such as is it watery, bloody, purulent, or foul smelling. Ask if the discharge is copious or scanty. Ask him if it worsens or improves with the time of day. Find out if the patient is using any medications, especially nose drops or nasal sprays. Ask the patient if he has been exposed to nasal irritants at home or at work. Find out if he experiences seasonal allergies. Ask about recent head injuries.

Physical assessment
Examine the patient's nose, checking air flow from each nostril. Evaluate the size, color, and condition of the turbinate mucosa, which is normally pale pink. Note if the mucosa is red, unusually pale, blue, or gray. Then examine the area beneath each turbinate. Be sure to palpate over the frontal, ethmoid, and maxillary sinuses for tenderness.

To differentiate nasal mucus from cerebrospinal fluid (CSF), collect a small amount of drainage on a glucose test strip. If CSF (which contains glucose) is present, the test result will be abnormal. Finally, using a nonirritating substance, be sure to test for anosmia.

Analysis

Rhinorrhea may result from a nasal, sinus, or systemic disorder, or from a basilar skull fracture. Rhinorrhea can also result from sinus or cranial surgery, excessive use of vasoconstricting nose drops or sprays, or inhalation of an irritant, such as tobacco smoke, dust, and fumes.

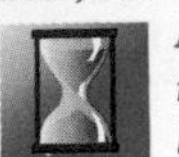

AGE ISSUE *In children, rhinorrhea may stem from choanal atresia, allergic or chronic rhinitis, acute ethmoiditis, or congenital syphilis. Assume that unilateral rhinorrhea and nasal obstruction is caused by a foreign body in the nose until proven otherwise.*

Throat pain

Throat pain, which is commonly known as a sore throat, refers to discomfort in any part of the pharynx that includes the nasopharynx, oropharynx, or hypopharynx. This common symptom ranges from a sensation of scratchiness to severe pain. It's commonly accompanied by ear pain because cranial nerves IX and X innervate the pharynx as well as the middle and external ear.

History

Ask the patient when he first noticed the pain and have him describe it. Find out if he has had throat pain before and if it was accompanied by fever, ear pain, or dysphagia. Review the patient's medical history for throat problems, allergies, and systemic disorders.

Physical assessment

Carefully examine the pharynx, noting redness, exudate, or swelling. Examine the oropharynx, using a warmed metal spatula or tongue blade, and the nasopharynx, using a warmed laryngeal mirror or a fiberoptic nasopharyngoscope. Laryngoscopic examination of the hypopharynx may be required. If necessary, spray the soft palate and pharyngeal wall with a local anesthetic to prevent gagging. Observe the tonsils for redness, swelling, or exudate. Obtain an exudate specimen for culture. Then examine the nose, using a nasal speculum. Also check the patient's ears, especially if he reports ear pain. Finally, palpate the neck and oropharynx for nodules or lymph node enlargement.

Analysis

Throat pain may result from infection, trauma, allergy, cancer, or a systemic disorder. It may also follow surgery and endotracheal intubation. Nonpathologic causes include dry mucous membranes associated with mouth breathing and laryngeal irritation associated with alcohol consumption, inhaling smoke or chemicals like ammonia, and vocal strain.

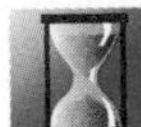

AGE ISSUE *In children, throat pain is a common complaint. Other pediatric causes of throat pain include acute epiglottiditis, herpangina, scarlet fever, acute follicular tonsillitis, and retropharyngeal abscess.*

8

Respiratory system

The respiratory system includes the airways, lungs, bony thorax, respiratory muscles, and central nervous system (CNS). These structures and the CNS work together to deliver oxygen to the bloodstream and remove excess carbon dioxide from the body.

Respiratory anatomy

Knowing the basic anatomy of the respiratory system will help you perform a comprehensive respiratory assessment and recognize any abnormalities. (See *Structures of the respiratory system,* page 172.)

Airways and lungs

The airways are divided into the upper and lower airways. The upper airways include the nasopharynx (nose), oropharynx (mouth), laryngopharynx, and larynx. Their purpose is to warm, filter, and humidify inhaled air. They also help to make sound and send air to the lower airways.

The epiglottis is a flap of tissue that closes over the top of the larynx when the patient swallows. It protects the patient from aspirating food or fluid into the lower airways. The larynx is located at the top of the trachea and houses the vocal cords. It's the transition point between the upper and lower airways.

The lower airways begin with the trachea, which then divides into the right and left mainstem bronchial tubes. The bronchial tubes divide into bronchi, which are lined with mucus-producing ciliated epithelium, one of the lungs' major defense systems.

The bronchi then divide into secondary bronchi, tertiary bronchi, terminal bronchioles, respiratory bronchioles, alveolar ducts and, finally, into the alveoli, the gas-

STRUCTURES OF THE RESPIRATORY SYSTEM

The major structures of the upper and lower airways are illustrated below.

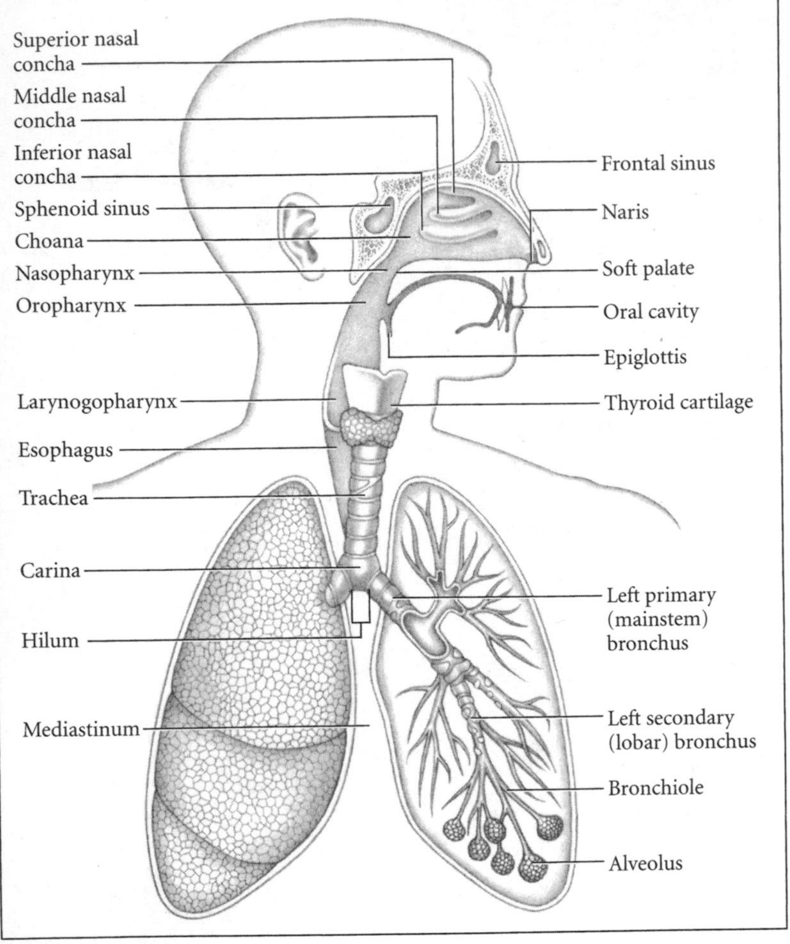

exchange units of the lungs. The lungs in an adult typically contain about 300 million alveoli.

Each lung is wrapped in a lining called the visceral pleura. The right lung is larger and has three lobes: upper, middle, and lower. The left lung is smaller and has only an upper and a lower lobe. The lungs share space in the thoracic cavity with the heart and great vessels, the trachea, the esophagus, and the bronchi. All areas of the thoracic cavity that come in contact with the lungs are lined with parietal pleura.

A small amount of fluid fills the area between the two layers of the pleura. That fluid, called pleural fluid, allows the layers of the pleura to slide smoothly over one another as the chest expands and contracts. The parietal pleura also contains nerve endings that emit pain signals when inflammation occurs.

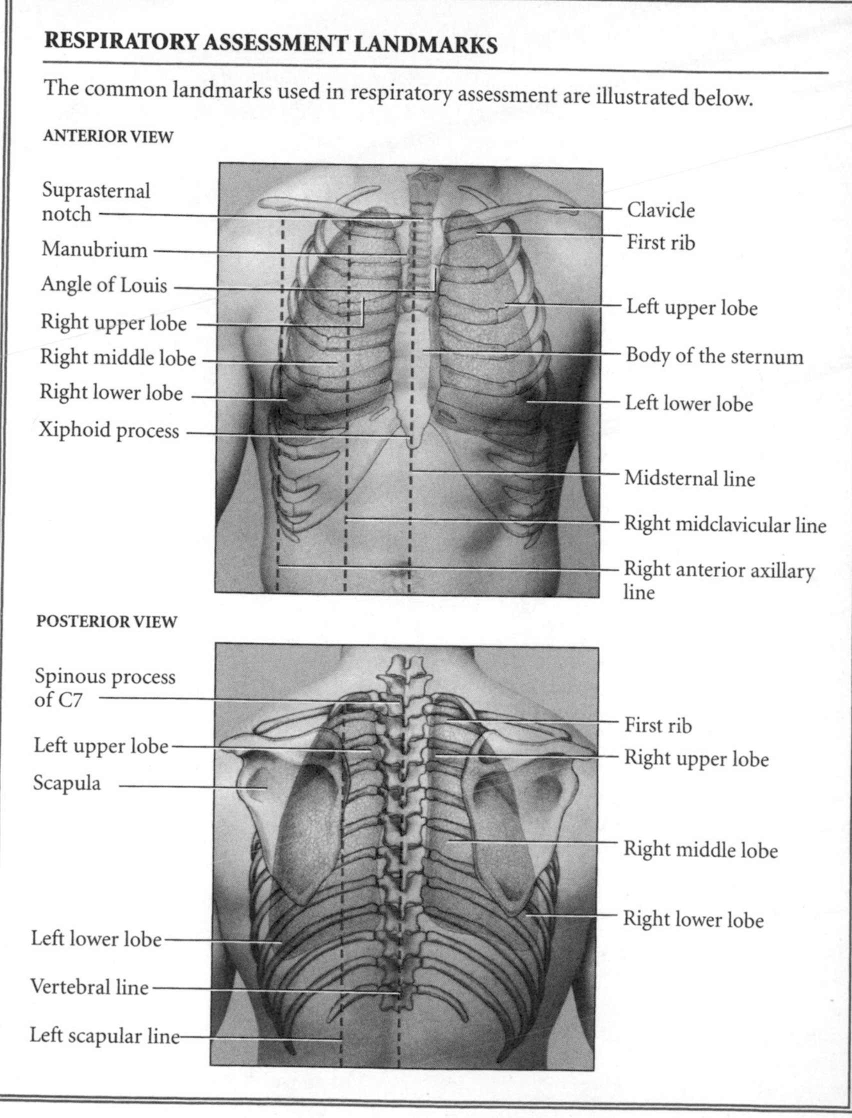

RESPIRATORY ASSESSMENT LANDMARKS

The common landmarks used in respiratory assessment are illustrated below.

Thorax

Composed of bone and cartilage, the thoracic cage supports and protects the lungs. The vertebral column and 12 pairs of ribs form the posterior portion of the thoracic cage. The ribs, the major portion of the thoracic cage, extend from the thoracic vertebrae toward the anterior thorax. Along with the vertebrae, they support and protect the thorax, permitting the lungs to expand and contract. Both are numbered from top to bottom. Posteriorly, certain landmarks are used as well to help identify specific vertebrae. In 90% of people, the seventh cervical vertebra (C7) is the most prominent vertebra on a flexed neck; for the remaining 10%, it's the first thoracic vertebra (T1). Thus, to locate a specific vertebra, count down along the vertebrae from C7 or T1. (See *Respiratory assessment landmarks.*)

The manubrium, sternum, xiphoid process, and ribs form the anterior thoracic

THE MECHANICS OF BREATHING

These illustrations show how mechanical forces, such as the movement of the diaphragm and intercostal muscles, produce a breath. A plus sign (+) indicates positive pressure, and a minus sign (-) indicates negative pressure.

At rest

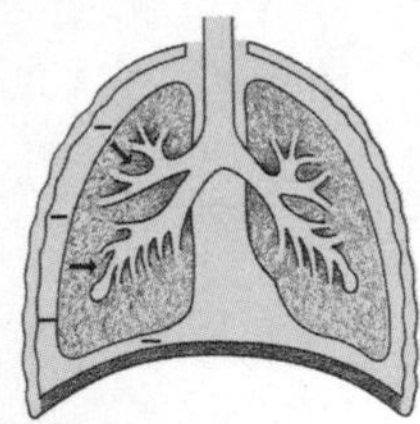

- Inspiratory muscles relax.
- Atmospheric pressure is maintained in the tracheobronchial tree.
- No air movement occurs.

Inspiration

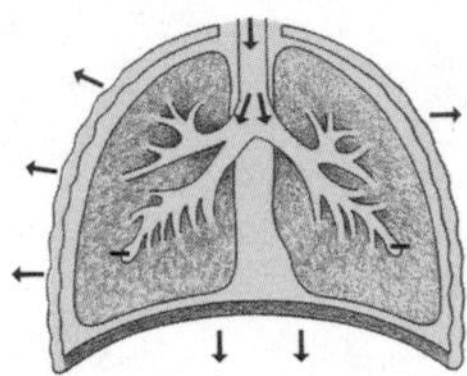

- Inspiratory muscles contract.
- The diaphragm decends.
- Negative alveolar pressure is maintained.
- Air moves into the lungs.

Expiration

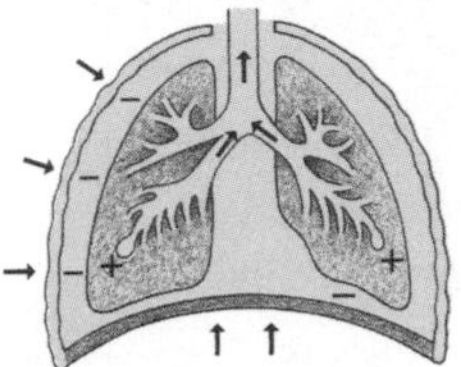

- Inspiratory muscles relax, causing lungs to recoil to their resting size and position.
- The diaphragm ascends.
- Positive alveolar pressure is maintained.
- Air moves out of the lungs.

cage, which has the additional duty of protecting the mediastinal organs that lie between the right and left pleural cavities. Ribs 1 through 7 attach directly to the sternum; ribs 8 through 10 attach to the cartilage of the preceding rib. The other two pairs of ribs are "free-floating"; they don't attach to any part of the anterior thoracic cage. Rib 11 ends anterolaterally, and rib 12 ends laterally. The lower parts of the rib cage (the costal margins) near the xiphoid process form the borders of the costal angle — an angle of about 90 degrees normally.

Above the anterior thorax is a depression called the suprasternal notch. Because this notch isn't covered by the rib cage like the rest of the thorax, it allows you to palpate the trachea and check aortic pulsation.

Respiratory muscles

The diaphragm and the external intercostal muscles are the primary muscles used in breathing. They contract when the patient inhales and relax when the patient exhales.

The respiratory center in the medulla initiates each breath by sending messages to the primary respiratory muscles over the phrenic nerve. Impulses from the phrenic nerve adjust the rate and depth of breathing, depending on the carbon dioxide and pH levels in the cerebrospinal fluid. (See *The mechanics of breathing.*)

Accessory inspiratory muscles also assist in breathing and include the trapezius, the sternocleidomastoid, and the scalenes, which combine to elevate the scapula, clavicle, sternum, and upper ribs. That elevation expands the front-to-back diameter of the chest when use of the diaphragm and intercostal muscles isn't effective.

Expiration occurs when the diaphragm and external intercostal muscles relax. If the patient has an airway obstruction, he may also use the abdominal muscles and internal intercostal muscles to exhale.

Respiratory physiology

The primary function of the respiratory system is gas exchange, which involves pulmonary circulation, respiration, ventilation, pulmonary perfusion, diffusion, and acid-base balance.

Pulmonary circulation

Oxygen-depleted blood enters the lungs from the pulmonary artery of the right ventricle, then it flows through the main pulmonary arteries into the pleural cavities and the main bronchi, where it continues to flow through progressively smaller vessels until it reaches the single-celled endothelial capillaries serving the alveoli. Here, oxygen and carbon dioxide diffusion takes place. After passing through the pulmonary capillaries, blood flows through progressively larger vessels, enters the main pulmonary veins, finally flowing into the left atrium.

Respiration

Effective respiration requires gas exchange in the lungs through external respiration and in the tissues through internal respiration. Three processes contribute to external respiration:

- ventilation — gas distribution into and out of the pulmonary airways
- pulmonary perfusion — blood flow from the right side of the heart, through the pulmonary circulation, and into the left side of the heart
- diffusion — gas movement from an area of greater to lesser concentration through a semipermeable membrane.

Internal respiration occurs only through diffusion. These processes are vital to maintain adequate oxygenation and acid-base balance.

Ventilation

Adequate ventilation depends on the nervous, musculoskeletal, and pulmonary systems for the requisite lung pressure changes. Any dysfunction in these systems increases the work of breathing, diminishing its effectiveness.

Nervous system effects. Although ventilation is largely involuntary, individuals can control its rate and depth. Involuntary breathing results from neurogenic stimulation of the respiratory center in the medulla and the pons of the brain stem. The medulla controls the rate and depth of respiration; the pons moderates the rhythm of the switch from inspiration to expiration. Specialized neurovascular tissue alters these phases of the breathing process automatically and instantaneously.

When carbon dioxide in the blood diffuses into the cerebrospinal fluid, specialized tissue in the respiratory center of the brain stem responds. At the same time, peripheral chemoreceptors in the aortic arch and the bifurcation of the carotid arteries respond to reduced oxygen levels in the blood. When carbon dioxide level rises or oxygen level falls noticeably, the respiratory center of the medulla initiates respiration.

Musculoskeletal effects. The adult thorax is a flexible structure — its shape can be altered by contracting the chest muscles. The medulla controls ventilation primarily by stimulating contraction of the diaphragm and the external intercostals, the major muscles of breathing. The diaphragm descends to expand the length of the chest cavity, while the external intercostals contract to expand the anteroposterior and lateral chest diameter. These actions of the musculoskeletal system produce changes in intrapulmonary pressure that cause inspiration.

Pulmonary effects. During inspiration, air flows through the right and left mainstem bronchi into increasingly smaller bronchi, then into bronchioles, alveolar ducts, and alveolar sacs, finally reaching the alveolar membrane. Many pulmonary effects can alter airflow distribution, including air flow pattern, volume and location of the functional reserve capacity (air retained in the alveoli that prevents their collapse during respiration), amount of intrapulmonary resistance, and presence of lung disease. If disrupted, airflow distribution will follow the path of least resistance. For example, an intrapulmonary obstruction or forced inspiration will cause an uneven distribution of air.

Normal breathing requires active inspiration and passive expiration. Forced breathing, as in cases of emphysema, demands active inspiration and expiration. It activates accessory muscles of respiration, which requires additional oxygen to work, resulting in less efficient ventilation with an increased workload.

WHAT HAPPENS IN VENTILATION-PERFUSION MISMATCH

Effective gas exchange depends on the relationship between ventilation and perfusion ($\dot{V}/\dot{Q}$) ratio. The diagrams shown here demonstrate what happens when the $\dot{V}/\dot{Q}$ ratio is normal and abnormal.

Normal ventilation and perfusion
When $\dot{V}/\dot{Q}$ are matched, unoxygenated blood from the venous system returns to the right ventricle through the pulmonary artery to the lungs, carrying carbon dioxide. The arteries branch into the alveolar capillaries. Gas exchange takes place in the alveolar capillaries.

From pulmonary artery
To pulmonary vein
Alveolus
Normal capillary

Inadequate perfusion (dead-space ventilation)
When the $\dot{V}/\dot{Q}$ ratio is high, as shown here, ventilation is normal, but alveolar perfusion is reduced or absent. Note the narrowed capillary, indicating poor perfusion. This typically results from a perfusion defect such as pulmonary embolism or a disorder that decreases cardiac output.

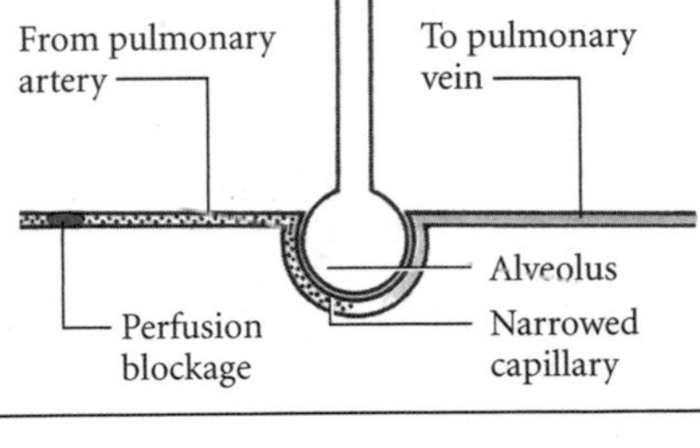

Blood with CO_2 Blood with O_2 Blood with CO_2 and O_2

Other alterations in airflow, such as changes in compliance (distensibility of the lungs and thorax) and resistance (interference with airflow in the tracheobronchial tree), can also increase oxygen and energy demands and lead to respiratory muscle fatigue.

Pulmonary perfusion

Optimal pulmonary perfusion aids external respiration and promotes efficient alveolar gas exchange. However, factors that reduce blood flow, such as a cardiac output that is less than average (5 L/minute) and elevated pulmonary and systemic vascular resistance, can interfere with gas transport to the alveoli. Also, abnormal or insufficient hemoglobin (Hb) picks up less oxygen than is needed for efficient gas exchange.

Gravity can affect oxygen and carbon dioxide transport by influencing pulmonary circulation. Gravity pulls more unoxygenated blood to the lower and middle lung lobes relative to the upper lobes, where most of the tidal volume also flows. As a result, neither ventilation nor perfusion is uniform throughout the lung. Areas of the lung where perfusion and ventilation are similar have good ventilation-perfusion matching. In such areas, gas exchange is most efficient. Areas of the lung that demonstrate ventilation-perfusion inequality result in less efficient gas exchange. (See *What happens in ventilation-perfusion mismatch.*)

Diffusion

In diffusion, molecules of oxygen and carbon dioxide move between the alveoli and the capillaries. Partial pressure — the pressure exerted by one gas in a mixture of gases — dictates the direction of movement, which is always from an area of greater concentration to one of lesser concentration. During diffusion, oxygen moves across the alveolar and capillary membranes, then dissolves in the plasma, and passes through the

Inadequate ventilation (shunt)
When the $\dot{V}/\dot{Q}$ ratio is low, pulmonary circulation is adequate, but not enough oxygen is available to the alveoli for normal diffusion. A portion of the blood flowing through the pulmonary vessels doesn't become oxygenated.

Inadequate ventilation and perfusion (silent unit)
The silent unit indicates an absence of ventilation and perfusion to the lung area. The silent unit may help compensate for a $\dot{V}/\dot{Q}$ imbalance by delivering blood flow to better-ventilated areas.

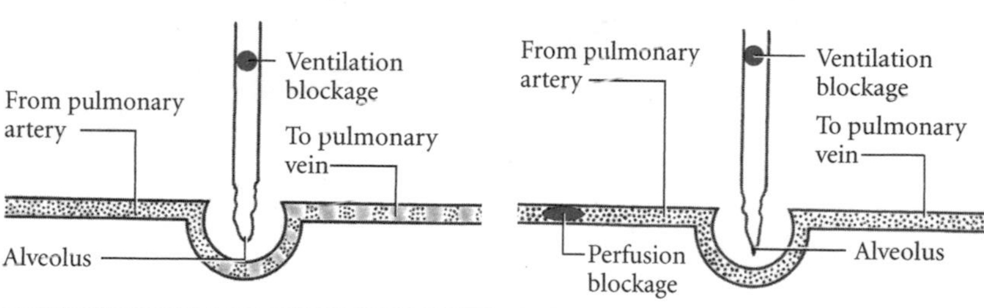

red blood cell (RBC) membrane. Carbon dioxide moves in the opposite direction.

Successful diffusion requires an intact alveolocapillary membrane. Both the alveolar epithelium and the capillary endothelium are composed of a single layer of cells. Between these layers are minute interstitial spaces filled with elastin and collagen. Normally, oxygen and carbon dioxide move easily through all of these layers. Oxygen moves from the alveoli into the bloodstream, where it's taken up by Hb in the RBCs. When there, it displaces carbon dioxide (the by-product of metabolism), which diffuses from the RBCs into the blood and then it moves to the alveoli. Most transported oxygen binds with Hb to form oxyhemoglobin, while a small portion dissolves in the plasma (measurable as the partial pressure of arterial oxygen [PaO_2]).

After oxygen binds to Hb, the RBCs travel to the tissues. At this point, the blood cells contain more oxygen, and the tissue cells contain more carbon dioxide. Internal respiration occurs during cellular diffusion, as RBCs release oxygen and absorb carbon dioxide. The RBCs then transport carbon dioxide back to the lungs for removal during expiration.

Acid-base balance

The lungs help maintain acid-base balance in the body by maintaining external and internal respiration. Oxygen collected in the lungs is transported to the tissues by the circulatory system, which exchanges it for the carbon dioxide produced by cellular metabolism. Because carbon dioxide is 20 times more soluble than oxygen, it dissolves in the blood, where most of it forms bicarbonate (base) and smaller amounts form carbonic acid (acid).

The lungs control bicarbonate levels by converting bicarbonate to carbon dioxide and water for excretion. In response to signals from the medulla, the lungs can change the rate and depth of ventilation. Such changes maintain acid-base balance by adjusting the amount of carbon dioxide that is lost. For example, in metabolic alkalosis, which results from excess bicarbonate retention, the rate and depth of ventilation decrease so that carbon dioxide is retained. This increases carbonic acid levels. In metabolic acidosis — a condition resulting from excess acid retention or excess bicarbonate loss — the lungs increase the rate and depth of ventilation to exhale excess carbon dioxide, thereby reducing carbonic acid levels.

A patient with inadequately functioning lungs can experience acid-base imbalances. For example, hypoventilation, which reduces the rate and depth of ventilation of the lungs, results in carbon dioxide retention causing respiratory acidosis. Conversely, hyperventilation, which increases the rate and depth of ventilation of the lungs, leads to increased exhalation of carbon dioxide and will result in respiratory alkalosis.

Health history

Build the patient's health history by asking him open-ended questions. If possible, ask these questions systematically to avoid overlooking important information. If necessary conduct the interview in several short sessions, depending on the severity of your patient's condition, and his expectations as well as staffing constraints.

During the interview, establish a rapport with the patient by explaining who you are and what you'll do. The quantity and quality of the information gathered depends on the relationship built with the patient. Try to gain his trust by being sensitive to his concerns and feelings. Be alert to nonverbal responses that support or contradict his verbal responses. He may, for example, deny chest pain verbally but reveal it through his facial expressions. If the patient's verbal and nonverbal responses contradict each other, explore this with him to clarify your assessment.

Chief complaint

Ask your patient to tell you about his chief complaint. Use such questions as "When did you first notice you weren't feeling well?" and "What has happened since then that brings you here today?" Because many respiratory disorders are chronic, be sure to ask him how the latest episode compared with the previous episode, and what relief measures were helpful or unhelpful.

Current health history

The current health history includes the patient's biographic data and an analysis of his symptoms. Determine the patient's age, gender, marital status, occupation, education, religion, and ethnic background. These factors provide clues to potential risks and to the patient's interpretation of his respiratory condition. Advanced age, for example, suggests physiologic changes such as decreased vital capacity. Alternatively, the patient's occupation may alert you to problems related to hazardous materials. Ask him for the name, address, and phone number of a relative who can be contacted in an emergency.

After obtaining biographic data, ask the patient to describe his symptoms chronologically. Concentrate on the symptoms:

- onset — the first occurrence of symptoms and if they appeared suddenly or gradually
- incidence — the frequency of his symptoms, for example, if the pain is constant, intermittent, steadily worsening, or crescendo-decrescendo
- duration — the time period of his symptoms; ask him to use precise terms to describe his answers, such as 30 minutes after meals, twice a day, or for 3 hours
- manner — the symptom changes over time.

Next, ask the patient to characterize his symptoms. Have him describe:

- aggravating factors — the cause of increased intensity, for example, if he has dyspnea, ask him how many blocks he can walk before he feels short of breath
- alleviating factors — the relieving measures; determine if he's using any home remedies, such as over-the-counter medications, alternative therapies, or a change in sleeping position
- associated factors — the other symptoms that occur at the same time as the primary symptom
- location — the area where he experiences the symptom; ask him to pinpoint it and determine if it radiates to other areas

EXPERT TECHNIQUE

GRADING DYSPNEA

To assess dyspnea as objectively as possible, ask your patient to briefly describe how various activities affect his breathing. Then document his response using the grading system.

Grade 0—not troubled by breathlessness except with strenuous exercise

Grade 1—troubled by shortness of breath when hurrying on a level path or walking up a slight hill

Grade 2—walks more slowly on a level path because of breathlessness than people of the same age or has to stop to breathe when walking on a level path at his own pace

Grade 3—stops to breathe after walking about 100 yards (91.5 m) on a level path

Grade 4—too breathless to leave the house or breathless when dressing or undressing

- quality—the feeling that accompanies the symptom and if he has experienced similar symptoms in the past; ask him to characterize the symptom in his own words and document his description, including the words he chooses to describe pain, for example, sharp, stabbing, or throbbing
- duration—the time the symptom lasts
- setting—the place where he was when the symptom occurred; ask him what he was doing and who was with him. Be sure to document the findings.

A patient with a respiratory disorder may complain of dyspnea, cough, sputum production, wheezing, and chest pain. Here are some helpful assessment techniques to gain information about each of these signs and symptoms.

Dyspnea

Dyspnea, or shortness of breath, occurs when breathing is inappropriately difficult for the activity that the patient is performing. When ventilation is disturbed and ventilatory demands exceed the actual or perceived capacity of the lungs to respond, the patient becomes short of breath. In addition, dyspnea is caused by decreased lung compliance, disturbances in the chest bellows system, airway obstruction, or exogenous factors such as obesity.

Obtain the patient's history of dyspnea by using several scales. Ask the patient to rate his usual level of dyspnea on a scale of 1 to 10, in which 1 means no dyspnea and 10 means the worst he has experienced. Then ask him to rate the level that day. Another method to assess dyspnea is to count the number of words the patient speaks between breaths. A normal individual can speak 10 to 12 words. A severely dyspneic patient may speak only 1 to 2 words per breath.

Other scales grade dyspnea as it relates to activity. Ask the patient what he does to relieve the dyspnea and how well those measures work. (See *Grading dyspnea.*)

To find out if the dyspnea stems from pulmonary disease, ask the patient about its onset and severity:

- A sudden onset may indicate an acute problem, such as pneumothorax or pulmonary embolus, or may also result from anxiety caused by hyperventilation.
- A gradual onset suggests a slow, progressive disorder, such as emphysema, whereas acute intermittent attacks may indicate asthma.

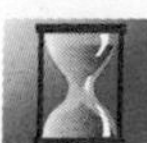

AGE ISSUE *Normally, an infant's respirations are abdominal, gradually changing to costal by age 7. Suspect dyspnea in an infant who breathes costally, in an older child who breathes abdominally, or in any child who uses neck or shoulder muscles to help in breathing.*

Orthopnea. Orthopnea is increased dyspnea when the patient is in a supine position.

It's traditionally measured in "pillows"—as in the number (usually one to three) of pillows needed to prop the patient before dyspnea resolves. A better method is to record the degree of head elevation at which dyspnea is relieved using a goniometer. This device is used by physical therapists to determine range of motion and may be used to measure a patient's orthopnea, for example, "relieved at 35 degrees."

Orthopnea is commonly associated with:

- pulmonary hypertension
- left-sided heart failure
- obesity
- diaphragmatic paralysis
- asthma
- chronic obstructive pulmonary disease.

Cough

If the patient is experiencing a cough, ask him these questions: Is the cough productive? If the cough is a chronic problem, has it changed recently? If so, how? What makes the cough better? What makes it worse?

Also investigate the characteristics of the cough:

- severe, it disrupts daily activities and causes chest pain or acute respiratory distress
- dry, signaling a cardiac condition
- hacking, signaling pneumonia
- congested, suggesting a cold, pneumonia, or bronchitis
- increased amounts of mucoid sputum, suggesting acute tracheobronchitis or acute asthma
- chronic productive with mucoid sputum, signaling asthma or chronic bronchitis
- changing sputum, from white to yellow or green, suggesting a bacterial infection
- occurring in the early morning, indicating chronic airway inflammation, possibly from cigarette smoke
- occurring in late afternoon, indicating exposure to irritants
- occurring in the evening, suggesting chronic postnasal drip or sinusitis.

AGE ISSUE *In children, evaluate a cough for these characteristics:*

- *barking, signaling croup*
- *nonproductive, indicating obstruction with a foreign body, asthma, pneumonia, or acute otitis media, or an early indicator of cystic fibrosis*
- *productive, accompanied by thick or excessive secretions, suggesting respiratory distress, asthma, bronchiectasis, bronchitis, cystic fibrosis, and pertussis.*

Sputum production

When a patient produces sputum, ask him to estimate the amount produced in teaspoons or some other common measurement. Find out what time of day he usually coughs and the color and consistency of his sputum. Ask if his sputum is a chronic problem and if it has recently changed. If it has, ask him how. Also ask if he coughs up blood; if so, find out how much and how often.

Hemoptysis. If a patient is experiencing hemoptysis (coughing up blood), this may result from violent coughing or from serious disorders, such as pneumonia, lung cancer, lung abscess, tuberculosis, pulmonary embolism, bronchiectasis, and left-sided heart failure. If the hemoptysis is mild (sputum streaked with blood), reassure the patient, making sure to ask him when he first noticed it and how often it occurs.

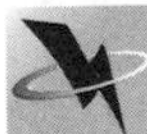

CRITICAL POINT *If hemoptysis is severe, causing frank bleeding, place the patient in a semirecumbent position, note pulse rate, blood pressure, and general condition. When the patient's condition stabilizes, ask whether he has ever experienced similar bleeding. (See* Hemoptysis or hematemesis?*)*

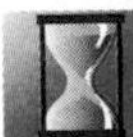

AGE ISSUE *If the elderly patient experiences hemoptysis, check his medication history for use of anticoagulants. Changes in medications, including over-the-counter and herbal supplements, or diet may be necessary because anticoagulants can affect blood clotting. In children, hemoptysis may stem from Goodpasture's syndrome, cystic fibrosis or, in rare cases, idiopathic primary pulmonary hemosiderosis. In rare cases, the cause is unknown in pulmonary hemorrhage occurring within the first 2 weeks of life; in such cases, the prognosis is poor.*

Wheezing

If a patient wheezes, initially determine the severity of the condition.

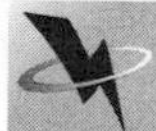

CRITICAL POINT *If the patient is in distress, immediately assess ABCs—airway, breathing, and circulation. Does he have an open airway? Is he breathing? Does he have a pulse? If these are absent, call for help and start cardiopulmonary resuscitation.*

Next, quickly check for signs of impending crisis:

- *Is the patient having difficulty breathing?*
- *Is he using accessory muscles to breathe? If chest excursion is less than the normal 1⅛" to 2" (3 to 5 cm), he'll use accessory muscles when he breathes. Look for shoulder elevation, intercostal muscle retraction, and use of scalene and sternocleidomastoid muscles.*
- *Has his level of consciousness diminished?*
- *Is he confused, anxious, or agitated?*
- *Does he change his body position to ease breathing?*
- *Does his skin look pale, diaphoretic, or cyanotic*

If the patient is not in acute distress, then ask him these questions: When does wheezing occur? What makes you wheeze? Do you wheeze loudly enough for others to hear it? What helps stop your wheezing?

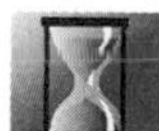

AGE ISSUE *Children are especially susceptible to wheezing due to their small airways, which allow for rapid obstruction.*

Chest pain

If the patient has chest pain, ask him where the pain is located. Ask him what the pain feels like, if it's sharp, stabbing, burning, or aching. Find out if it radiates to another area in his body and if so, find out where. Ask the patient how long the pain lasts, what causes it to occur, and what makes it better.

When the patient is describing his chest pain, attempt to determine the type of pain he's experiencing:

- substernal pain, which is sharp, stabbing pain in the middle of his chest, indicating spontaneous pneumothorax
- tracheal pain, which is a burning sensation that intensifies with deep breathing or coughing, suggesting oxygen toxicity or aspiration
- esophageal pain, which is a burning sensation that intensifies with swallowing, indicating local inflammation
- pleural pain, associated with pulmonary infarction, pneumothorax, or pleurisy, which is a stabbing, knifelike pain that increases with deep breathing or coughing
- chest wall pain, which is localized and tender, indicating an infection or inflammation of the chest wall, intercostal nerves, or intercostal muscles, or possibly, blunt chest trauma.

Regardless of the type of pain the patient describes, remember to assess associated factors, such as breathing, body position, and ease or difficulty of movement.

HEMOPTYSIS OR HEMATEMESIS?

If a patient begins bleeding from his mouth, determine if he's experiencing hemoptysis, which is coughing up blood from the lungs; hematemesis, which is vomiting blood from the stomach; or bleeding from a site in the upper respiratory tract. Compare the conditions based on the signs and symptoms listed here.

Hemoptysis

- Bright red or pink, frothy blood
- Blood mixed with sputum
- Negative litmus paper test of blood (paper remains blue)

Hematemesis

- Dark red blood, possibly with coffee-ground appearance
- Blood mixed with food
- Positive litmus paper test of blood (paper turns pink)

Upper respiratory tract bleeding

Oral sources

- Blood mixed with saliva
- Evidence of mouth or tongue laceration
- Negative litmus test

Nasal or sinus source

- Tickling sensation in nasal passages
- Sniffing behavior

Past health history

The information gained from the patient's past health history helps in understanding his current symptoms. It also helps to identify patients at risk for developing respiratory difficulty.

First, focus on identifying previous respiratory problems, such as asthma and emphysema. A history of these disorders provides instant clues to the patient's current condition. Then ask about childhood illnesses.

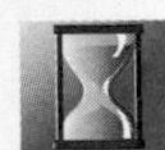

AGE ISSUE *Infantile eczema, atopic dermatitis, or allergic rhinitis, for example, may precipitate current respiratory problems such as asthma.*

Obtain an immunization history, especially of influenza and pneumococcal vaccination, which may provide clues about the potential for respiratory disease. A travel history may be useful and should include dates, destinations, and length of stay.

Next, ask what problems caused the patient to see a health care provider or required hospitalization in the past. Again, pay particular attention to respiratory problems. For example, chronic sinus infection or postnasal discharge may lead to recurrent bronchitis, and repeated episodes of pneumonia involving the same lung lobe may accompany bronchogenic carcinoma.

Ask the patient to describe the prescribed treatment, whether he followed the treatment plan, and whether the treatment helped. Determine whether he has suffered any traumatic injuries. If he has, note when they occurred and how they were treated.

The history should also include brief personal details. Ask the patient if he smokes; if he does, ask when he started and how many cigarettes he smokes per day. By calculating his smoking in pack-years, you can assess his risk of respiratory disease. To estimate pack-years, use this simple formula: number of packs smoked per day multiplied by the number of years the patient has smoked. For example, a patient who has smoked 2 packs of cigarettes per day for 42 years has accumulated 84 pack-years.

Remember to ask about alcohol use and about his diet because nutritional status commonly influences a patient's risk of respiratory infection.

Family history

Obtaining a family history helps determine whether a patient is at risk for hereditary or infectious respiratory diseases. First, ask if any of his immediate blood relatives, such as parents, siblings, and children, have had cancer, sickle cell anemia, heart disease, or a chronic illness, such as asthma and emphysema. Remember that diabetes can lead to cardiac, and possibly respiratory, problems. If an immediate relative has one or more of these disorders, ask for more information about the patient's maternal and paternal grandparents, aunts, and uncles.

Be sure to determine whether the patient lives with anyone who has an infectious disease, such as influenza and tuberculosis.

Psychosocial history

Ask your patient about his psychosocial history to assess his lifestyle. Be sure to cover his home, community, and other environmental factors that might influence how he deals with his respiratory problems. For instance, people who work in mining, construction, or chemical manufacturing are commonly exposed to environmental irritants. Also ask about interpersonal relationships, mental health status, stress management, and coping style. Keep in mind that a patient's sexual habits or drug use may be connected with acquired immunodeficiency syndrome-related pulmonary disorders.

Physical assessment

Any patient can develop a respiratory disorder. Using a systematic assessment enables the health care provider to detect subtle or obvious respiratory changes. The depth of the assessment will depend on several factors, including the patient's primary health problem and his risk of developing respiratory complications.

A physical examination of the respiratory system follows four steps: inspection, palpation, percussion, and auscultation. Before you begin, make sure the examination room is well lit and warm.

Make a few observations about the patient as soon as you enter the room. Note how he's seated, which will most likely be the position most comfortable for him. Take note of his level of awareness and general appearance. Does he appear relaxed? Anxious? Uncomfortable? Is he having trouble breathing? Include those observations in your final assessment.

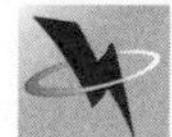

CRITICAL POINT *Assess the patient's ability to speak. If he's unable to speak, suspect a complete airway obstruction.*

When ready to begin the physical assessment, seat the patient in a position that allows access to the anterior and posterior thorax. Provide an examination gown that offers easy access to the chest and back without requiring unnecessary exposure. Make sure the patient isn't cold because shivering may alter breathing patterns.

If the patient can't sit up, place him in the semi-Fowler position to assess the anterior chest wall and the side-lying position to assess the posterior thorax. Keep in mind that these positions may cause some distortion of findings.

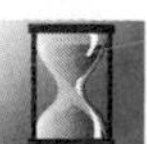

AGE ISSUE *If the patient is an infant or a small child, assess him while he's seated on the parent's lap.*

When performing the physical assessment, it may be easier to inspect, palpate, percuss, and auscultate the anterior chest before the posterior. However, this section covers inspection of the entire chest, then palpation, percussion, and auscultation of the entire chest.

Chest inspection

To assess respiratory function, determine the rate, rhythm, and quality of the patient's respirations and inspect his chest configuration, tracheal position, chest symmetry, skin condition, nostrils (for flaring), and accessory muscle use. Accomplish this by observing the patient's breathing and inspecting his anterior and posterior thorax. Note all abnormal findings.

Respiratory pattern

To find the patient's respiratory rate, count for a full minute—longer if you note abnormalities. Don't tell him what you're doing, or he might alter his natural breathing pattern. Adults normally breathe at a rate of 12 to 20 breaths/minute.

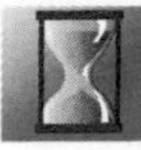

AGE ISSUE *An infant's breathing rate may reach about 40 breaths/minute.*

The respiratory pattern should be even, coordinated, and regular, with occasional sighs. The normal ratio of inspiration to expiration (I:E) is about 1:2.

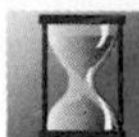

AGE ISSUE *Men, children, and infants usually use abdominal, or diaphragmatic, breathing. Athletes and singers do as well. Most women, however, usually use chest, or intercostal breathing.*

Paradoxical, or uneven, movement of the chest wall may appear as an abnormal collapse of part of the chest wall when the patient inhales or an abnormal expansion when the patient exhales. In either case, this uneven movement indicates a loss of normal chest-wall function.

When the patient inhales, his diaphragm should descend and the intercostal muscles should contract. This dual motion causes the abdomen to push out and the lower ribs to expand laterally. When the patient exhales, his abdomen and ribs return to their resting position. The upper chest shouldn't move much. Accessory muscles may hypertrophy, indicating frequent use.

Identifying abnormal respiratory patterns can help assess more completely a patient's respiratory status and his overall condition. (See *Recognizing abnormal respiratory patterns,* page 184.)

When examining the patient, be alert for these respiratory abnormalities:

- Frequent use of accessory muscles—indicates a respiratory problem, particularly when the patient purses his lips and flares his nostrils when breathing.
- Tachypnea—a respiratory rate greater than 20 breaths/minute with shallow breathing, which is commonly seen in patients with restrictive lung disease, pain, sepsis, obesity, or anxiety. Fever may be another cause. The respiratory rate may increase by 4 breaths/minute for every 1° F (0.6° C) rise in body temperature.
- Bradypnea—a respiratory rate below 10 breaths/minute, which is commonly noted just before a period of apnea or full respiratory arrest. Patients with bradypnea might have central nervous system (CNS) depression as a result of excessive sedation, tissue damage, or diabetic coma, which all depress the brain's respiratory control center. (The respiratory rate normally decreases during sleep.)

RECOGNIZING ABNORMAL RESPIRATORY PATTERNS

To better recognize abnormal respiratory patterns, illustrated below are typical characteristics of the more common ones.

Tachypnea
Shallow breathing with increased respiratory rate

Bradypnea
Decreased rate but regular breathing

Apnea
Absence of breathing; may be periodic

Hyperpnea
Deep breathing at a normal rate

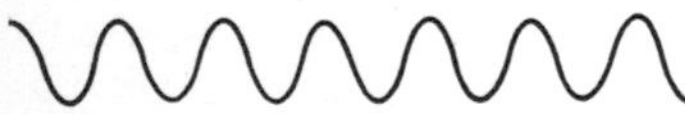

Kussmaul's respirations
Rapid, deep breathing without pauses; in adults, more than 20 breaths/minute; breathing usually sounds labored with deep breaths that resemble sighs

Cheyne-Stokes respirations
Breaths that gradually become faster and deeper than normal, then slower, during a 30- to 170-second period; alternates with 20- to 60-second periods of apnea

Biot's respirations
Rapid, deep breathing with abrupt pauses between each breath; equal depth to each breath

- Apnea — the absence of breathing where periods may be short and occur sporadically during Cheyne-Stokes respirations, Biot's respirations, or other abnormal respiratory patterns.

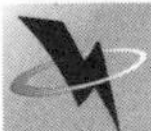

CRITICAL POINT *Apnea in patients may be life-threatening if the periods last long enough.*

- Hyperpnea — characterized by deep breathing, which occurs in patients who exercise or who have anxiety, pain, or metabolic acidosis. In a comatose patient, hyperpnea may indicate hypoxia or hypoglycemia.
- Kussmaul's respirations — rapid, deep, sighing breaths, which occur in patients with metabolic acidosis, especially when associated with diabetic ketoacidosis.
- Cheyne-Stokes respirations — a regular pattern of variations in the rate and depth of breathing where deep breaths alternate with short periods of apnea. This respiratory pattern is seen in patients with heart failure, kidney failure, or CNS damage.

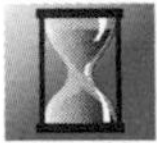

AGE ISSUE *In children and elderly patients during sleep, Cheyne-Stokes respirations may be normal.*

- Biot's respirations — rapid deep breaths that alternate with abrupt periods of apnea, which are an ominous sign of severe CNS damage.

Anterior thorax

After assessing respiration, inspect the anterior thorax for structural deformities such as a concave or convex curvature of the anterior chest wall over the sternum. Inspect between and around the ribs for visible sinking of soft tissues (retractions). Assess the patient's respiratory pattern for symmetry. Look for abnormalities in skin color or alterations in muscle tone. For future documentation, note the location of abnormalities according to regions delineated by imaginary lines on the thorax.

Initially inspect the chest wall to identify the shape of the thoracic cage. In an adult, the thorax should have a greater diameter laterally (from side to side) than anteroposteriorly (from front to back).

Note the angle between the ribs and the sternum at the point immediately above the xiphoid process. This angle, called the sternocostal angle, should be less than 90 degrees in an adult; it widens if the chest wall is chronically expanded, as in cases of increased anteroposterior diameter, or barrel chest.

To inspect the anterior chest for symmetry of movement, have the patient lie in a supine position. Stand at the foot of the bed and carefully observe the patient's quiet and deep breathing for equal expansion of the chest wall.

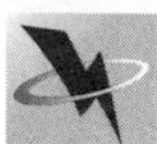

CRITICAL POINT *Watch for abnormal collapse of part of the chest wall during inspiration, along with abnormal expansion of the same area during expiration, which signals paradoxical movement—a loss of normal chest wall function. Also check whether one portion of the chest wall lags behind the others as the chest moves, which may indicate an obstruction in the patient's lung disease.*

Next, check for use of accessory muscles for respiration by observing the sternocleidomastoid, scalene, and trapezius muscles in the shoulders and neck. During normal inspiration and expiration, the diaphragm and external intercostal muscles should easily maintain the breathing process.

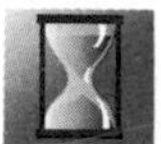

AGE ISSUE *In elderly patients, hypertrophy of any of the accessory muscles may indicate frequent abnormal use—although hypertrophy may be normal in a well-conditioned athlete.*

Note the position the patient assumes to breathe. A patient who depends on accessory muscles may assume a "tripod position," where he rests his arms on his knees or on the sides of a chair and supports his head.

Observe the patient's skin on the anterior chest for any unusual color, lumps, or lesions, and note the location of any abnormality. Unless the patient has been exposed to significant sun or heat, the skin color of the chest should match the rest of the patient's complexion. A skin abnormality may reflect problems in the underlying structure, so note the location of underlying ribs and other bones, cartilage, and lung lobes. Also check for any chest wall scars from previous surgeries. If the patient didn't mention past surgery during the health history, ask about it now.

Posterior thorax

To inspect the posterior thorax, observe the patient's breathing again. If he can't sit in a backless chair or lean forward against a supporting structure, direct him to lie in a lateral position. Be aware that this may distort the findings in some situations. If the patient is obese, findings may be distorted because he may be unable to fully expand the lower lung from the lateral position, leaving breath sounds on that side diminished.

Assess the posterior chest wall for the same characteristics as the anterior: chest structure, respiratory pattern, symmetry of expansion, skin color and muscle tone, and accessory muscle use. During the examination for chest wall abnormalities, keep in mind that the patient might have completely normal lungs and that the lungs might be cramped within the chest. The patient might have a smaller-than-normal lung capacity and limited exercise tolerance, and he may more easily develop respiratory failure from a respiratory tract infection. Other chest wall abnormalities include:

- A barrel chest, which looks like its name implies, is characterized by an abnormally round and bulging chest, with a greater-than-normal front-to-back diameter. It occurs as a result of chronic obstructive pulmonary disease, indicating that the lungs have lost their elasticity and that the diaphragm is flattened. The patient typically uses accessory muscles when he inhales and easily becomes breathless. You'll also note kyphosis of the thoracic spine, ribs that run horizontally rather than tangentially, and a prominent sternal angle.

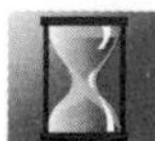

AGE ISSUE *In infants and elderly patients, barrel chest may be normal.*

- Pigeon chest, or pectus carinatum, is characterized by a chest with a sternum that protrudes beyond the front of the abdomen. The displaced sternum increases the front-to-back diameter of the chest.
- Funnel chest, or pectus excavatum, is characterized by a funnel-shaped depression on all or part of the sternum. The shape of the chest may interfere with respiratory and cardiac function. If cardiac compression occurs, you may hear a murmur.
- Thoracic kyphoscoliosis is characterized by the patient's spine curving to one side with the vertebrae rotated. Because the rotation distorts lung tissues, you may have a more difficult time assessing respiratory status. (See *Identifying chest deformities,* pages 186 and 187.)

IDENTIFYING CHEST DEFORMITIES

When inspecting the patient's chest, note deviations in size and shape. These illustrations show a normal adult chest, along with four common chest deformities.

NORMAL ADULT CHEST
No structural deformities or visible retractions

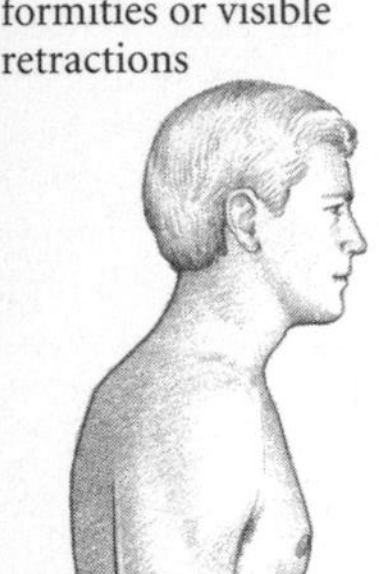

BARREL CHEST
Increased anteroposterior diameter

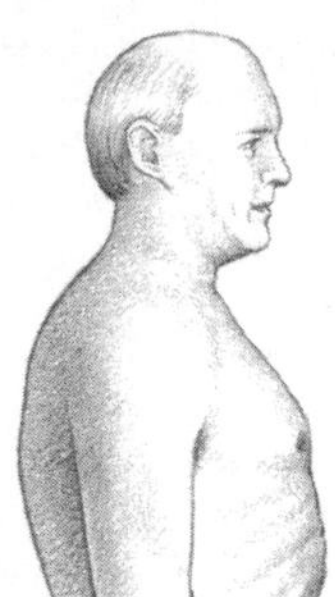

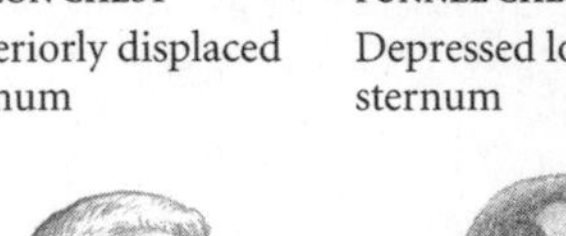

PIGEON CHEST
Anteriorly displaced sternum

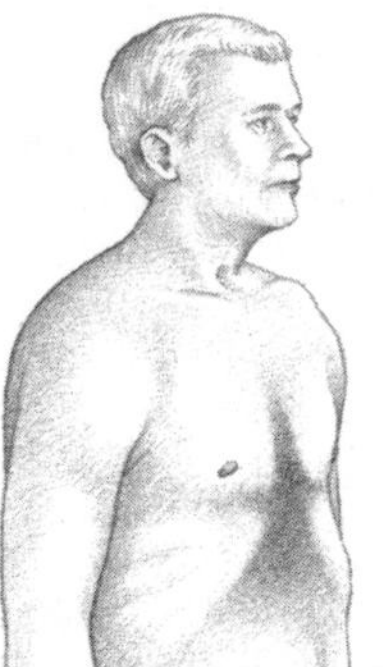

FUNNEL CHEST
Depressed lower sternum

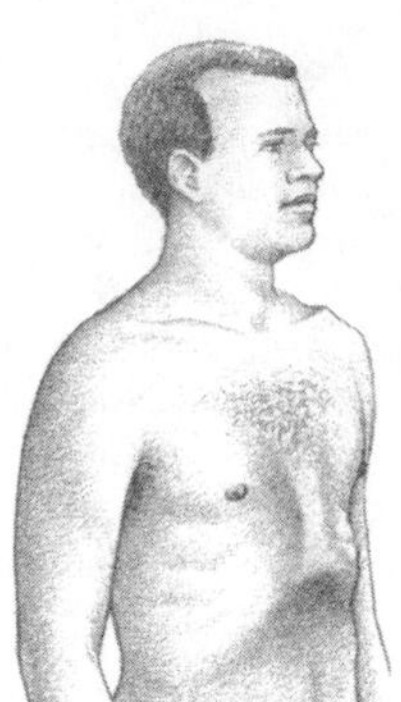

Inspection of related structures

Inspecting the patient's related structures, such as the skin and nails, will provide an overview of the patient's clinical status along with an assessment of his peripheral oxygenation. A dusky or bluish tint (cyanosis) to the patient's skin may indicate decreased Hb oxygen saturation. Distinguishing central from peripheral cyanosis is important:

- Central cyanosis results from hypoxemia and may appear in patients with right-to-left cardiac shunting or a pulmonary disease that causes hypoxemia, such as chronic bronchitis. It appears on the skin; the mucous membranes of the mouth, lips, and conjunctivae; or in other highly vascular areas, such as the earlobes, tip of the nose, and nail beds.
- Peripheral cyanosis, typically seen in patients exposed to the cold, results from vasoconstriction, vascular occlusion, or reduced cardiac output and appears in the nail beds, nose, ears, and fingers. Note that unlike central cyanosis, it doesn't affect the mucous membranes. Peripheral cyanosis indicates oxygen depletion in non-perfused areas of the body because oxyhemoglobin reduced by metabolism isn't replaced by fresh blood.

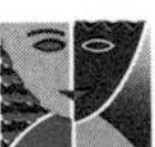

CULTURAL INSIGHT *A dark-skinned patient may be more difficult to assess for central cyanosis. In this patient, inspect the oral mucous membranes and lips, which will appear ashen gray rather than bluish. Facial skin may appear pale gray or ashen in a cyanotic black-skinned patient and yellowish brown in a cyanotic brown-skinned patient.*

Next, assess the patient's nail beds and toes for abnormal enlargement. Abnormal enlargement of the patient's nail beds and toes is called clubbing, which results from chronic tissue hypoxia. Nail thinning accompanied by an abnormal alteration of the angle of the finger and toe bases distinguishes clubbing. (See *Checking for clubbed fingers.*)

Chest palpation

Careful palpation of the trachea and the anterior and posterior thorax helps to detect structural and skin abnormalities, areas of pain, and chest asymmetry.

Trachea and anterior thorax

First, palpate the trachea for position. (See *Palpating the trachea,* page 188.)

Palpation of the patient's trachea may reveal that:

THORACIC KYPHOSCOLIOSIS

Raised shoulder and scapula, thoracic convexity, and flared interspaces

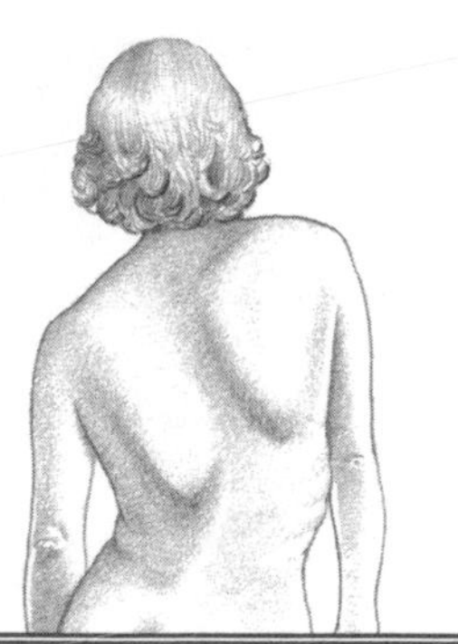

■ the trachea isn't midline, possibly resulting from atelectasis (collapsed lung tissue), thyroid enlargement, or pleural effusion (fluid accumulation in the air spaces of the lungs)

■ a tumor or pneumothorax (collapsed lung) may have also displaced the trachea to one side.

Observe the patient to determine whether he uses accessory neck muscles to breathe. Next, palpate the suprastemal notch. In most patients, the arch of the aorta lies close to the surface just behind the suprasternal notch. Use your fingertips to gently evaluate the strength and regularity of the patient's aortic pulsations in this area. Then palpate the thorax to assess the skin and underlying tissues for density. (See *Palpating the thorax,* page 188.)

Gentle palpation shouldn't be painful, so assess any complaints of pain for localization, radiation, and severity. Be especially careful to palpate any areas that looked abnormal during inspection. If necessary, support the patient during the procedure with one hand while using the other hand to palpate one side at a time, continuing to compare sides. Note any unusual findings, such as masses, crepitus, skin irregularities, and painful areas. The chest wall should feel smooth, warm, and dry.

EXPERT TECHNIQUE

CHECKING FOR CLUBBED FINGERS

To assess the patient for chronic tissue hypoxia, check his fingers for clubbing. Normally, the angle between the fingernail and the point where the nail enters the skin is about 160 degrees, as shown. Clubbing occurs when that angle increases to 180 degrees or more, as shown.

NORMAL FINGER

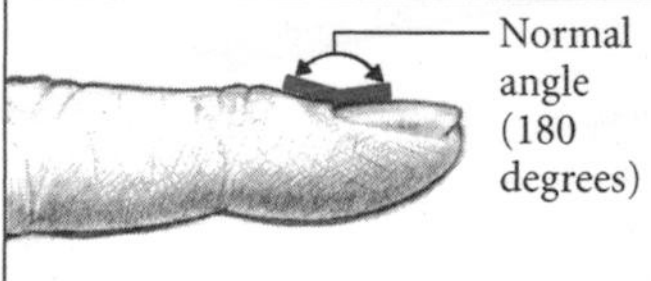

CLUBBED FINGER

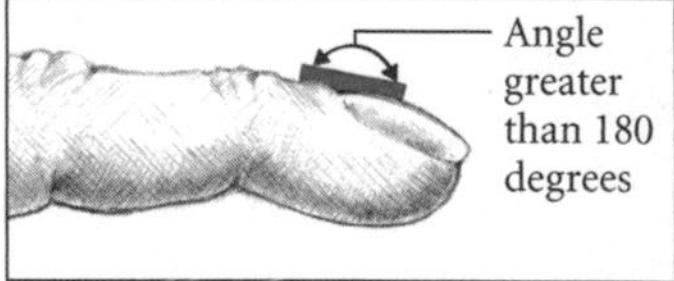

If the patient has subcutaneous air in the chest, this indicates crepitus, an abnormal condition that feels like puffed-rice cereal crackling under the skin and indicates that air is leaking from the airways or lungs. If a patient has a chest tube, you may find a small amount of subcutaneous air around the insertion site.

CRITICAL POINT *If the patient has no chest tube or the area of crepitus is getting larger, immediately alert the health care provider.*

If the patient complains of chest pain, attempt to determine the cause by palpating the anterior chest.

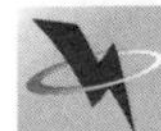

CRITICAL POINT *Increased pain during palpation may be caused by certain conditions—such as musculoskeletal pain, an irritation of the nerves covering the xiphoid process, and an inflammation of the cartilage connecting the bony*

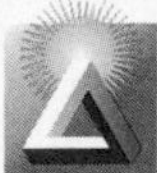

EXPERT TECHNIQUE

PALPATING THE TRACHEA

To palpate the trachea, stand in front of the patient and place one thumb on either side of the trachea above the suprasternal notch. Gently slide both thumbs, at equal speed, along the upper edge of the patient's clavicle until you reach the sternocleidomastoid muscle. Each thumb should cover an equal distance, indicating a midline trachea.

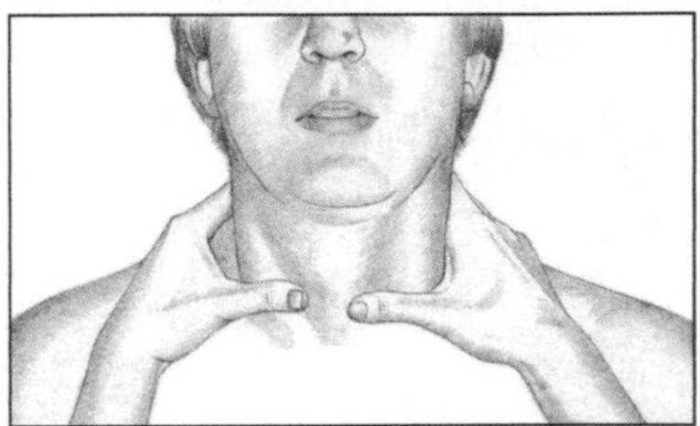

EXPERT TECHNIQUE

PALPATING THE THORAX

To palpate the thorax, place the palm of your hand (or hands) lightly over the thorax, as shown. Palpate for tenderness, alignment, bulging, or retractions of the chest and intercostal spaces. Assess the patient for crepitus, especially around drainage sites. Repeat this procedure on the patient's back.

Next, use the pads of your lingers, as shown, to palpate the front and back of the thorax. Pass your fingers over the ribs and any scars, lumps, lesions, or ulcerations. Note the skin temperature, turgor, and moisture. Also note tenderness or bony or subcutaneous crepitus. The muscles should feel firm and smooth.

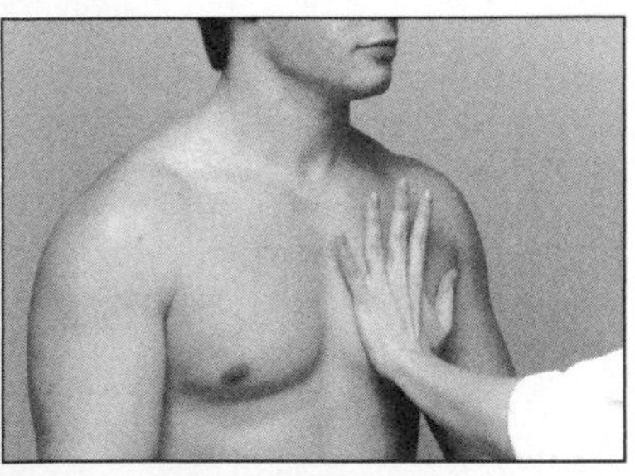

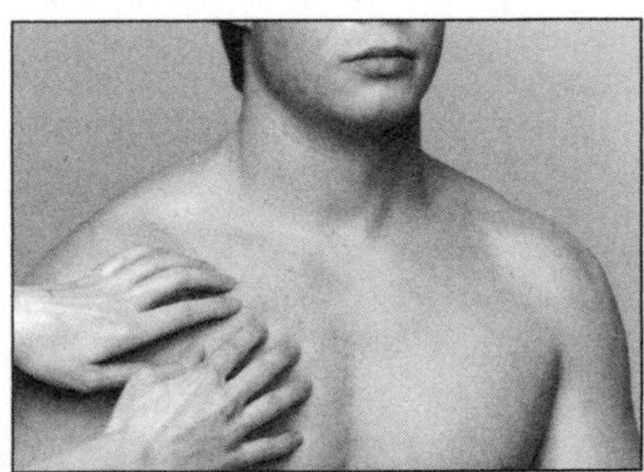

ribs to the sternum (costochondritis). These conditions may also produce pain during inspiration, causing the patient to breathe shallowly to decrease his discomfort. Keep in mind that palpation doesn't worsen pain caused by cardiac or pulmonary disorders, such as angina and pleurisy.

Next, palpate the costal angle. The area around the xiphoid process contains many nerve endings, so be gentle to avoid causing pain.

If a patient frequently uses the internal intercostal muscles to breathe, these muscles will eventually pull the chest cavity upward and outward. If this has occurred, the costal angle will be greater than the normal 90 degrees.

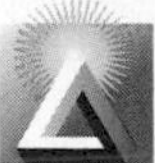

EXPERT TECHNIQUE

PALPATING THE THORAX FOR TACTILE FREMITUS

When checking the back of the thorax for tactile fremitus, ask the patient to fold his arms across his chest. This movement shifts the scapulae out of the way.

Palpation

Check for tactile fremitus by lightly placing your open palms on both sides of the patient's back, as shown, without touching his back with your fingers. Ask the patient to repeat the phrase "ninety-nine" loud enough to produce palpable vibrations. Then palpate the front of the chest using the same hand positions.

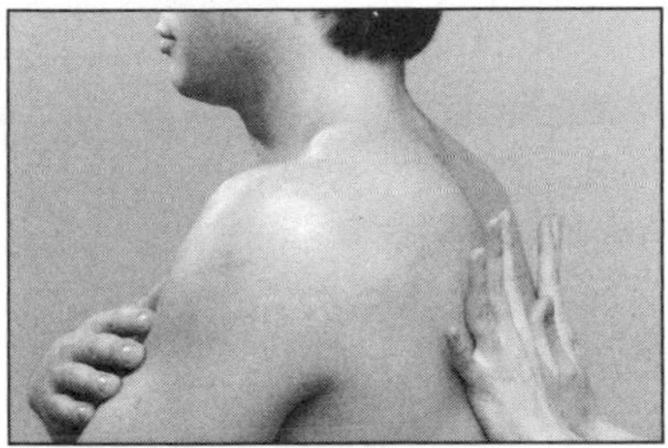

Interpretation

Vibrations that feel more intense on one side than the other indicate tissue consolidation on that side. Less intense vibrations may indicate emphysema, pneumothorax, or pleural effusion. Faint or no vibrations in the upper posterior thorax may indicate bronchial obstruction or a fluid-filled pleural space.

To evaluate how symmetrical the patient's chest wall is and how much it expands, place both hands on the front of the chest wall, with thumbs touching each other at the second intercostal space. As the patient inhales deeply, watch the thumbs. They should separate simultaneously and equally to a distance several centimeters away from the sternum. Repeat the measurement at the fifth intercostal space. The same measurement may be made on the back of the chest near the tenth rib.

During chest palpation, be alert for these findings in the patient's chest:

- asymmetrical expansion possibly due to pleural effusion, atelectasis, pneumonia, or pneumothorax
- decreased expansion at the level of the diaphragm secondary to emphysema, respiratory depression, diaphragm paralysis, atelectasis, obesity, or ascites
- absent or delayed chest movement during respiratory excursion, indicating previous surgical removal of the lung, complete or partial obstruction of the airway or underlying lung, or diaphragmatic dysfunction on the affected side.

Posterior thorax

Palpate the posterior thorax in a similar manner, using the palmar surface of the fingertips of one or both hands. During the process, identify bony structures, such as the vertebrae and the scapulae.

To determine the location of abnormalities, identify the first thoracic vertebra (with the patient's head tipped forward) and count the number of spinous processes from this landmark to the abnormal finding. Use this reference point for documentation. Also identify the inferior scapular tips and medial borders of both bones to define the margins of the upper and lower lung lobes posteriorly. Locate and describe all abnormalities in relation to these landmarks. Remember to evaluate abnormalities, such as use of accessory muscles and complaints of pain.

Tactile fremitus. Because sound travels more easily through solid structures than through air, checking for tactile fremitus (the palpation of vocalizations) helps you learn about the contents of the patient's lungs. (See *Palpating the thorax for tactile fremitus.*)

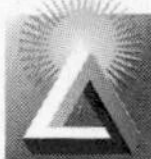

EXPERT TECHNIQUE

PERCUSSING THE CHEST

To percuss the chest, hyperextend the middle finger of your left hand if you're right-handed and the middle finger of your right hand if you're left-handed. Place your hand firmly on the patient's chest. Use the tip of the middle finger of your dominant hand — your right hand if you're right-handed, left hand if you're left-handed — to tap on the middle finger of your other hand just below the distal joint (as shown).

The movement should come from the wrist of your dominant hand, not your elbow or upper arm. Keep the fingernail you use for tapping short so you won't hurt yourself. Follow the standard percussion sequence over the front and back chest walls.

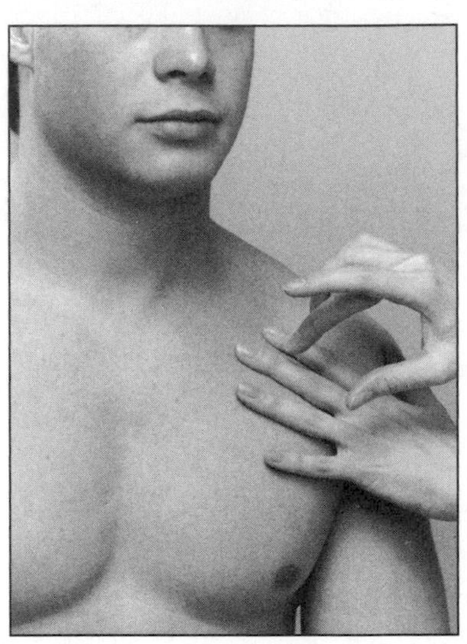

The patient's vocalization should produce vibrations of equal intensity on both sides of the chest. Normally, vibrations should occur in the upper chest, close to the bronchi, and then decrease and finally disappear toward the periphery of the lungs.

Conditions that restrict air movement, such as pneumonia, pleural effusion, and chronic obstructive pulmonary disease with overinflated lungs, cause decreased tactile fremitus. Conditions that consolidate tissue or fluid in a portion of the pleural area, such as a lung tumor, pneumonia, and pulmonary fibrosis, increase tactile fremitus. A grating feeling when palpating the patient's chest may signify a pleural friction rub.

Chest percussion

Percuss the patient's chest to find the boundaries of the lungs; to determine whether the lungs are filled with air, fluid, or solid material; and to evaluate the distance the diaphragm travels between the patient's inhalation and exhalation. (See *Percussing the chest.*)

Percussion allows you to assess structures as deep as 3″ (7.6 cm). You'll hear different percussion sounds in different areas of the chest. (See *Percussion sounds.*)

You may also hear different sounds after certain treatments. For instance, if your patient has atelectasis and you percuss his chest before chest physiotherapy, you'll hear a high-pitched, dull, soft sound. After physiotherapy, you should hear a low-pitched, hollow sound. In all cases, make sure you use other assessment techniques to confirm percussion findings.

You'll hear resonant sounds over normal lung tissue, which you should find over most of the chest. In the left front chest, from the third or fourth intercostal space at the sternum to the third or fourth intercostal space at the midclavicular line, you should hear a dull sound. Percussion is dull here because that's the space occupied by the heart. Resonance resumes at the sixth intercostal space. The sequence of sounds in the back is slightly different. (See *Percussion sequences.*)

PERCUSSION SOUNDS

This chart describes percussion sounds and their clinical significance. To master the different percussion sounds, practice on yourself, your patients, and any other person willing to help.

Sound	Description	Clinical significance
Flat	Short, soft, high-pitched, extremely dull, found over the thigh	Consolidation as in atelectasis and extensive pleural effusion
Dull	Medium in intensity and pitch, moderate length, thudlike, found over the liver	Solid area as in pleural effusion, mass, or lobar pneumonia
Resonant	Long, loud, low-pitched, hollow	Normal lung tissue, bronchitis
Hyperresonant	Very loud, lower-pitched, found over the stomach	Hyperinflated lung as in emphysema or pneumothorax
Tympanic	Loud, high-pitched, moderate length, musical, drumlike, found over a puffed-out cheek	Air collection as in a gastric air bubble or air in the intestines, large pneumothorax

EXPERT TECHNIQUE

PERCUSSION SEQUENCES

When percussing the lungs, follow these percussion sequences to distinguish between normal and abnormal sounds in the patient's lungs. Remember to compare sound variations from one side with the other as you proceed. Carefully document abnormal sounds you hear and include their locations. You'll follow the same sequences for auscultation.

ANTERIOR

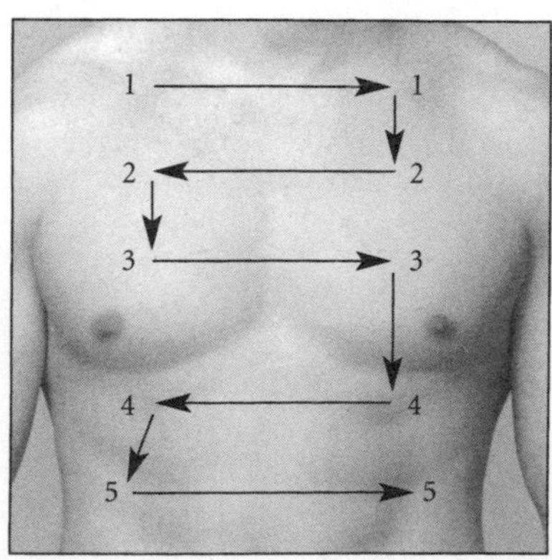

POSTERIOR

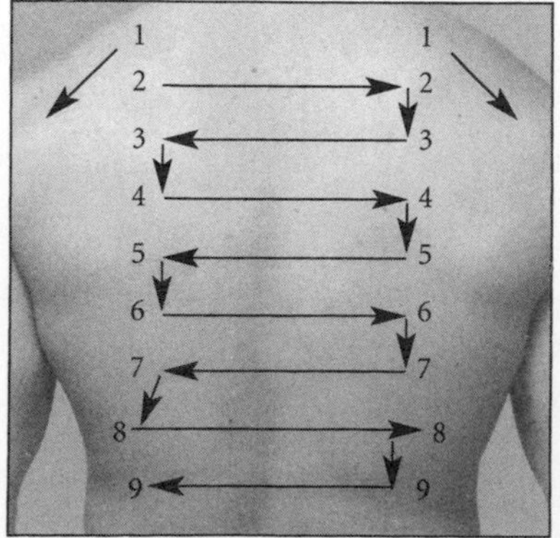

EXPERT TECHNIQUE

MEASURING DIAPHRAGMATIC MOVEMENT

You can measure how far the diaphragm moves by first asking the patient to exhale. Percuss the back on one side to locate the upper edge of the diaphragm, the point at which normal lung resonance changes to dullness. Use a pen to mark the spot indicating the position of the diaphragm at full expiration on that side of the back.

Then ask the patient to inhale as deeply as possible. Percuss the back when the patient has breathed in fully until you locate the diaphragm. Use the pen to mark this spot as well. Repeat on the opposite side of the back.

Use a ruler or tape measure to determine the distance between the marks. The distance, normally 1¼″ to 2″ (3 to 5 cm) long, should be equal on both the right and left sides

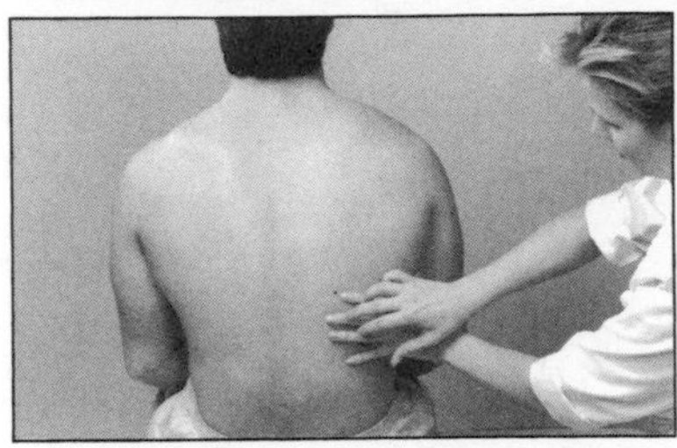

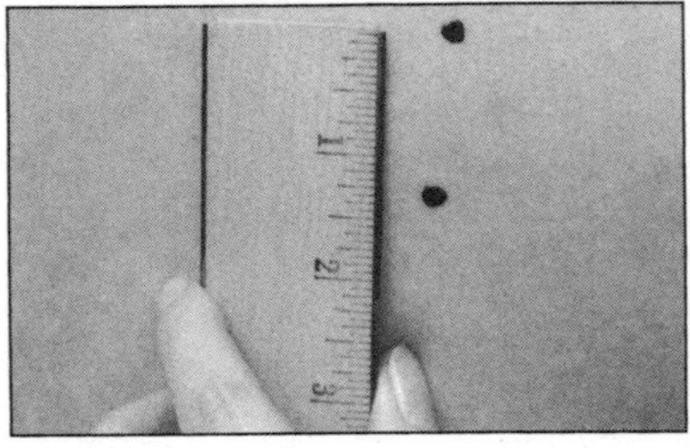

Hyperresonance during percussion indicates an area of increased air in the lung or pleural space that's associated with pneumothorax, acute asthma, bullous emphysema (large holes in the lungs from alveolar destruction), and gastric distention that pushes up on the diaphragm. Abnormal dullness during percussion indicates areas of decreased air in the lungs that's associated with pleural fluid, consolidation, atelectasis, or a tumor.

Chest percussion also allows assessment of the amount of diaphragmatic movement during inspiration and expiration. The normal diaphragm descends 2″ to 2½″ (5 to 6 cm) when the patient inhales. (See *Measuring diaphragmatic movement.*) The diaphragm doesn't move as far in a patient with emphysema, respiratory depression, diaphragm paralysis, atelectasis, obesity, or ascites.

Chest auscultation

As air moves through the bronchial tubes, it creates sound waves that travel to the chest wall. The sounds produced by breathing change as air moves from larger airways to smaller airways. Sounds also change if they pass through fluid, mucus, or narrowed airways. Chest auscultation helps you to determine the condition of the alveoli and surrounding pleura.

Auscultation sites are the same as percussion sites. Listen to a full inspiration and a full expiration at each site, using the diaphragm of the stethoscope. Ask the patient to breathe through his mouth; nose breathing alters the pitch of breath sounds.

To auscultate for breath sounds, press the stethoscope firmly against the patient's skin. Remember that listening through clothing or dry chest hair may result in hearing unusual and deceptive sounds. If the patient has abundant chest hair, mat it down with a damp washcloth so the hair doesn't make sounds like crackles.

Normal breath sounds

Four types of breath sounds are heard over normal lungs. The type of sound you hear depends on where you listen. (See *Qualities*

QUALITIES OF NORMAL BREATH SOUNDS

Breath sound	Quality	Inspiration-expiration ratio	Location
Tracheal	Harsh, high-pitched	I about = E	Over the treachea
Bronchial	Loud, high-pitched	I < E	Over the manubrium
Bronchovesicular	Medium in loudness and pitch	I = E	Next to the sternum, between scapula
Vesicular	Soft, low-pitched	I > E	Over most of both lungs

of normal breath sounds. Also see *Locations of normal breath sounds,* page 194.)

- Tracheal breath sounds are harsh, high-pitched, and discontinuous sounds heard over the trachea. They occur when a patient inhales or exhales.
- Bronchial breath sounds are loud, high-pitched sounds normally heard over the manubrium. They're discontinuous, and they're loudest when the patient exhales.
- Bronchovesicular sounds are medium-pitched, continuous sounds. They're heard when the patient inhales or exhales and are best heard over the upper third of the sternum and between the scapulae.
- Vesicular sounds are soft, low-pitched sounds heard over the remainder of the lungs. They're prolonged when the patient inhales and shortened during exhalation in about a 3:1 ratio.

If you hear diminished but normal breath sounds in both lungs, the patient may have emphysema, atelectasis, severe bronchospasm, or shallow breathing. If breath sounds are heard in one lung only, the patient may have pleural effusion, pneumothorax, a tumor, or mucus plugs in the airways.

Classify each breath sound according to its intensity, location, pitch, duration, and characteristic. Note whether the sound occurs when the patient inhales, exhales, or both. If you hear a sound in an area other than where you would expect to hear it, consider the sound abnormal.

For instance, bronchial or bronchovesicular breath sounds found in an area where vesicular breath sounds would normally be heard indicates that the alveoli and small bronchioles in that area might be filled with fluid or exudate, as in pneumonia and atelectasis. You won't hear vesicular sounds in those areas because no air is moving through the small airways.

Examination may reveal abnormal breath sounds, including:

- louder than normal over areas of consolidation because solid tissue transmits sound better than air or fluid
- quieter than normal if pus, fluid, or air fills the pleural space
- diminished or absent if a foreign body or secretions obstruct a bronchus, over lung tissue located distal to the obstruction
- adventitious sounds anywhere in the lungs, which include fine and coarse crackles, wheezes, rhonchi, stridor, and pleural friction rub
- crackles, which are caused by collapsed or fluid-filled alveoli popping open when the patient inhales and are classified as either fine or coarse and usually don't clear with coughing (see *Types of crackles*, page 195)
- wheezes, which are high-pitched sounds heard on exhalation when airflow is blocked (As severity of the block increases, they may also be heard when the patient inhales. The sound of a wheeze doesn't change with coughing. Patients may wheeze as a result of asthma, infection, heart failure, or airway obstruction from a tumor or foreign body.)

LOCATIONS OF NORMAL BREATH SOUNDS

These photographs show the normal locations of different types of breath sounds.

ANTERIOR THORAX

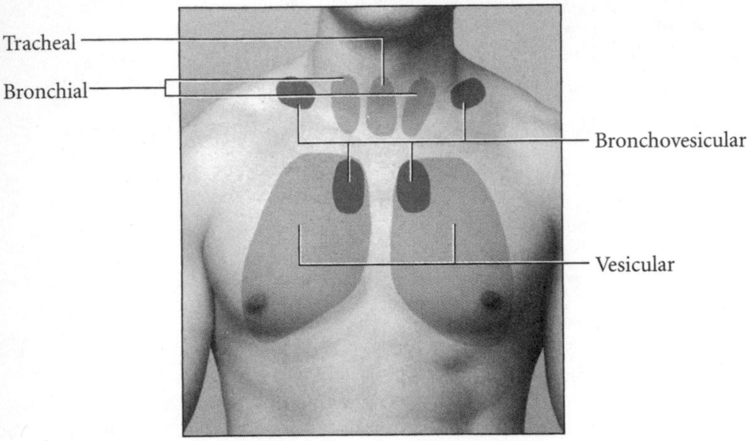

Tracheal

Bronchial

Bronchovesicular

Vesicular

POSTERIOR THORAX

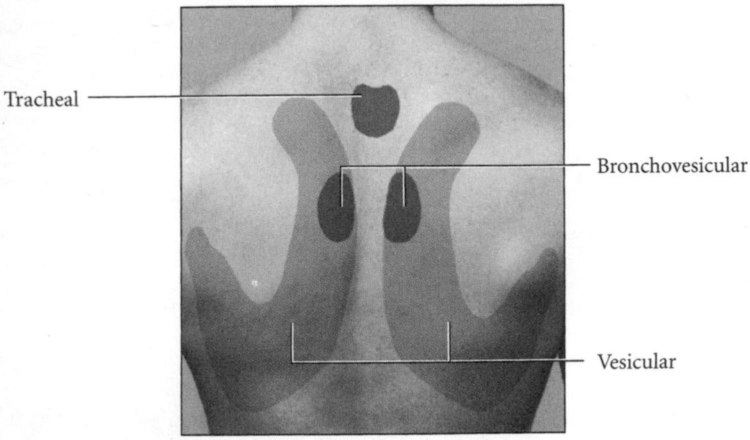

Tracheal

Bronchovesicular

Vesicular

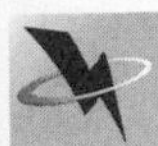

CRITICAL POINT *If your patient is having an acute asthma attack, the absence of wheezing sounds may not mean that the attack is over. When bronchospasm and mucosal swelling become severe, little air can move through the patient's airways. As a result, you won't hear wheezing. If all other assessment criteria—labored breathing, prolonged expiratory time, accessory muscle use—point to acute bronchial obstruction, maintain the patient's airway and give oxygen, as ordered. The patient may begin wheezing again when the airways open more.*

■ rhonchi, which are low-pitched, snoring, rattling sounds heard on exhalation, though they may also be heard inhalation,change sound or disappear with coughing when fluid partially blocks the large airways

- stridor, which is a loud, high-pitched crowing sound heard, usually without a stethoscope, during inspiration (louder in the neck than over the chest wall) and is caused by an obstruction in the upper airway and warrants immediate medical attention
- pleural friction rub, which is a low-pitched, grating, rubbing sound heard when the patient inhales and exhales that's caused by pleural inflammation of the two layers of pleura rubbing together. (The patient may complain of pain in areas where the rub is heard.)

Vocal fremitus

Vocal fremitus is the sound that chest vibrations produce as the patient speaks. Abnormal voice sounds—the most common of which are bronchophony, egophony, and whispered pectoriloquy—may occur over areas that are consolidated. Ask the patient to repeat the words listed below beside each abnormal sound, while you listen. Auscultate over an area where you hear vesicular sounds and then again over an area where you hear bronchial breath sounds.

Bronchophony. Ask the patient to say "ninety-nine" or "blue moon." Over normal lung tissue, the words sound muffled. Over consolidated areas, the words sound unusually loud.

Egophony. Ask the patient to say the letter "e." Over normal lung tissue, the sound is muffled. Over consolidated lung tissue, it will sound like the letter "a."

Whispered pectoriloquy. Ask the patient to whisper "1, 2, 3." Over normal lung tissue, the numbers will be almost indistinguishable. Over consolidated lung tissue, the numbers will be loud and clear.

A patient with abnormal findings during a respiratory assessment may be further evaluated using such diagnostic tests as arterial blood gas analysis or pulmonary function tests.

TYPES OF CRACKLES

When assessing the patient's lungs, it's critical to differentiate the characteristics of fine from coarse crackles.

Fine crackles

These characteristics distinguish fine crackles:

- Occur when the patient stops inhaling and alveoli "pop" open
- Are usually heard in lung bases
- Sound like a piece of hair being rubbed between the fingers or like Velcro being pulled apart
- Occur in restrictive diseases, such as pulmonary fibrosis, asbestosis, silicosis, atelectasis, congestive heart failure, and pneumonia
- Are soft, high-pitched, and very brief sounds unaffected by coughing

Coarse crackles

These characteristics distinguish coarse crackles:

- Are somewhat louder, lower in pitch, and not as brief as fine crackles
- Are heard primarily in the trachea and bronchi
- Are usually clear or diminish after coughing
- Occur when the patient starts to inhale; may be present when the patient exhales
- Mmay be heard through the lungs and even at the mouth
- Sound more like bubbling or gurgling, as air moves through secretions in larger airways
- Occur in chronic obstructive pulmonary disease, bronchiectasis, pulmonary edema, and with severely ill patients who can't cough; also called "death rattle"

Abnormal findings

A patient's chief complaint may stem from any of the number of signs and symptoms related to the respiratory system. Common findings include coughing, crackles, crepitus, cyanosis, dyspnea, hemoptysis, rhonchi, stridor, and wheezing. The following history, physical examination, and analysis summaries will help you assess each one quickly and accurately. After obtaining further information, begin to interpret the findings. (See *Respiratory system: Interpreting your findings.*)

Coughing

A cough is a sudden, noisy, forceful expulsion of air from the lungs and may be productive, nonproductive, or barking. Coughing is a necessary protective mechanism that clears airway passages. The cough reflex generally occurs when mechanical, chemical, thermal, inflammatory, or psychogenic stimuli activate cough receptors.

History

Ask the patient when the cough began and whether any body position, time of day, or specific activity affects it. Ask him if there's pain associated with the cough. Ask him to describe the cough, such as harsh, brassy, dry, or hacking.

If the cough is productive, find out how much sputum the patient is coughing up each day. Ask at what time of day he coughs up the most sputum. Find out if sputum production has any relationship to what or when he eats, where he is, or what he's doing. Also ask about the color, odor, and consistency of the sputum.

Ask about cigarette, drug, and alcohol use and whether his weight or appetite has changed. Find out if he has a history of asthma, allergies, or respiratory disorders, and ask about recent illnesses, surgery, or trauma. Find out what medications he's taking and if he works around chemicals or respiratory irritants such as silicone.

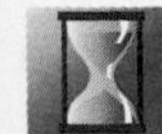

AGE ISSUE *If a child presents with a barking cough, ask his parents if he had any previous episodes of croup syndrome. Also ask the parents if the coughing improves upon exposure to cold air and what other signs and symptoms the child has.*

Physical assessment

Check the depth and rhythm of the patient's respirations, and note if wheezing or "crowing" noises occur with breathing. Feel the patient's skin: Is it cold, clammy, or dry?

Check his nose and mouth for congestion, inflammation, drainage, or signs of infection. Note breath odor as halitosis can be a sign of pulmonary infection. Inspect the neck for vein distention and tracheal deviation, and palpate for masses or enlarged lymph nodes.

Observe the patient's chest for accessory muscle use, retractions, and uneven chest expansion. Percuss for dullness, tympany, or flatness. Finally, auscultate for pleural friction rub and abnormal breath sounds, such as rhonchi, crackles, or wheezes.

Analysis

Coughing usually indicates a respiratory disorder. Evaluating a cough isn't an easy task because the cause can range from trivial (postnasal drip) to life-threatening (severe asthma or lung cancer).

A severe cough can disrupt daily activities and cause chest pain or acute respiratory distress. An early morning cough may indicate chronic airway inflammation, possibly from cigarette smoke. A late afternoon cough may indicate exposure to irritants. An evening cough may suggest chronic postnasal drip or sinusitis. A dry cough may signal a cardiac condition; a hacking cough, pneumonia; and a congested cough, a cold, pneumonia, or bronchitis.

Increasing amounts of mucoid sputum may suggest acute tracheobronchitis or acute asthma. If the patient has a chronic productive cough with mucoid sputum, suspect asthma or chronic bronchitis. If the sputum changes from white to yellow or green, suspect a bacterial infection.

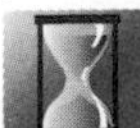

AGE ISSUE *In children, a barking cough is characteristic of croup. A nonproductive cough may indicate obstruction with a foreign body, asthma, pneumonia, or acute otitis media, or it may be an early indicator of cystic fibrosis. Because a child's airway is narrow, a productive cough can quickly develop airway occlusion and respiratory distress from thick or excessive secretions. Causes include asthma, bronchiectasis, bronchitis, cystic fibrosis, and pertussis. For elderly patients, always ask about productive or*

(Text continues on page 201.)

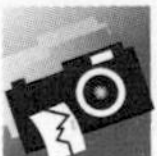

CLINICAL PICTURE

RESPIRATORY SYSTEM: INTERPRETING YOUR FINDINGS

After you assess the patient, a group of findings may lead you to a particular disorder of the respiratory system. The chart below shows some common groups of findings for major signs and symptoms related to a respiratory assessment, along with their probable causes.

Sign or symptom and findings	Probable cause
Cough	
▪ Nonproductive cough ▪ Pleuritic chest pain ▪ Dyspnea ▪ Tachypnea ▪ Anxiety ▪ Decreased vocal fremitus ▪ Tracheal deviation toward the affected side	Atelectasis
▪ Productive cough with small amounts of purulent (or mucopurulent), blood-streaked sputum or large amounts of frothy sputum ▪ Dyspnea ▪ Anorexia ▪ Fatigue ▪ Weight loss ▪ Wheezing ▪ Clubbing	Lung cancer
▪ Nonproductive cough ▪ Dyspnea ▪ Pleuritic chest pain ▪ Decreased chest motion ▪ Pleural friction rub ▪ Tachypnea ▪ Tachycardia ▪ Flatness on percussion ▪ Egophony	Pleural effusion
Crackles	
▪ Diffuse, fine to coarse crackles commonly in dependent lung areas ▪ Cyanosis ▪ Nasal flaring ▪ Tachypnea ▪ Tachycardia ▪ Grunting respirations ▪ Rhonchi ▪ Dyspnea ▪ Anxiety ▪ Decreased level of consciousness (LOC)	Acute respiratory distress syndrome (ARDS)
▪ Coarse crackles usually at lung bases ▪ Prolonged expirations ▪ Wheezing ▪ Rhonchi ▪ Exertional dyspnea ▪ Tachypnea ▪ Persistent productive cough ▪ Clubbing ▪ Cyanosis	Chronic bronchitis
▪ Diffuse, fine to coarse, moist crackles ▪ Productive cough with purulent sputum ▪ Dyspnea ▪ Wheezing ▪ Orthopnea ▪ Fever ▪ Malaise ▪ Mucous membrane irritation	Chemical pneumonitis

(continued)

RESPIRATORY SYSTEM: INTERPRETING YOUR FINDINGS *(continued)*

Sign or symptom and findings	Probable cause
Crackles *(continued)*	
■ Moist or coarse crackles ■ Productive cough ■ Chills ■ Sore throat ■ Slight fever ■ Muscle and back pain ■ Substernal tightness ■ Rhonchi ■ Wheezing	Tracheobronchitis
Crepitation, subcutaneous	
■ Crepitation over eyelid and orbit ■ Periorbital ecchymoses ■ Swollen eyelid ■ Facial edema ■ Diplopia ■ Hyphema ■ Possible dilated or unreactive pupil on affected side	Orbital fracture
■ Crepitation in upper chest and neck ■ Unilateral chest pain, increasing on inspiration ■ Dyspnea ■ Anxiety ■ Restlessness ■ Tachypnea ■ Cyanosis ■ Tachycardia ■ Accessory muscle use ■ Asymmetrical chest expansion ■ Nonproductive cough	Pneumothorax
Crepitation, subcutaneous *(continued)*	
■ Abrupt crepitation of neck and anterior chest wall ■ Severe dyspnea with nasal flaring ■ Tachycardia ■ Accessory muscle use ■ Hypotension ■ Cyanosis ■ Extreme anxiety ■ Hemoptysis ■ Mediastinal emphysema	Tracheal rupture
Cyanosis	
■ Central cyanosis, possibly aggravated by exertion ■ Exertional dyspnea ■ Productive cough with thick sputum ■ Anorexia ■ Weight loss ■ Pursed-lip breathing ■ Tachypnea ■ Wheezing ■ Hyperresonant lung sounds ■ Barrel chest ■ Clubbing	Chronic obstructive pulmonary disease

RESPIRATORY SYSTEM: INTERPRETING YOUR FINDINGS *(continued)*

Sign or symptom and findings	Probable cause
Cyanosis *(continued)*	
▪ Chronic central cyanosis ▪ Fever ▪ Weakness ▪ Weight loss ▪ Anorexia ▪ Dyspnea ▪ Chest pain ▪ Hemoptysis ▪ Possible atelectasis ▪ Decreased diaphragmatic excursion ▪ Asymmetrical chest expansion ▪ Dullness on percussion ▪ Diminished breath sounds	Lung cancer
▪ Acute central cyanosis ▪ Dyspnea ▪ Orthopnea ▪ Frothy blood-tinged sputum ▪ Tachycardia ▪ Tachypnea ▪ Dependent crackles ▪ Ventricular gallop ▪ Cold, clammy skin ▪ Hypotension ▪ Weak thready pulse ▪ Confusion	Pulmonary edema
▪ Acute peripheral cyanosis in hands and feet ▪ Cold, clammy pale extremities ▪ Lethargy ▪ Confusion ▪ Increased capillary refill time ▪ Rapid weak pulse	Shock
Dyspnea	
▪ Acute dyspnea ▪ Tachypnea ▪ Crackles and rhonchi in both lung fields ▪ Intercostal and suprasternal retractions ▪ Restlessness ▪ Anxiety ▪ Tachycardia	ARDS
▪ Progressive exertional dyspnea ▪ History of smoking ▪ Barrel chest ▪ Accessory muscle hypertrophy ▪ Diminished breath sounds ▪ Pursed-lip breathing ▪ Prolonged expiration ▪ Anorexia ▪ Weight loss	Emphysema
▪ Acute dyspnea ▪ Pleuritic chest pain ▪ Tachycardia ▪ Decreased breath sounds ▪ Low-grade fever ▪ Dullness or percussion ▪ Cool, clammy skin	Pulmonary embolism

(continued)

RESPIRATORY SYSTEM: INTERPRETING YOUR FINDINGS *(continued)*

Sign or symptom and findings	Probable cause
Hemoptysis	
■ Sputum ranging from pink to dark brown ■ Productive cough ■ Dyspnea ■ Chest pain ■ Crackles on auscultation ■ Chills ■ Fever	Pneumonia
■ Frothy, blood-tinged pink sputum ■ Severe dyspnea ■ Orthopnea ■ Gasping ■ Diffuse crackles ■ Cold, clammy skin ■ Anxiety	Pulmonary edema
■ Blood streaked or blood-tinged sputum ■ Chronic productive cough ■ Fine crackles after coughing ■ Dyspnea ■ Dullness to percussion ■ Increased tactile fremitus	Pulmonary tuberculosis
Rhonchi	
■ Accompanied by crackles ■ Rapid, shallow respirations ■ Dyspnea ■ Hypoxemia ■ Retractions ■ Diaphoresis ■ Restlessness ■ Apprehension ■ Decreased LOC	ARDS
Rhonchi *(continued)*	
■ Sonorous rhonchi ■ Wheezing ■ Chills ■ Sore throat ■ Low-grade fever ■ Muscle and back pain ■ Substernal tightness	Bronchitis
■ Sonorous rhonchi with faint, high-pitched wheezing ■ Weight loss ■ Mild chronic productive cough with scant sputum ■ Exertional dyspnea ■ Accessory muscle use on inspiration ■ Grunting expirations ■ Anorexia ■ Barrel chest ■ Peripheral cyanosis	Emphysema
Stridor	
■ Upper airway edema and laryngospasm ■ Nasal flaring ■ Wheezing ■ Accessory muscle use ■ Intercostals retractions ■ Dyspnea ■ Nasal congestion	Anaphylaxis

RESPIRATORY SYSTEM: INTERPRETING YOUR FINDINGS *(continued)*

Sign or symptom and findings	Probable cause
Stridor *(continued)*	
■ Sudden stridor ■ Dry paroxysmal coughing ■ Gagging or choking ■ Hoarseness ■ Tachycardia ■ Wheezing ■ Tachypnea ■ Intercostal muscle retractions ■ Diminished breath sounds ■ Cyanosis ■ Shallow respirations	Aspiration of a foreign body
■ Erythematous epiglottiditis ■ Fever ■ Sore throat ■ Crouplike cough	Epiglottiditis
Wheezing	
■ Sudden onset of wheezing ■ Stridor ■ Dry, paroxysmal cough ■ Gagging ■ Hoarseness ■ Decreased breath sounds ■ Dyspnea ■ Cyanosis	Aspiration of a foreign body
Wheezing *(continued)*	
■ Audible wheezing on expiration ■ Prolonged expiration ■ Apprehension ■ Intercostal and supraclavicular retractions ■ Rhonchi ■ Nasal flaring ■ Tachypnea	Asthma
■ Wheezing ■ Coarse crackles ■ Hacking cough that later becomes productive ■ Dyspnea ■ Barrel chest ■ Clubbing ■ Edema ■ Weight gain	Chronic bronchitis

nonproductive cough because either can indicate serious acute or chronic illness.

Crackles

A common finding in patients with certain pulmonary and cardiovascular disorders, crackles are nonmusical clicking or rattling noises heard during auscultation of breath sounds. They usually occur during inspiration and recur constantly from one respiratory cycle to the next. They can be unilateral or bilateral, moist or dry. They're characterized by their pitch, loudness, location, persistence, and occurrence during the respiratory cycle.

History

Determine if the patient is in acute respiratory distress or is experiencing airway obstruction. Quickly take the patient's vital signs and check the depth and rhythm of respirations. If he's struggling to breathe, check for increased accessory muscle use and chest wall motion, retractions, stridor, or nasal flaring. Provide supplemental oxygen. Endotracheal intubation may be necessary.

If the patient also has a cough, ask when it began and if it's constant or intermittent. Find out what the cough sounds like and whether he's coughing up sputum or blood. If the cough is productive, determine the sputum's consistency, amount, odor, and color.

Ask the patient if he has any pain and where it's located. Find out when he first noticed it and if it radiates to other areas. Also ask the patient if movement, coughing, or breathing worsens or helps to relieve his pain. Note the patient's position, for instance, if he's lying still or moving about restlessly.

Obtain a brief medical history. Find out if the patient has cancer or any known respiratory or cardiovascular problems. Ask about recent surgery, trauma, or illness. Ask him if he smokes or drinks alcohol. Find out if he's experiencing hoarseness or difficulty swallowing. Ask about which medications he's taking. Also ask about recent weight loss, anorexia, nausea, vomiting, fatigue, weakness, vertigo, and syncope. Find out if the patient has been exposed to irritants, such as vapors, fumes, or smoke.

Physical assessment

Perform a physical examination. Examine the patient's nose and mouth for signs of infection, such as inflammation or increased secretions. Note his breath odor because halitosis could indicate pulmonary infection.

Check his neck for masses, tenderness, swelling, lymphadenopathy, or venous distention. Inspect the patient's chest for abnormal configuration or uneven expansion. Percuss for dullness, tympany, or flatness. Auscultate his lungs for other abnormal, diminished, or absent breath sounds. Listen to his heart for abnormal sounds, and check his hands and feet for edema or clubbing.

Analysis

Crackles indicate abnormal movement of air through fluid-filled airways. They can be irregularly dispersed, as in pneumonia, or localized, as in bronchiectasis. A few basilar crackles can be heard in normal lungs after prolonged shallow breathing. These normal crackles clear with a few deep breaths. Usually, crackles indicate the degree of an underlying illness. When crackles result from a generalized disorder, they usually occur in the less distended and more dependent areas of the lungs such as the lung bases when the patient is standing. Crackles due to air passing through inflammatory exudate may not be audible if the involved portion of the lung isn't being ventilated because of shallow respirations.

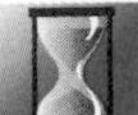

AGE ISSUE *In infants or children, crackles may indicate a serious respiratory or cardiovascular disorder. Pneumonia produces diffuse, sudden crackles in children. Esophageal atresia and tracheoesophageal fistula can cause bubbling, moist crackles due to aspiration of food or secretions into the lungs—especially in neonates. Pulmonary edema causes fine crackles at the base of the lungs, and bronchiectasis produces moist crackles. Cystic fibrosis produces widespread, fine to coarse inspiratory crackles and wheezing in infants. Sickle cell anemia may produce crackles when it causes pulmonary infarction or infection.*

Crackles that clear after deep breathing may indicate mild basilar atelectasis. In older patients, auscultate lung bases before and after auscultating apices.

Crepitation, subcutaneous

When bubbles of air or other gases such as carbon dioxide are trapped in subcutaneous tissue, palpation or stroking of the skin produces a crackling sound called subcutaneous crepitation or subcutaneous emphysema. The bubbles feel like small, unstable nodules and aren't painful, even though subcutaneous crepitation is commonly associated with painful disorders. Usually, the affected tissue is visibly edematous; this can lead to life-threatening airway occlusion if the edema affects the neck or upper chest.

History

Because subcutaneous crepitation can indicate a life-threatening disorder, perform a rapid initial evaluation and intervene if necessary. Ask the patient if he's experiencing pain or having difficulty breathing. If he's in pain, find out where the pain is located, how severe it is, and when it began. Ask about recent thoracic surgery, diagnostic tests, and respiratory therapy, or a history of trauma or chronic pulmonary disease.

Physical assessment
When the patient's condition permits, palpate the affected skin to evaluate the location and extent of subcutaneous crepitation and to obtain baseline information. Repalpate frequently to determine if the subcutaneous crepitation is increasing.

Analysis
The air or gas bubbles enter the tissues through open wounds from the action of anaerobic microorganisms or from traumatic or spontaneous rupture or perforation of pulmonary or GI organs.

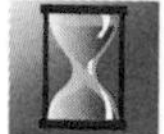
AGE ISSUE *Children may develop subcutaneous crepitation in the neck from ingestion of corrosive substances that perforate the esophagus.*

Cyanosis
Cyanosis — a bluish or bluish-black discoloration of the skin and mucous membranes — results from excessive concentration of unoxygenated Hb in the blood. This common sign may develop abruptly or gradually. It can be classified as central or peripheral, although the two types may coexist.

History
If cyanosis accompanies less-acute conditions, perform a thorough examination. Begin with a health history, focusing on pulmonary, cardiac, and hematologic disorders. Ask about previous surgeries. Ask the patient if he has a cough and if it's productive. If so, have the patient describe the sputum. Ask about sleep apnea. Find out if the patient sleeps with his head propped up on pillows. Also ask about nausea, anorexia, and weight loss.

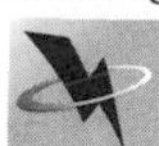
CRITICAL POINT *If the patient displays sudden, localized cyanosis and other signs of arterial occlusion, protect the affected limb from injury; however, don't massage the limb. If you see central cyanosis stemming from a pulmonary disorder or shock, perform a rapid evaluation. Take immediate steps to maintain ABCs.*

Physical assessment
Begin the physical examination by taking vital signs. Inspect the skin and mucous membranes to determine the extent of cyanosis. Ask the patient when he first noticed the cyanosis and if it subsides and recurs. Find out if it's aggravated by cold, smoking, or stress, and alleviated by massage or rewarming. Check the skin for coolness, pallor, redness, pain, and ulceration. Also note clubbing.

Next, evaluate the patient's level of consciousness. Ask about headaches, dizziness, or blurred vision. Then test his motor strength. Ask about pain in the arms and legs, especially with walking, and about abnormal sensations, such as numbness, tingling, and coldness.

Ask the patient about chest pain and its severity. Ask him to identify any aggravating and alleviating factors. Palpate peripheral pulses, and test capillary refill time. Also note edema. Auscultate heart rate and rhythm, especially noting gallops and murmurs. Also auscultate the abdominal aorta and femoral arteries to detect any bruits.

Evaluate respiratory rate and rhythm. Check for nasal flaring and use of accessory muscles. Inspect the patient for asymmetrical chest expansion or barrel chest. Percuss the lungs for dullness or hyperresonance, and auscultate for decreased or adventitious breath sounds.

Inspect the abdomen for ascites, and test for shifting dullness or fluid wave. Percuss and palpate for liver enlargement and tenderness.

Analysis
Central cyanosis reflects inadequate oxygenation of systemic arterial blood caused by right-to-left cardiac shunting, pulmonary disease, or hematologic disorders. It may occur anywhere on the skin and also on the mucous membranes of the mouth, lips, and conjunctiva.

Peripheral cyanosis reflects sluggish peripheral circulation caused by vasoconstriction, reduced cardiac output, or vascular occlusion. It may be widespread or may occur locally in one extremity; however, it doesn't affect mucous membranes. Typically, peripheral cyanosis appears on exposed areas, such as the fingers, nail beds, feet, nose, and ears.

Although cyanosis is an important sign of pulmonary and cardiovascular disorders, it isn't always an accurate gauge of oxygenation. Several factors contribute to its development: Hb concentration and oxygen saturation, cardiac output, and partial pressure of arterial oxygen (PaO_2). Cyanosis is usually undetectable until the oxygen saturation of Hb falls below 80%. Severe cyanosis is quite obvious, whereas mild cyanosis is more difficult to detect, even in natural, bright light.

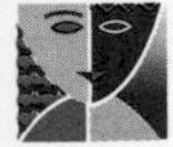

CULTURAL INSIGHT *In dark-skinned patients, cyanosis is most apparent in the mucous membranes and nail beds.*

Transient, nonpathologic cyanosis may result from environmental factors. For example, peripheral cyanosis may result from cutaneous vasoconstriction following a brief exposure to cold air or water. Central cyanosis may result from reduced PaO_2 at high altitudes.

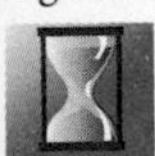

AGE ISSUE *Children are afflicted with many of the same pulmonary disorders responsible for cyanosis in adults. In addition, central cyanosis may result from cystic fibrosis, asthma, airway obstruction by a foreign body, acute laryngotracheobronchitis, or epiglottiditis. It may also result from a congenital heart defect such as transposition of the great vessels that causes right-to-left intracardiac shunting. In children, circumoral cyanosis may precede generalized cyanosis. In infants, acrocyanosis (also called "glove and bootee" cyanosis) may occur due to excessive crying or exposure to cold. Elderly patients commonly have reduced tissue perfusion; therefore, peripheral cyanosis can present even with a slight decrease in cardiac output or systemic blood pressure.*

Dyspnea

Commonly a symptom of cardiopulmonary dysfunction, dyspnea is the sensation of difficult or uncomfortable breathing. It's usually reported as shortness of breath. The severity varies greatly and is typically unrelated to the severity of the underlying cause.

Dyspnea may arise suddenly or slowly and may subside rapidly or persist for years.

History

If your patient complains of dyspnea, ask if it began suddenly or gradually. Find out if it's constant or intermittent and when the attack began. Ask if it occurs during activity or while at rest. If the patient has had dyspneic attacks before, ask if they're increasing in severity. Ask him to identify what aggravates or alleviates these attacks. Find out if he has a productive or nonproductive cough or chest pain.

Ask about recent trauma, and note a history of upper respiratory tract infections, deep vein phlebitis, or other disorders. Ask the patient if he smokes or is exposed to toxic fumes or irritants in his occupation.

Find out if he has orthopnea (dyspnea when in a supine position), paroxysmal nocturnal dyspnea (dyspnea during sleep), or progressive fatigue.

Physical assessment

During the physical examination, look for signs of chronic dyspnea such as accessory muscle hypertrophy, especially in the shoulders and neck. Also look for pursed-lip exhalation, clubbing, peripheral edema, barrel chest, diaphoresis, and neck vein distention. Auscultate for crackles, abnormal heart sounds or rhythms, egophony, bronchophony, and whispered pectoriloquy. Then palpate the abdomen for hepatomegaly.

Analysis

Most people normally experience dyspnea when they overexert themselves, and its severity depends on their physical condition. In a healthy person, dyspnea is quickly relieved by rest. Pathologic causes of dyspnea include pulmonary, cardiac, neuromuscular, and allergic disorders. In addition, anxiety may cause dyspnea.

Dyspnea occurs when ventilation is disturbed. When ventilatory demands exceed the actual or perceived capacity of the lungs to respond, the patient becomes short of breath. Decreased lung compliance, a disturbance in the chest bellows system, an airway obstruction, or obesity can increase the work of breathing.

When evaluating dyspnea determine whether it stems from pulmonary or cardiac disease; then evaluate the degree of impairment the dyspnea has caused.

Your questions about the onset and severity of your patient's dyspnea should prove helpful. A sudden onset may indicate an acute problem, such as pneumothorax or pulmonary embolus. Sudden dyspnea may also result from anxiety caused by hyperventilation. A gradual onset suggests a slow, progressive disorder, such as emphysema, whereas acute intermittent attacks may indicate asthma.

Precipitating factors also help pinpoint the cause. For instance, paroxysmal nocturnal dyspnea or orthopnea may stem from a chronic lung disorder or a cardiac disorder, such as left-sided heart failure. Dyspnea aggravated by activity suggests poor ventilation and perfusion or inefficient breathing mechanisms.

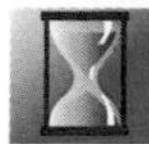

AGE ISSUE *Elderly patients with dyspnea related to chronic illness may not initially be aware of a significant change in their breathing pattern.*

Hemoptysis

Hemoptysis is the expectoration of blood or bloody sputum from the lungs or tracheobronchial tree. It's sometimes confused with bleeding from the mouth, throat, nasopharynx, or GI tract.

History

If your patient complains of hemoptysis, ask if it's mild and when it began. Find out if the patient has ever coughed up blood before. Ask him about how much blood he's coughing up now and how often.

Ask about a history of pulmonary, cardiac, or bleeding disorders. If he's receiving anticoagulant therapy, find out the drug, its dosage and schedule, and the duration of therapy. Find out if he's taking other prescription drugs and if he smokes.

Physical assessment

Examine the patient's nose, mouth, and pharynx to determine the source of the bleeding. Inspect the configuration of his chest, and look for abnormal movement during breathing, use of accessory muscles, and retractions. Observe respiratory rate, depth, and rhythm. Examine the skin for lesions.

Next, palpate the patient's chest for diaphragm level and for tenderness, respiratory excursion, fremitus, and abnormal pulsations; then percuss for flatness, dullness, resonance, hyperresonance, and tympany. Finally, auscultate the lungs, noting especially the quality and intensity of breath sounds. Also auscultate for heart murmurs, bruits, and pleural friction rubs.

Obtain a sputum sample and examine it for overall quantity; for the amount of blood it contains; and for its color, odor, and consistency.

Analysis

Commonly frothy because it's mixed with air, hemoptysis is typically bright red with an alkaline pH. Expectoration of 200 ml of blood in a single episode suggests severe bleeding, whereas expectoration of 400 ml in 3 hours or more than 600 ml in 16 hours signals a life-threatening crisis.

Hemoptysis usually results from chronic bronchitis, lung cancer, or bronchiectasis. However, it may also result from inflammatory, infectious, cardiovascular, and coagulation disorders or, in rare cases, from a ruptured aortic aneurysm. In up to 15% of patients, the cause is unknown. The most common causes of massive hemoptysis are lung cancer, bronchiectasis, active tuberculosis, and cavitary pulmonary disease from necrotic infections or tuberculosis.

Rhonchi

Rhonchi are continuous adventitious breath sounds detected by auscultation. They're usually louder and lower-pitched than crackles — more like a hoarse moan or a deep snore — though they may be described as rattling, sonorous, bubbling, rumbling, or musical. However, sibilant rhonchi, or wheezes, are high pitched.

History

When obtaining the health history, ask these related questions: Does the patient smoke? If so, obtain a history in pack-years. Has he recently lost weight or felt tired or weak? Does he have asthma or other pulmonary disorder? Is he taking any prescription or over-the-counter drugs?

Physical assessment

If you auscultate rhonchi, take the patient's vital signs, including oxygen saturation, and be alert for signs of respiratory distress. Characterize the patient's respirations as rapid or slow, shallow or deep, and regular or irregular. Inspect the chest, noting the use of accessory muscles. Observe if the patient is audibly wheezing or gurgling. Auscultate for other abnormal breath sounds, such as crackles and a pleural friction rub. If you detect these sounds, note their location. Note if breath sounds are diminished or absent.

Next, percuss the chest. If the patient has a cough, note its frequency and characterize its sound. If it's productive, examine the sputum for color, odor, consistency, and blood.

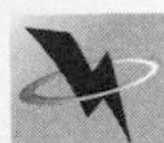

CRITICAL POINT *During the examination, keep in mind that thick or excessive secretions, bronchospasm, or inflammation of mucous membranes may lead to airway obstruction. If necessary, suction the patient and keep equipment available for inserting an artificial airway. Keep a bronchodilator available to treat bronchospasm.*

Analysis
Rhonchi are heard over large airways such as the trachea. They can occur in a patient with a pulmonary disorder when air flows through passages that have been narrowed by secretions, a tumor or foreign body, bronchospasm, or mucosal thickening. The resulting vibration of airway walls produces the rhonchi.

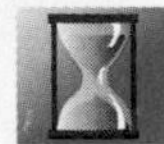

AGE ISSUE *In children, rhonchi can result from bacterial pneumonia, cystic fibrosis, and croup. Because a respiratory tract disorder may begin abruptly and progress rapidly in an infant or a child, observe closely for signs of airway obstruction.*

Stridor
A loud, harsh, musical respiratory sound, stridor results from an obstruction in the trachea or larynx. Usually heard during inspiration, this sign may also occur during expiration in severe upper airway obstruction.

History
When the patient's condition permits, obtain a health history from him or a family member. First, find out when the stridor began and if he has had it before. Ask if he has had an upper respiratory tract infection and, if so, how long has he had it.

Ask about a history of allergies, tumors, and respiratory and vascular disorders. Note recent exposure to smoke or noxious fumes or gases. Next, explore associated signs and symptoms. Find out if the stridor occurs with pain or a cough.

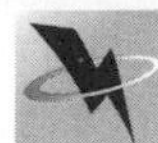

CRITICAL POINT *If you hear stridor, quickly check the patient's vital signs including oxygen saturation and examine him for other signs of partial airway obstruction—choking or gagging, tachypnea, dyspnea, shallow respirations, intercostal retractions, nasal flaring, tachycardia, cyanosis, and diaphoresis. Be aware that abrupt cessation of stridor signals complete obstruction in which the patient has inspiratory chest movement but absent breath sounds. He may be unable to talk and can quickly become lethargic and lose consciousness. In this case, begin measures to clear the obstruction.*

Physical assessment
Examine the patient's mouth for excessive secretions, foreign matter, inflammation, and swelling. Assess his neck for swelling, masses, subcutaneous crepitation, and scars. Observe the patient's chest for delayed, decreased, or asymmetrical chest expansion. Auscultate for wheezes, rhonchi, crackles, rubs, and other abnormal breath sounds. Percuss for dullness, tympany, or flatness. Finally, note any burns or signs of trauma, such as ecchymoses and lacerations.

Analysis
Stridor may begin as low-pitched "croaking" and progress to high-pitched "crowing" as respirations become more vigorous. Life-threatening upper airway obstruction can stem from foreign-body aspiration, increased secretions, intraluminal tumor, localized edema or muscle spasms, and external compression by a tumor or aneurysm.

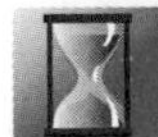

AGE ISSUE *In children, stridor is a major sign of airway obstruction. Quick intervention is needed to prevent total airway obstruction. This emergency can happen more rapidly in a child because his airway is narrower than an adult's. Causes of stridor include foreign-body aspiration, croup syndrome, laryngeal diphtheria, pertussis, retropharyngeal abscess, and congenital abnormalities of the larynx.*

Wheezing
Wheezes are adventitious breath sounds with a high-pitched, musical, squealing,

creaking, or groaning quality. When they originate in the large airways, they can be heard by placing an unaided ear over the chest wall or at the mouth. When they originate in the smaller airways, they can be heard by placing a stethoscope over the anterior or posterior chest. Unlike crackles and rhonchi, wheezes can't be cleared by coughing.

History

Ask the patient what triggers his wheezing. Find out if he has asthma or allergies, if he smokes or has a history of pulmonary, cardiac, or circulatory disorders, or if he has cancer.

Ask the patient if he recently had surgery, illness, or trauma, or changes in appetite, weight, exercise tolerance, or sleep patterns. Find out which drugs he's currently taking and which ones has he taken in the past. Also find out if he has been exposed to toxic fumes or respiratory irritants.

If he has a cough, ask how it sounds, when it occurs, and how often it occurs. Find out if he has paroxysms of coughing and if the cough is dry, sputum producing, or bloody.

Ask the patient if he's experiencing chest pain. If so, determine its quality, onset, duration, intensity, and radiation. Find out if it increases with breathing, coughing, or certain positions.

Physical assessment

Examine the patient's nose and mouth for congestion, drainage, or signs of infection, such as halitosis. If he produces sputum, obtain a sample for examination. Check for cyanosis, pallor, clamminess, masses, tenderness, swelling, distended neck veins, and enlarged lymph nodes. Inspect his chest for abnormal configuration and asymmetrical motion, and determine if the trachea is midline. Percuss for dullness or hyperresonance, and auscultate for crackles, rhonchi, or pleural friction rubs. Note absent or hypoactive breath sounds, abnormal heart sounds, gallops, or murmurs. Also note arrhythmias, bradycardia, or tachycardia.

Analysis

Usually, prolonged wheezing occurs during expiration when bronchi are shortened and narrowed. Causes of airway narrowing include bronchospasm; mucosal thickening or edema; partial obstruction from a tumor, a foreign body, or secretions; and extrinsic pressure, as in tension pneumothorax or goiter. With airway obstruction, wheezing occurs during inspiration.

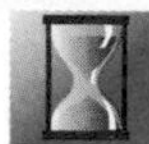

AGE ISSUE *Children are especially susceptible to wheezing because their small airways allow rapid obstruction. Primary causes of wheezing include bronchospasm, mucosal edema, and accumulation of secretions. These may occur with such disorders as cystic fibrosis, acute bronchiolitis, and pulmonary hemosiderosis, or foreign-body aspiration.*

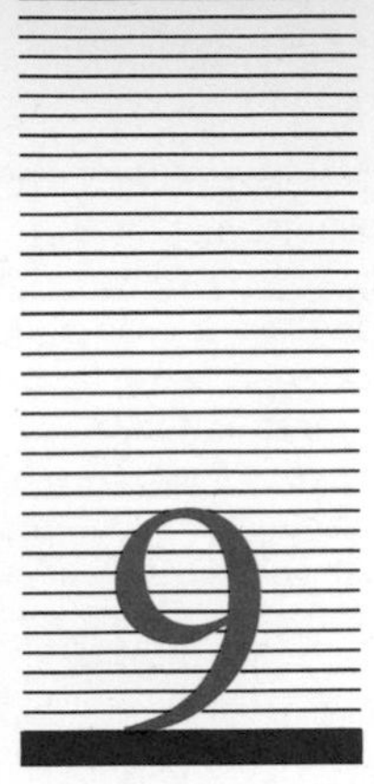

Cardiovascular system

Although people are living longer, they're increasingly living with chronic conditions or the sequelae of acute ones. Regardless of the practice setting, you'll be dealing with cardiovascular patients more often. To provide effective care for these patients, a clear understanding of cardiovascular anatomy and physiology, assessment techniques, and how to interpret the findings is essential.

Cardiovascular anatomy

The cardiovascular system plays an important role in the body. It delivers oxygenated blood to tissues and removes waste products. The heart pumps blood to all organs and tissues of the body. The autonomic nervous system controls how the heart pumps. The vascular network — the arteries and veins — carries blood throughout the body, keeps the heart filled with blood, and maintains blood pressure.

Structures of the heart

The heart is a hollow, muscular organ about the size of a closed fist. It's about 5″ (12.5 cm) long and 3½″ (9 cm) in diameter at its widest point. It weighs 1 to 1¼ lb (454 to 567 g). The heart is located between the lungs in the mediastinum, behind and to the left of the sternum.

The heart spans the area from the second to the fifth intercostal space. The right border of the heart lines up with the right border of the sternum. The left border lines up with the left midclavicular line. The exact position of the heart may vary slightly with each patient. Leading into and out of the heart are the great vessels that include the inferior vena cava, the superior vena cava,

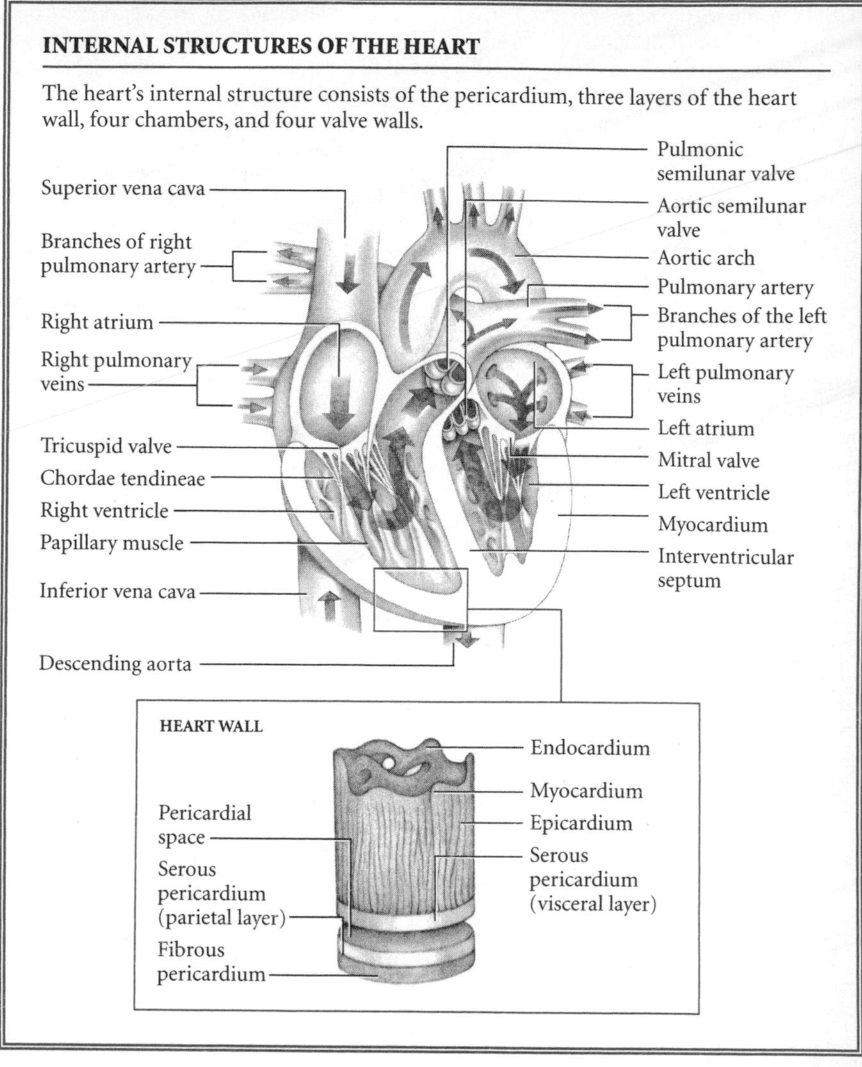

INTERNAL STRUCTURES OF THE HEART

The heart's internal structure consists of the pericardium, three layers of the heart wall, four chambers, and four valve walls.

the aorta, the pulmonary artery, and four pulmonary veins.

Heart wall

The heart wall consists of three layers. A thick myocardium, composed of interlacing bundles of cardiac muscle fibers, forms most of the heart wall. A thin layer of endothelial tissue forms the inner endocardium. The epicardium makes up the outside layer.

The pericardium is a fibroserous sac that surrounds the heart and the roots of the great vessels. It consists of the serous pericardium and the fibrous pericardium. The serous pericardium consists of the parietal layer, which lines the inside of the fibrous pericardium, and the visceral layer, which adheres to the surface of the heart. The fibrous pericardium is a thicker layer that's fibrous in nature. This layer protects the heart. The space between the two layers, called the pericardial space, contains 10 to 30 ml of serous fluid, which prevents friction between the layers as the heart pumps. (See *Internal structures of the heart.*)

Heart chambers

The heart contains four hollow chambers: two atria and two ventricles. The right atrium lies in front and to the right of the left atrium. It receives blood from the superior and inferior venae cavae. The left atrium, smaller but with thicker walls than the right atrium, forms the uppermost part of the heart's left border, extending to the left of and behind the right atrium. It receives blood from the pulmonary veins. The interatrial septum separates the left and right atria.

The right and left ventricles make up the two lower chambers. Both are large and thick-walled. The right ventricle lies behind the sternum and forms the largest part of the sternocostal surface and inferior border of the heart. The left ventricle is larger than the right because it must contract with enough force to eject blood into the aorta and the rest of the body. This ventricle forms the apex and most of the left border of the heart and its diaphragmatic surface.

Blood vessels

Deoxygenated venous blood returns to the right atrium through three vessels: the superior vena cava, inferior vena cava, and coronary sinus. Blood from the upper body returns to the heart through the superior vena cava. Blood in the lower body returns through the inferior vena cava, and blood from the heart muscle itself returns through the coronary sinus. All of the blood from those vessels empties into the right atrium.

Blood in the right atrium empties into the right ventricle and is then ejected through the pulmonic valve into the pulmonary artery when the ventricle contracts. The blood then travels to the lungs to be oxygenated.

From the lungs, blood travels to the left atrium through the pulmonary veins. The left atrium empties the blood into the left ventricle, which then pumps the blood through the aortic valve into the aorta and throughout the body with each contraction. Because the left ventricle pumps blood against a much higher pressure than the right ventricle, its wall is three times thicker.

Heart valves

Valves in the heart keep blood flowing in only one direction through the heart—preventing blood from traveling the wrong way. Healthy valves open and close passively as a result of pressure changes within the four heart chambers.

Valves between the atria and ventricles are called atrioventricular valves and include the tricuspid valve on the right side of the heart and the mitral valve on the left. The pulmonic valve, located between the right ventricle and pulmonary artery, and the aortic valve, located between the left ventricle and the aorta, are called semilunar valves.

Each valve's leaflets, or cusps, are anchored to the heart wall by cords of fibrous tissue. Those cords, called *chordae tendineae,* are controlled by papillary muscles. The cusps of the valves act to maintain tight closure. The tricuspid valve has three cusps, the mitral valve has two, and the semilunar valves each have three cusps.

Cardiovascular physiology

The autonomic nervous system (ANS) controls how the heart pumps by an electrical conduction system, which regulates myocardial contraction. This system includes the nerve fibers of the ANS and specialized nerves and fibers in the heart. The ANS involuntarily increases or decreases heart action to meet the individual's metabolic needs. (See *Cardiac conduction.*)

Both sympathetic and parasympathetic nerves participate in the control of cardiac function. With the body at rest, the parasympathetic nervous system controls the heart through branches of the vagus nerve (cranial nerve X). Heart rate and electrical impulse propagation are very slow.

In times of activity or stress, the sympathetic nervous system takes control. It stimulates the heart's nerves and fibers to fire and conduct more rapidly and the ventricles to contract more forcefully.

Pacemaker cells

Myocardial cells have specialized pacemaker cells that allow electrical impulse conduction. Pacemaker cells control heart rate and rhythm, a property known as automaticity. However, any myocardial muscle cell can

CARDIAC CONDUCTION

In the heart's conduction system, specialized fibers spread an impulse quickly throughout the heart's muscle cell network, causing a generalized contraction. This illustration shows the elements of the cardiac conduction system.

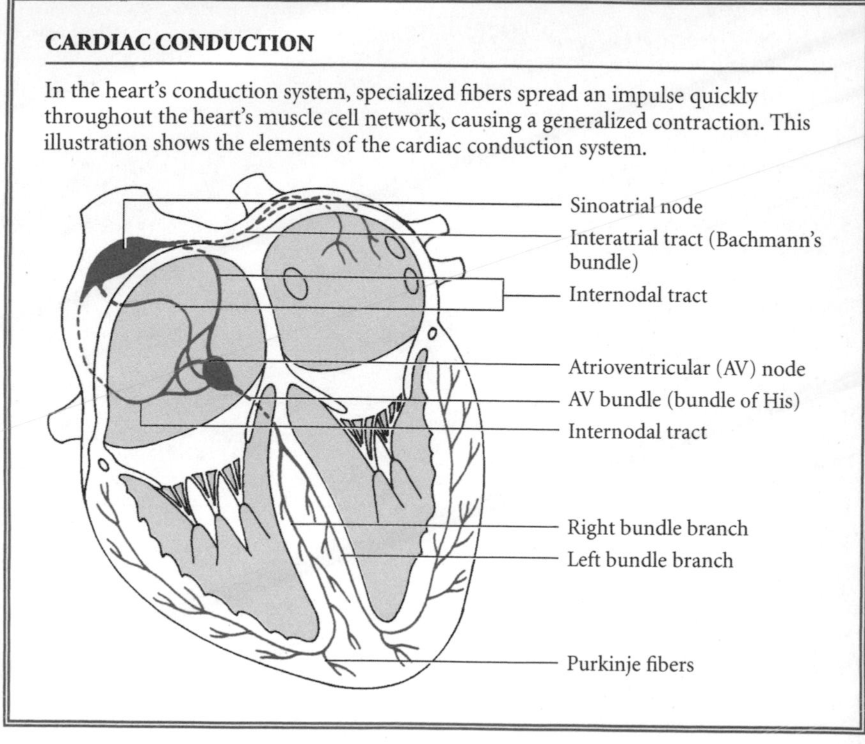

control the rate and rhythm of contractions under certain circumstances.

Normally, the sinoatrial (SA) node, located on the endocardial surface of the right atrium, near the superior vena cava, paces the heart. SA node firing spreads an impulse throughout the right and left atria, by way of internodal pathways, resulting in atrial contraction.

The atrioventricular (AV) node, which is located low in the septal wall of the right atrium immediately above the coronary sinus opening, takes up impulse conduction. Normally, the AV node forms the only electrical connection between the atria and ventricles. It initially slows the impulse, delaying ventricular activity and allowing blood to fill from the atria. Then conduction speeds through the AV node and a network of fibers called the bundle of His.

The bundle of His arises in the AV node and continues along the right interventricular septum. It divides in the ventricular septum to form the right and left bundle branches. Its fibers rapidly spread the impulse throughout both ventricles.

Purkinje fibers, the distal portions of the left and right bundle branches, fan across the subendocardial surface of the ventricles from the endocardium through the myocardium. As the impulse spreads throughout the distal conduction system, it prompts ventricular contraction.

Cardiac cycle

The cardiac cycle describes the period from the beginning of one heartbeat to the beginning of the next. During this cycle, electrical and mechanical events must occur in the proper order and to the proper degree to provide adequate blood flow to all body parts. Basically, the cardiac cycle has two phases, systole and diastole.

Systole

At the beginning of systole, the ventricles contract, increasing pressure and forcing the mitral and tricuspid valves shut. This valvular closing prevents blood backflow into the

PHASES OF THE CARDIAC CYCLE

The cardiac cycle is a coordinated sequence of events that controls blood flow through the heart's chambers and valves. It consists of two phases: systole and diastole.

In the top illustration, which shows systolic events, the arrows indicate ventricular contraction, the opening of the aortic and pulmonic valves, and the ejection of blood into the aorta and pulmonary artery.

In the bottom illustration, which shows diastolic events, the arrows indicate ventricular relaxation, the opening of the tricuspid and mitral valves, and the flow of blood into the ventricles.

Events on the heart's right side occur a fraction of a second after events on the left side because right-sided pressure is lower.

SYSTOLE

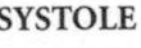

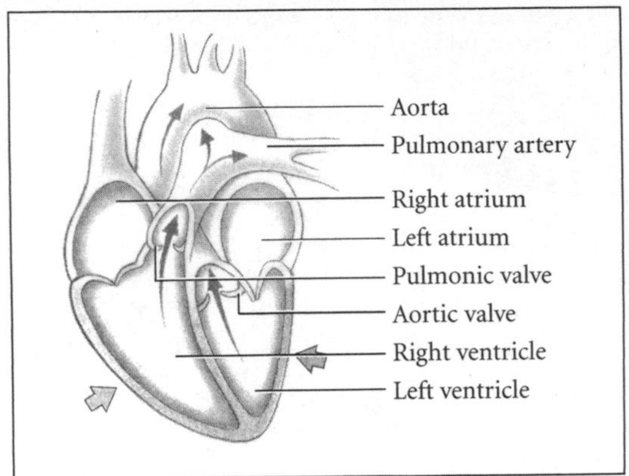

DIASTOLE

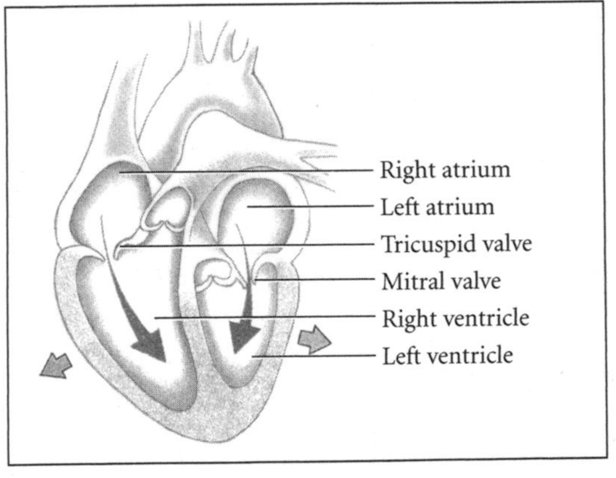

atria and coincides with the first heart sound (S_1), also known as the *"lub"* of "lub-dub." As the ventricles contract, ventricular pressure builds until it exceeds that in the pulmonary artery and the aorta. Then the aortic and pulmonary semilunar valves open, and the ventricles eject blood into the aorta and the pulmonary artery.

Diastole

When the ventricles empty and relax, ventricular pressure falls below that in the pulmonary artery and the aorta. At the beginning of diastole, the semilunar valves close to prevent backflow into the ventricles. This coincides with the second heart sound, S_2, also known as the *"dub"* of *"lub-dub."*

As the ventricles relax the mitral and tricuspid valves open and blood begins to flow into the ventricles from the atria. When the ventricles become full, near the end of diastole, the atria contract to send the remaining blood to the ventricles. Then a new cardiac cycle begins as the heart enters systole again. (See *Phases of the cardiac cycle.*)

Cardiac output and stroke volume

Cardiac output refers to the amount of blood the heart pumps in 1 minute. Stroke volume, the amount of blood ejected with each beat multiplied by the number of beats per minute, determines cardiac output. Stroke volume depends on three major factors:

- preload — the stretching of heart muscle fibers caused by blood volume in the ventricles at the end of diastole
- afterload — the pressure that the ventricular muscles must generate to overcome the higher pressure in the aorta
- contractility — the myocardium's inherent ability to contract normally.

Understanding the cardiac cycle can help to assess the heart's hemodynamics. Many cardiac dysfunctions cause abnormal findings that correlate with specific events in the cardiac cycle. (See *Understanding preload and afterload.*)

Functions of the vascular system

About 60,000 miles of arteries, arterioles, capillaries, venules, and veins keep blood circulating to and from every functioning cell in the body. This network has two branches that include the pulmonary circulation and systemic circulation. (See *Major blood vessels,* page 214.)

Pulmonary circulation

Pulmonary circulation refers to blood that travels to the lungs to pick up oxygen and liberate carbon dioxide. It works as follows:

- Deoxygenated blood travels from the right ventricle through the pulmonic valve into the pulmonary arteries.
- Blood passes through progressively smaller arteries and arterioles into the capillaries of the lungs.
- Blood reaches the alveoli and exchanges carbon dioxide for oxygen.
- The oxygenated blood then returns via venules and veins to the pulmonary veins, which carry it back to the left atrium of the heart.

Systemic circulation

Through the systemic circulation, blood carries oxygen and other nutrients to body cells and transports waste products for excretion. At specific sites, the pumping action of the heart that forces blood through the arteries becomes palpable. This regular expansion and contraction of the arteries is called the pulse.

UNDERSTANDING PRELOAD AND AFTERLOAD

Preload refers to a passive stretching force exerted on the ventricular muscle at end diastole by the amount of blood in the chamber. According to Starling's law, the more cardiac muscles are stretched in diastole, the more forcefully they contract in systole.

Afterload refers to the pressure the ventricular muscles must generate to overcome the higher pressure in the aorta. Normally, end-diastolic pressure in the left ventricle is 5 to 10 mm Hg; in the aorta, however, it's 70 to 80 mm Hg. This difference means that the ventricle must develop enough pressure to force open the aortic valve.

PRELOAD

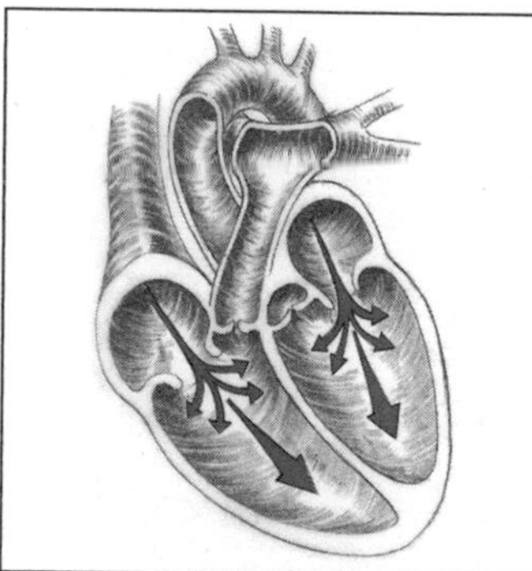

AFTERLOAD

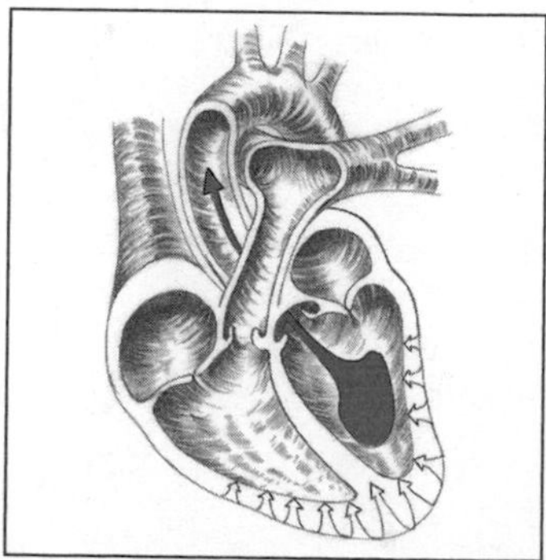

MAJOR BLOOD VESSELS

This illustration shows the body's major arteries and veins.

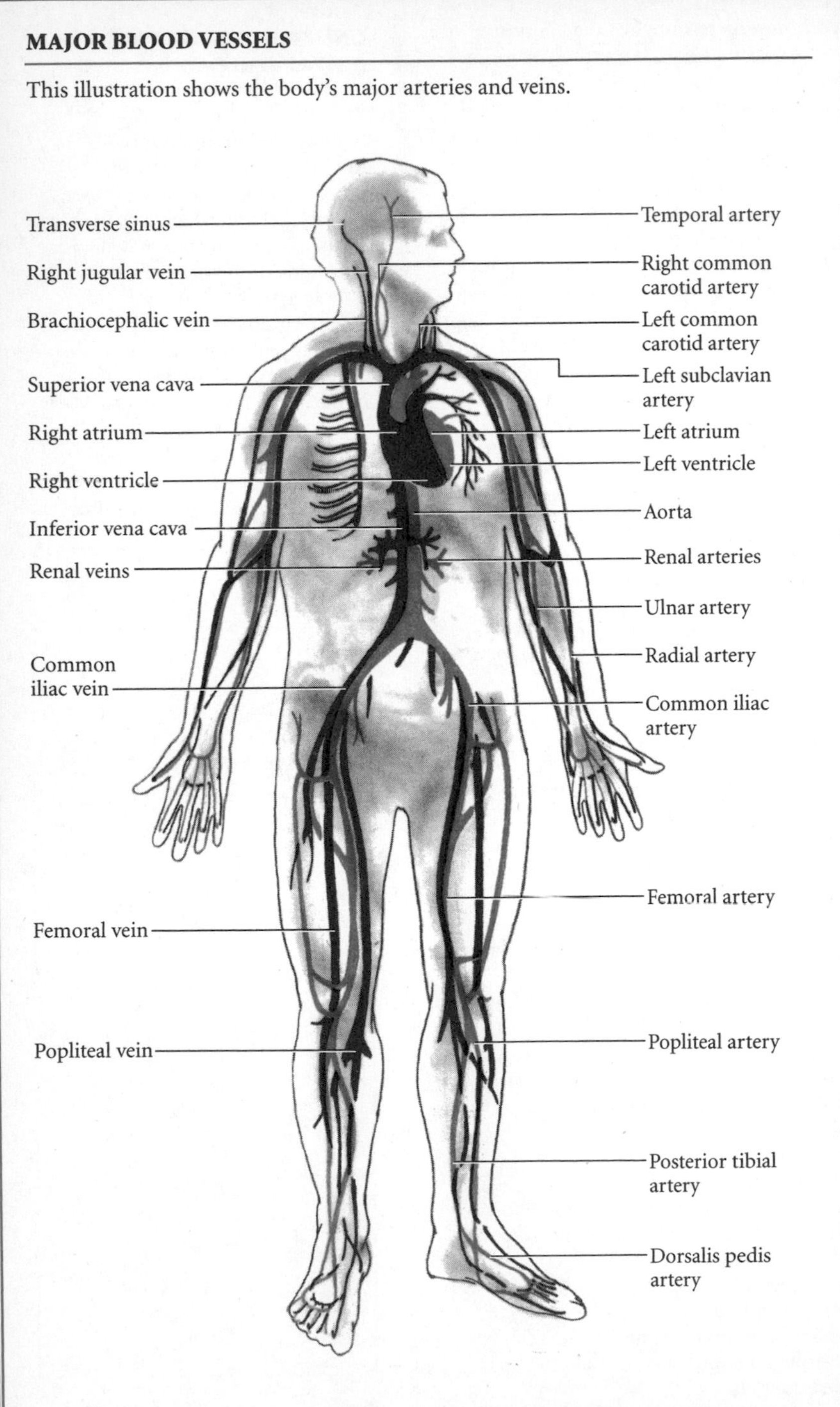

The major artery — the aorta — branches into vessels that supply blood to specific organs and areas of the body. The left common carotid, left subclavian, and innominate arteries arise from the arch of the aorta and supply blood to the brain, arms, and upper chest. As the aorta descends through the thorax and abdomen, its branches supply blood to the GI and genitourinary organs, spinal column, and lower chest and abdominal muscles. Then the aorta divides into the iliac arteries, which further divide into femoral arteries.

As the arteries divide into smaller units, the number of vessels increase dramatically, thereby increasing the area of perfusion. Arteries are thick-walled because they transport blood under high pressure. Arterial walls contain a tough, elastic layer to help propel blood through the arterial system. At the end of the arterioles and the beginning of the capillaries, strong sphincters control blood flow into the tissues. These sphincters dilate to permit more flow when needed, close to shunt blood to other areas, or constrict to increase blood pressure.

Although the capillary bed contains the smallest vessels, it supplies blood to the largest area. Capillary pressure is extremely low to allow for the exchange of nutrients, oxygen, and carbon dioxide with body cells. From the capillaries, blood flows into venules and, eventually, into veins. About 5% of the circulating blood volume at any given moment is contained within the capillary network.

Nearly all veins carry oxygen-depleted blood, the sole exception being the pulmonary vein, which carries oxygenated blood from the lungs to the left atrium. Veins serve as a large reservoir for circulating blood. Valves in the veins prevent blood backflow, and the pumping action of skeletal muscles assists venous return. The wall of a vein is thinner and more pliable than the wall of an artery. That pliability allows the vein to accommodate variations in blood volume. The veins merge until they form two main branches — the superior and inferior venae cavae — that return blood to the right atrium.

Coronary circulation

Blood flowing through the heart's chambers doesn't exchange oxygen and other nutrients with the myocardial cells. Instead, a specialized part of the systemic circulation, the coronary circulation, supplies blood to the heart. (See *The heart's blood supply,* page 216.)

Pulses

Arterial pulses are pressure waves of blood generated by the pumping action of the heart. All vessels in the arterial system have pulsations, but the pulsations can be felt only where an artery lies near the skin. You can palpate for these peripheral pulses: temporal, carotid, brachial, radial, ulnar, femoral, popliteal, posterior tibial, and dorsalis pedis.

Health history

To obtain a health history of a patient's cardiovascular system, begin by introducing yourself and explaining what will occur during the health history and physical examination. To take an effective history, establish rapport with the patient. Ask open-ended questions and listen carefully to responses. Closely observe the patient's nonverbal behavior.

Chief complaint

A patient with a cardiovascular problem typically cites specific complaints, such as:

- chest pain
- irregular heartbeat or palpitations
- shortness of breath on exertion, lying down, or at night
- cough
- cyanosis or pallor
- weakness
- fatigue
- unexplained weight change
- swelling of the extremities
- dizziness
- headache
- high or low blood pressure
- peripheral skin changes, such as decreased hair distribution, skin color changes, or a thin, shiny appearance to the skin
- pain in the extremities, such as leg pain or cramps.

Ask the patient how long he has had the problem, how it affects his daily routine, and when it began. Find out about any asso-

THE HEART'S BLOOD SUPPLY

The heart relies on the coronary arteries and their branches to supply itself with oxygenated blood, and on the cardiac veins to remove oxygen-depleted blood. During left ventricular systole, blood is ejected into the aorta. During diastole, blood flows into the coronary ostia and then through the coronary arteries to nourish the heart muscle.

The right coronary artery supplies blood to the right atrium (including the sinoatrial and atrioventricular nodes of the conduction system), part of the left atrium, most of the right ventricle, and the inferior part of the left ventricle.

The left coronary artery, which splits into the anterior descending and circumflex arteries, supplies blood to the left atrium, most of the left ventricle, and most of the interventricular septum. Many collateral arteries connect the branches of the right and left coronary arteries.

The cardiac veins lie superficial to the arteries. The largest vein, the coronary sinus, lies in the posterior part of the coronary sulcus and opens into the right atrium. Most of the major cardiac veins empty into the coronary sinus, except for the anterior cardiac veins, which empty into the right atrium.

ANTERIOR VIEW

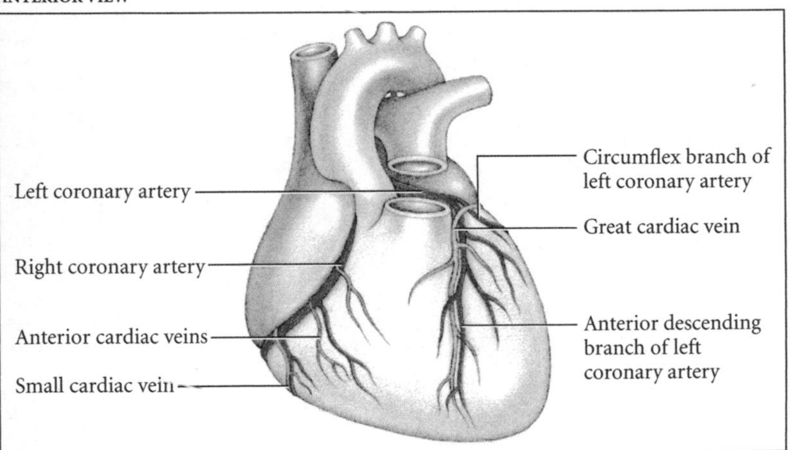

POSTERIOR VIEW

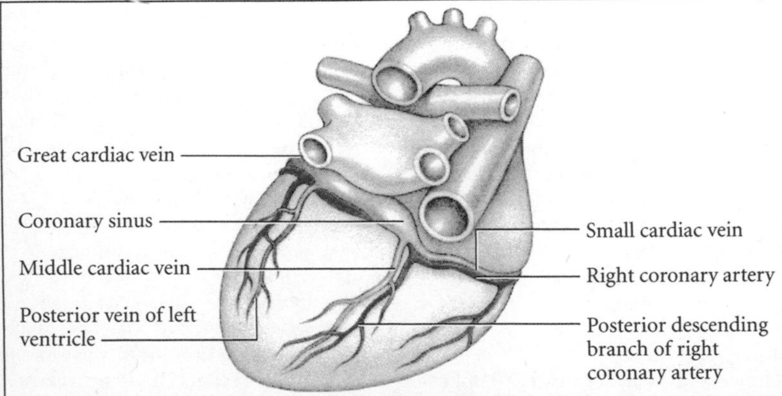

ciated signs and symptoms. Ask about the location, radiation, intensity, and duration of any pain and any precipitating, exacerbating, or relieving factors. Ask him to rate the pain on a scale of 1 to 10, in which 1 means negligible and 10 means the worst pain imaginable. (See *Understanding chest pain,* pages 218 and 219.)

Let the patient describe his problem in his own words. Avoid leading questions. Use familiar expressions rather than medical terms whenever possible. If the patient isn't in distress, ask questions that require more than a yes-or-no response. Try to obtain as accurate a description as possible of any chest pain.

AGE ISSUE *Even a child old enough to talk may have difficulty describing chest pain, so be alert for nonverbal clues, such as restlessness, facial grimaces, or holding of the painful area. Ask the child to point to the area and then to where the pain goes (to find out if it's radiating). Determine the pain's severity by asking the parents if the pain interferes with the child's normal activities and behavior. Because elderly patients have a higher risk of developing life-threatening conditions—such as a myocardial infarction (MI), angina, and aortic dissection—carefully evaluate chest pain in these patients.*

Current health history

Besides checking for pain, also ask the patient the following questions.

- Are you ever short of breath? If so, what activities cause you to be short of breath? Orthopnea or dyspnea that occurs when the patient is lying down and improves when he sits up, suggests left ventricular heart failure or mitral stenosis. It can also accompany obstructive lung disease.
- Do you feel dizzy or fatigued?

AGE ISSUE *When evaluating a child for fatigue, ask his parents if they have noticed any changes in his activity level. Fatigue without an organic cause occurs normally during accelerated growth phases in preschool-age and prepubescent children. In the elderly patient, always ask about fatigue because this symptom may be insidious and mask a more serious underlying condition.*

- Do your rings or shoes feel tight?
- Do your ankles swell? (Pregnant patients, especially those in the third trimester or those who stand for long periods of time may report ankle edema. This is a common discomfort of pregnancy.)
- Have you noticed changes in color or sensation in your legs? If so, what are those changes?
- If you have sores or ulcers, how quickly do they heal?
- Do you stand or sit in one place for long periods at work?
- How many pillows do you sleep on at night? (See *Key questions for assessing cardiac function,* page 220.)

Past health history

Ask the patient about any history of cardiac-related disorders, such as hypertension, rheumatic fever, scarlet fever, diabetes mellitus, hyperlipidemia, congenital heart defects, and syncope. Other questions to ask include:

- Have you ever had severe fatigue not caused by exertion?
- Are you taking any prescription, over-the-counter, or illicit drugs?
- Are you allergic to any drugs, foods, or other products? If yes, describe the reaction you experienced.

In addition, ask the female patient:

- Have you begun menopause?
- Do you use hormonal contraceptives or estrogen?
- Have you experienced any medical problems during pregnancy? Have you ever had pregnancy-induced hypertension?

Family history

Information about the patient's blood relatives may suggest a specific cardiac problem. Ask him if anyone in his family has ever had hypertension, MI, cardiomyopathy, diabetes mellitus, coronary artery disease (CAD), vascular disease, hyperlipidemia, or sudden death.

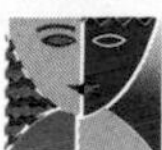

CULTURAL INSIGHT *As you analyze a patient's problems, remember that age, gender, and race are essential considerations in identifying the risk for cardiovascular disorders. For example, CAD most commonly affects White men between ages 40 and 60. Hypertension occurs most commonly in Blacks. Women are also vulnerable to heart disease, especially postmeno-*

UNDERSTANDING CHEST PAIN

This chart outlines the different types of chest pain including their location, exacerbating factors, causes, and alleviating measures. Use this chart to accurately assess your patients with chest pain.

Description	Location
Aching, squeezing, pressure, heaviness, burning pain; usually subsides within 10 minutes	Substernal; may radiate to jaw, neck, arms, and back
Tightness or pressure; burning, aching pain; possibly accompanied by dyspnea, diaphoresis, weakness, anxiety, or nausea; sudden onset; lasts ½ to 2 hours	Typically across chest but may radiate to jaw, neck, arms, or back
Sharp and continuous; may be accompanied by friction rub; sudden onset	Substernal; may radiate to neck or left arm
Excruciating, tearing pain; may be accompanied by blood pressure difference between right and left arm; sudden onset	Retrosternal, upper abdominal, or epigastric; may radiate to back, neck, or shoulders
Sudden, stabbing pain; may be accompanied by cyanosis, dyspnea, or cough with hemoptysis	Over lung area
Sudden and severe pain; sometimes accompanied by dyspnea, increased pulse rate, decreased breath sounds, or deviated trachea	Lateral thorax
Dull, pressurelike, squeezing pain	Substernal, epigastric areas
Sharp, severe pain	Lower chest or upper abdomen
Burning feeling after eating sometimes accompanied by hematemesis or tarry stools; sudden onset that generally subsides within 15 to 20 minutes	Epigastric
Gripping, sharp pain; possibly nausea and vomiting	Right epigastric or abdominal areas; possible radiation to shoulders
Continuous or intermittent sharp pain; possibly tender to touch; gradual or sudden onset	Anywhere in chest
Dull or stabbing pain usually accompanied by hyperventilation or breathlessness; sudden onset; lasting less than 1 minute or as long as several days	Anywhere in chest

pausal women and those with diabetes mellitus.

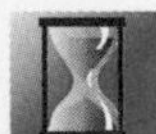

AGE ISSUE *Many elderly people have increased systolic blood pressure because of an increase in the rigidity of blood vessel walls with age. Overall, elderly people have a higher incidence of cardiovascular disease than younger people.*

Exacerbating factors	Causes	Alleviating measures
Eating, physical effort, smoking, cold weather, stress, anger, hunger, lying down	Angina pectoris	Rest, nitroglycerin (*Note:* Unstable angina appears even at rest.)
Exertion, anxiety	Acute myocardial infarction	Opioid analgesics such as morphine, nitroglycerin
Deep breathing, lying in a supine position	Pericarditis	Sitting up, leaning forward, anti-inflammatory drugs
Not applicable	Dissecting aortic aneurysm	Analgesics, surgery
Inspiration	Pulmonary embolus	Analgesics
Normal respiration	Pneumothorax	Analgesics, chest tube insertion
Food, cold liquids, exercise	Esophageal spasm	Nitroglycerin, calcium channel blockers
Eating a heavy meal, bending, lying down	Hiatal hernia	Antacids, walking, semi-Fowler's position
Lack of food or highly acidic foods	Peptic ulcer	Food, antacids
Eating fatty foods, lying down	Cholecystitis	Rest and analgesics, surgery
Movement, palpation	Chest-wall syndrome	Time, analgesics, heat applications
Increased respiratory rate, stress or anxiety	Acute anxiety	Slowing of respiratory rate, stress relief

Psychosocial history

Obtain information about your patient's occupation, educational background, living arrangements, daily activities, and family relationships.

Also obtain information about:

- stress and how he deals with it
- current health habits, such as smoking, alcohol intake, caffeine intake, exercise, and dietary intake of fat and sodium

KEY QUESTIONS FOR ASSESSING CARDIAC FUNCTION

These questions and statements will help you to assess your patient's cardiac function more accurately:

- Are you still in pain? Where's it located? Point to where you feel it.
- Describe what the pain feels like. (If the patient needs prompting, ask if he feels a burning, tightness, or squeezing sensation in his chest.)
- Does the pain radiate to any other part of your body? Your arm? Neck? Back? Jaw?
- When did the pain begin? What relieves it? What makes it feel worse?
- Tell me about any other feelings you're experiencing. (If the patient needs prompting, suggest nausea, dizziness, or sweating.)
- Tell me about any feelings of shortness of breath. Does a particular body position seem to bring this on? Which one? How long does any shortness of breath last? What relieves it?
- Has sudden breathing trouble ever awakened you from sleep? Tell me more about this.
- Do you ever wake up coughing? How often? Have you ever coughed up blood?
- Does your heart ever pound or skip a beat? If so, when does this happen?
- Do you ever get dizzy or faint? What seems to bring this on?
- Tell me about any swelling in your ankles or feet. At what time of day? Does anything relieve the swelling?
- Do you urinate more frequently at night?
- Tell me how you feel while you're doing your daily activities. Have you had to limit your activities or rest more often while doing them?

- environmental or occupational considerations
- activities of daily living.

During the history-taking session, note the appropriateness of the patient's responses, his speech clarity, and his mood to aid in better identifying changes later.

Physical assessment

Cardiovascular disease affects people of all ages and can take many forms. Using a consistent, methodical approach to your assessment will help you identify abnormalities. The key to accurate assessment is regular practice, which will help improve technique and efficiency.

Before assessing the patient's cardiovascular system, assess the factors that reflect cardiovascular function. These include vital signs, general appearance, and related body structures.

Wash your hands and gather the necessary equipment. Choose a private room. Adjust the thermostat, if necessary; cool temperatures may alter the patient's skin temperature and color, heart rate, and blood pressure. Make sure the room is quiet. If possible, close the door and windows and turn off radios and noisy equipment.

Combine parts of the physical assessment, as needed, to conserve time and the patient's energy. If a female patient feels embarrassed about exposing her chest, explain each assessment step beforehand, use drapes appropriately, and expose only the area being assessed. If the patient experiences cardiovascular difficulties, alter the order of the assessment as needed.

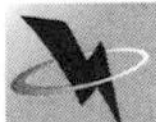

CRITICAL POINT *If the patient develops chest pain and dyspnea, quickly check his vital signs and then auscultate the heart.*

Vital sign assessment

Assessing vital signs includes measurement of temperature, blood pressure, pulse rate, and respiratory rate.

Temperature measurement

Temperature is measured and documented in degrees Fahrenheit (° F) or degrees Celsius (° C). Choose the method of obtaining the patient's temperature (oral, tympanic, rectal, or axillary) based on the patient's age and condition. Normal body temperature ranges from 96.8° F to 99.5° F (36° C to 37.5° C).

If the patient has a fever, anticipate these possibilities:

- cardiovascular inflammation or infection
- heightened cardiac workload (Assess a febrile patient with heart disease for signs of increased cardiac workload such as tachycardia.)
- myocardial infarction (MI) or acute pericarditis (mild to moderate fever usually occurs 2 to 5 days after an MI when the healing infarct passes through the inflammatory stage)
- infections, such as infective endocarditis, which causes fever spikes (high fever).

In patients with lower than normal body temperatures, findings include poor perfusion and certain metabolic disorders.

Blood pressure measurement

First, palpate and then auscultate the blood pressure in an arm or a leg. Wait 3 to 5 minutes between measurements. Normally, blood pressure readings are less than 140/90 mm Hg in a resting adult and 78/46 to 114/78 mm Hg in a young child. (See *Ensuring accurate blood pressure measurement,* page 222.)

Emotional stress caused by physical examination may elevate blood pressure. If the patient's blood pressure is high, allow him to relax for several minutes and then measure again to rule out stress.

When assessing a patient's blood pressure for the first time, take measurements in both arms.

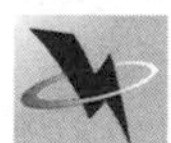

CRITICAL POINT *A difference of 10 mm Hg or more between the patient's arms may indicate thoracic outlet syndrome or other forms of arterial obstruction.*

If blood pressure is elevated in both arms, measure the pressure in the thigh. Wrap a large cuff around the patient's upper leg at least 1″ (2.5 cm) above the knee. Place the stethoscope over the popliteal artery, located on the posterior surface slightly above the knee joint. Listen for sounds when the bladder of the cuff is deflated.

High blood pressure in the patient's arms with normal or low pressure in the legs suggests aortic coarctation.

Pulse pressure determination

To calculate the patient's pulse pressure, subtract the diastolic pressure from the systolic pressure. This reflects arterial pressure during the resting phase of the cardiac cycle and normally ranges from 30 to 50 mm Hg.

Rising pulse pressure is seen with:

- increased stroke volume, which occurs with exercise, anxiety, and bradycardia
- declined peripheral vascular resistance or aortic distention, which occurs with anemia, hyperthyroidism, fever, hypertension, aortic coarctation, and aging.

Diminishing pulse pressure occurs with:

- mitral or aortic stenosis, which occurs with mechanical obstruction
- constricted peripheral vessels, which occurs with shock
- declined stroke volume, which occurs with heart failure, hypovolemia, cardiac tamponade, or tachycardia.

Radial pulse assessment

If you suspect cardiac disease, palpate the radial pulse for 1 full minute to detect arrhythmias. Normally, an adult's pulse ranges from 60 to 100 beats/minute. Its rhythm should feel regular, except for a subtle slowing on expiration, caused by changes in intrathoracic pressure and vagal response. Note whether the pulse feels weak, normal, or bounding.

Respiration evaluation

Observe for eupnea — a regular, unlabored, and bilaterally equal breathing pattern. In patients with irregular breathing, altered patterns may indicate:

- tachypnea with low cardiac output
- dyspnea, a possible indicator of heart failure (not evident at rest; however, pausing occurs after only a few words to take breaths)
- Cheyne-Stokes respirations, possibly accompanying severe heart failure (seen especially with coma)
- shallow breathing, possibly seen with acute pericarditis (deep respirations occur in an attempt to reduce the pain associated with deep respirations).

General appearance assessment

Begin by observing the patient's general appearance, particularly noting weight and muscle composition. Is he well developed,

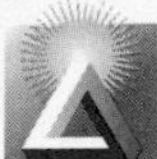

EXPERT TECHNIQUE

ENSURING ACCURATE BLOOD PRESSURE MEASUREMENT

When taking the patient's blood pressure, begin by applying the cuff properly, as shown here. Then be alert for these common problems to avoid recording an inaccurate blood pressure measurement.

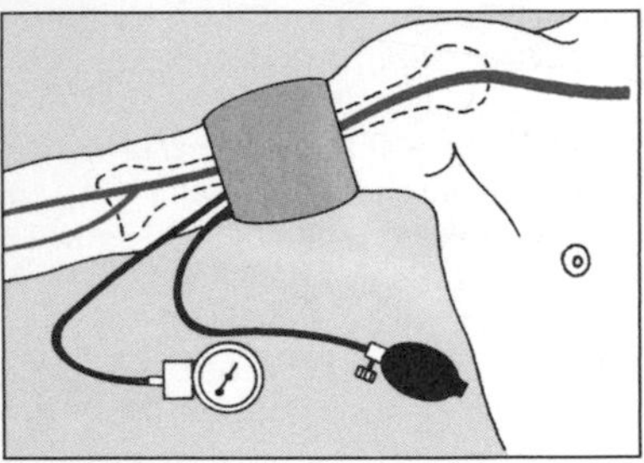

■ *Wrong-sized cuff.* Select the appropriate-sized cuff for the patient. This ensures that adequate pressure is applied to compress the brachial artery during cuff inflation. If the cuff bladder is too narrow, a false-high reading will be obtained; too wide, a false-low reading. The cuff bladder width should be about 40% of the circumference of the midpoint of the limb; bladder length should be twice the width. If the arm circumference is less than 13″ (33 cm), select a regular-sized cuff; if it's between 13″ and 16″ (33 to 40.5 cm), a large-sized cuff; if it's more than 16″, a thigh cuff. Pediatric cuffs are also available.

■ *Slow cuff deflation, causing venous congestion in the extremity.* Don't inflate the cuff more slowly than 2 mm Hg/heartbeat because you'll get a false-high reading.

■ *Cuff wrapped too loosely, reducing its effective width.* Tighten the cuff to avoid a false-high reading.

■ *Mercury column not read at eye level.* Read the mercury column at eye level. If the column is below eye level, you may record a false-low reading; if it's above eye level, a false-high reading.

■ *Poorly timed measurement.* Don't take the patient's blood pressure if he appears anxious or has just eaten or been ambulated; you'll get a false-high reading.

■ *Incorrect position of the arm.* Keep the patient's arm level with his heart to avoid a false-low reading.

■ *Failure to notice an ausculatory gap* (sound fades out for 10 to 15 mm Hg then returns). To avoid missing the top Korotkoff sounds, stimulate systolic pressure by palpation first.

■ *Inaudibility of feeble sounds.* Before reinflating the cuff, have the patient raise his arm to reduce venous pressure and amplify low-volume sounds. After inflating the cuff, lower the patient's arm; then deflate the cuff and listen. Alternatively, with the patient's arm positioned at heart level, inflate the cuff and have the patient make a fist. Have him rapidly open and close his hand 10 times before you begin to deflate the cuff; then listen. Be sure to document that the blood pressure reading was augmented.

well nourished, alert, and energetic? Document any departures from normal. Does the patient appear older than his chronological age or seem unusually tired or slow-moving? Does the patient appear comfortable or does he seem anxious or in distress?

Height and body weight measurement

Accurately measure and record the patient's height and weight. These measurements will help determine risk factors, calculate hemodynamic indexes (such as cardiac index), guide treatment plans, determine medication dosages, assist with nutritional counseling, and detect fluid overload. Fluctuations in weight may prove significant, especially when extreme.

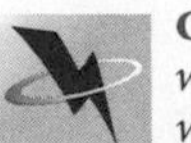

CRITICAL POINT *Extreme weight fluctuation, for instance, would occur if the patient with developing heart failure gains several pounds overnight.*

Next, assess for cachexia — weakness and muscle wasting. Observe the amount of muscle bulk in the upper arms, thighs, and chest wall. For a more precise measurement, calculate the percentage of body fat. For men, this should be 12%; for women, it should be 18%. Loss of the body's energy stores slows healing and impairs immune function.

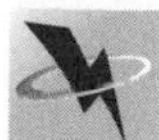

CRITICAL POINT *A patient with chronic cardiac disease may develop cachexia, losing body fat and muscle mass. However, be aware that edema may mask these effects.*

Skin assessment

Note the patient's skin color, temperature, turgor, and texture. Because normal skin color can vary widely among patients, ask him if his current skin tone is normal. Then inspect the skin color and note any cyanosis. Two types of cyanosis can occur in patients:

- central cyanosis, suggesting reduced oxygen intake or transport from the lungs to the bloodstream, which may occur with heart failure
- peripheral cyanosis, suggesting constriction of peripheral arterioles, a natural response to cold or anxiety or a result of hypovolemia, cardiogenic shock, or a vasoconstrictive disease.

Examine the underside of the tongue, buccal mucosa, and conjunctiva for signs of central cyanosis. Inspect the lips, tip of the nose, earlobes, and nail beds for signs of peripheral cyanosis. The color range for normal mucous membranes is narrower than that for the skin; therefore, it provides a more accurate assessment.

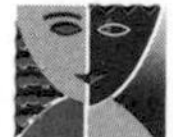

CULTURAL INSIGHT *In a dark-skinned patient, inspect the oral mucous membranes, such as the lips and gingivae, which normally appear pink and moist but would appear ashen if cyanotic.*

When evaluating the patient's skin color, also observe for flushing, pallor, and rubor. Flushing of a patient's skin can result from medications, excess heat, anxiety, or fear. Pallor can result from anemia or increased peripheral vascular resistance caused by atherosclerosis. Dependent rubor may be a sign of chronic arterial insufficiency.

Next, assess the patient's perfusion by evaluating the arterial flow adequacy. With the patient lying down, elevate one of the patient's legs 12″ (30.5 cm) above heart level for 60 seconds. Next, tell him to sit up and dangle both legs. Compare the color of both legs. The leg that was elevated should show mild pallor compared with the other leg. Color should return to the pale leg in about 10 seconds, and the veins should refill in about 15 seconds. Suspect arterial insufficiency if the patient's foot shows marked pallor, delayed color return that ends with a mottled appearance, delayed venous filling, or marked redness.

Next, touch the patient's skin. It should feel warm and dry. If the patient's skin is cool and clammy, this results from vasoconstriction, which occurs when cardiac output is low such as during shock. Warm, moist skin results from vasodilation, which occurs when cardiac output is high — for example, during exercise.

Evaluate skin turgor by grasping and raising the skin between two fingers and then letting it go. Normally, the skin immediately returns to its original position. If the patient's skin is taut and shiny and can't be grasped, this may result from ascites or the marked edema that accompanies heart failure. Skin that doesn't immediately return to the original position exhibits tenting, a sign of decreased skin turgor, which may result from dehydration, especially if the patient takes diuretics. It may also result from age, malnutrition, or an adverse reaction to corticosteroid treatment.

Observe the skin for signs of edema. Inspect the patient's arms and legs for symmetrical swelling. Because edema usually affects lower or dependent areas of the body first, be especially alert when assessing the arms, hands, legs, feet, and ankles of an ambulatory patient or the buttocks and sacrum of a bedridden patient. Determine the type of edema (pitting or nonpitting), its location, its extent, and its symmetry (unilateral or symmetrical). If the patient has pitting edema, assess the degree of pitting.

Edema can result from heart failure or venous insufficiency caused by varicosities or thrombophlebitis. Chronic right-sided heart failure may even cause ascites, which leads to generalized edema and abdominal distention. Venous compression may result in localized edema along the path of the compressed vessel.

While inspecting the patient's skin, note the location, size, number, and appearance of any lesions. Dry, open lesions on the patient's lower extremities accompanied by pallor, cool skin, and lack of hair growth signify arterial insufficiency, possibly caused by arterial peripheral vascular disease. Wet, open lesions with red or purplish edges that appear on the patient's legs may result from the venous stasis associated with venous peripheral vascular disease.

Extremity assessment

Inspect the hair on the patient's arms and legs. Hair should be distributed symmetrically and should grow thicker on the anterior surface of the arms and legs. If the patient's hair isn't thicker on the anterior of the surface of the arms and legs, it may indicate diminished arterial blood flow to these extremities.

Note whether the length of the arms and legs is proportionate to the length of the trunk. A patient with long, thin arms and legs may have Marfan syndrome, a congenital disorder that causes cardiovascular problems, such as aortic dissection, aortic valve incompetence, and cardiomyopathy.

Fingernail assessment

Fingernails normally appear pinkish with no markings. A bluish color in the nail beds indicates peripheral cyanosis.

Estimate the rate of peripheral blood flow, assess the capillary refill in the patient's fingernails (or toenails) by applying pressure to the nail for 5 seconds, then assessing the time it takes for color to return. In a patient with a good arterial supply, color should return in less than 3 seconds.

Delayed capillary refill in the patient's fingernails suggests reduced circulation to that area, a sign of low cardiac output that may lead to arterial insufficiency.

Assess the angle between the nail and the cuticle. An angle of 180 degrees or greater indicates finger clubbing. Check for enlarged fingertips with spongy, slightly swollen nail bases. Normally, the nail bases feel firm, but in early clubbing, they're spongy. Finger clubbing commonly indicates chronic tissue hypoxia.

The shape of the patient's nails should be smooth and rounded. A concave depression in the middle of a thin nail indicates koilonychia (spoon nail), a sign of iron deficiency anemia or Raynaud's disease, whereas thick, ridged nails can result from arterial insufficiency.

Finally, check for splinter hemorrhages—small, thin, red or brown lines that run from the base to the tip of the nail. Splinter hemorrhages develop in patients with bacterial endocarditis.

Eye assessment

Inspect the eyelids for xanthelasma—small, slightly raised, yellowish plaques that usually appear around the inner canthus. The plaques that occur in xanthelasma result from lipid deposits and may signal severe hyperlipidemia, a risk factor of cardiovascular disease.

Next, observe the color of the patient's sclerae. Yellowish sclerae may be the first sign of jaundice, which occasionally results from liver congestion caused by right-sided heart failure.

Next, check for arcus senilis—a thin grayish ring around the edge of the cornea. A normal occurrence in older patients, arcus senilis can indicate hyperlipidemia in patients younger than age 65.

Using an ophthalmoscope, examine the retinal structures, including the retinal vessels and background. The retina is normally light yellow to orange, and the background should be free from hemorrhages and exudates. Structural changes, such as narrowing or blocking of a vein where an arteriole crosses over, indicate hypertension. Soft exudates may suggest hypertension or subacute bacterial endocarditis.

Head movement assessment

Assess the patient's head at rest and be alert for abnormal positioning or movements. Also check range of motion and rotation of the neck.

A slight, rhythmic bobbing of the patient's head in time with his heartbeat (Musset's sign) may accompany the high backpressure caused by aortic insufficiency or aneurysm.

Heart assessment

Ask the patient to remove all clothing except his underwear and to put on an examination gown. Have the patient lie on his back, with the head of the examination table at a 30- to 45-degree angle. Stand on the patient's right side if you're right-handed or his left side if you're left-handed so you can auscultate more easily.

As with assessment of other body systems, inspect, palpate, percuss, and auscultate when assessing the heart.

Inspection

First, inspect the patient's chest and thorax. Expose the anterior chest and observe its general appearance. Normally, the lateral diameter is twice the anteroposterior diameter. Note any deviations from typical chest shape.

Note landmarks you can use to describe your findings as well as structures underlying the chest wall. (See *Identifying cardiovascular landmarks,* page 226.)

Look for pulsations, symmetry of movement, retractions, or heaves. A heave is a strong outward thrust of the chest wall and occurs during systole.

Position a light source, such as a flashlight or gooseneck lamp, so that it casts a shadow on the patient's chest. Note the location of the apical impulse. This is also usually the point of maximum impulse (PMI) and should be located in the fifth intercostal space medial to the left midclavicular line. The apical impulse gives an indication of how well the left ventricle is working because it corresponds to the apex of the heart. The impulse can be seen in about 50% of adults.

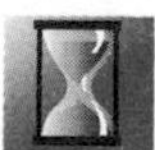

AGE ISSUE *In children and patients with thin chest walls, the apical impulse is noted more easily. In these patients, you may see slight sternal movement and pulsations over the pulmonary arteries or the aorta as well as visible pulsations in the epigastric area. To find the apical impulse in a woman with large breasts, displace the breasts during the examination.*

On inspection, irregularities in the patient's heart may be noted. Some of these can impair cardiac output by preventing chest expansion and inhibiting heart muscle movement, including:

- barrel chest, indicated by a rounded thoracic cage caused by chronic obstructive pulmonary disease
- pectus excavatum, indicated by a depressed sternum
- scoliosis, which is a lateral curvature of the spine
- pectus carinatum, indicated by a protruding sternum
- kyphosis, which is a convex curvature of the thoracic spine
- retractions, indicated by visible indentations of the soft tissue covering the chest wall, or the use of accessory muscles to breathe, which typically results from a respiratory disorder, but may also indicate congenital heart defect or heart failure
- visible pulsation to the right of the sternum, a possible indication of aortic aneurysm
- pulsation in the sternoclavicular or epigastric area, a possible indication of aortic aneurysm
- sustained, forceful apical impulse, a possible indication of left ventricular hypertrophy, which increases blood pressure and may cause cardiomyopathy and mitral insufficiency
- laterally displaced apical impulse, a possible sign of left ventricular hypertrophy.

Palpation

Maintain a gentle touch when palpating so you won't obscure pulsations or similar findings. Follow a systematic palpation sequence covering the sternoclavicular, aortic, pulmonary right ventricular, left ventricular (apical), and epigastric areas. Use the pads of the fingers to effectively assess large pulse sites. Finger pads prove especially sensitive to vibrations.

Start at the sternoclavicular area and move methodically through the palpation sequence down to the epigastric area. At the sternoclavicular area, you may feel pulsation of the aortic arch, especially in a thin or average-build patient. In a thin patient, you may palpate a pulsation in the abdominal aorta over the epigastric area.

Using the ball of your hand, then your fingertips, palpate over the precordium to find the apical impulse. Note heaves or thrills, fine vibrations that feel like the purring of a cat. (See *Assessing the apical impulse,* page 227.)

Keep in mind that the apical impulse may be difficult to palpate in obese and pregnant patients and in patients with thick chest walls.

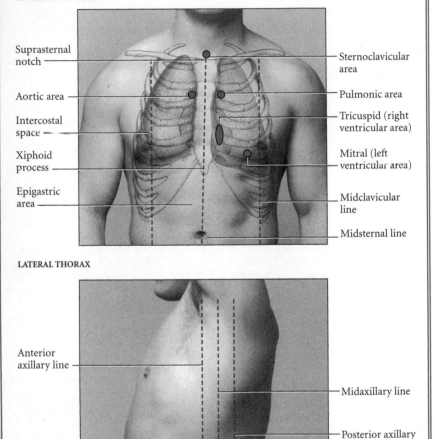

EXPERT TECHNIQUE

IDENTIFYING CARDIOVASCULAR LANDMARKS

The anterior and lateral views of the thorax shown here identify where to locate critical landmarks while performing the cardiovascular assessment.

ANTERIOR THORAX

Suprasternal notch
Aortic area
Intercostal space
Xiphoid process
Epigastric area
Sternoclavicular area
Pulmonic area
Tricuspid (right ventricular area)
Mitral (left ventricular area)
Midclavicular line
Midsternal line

LATERAL THORAX

Anterior axillary line
Midaxillary line
Posterior axillary line

If it's difficult to palpate with the patient lying on his back, have him lie on his left side or sit upright. It may also be helpful to have the patient exhale completely and hold his breath for a few seconds.

Palpation of the patient's heart may reveal:

- apical impulse that exerts unusual force and lasts longer than one-third of the cardiac cycle — a possible indication of increased cardiac output
- displaced or diffuse impulse — a possible indication of left ventricular hypertrophy

- pulsation in the aortic, pulmonary, or right ventricular area — a sign of chamber enlargement or valvular disease
- pulsation in the sternoclavicular or epigastric area — a sign of aortic aneurysm
- palpable thrill or fine vibration — an indication of blood flow turbulence, usually related to valvular dysfunction (Determine how far the thrill radiates and make a mental note to listen for a murmur at this site during auscultation.)
- heave or a strong outward thrust during systole along the left sternal border — an indication of right ventricular hypertrophy
- heave over the left ventricular area — a sign of a ventricular aneurysm (A thin patient may experience a heave with exercise, fever, or anxiety because of increased cardiac output and more forceful contraction.)
- displaced PMI — a possible indication of left ventricular hypertrophy caused by volume overload from mitral or aortic stenosis, septal defect, acute MI, or other disorder.

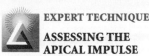

EXPERT TECHNIQUE

ASSESSING THE APICAL IMPULSE

The apical impulse is associated with the first heart sound and carotid pulsation. To ensure that you're feeling the apical impulse and not a muscle spasm or some other pulsation, use one hand to palpate the patient's carotid artery and the other to palpate the apical impulse. Then compare the timing and regularity of the impulses. The apical impulse should roughly coincide with the carotid pulsation.

Note the amplitude, size, intensity, location, and duration of the apical impulse. You should feel a gentle pulsation in an area about ½″ to ¾″ (1.5 to 2 cm) in diameter.

Percussion

Although percussion isn't as useful as other methods of assessment, this technique may help in locating cardiac borders. Begin percussing at the anterior axillary line, and percuss toward the sternum along the fifth intercostal space.

The sound changes from resonance to dullness over the left border of the heart, normally at the midclavicular line. If the cardiac border extends to the left of the midclavicular line, the patient's heart — and especially the left ventricle — may be enlarged.

The right border of the heart is usually aligned with the sternum and can't be percussed. In obese patients, percussion may be difficult because of the fat overlying the chest, or in female patients, because of breast tissue. In these cases, a chest X-ray can be used to provide information about the heart border.

Auscultation

Auscultating for heart sounds provides a great deal of information about the heart. Cardiac auscultation requires a methodical approach and plenty of practice. Begin by warming the stethoscope in your hands, and then identify the sites where you'll auscultate: over the four cardiac valves and at Erb's point, the third intercostal space at the left sternal border. Use the bell to hear low-pitched sounds and the diaphragm to hear high-pitched sounds. (See *Auscultation sites*, page 228.)

Auscultate for heart sounds with the patient in three positions: lying on his back with the head of the bed raised 30 to 45 degrees, sitting up, and lying on his left side. Use a zigzag pattern over the precordium, either auscultating from the base to the apex or the apex to the base. Whichever approach you use, be consistent.

Use the diaphragm of the stethoscope to listen as you go in one direction; use the bell as you come back in the other direction. Be sure to listen over the entire precordium, not just over the valves. Note the heart rate and rhythm.

Always identify the first heart sound (S_1) and the second heart sound (S_2), and then listen for adventitious sounds, such as third (S_3) and fourth heart sounds (S_4), murmurs, and rubs.

Auscultation for normal heart sounds. Start auscultating at the aortic area where S_2 is loudest. S_2 is best heard at the base of the heart at the end of ventricular systole. This

AUSCULTATION SITES

When auscultating for heart sounds, place the stethoscope over four different sites. Follow the same auscultation sequence during every cardiovascular assessment:

- Place the stethoscope in the second intercostal space along the right sternal border, as shown. In the aortic area, blood moves from the left ventricle during systole, crossing the aortic valve and flowing through the aortic arch.
- Move to the pulmonic area, located in the second intercostal space at the left sternal border. In the pulmonic area, blood ejected from the right ventricle during systole crosses the pulmonic valve and flows through the main pulmonary artery.
- In the third auscultation site, assess the tricuspid area, which lies in the fifth intercostal space along the left sternal border. In the tricuspid area, sounds reflect blood movement from the right atrium across the tricuspid valve, filling the right ventricle during diastole.
- Finally, listen in the mitral area, located in the fifth intercostal space near the midclavicular line. (If the patient's heart is enlarged, the mitral area may be closer to the anterior axillary line.) In the mitral (apical) area, sounds represent blood flow across the mitral valve and left ventricular filling during diastole.

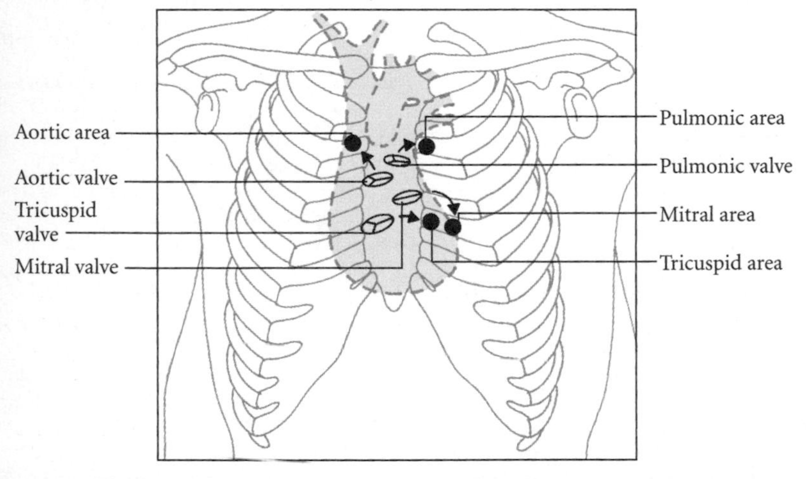

sound corresponds to closure of the pulmonic and aortic valves and is generally described as sounding like dub. It's a shorter, higher-pitched, louder sound than S_1. When the pulmonic valve closes later than the aortic valve during inspiration, you'll hear a split S_2.

From the base of the heart, move to the pulmonic area and down to the tricuspid area. Then move to the mitral area, where S_1 is the loudest. S_1 is best heard at the apex of the heart. This sound corresponds to closure of the mitral and tricuspid valves and is generally described as sounding like "lub." It's low-pitched and dull. S_1 occurs at the beginning of ventricular systole. It may be split if the mitral valve closes just before the tricuspid.

Auscultation may detect S_1 and S_2 that are accentuated, diminished, or inaudible. These abnormalities may result from pressure changes, valvular dysfunctions, and conduction defects. A prolonged, persistent, or reversed split sound may result from a mechanical or electrical problem.

Auscultation for abnormal heart sounds. Auscultation may reveal an S_3, an S_4, or both. Other abnormal sounds include a summation gallop, click, opening snap, rubs, and murmur.

S_3. Also known as a *ventricular gallop,* S_3 is a low-pitched noise that's best heard by placing the bell of the stethoscope at the apex of the heart. Its rhythm resembles a horse galloping, and its cadence resembles the word "Ken-tuc-ky" (lub-dub-by). Listen for S_3 with the patient in a supine or left-lateral decubitus position.

S_3 usually occurs during early diastole to middiastole, at the end of the passive-filling phase of either ventricle. Listen for this sound immediately after S_2. It may signify that the ventricle isn't compliant enough to accept the filling volume without additional force. If the right ventricle is noncompliant, the sound will occur in the tricuspid area; if the left ventricle is noncompliant, in the mitral area. A heave may be palpable when the sound occurs.

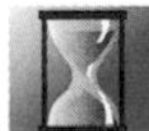

AGE ISSUE *In a child or young adult, S_3 may occur normally. It may also occur during the last trimester of pregnancy. In a patient over age 30, it usually indicates a disorder, such as right-sided heart failure, left-sided heart failure, pulmonary congestion, intracardiac shunting of blood, MI, anemia, or thyrotoxicosis.*

S_4. S_4 is an abnormal heart sound that occurs late in diastole, just before the pulse upstroke. It immediately precedes the S_1 of the next cycle and is associated with acceleration and deceleration of blood entering a chamber that resists additional filling. Known as the atrial or presystolic gallop, it occurs during atrial contraction.

S_4 shares the same cadence as the word "Ten-nes-see" (le-lub-dub). Heard best with the bell of the stethoscope and with the patient in a supine position, S_4 may occur in the tricuspid or mitral area, depending on which ventricle is dysfunctional.

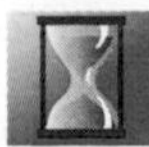

AGE ISSUE *In elderly patients, S_4 commonly appears with age-related systolic hypertension and aortic stenosis.*

Although rare, S_4 may occur normally in a young patient with a thin chest wall. More commonly, it indicates cardiovascular disease, such as acute MI, hypertension, CAD, cardiomyopathy, angina, anemia, elevated left ventricular pressure, or aortic stenosis. If the sound persists, it may indicate impaired ventricular compliance or volume overload.

SUMMATION GALLOP. Occasionally, a patient may have both S_3 and S_4. Auscultation may reveal two separate abnormal heart sounds and two normal sounds. Usually, the patient has tachycardia and diastole is shortened. S_3 and S_4 occur so close together that they appear to be one sound—a summation gallop.

CLICKS. Clicks are high-pitched abnormal heart sounds that result from tensing of the chordae tendineae structures and mitral valve cusps. Initially, the mitral valve closes securely, but a large cusp prolapses into the left atrium. The click usually precedes a late systolic murmur caused by regurgitation of a little blood from the left ventricle into the left atrium. Clicks occur in 5% to 10% of young adults and affect more women than men.

To detect the high-pitched click of mitral valve prolapse in the patient, place the stethoscope diaphragm at the apex and listen during midsystole to late systole. To enhance the sound, change the patient's position to sitting or standing, and listen along the lower left sternal border.

SNAPS. Upon placing the stethoscope diaphragm dial to the apex along the lower left sternal border, you may detect an opening snap immediately after S_2. The snap resembles the normal S_1 and S_2 in quality; its high pitch helps differentiate it from an S_3. Because the opening snap may accompany mitral or tricuspid stenosis, it usually precedes a middiastolic to late diastolic murmur—a classic sign of stenosis. It results from the stenotic valve attempting to open.

RUBS. To detect a pericardial friction rub, use the diaphragm of the stethoscope to auscultate in the third left intercostal space along the lower left sternal border. Listen for a harsh, scratchy, scraping, or squeaking sound that occurs throughout systole, diastole, or both. To enhance the sound, have

EXPERT TECHNIQUE

GRADING MURMURS

Use the system outlined here to grade the intensity of a murmur. When recording your findings, use Roman numerals as part of a fraction, always with VI as the denominator. For instance, a grade III murmur would be recorded as "grade III/VI."

- Grade I is barely audible.
- Grade II is audible but quiet and soft.
- Grade III is moderately loud, without a thrust or thrill.
- Grade IV is loud, with a thrill.
- Grade V is very loud, with a thrust or a thrill.
- Grade VI is loud enough to be heard before the stethoscope comes into contact with the patient's chest.

the patient sit upright and lean forward or exhale. A rub usually indicates pericarditis.

MURMURS. Longer than a heart sound, a murmur occurs as a vibrating, blowing, or rumbling noise. Just as turbulent water in a stream babbles as it passes through a narrow point, turbulent blood flow produces a murmur.

If you detect a murmur, identify where it's loudest, pinpoint the time it occurs during the cardiac cycle, and describe its pitch, pattern, quality, intensity, and implications.

Location and timing. Murmurs may occur in any cardiac auscultatory site and may radiate from one site to another. To identify the radiation area, auscultate from the site where the murmur seems loudest to the farthest site it's still heard. Note the anatomic landmark of this farthest site.

Determine if the murmur occurs during systole (between S_1 and S_2) or diastole (between S_2 and the next S_1). Pinpoint when in the cardiac cycle the murmur occurs—for example, during middiastole or late systole. A murmur that is heard throughout systole is called holosystolic or pansystolic, while a murmur heard throughout diastole is called a pandiastolic murmur. Occasionally murmurs occur during both portions of the cycle, known as continuous murmur.

Pitch. Depending on rate and pressure of blood flow, pitch may be high, medium, or low. You can best hear a low-pitched murmur with the bell of the stethoscope, a high-pitched murmur with the diaphragm, and a medium-pitched murmur with both.

Pattern. Crescendo occurs when the velocity of blood flow increases and the murmur becomes louder. Decrescendo occurs when velocity decreases and the murmur becomes quieter. A crescendo-decrescendo pattern describes a murmur with increasing loudness followed by increasing softness.

Quality. The volume of blood flow, the force of the contraction, and the degree of valve compromise all contribute to murmur quality. Terms used to describe quality include musical, blowing, harsh, rasping, rumbling, or machinelike.

Intensity. Use a standard, six-level grading scale to describe the intensity of the murmur. (See *Grading murmurs.*)

Implications. An innocent or functional murmur may appear in a patient without heart disease. Best heard in the pulmonic area, it occurs early in systole and seldom exceeds grade II in intensity. When the patient changes from a supine to a sitting position, the murmur may disappear. If fever, exercise, anemia, anxiety, pregnancy, or other factors increase cardiac output, the murmur may increase in intensity.

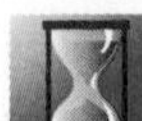

AGE ISSUE *Innocent murmurs affect up to 25% of all children but usually disappear by adolescence. Similarly, elderly patients who experience changes in the aortic valve structures and the aorta also experience a nonpathologic murmur. This murmur occurs as a short systolic murmur, best heard at the left sternal border.*

Pathologic murmurs in a patient may occur during systole or diastole and may affect any heart valve. These murmurs may result from valvular stenosis (inability of the heart valves to open properly), valvular insuffi-

EXPERT TECHNIQUE

POSITIONING THE PATIENT FOR AUSCULTATION

Forward-leaning position
The forward-leaning position is best suited for hearing high-pitched sounds related to semilunar valve problems, such as aortic and pulmonic valve murmurs. To auscultate for these sounds, place the diaphragm of the stethoscope over the aortic and pulmonic areas in the right and left second intercostal spaces, as shown.

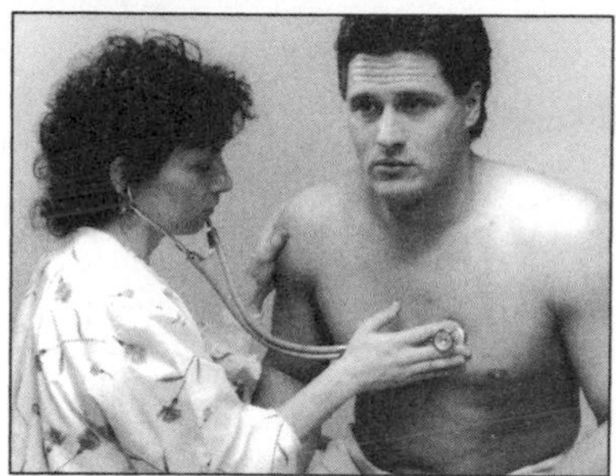

Left lateral recumbent position
The left lateral recumbent position is best suited for hearing low-pitched sounds, such as mitral valve murmurs and extra heart sounds. To hear these sounds, place the bell of the stethoscope over the apical area, as shown.

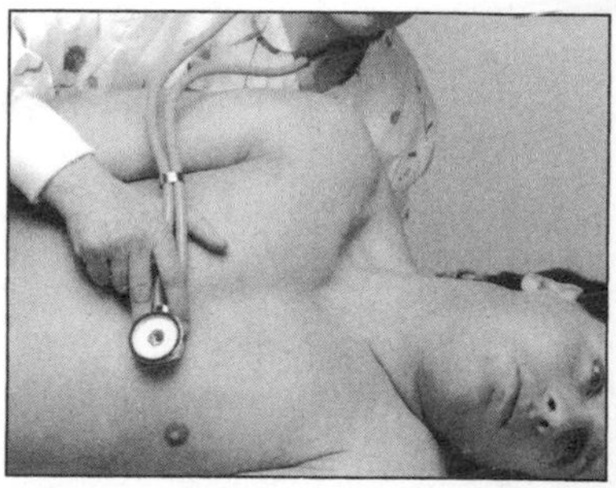

ciency (inability of the heart valves to close properly, allowing regurgitation of blood), or a septal defect (a defect in the septal wall separating two heart chambers).

The best way to hear murmurs is with the patient sitting up and leaning forward. You can also have him lie on his left side. (See *Positioning the patient for auscultation*. Also see *Identifying heart murmurs*, page 232.)

Vascular assessment

Assessment of the vascular system is an important part of a full cardiovascular assessment. Examination of the patient's arms and legs can reveal arterial or venous disorders. Examine the patient's arms when you take his vital signs. Check the legs later during the physical examination, when the patient is lying on his back. Remember to evaluate leg veins when the patient is standing.

Inspection

Start the vascular assessment in the same way as starting the cardiac assessment—by making general observations. Are the patient's arms equal in size? Are the legs symmetrical?

Inspect the patient's skin color. Note how body hair is distributed. Note lesions, scars, clubbing, and edema of the extremities. If the patient is bedridden, check the sacrum for swelling. Examine the fingernails and toenails for abnormalities.

Upon inspection of the patient's vascular system, note these irregularities, including:

- cyanosis, pallor, or cool or cold skin, indicating poor cardiac output and tissue perfusion
- warm skin caused by fever or increased cardiac output
- absence of body hair on the patient's arms or legs, indicating diminished arterial blood flow to those areas (See *Differentiating arterial and chronic venous insufficiency*, page 233.)
- swelling or edema, indicating heart failure or venous insufficiency, or varicosities or thrombophlebitis
- ascites and generalized edema suggesting chronic right-sided heart failure

IDENTIFYING HEART MURMURS

Heart murmurs can occur as a result of various conditions and have wide-ranging characteristics. Here's a list of some conditions and their associated murmurs

Aortic stenosis
In a patient with aortic stenosis, the aortic valve has calcified and restricts blood flow, causing a midsystolic, low-pitched, harsh murmur that radiates from the valve to the carotid artery. The murmur shifts from crescendo to decrescendo and back.

The crescendo-decrescendo murmur of aortic stenosis results from the turbulent, highly pressured flow of blood across stiffened leaflets and through a narrowed opening.

Pulmonic stenosis
During auscultation, listen for a murmur near the pulmonic valve. In a patient with this type of murmur it might indicate pulmonic stenosis, a condition in which the pulmonic valve has calcified and interferes with the flow of blood out of the right ventricle. The murmur is medium-pitched, systolic, and harsh and shifts from crescendo to decrescendo and back. The murmur is caused by turbulent blood flow across a stiffened, narrowed valve.

Aortic insufficiency
In a patient with aortic insufficiency, the blood flows backward through the aortic valve and causes a high-pitched, blowing, decrescendo, diastolic murmur. The murmur radiates from the aortic valve area to the left sternal border.

Pulmonic insufficiency
In a patient with pulmonic insufficiency, the blood flows backward through the pulmonic valve, causing a blowing, diastolic, decrescendo murmur at Erb's point (at the left sternal border of the third intercostal space). If the patient has a higher than normal pulmonary pressure, the murmur is high-pitched. If not, it will be low-pitched.

Mitral stenosis
In a patient with mitral stenosis, the mitral valve has calcified and is blocking blood flow out of the left atrium. Listen for a low-pitched, rumbling, crescendo-decrescendo murmur in the mitral valve area. This murmur results from turbulent blood flow across the stiffened, narrowed valve.

Mitral insufficiency
In a patient with mitral insufficiency, blood regurgitates into the left atrium. The regurgitation produces a high-pitched, blowing murmur throughout systole (pansystolic or holosystolic). The murmur may radiate from the mitral area to the left axillary line. You can hear it best at the apex.

Tricuspid stenosis
In a patient with tricuspid stenosis, the tricuspid valve has calcified and is blocking blood flow through the valve from the right atrium. Listen for a low, rumbling, crescendo-decrescendo murmur in the tricuspid area. The murmur results from turbulent blood flow across the stiffened, narrowed valvular leaflets.

Tricuspid insufficiency
In a patient with tricuspid insufficiency, blood regurgitates into the right atrium. This backflow of blood through the valve causes a high-pitched, blowing murmur throughout systole in the tricuspid area. The murmur becomes louder when the patient inhales.

DIFFERENTIATING ARTERIAL AND CHRONIC VENOUS INSUFFICIENCY

Assessment findings differ in patients with arterial insufficiency and those with chronic venous insufficiency. These illustrations show those differences.

Arterial insufficiency
In a patient with arterial insufficiency, pulses may be decreased or absent. His skin will be cool, pale, and shiny, and he may have pain in his legs and feet. Ulcerations typically occur in the area around the toes, and the foot usually turns deep red when dependent. Nails may be thick and ridged.

Chronic venous insufficiency
In a patient with chronic venous insufficiency, check for ulcerations around the ankle. Pulses are present but may be difficult to find because of edema. The foot may become cyanotic when dependent.

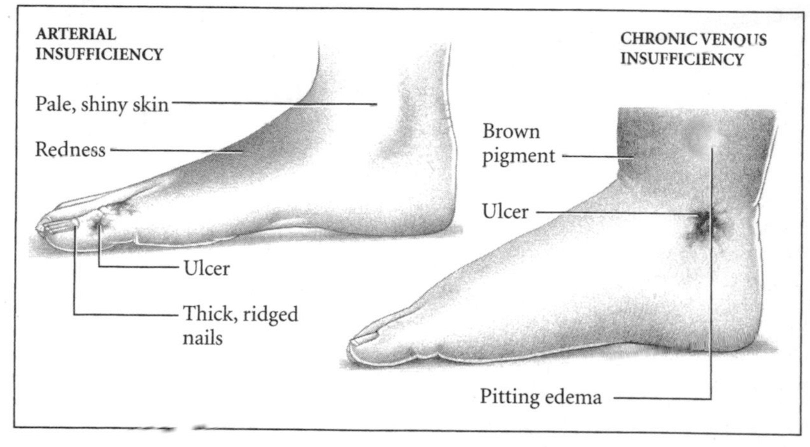

■ localized swelling due to compressed veins
■ lower leg swelling indicating right-sided heart failure.

Observe the vessels in the patient's neck. The carotid artery should appear as a brisk, localized pulsation. The internal jugular vein has a softer, undulating pulsation. The carotid pulsation doesn't decrease when the patient is upright, when he inhales, or when you palpate the carotid. The internal jugular pulsation, on the other hand, changes in response to position, breathing, and palpation.

Check carotid artery pulsations. Are they weak or bounding? Inspect the jugular veins. Inspection of these vessels can provide information about blood volume and pressure in the right side of the heart.

To check the jugular pulse, have the patient lie on his back. Elevate the head of the bed 30 to 45 degrees, and turn the patient's head slightly away from you. Normally, the highest pulsation occurs no more than 1½" (4 cm) above the sternal notch.

If the patient's pulsations appear higher, this indicates elevation in central venous pressure and jugular vein distention. Characterize this distention as mild, moderate, or severe. Determine the level of distention in fingerbreadths above the clavicle or in relation to the jaw or clavicle. Also note the amount of distention in relation to head elevation. (See *Evaluating jugular vein distention,* page 234.)

EXPERT TECHNIQUE

EVALUATING JUGULAR VEIN DISTENTION

With the patient in a supine position, position him so that you can visualize jugular vein with pulsations reflected from the right atrium. Elevate the head of the bed 45 to 50 degrees. (In the normal patient, veins distend only when the patient lies flat.) Next, locate the angle of Louis (sternal notch) — the reference point for measuring venous pressure. To do so, palpate the clavicles where they join the sternum (the suprasternal notch). Place your first two fingers on the suprasternal notch. Then, without lifting them from the skin, slide them down the sternum until you feel a bony protuberance — this is the angle of Louis.

Find the internal jugular vein, which indicates venous pressure more reliably than the external jugular vein. Shine a penlight across the patient's neck to create shadows that highlight his venous pulse. Be sure to distinguish jugular vein pulsations from carotid artery pulsations. One way to do this is to palate the vessel: Arterial pulsations continue, whereas venous pulsations disappear with light finger pressure. Also, venous pulsations increase or decrease with changes in body position; arterial pulsations remain constant.

Next, locate the highest point along the vein where you can see pulsations. Using a centimeter ruler, measure the distance between the highest point and the sternal notch. Record this finding as well as the angle at which the patient was lying. A finding greater than 1¼″ to 1½″ (3 to 4 cm) above the sternal notch, with the head of the bed at a 45-degree angle, indicates jugular vein distention.

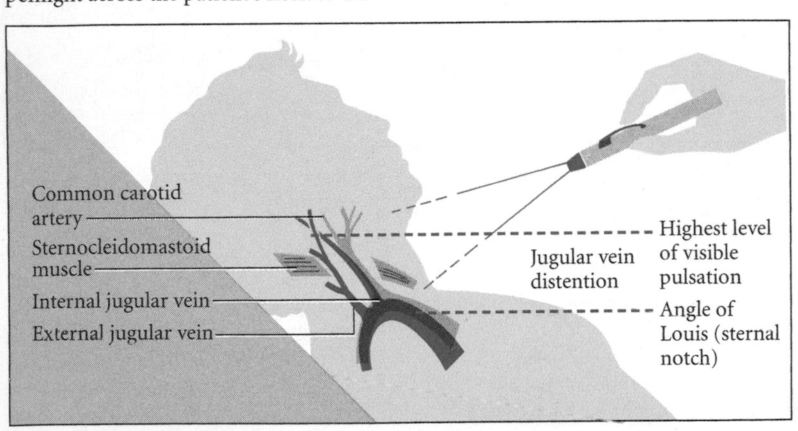

Palpation

The first step in palpating the vascular system is to assess skin temperature, texture, and turgor. Then check capillary refill time by assessing the nail beds on the fingers and toes. Refill time should be no more than 3 seconds, or long enough to say "capillary refill."

Palpate the patient's arms and legs for temperature and edema. Edema is graded on a four-point scale. If your finger leaves a slight imprint, the edema is recorded as +1. If your finger leaves a deep imprint that only slowly returns to normal, the edema is recorded as +4. (See *Edema: Pitting or nonpitting?*)

Palpate for arterial pulses by gently pressing with the pads of your index and middle fingers. Start at the top of the patient's body at the temporal artery, and work your way down. Check the carotid, brachial, radial, femoral, popliteal, posterior tibial, and dorsalis pedis pulses. Palpate for the pulse on each side, comparing pulse volume and symmetry.

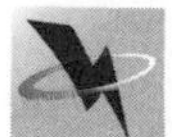

CRITICAL POINT *Don't palpate both carotid arteries at the same time or press too firmly. If you do, the patient may faint or become bradycardic.*

Put on gloves for the examination when you palpate the femoral arteries.

All pulses should be regular in rhythm and equal in strength. Pulses are graded on the following scale: 4+ is bounding, 3+ is increased, 2+ is normal, 1+ is weak, and 0 is absent. (See *Assessing arterial pulses,* page 236.)

A weak arterial pulse may indicate decreased cardiac output or increased peripheral vascular resistance, both of which point to arterial atherosclerotic disease.

Strong or bounding pulsations usually occur in a patient with a condition that causes increased cardiac output, such as hypertension, hypoxia, anemia, exercise, or anxiety. (See *Identifying pulse waveforms,* page 237.)

Auscultation

After you palpate, use the bell of the stethoscope to begin auscultating the vascular system; then follow the palpation sequence and listen over each artery. You shouldn't hear sounds over the carotid arteries. A hum, or bruit, sounds like buzzing or blowing and could indicate arteriosclerotic plaque formation.

Assess the upper abdomen for abnormal pulsations, which could indicate the presence of an abdominal aortic aneurysm. Finally, auscultate for the femoral and popliteal pulses, checking for a bruit or other abnormal sounds.

If you hear a bruit during arterial auscultation, the patient may have occlusive arterial disease or an arteriovenous fistula. Various high cardiac output conditions — such as anemia, hyperthyroidism, and pheochromocytoma — may also cause bruits.

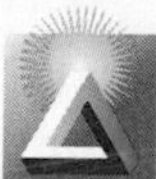

EXPERT TECHNIQUE

EDEMA: PITTING OR NONPITTING?

To differentiate pitting from nonpitting edema, press your finger against a swollen area for 5 seconds, then quickly remove it.

With pitting edema, pressure forces fluid into the underlying tissues, causing an indentation that slowly fills. To determine the severity of pitting edema, estimate the indentation's depth in centimeters: 1+ (1 cm), 2+ (2 cm), 3+ (3 cm), or 4+ (4 cm).

With nonpitting edema, pressure leaves no indentation because fluid has coagulated in the tissues. Typically, the skin feels unusually tight and firm.

PITTING EDEMA (4+)

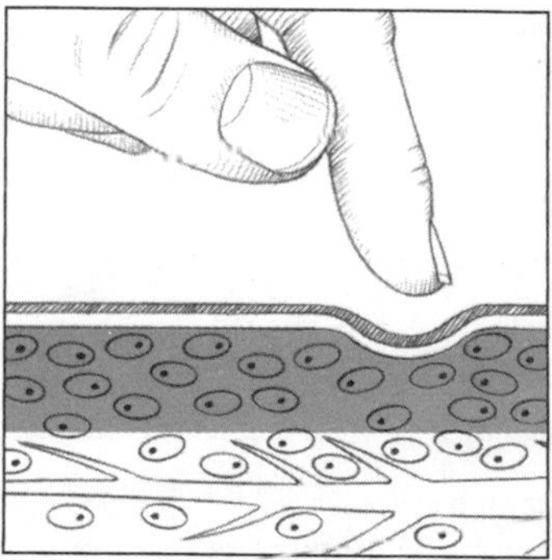

NONPITTING EDEMA

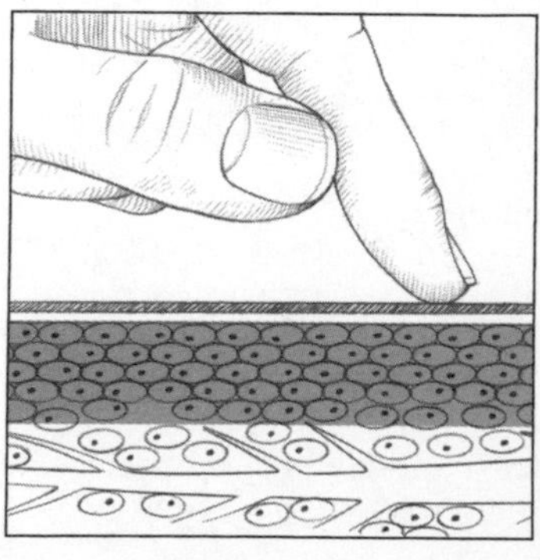

EXPERT TECHNIQUE

ASSESSING ARTERIAL PULSES

To assess arterial pulses, apply pressure with your index and middle fingers. These illustrations show where to position your fingers when palpating for various arterial pulses.

Carotid pulse
Lightly place your fingers just medial to the trachea and below the jaw angle. Never palpate both carotid arteries at the same time.

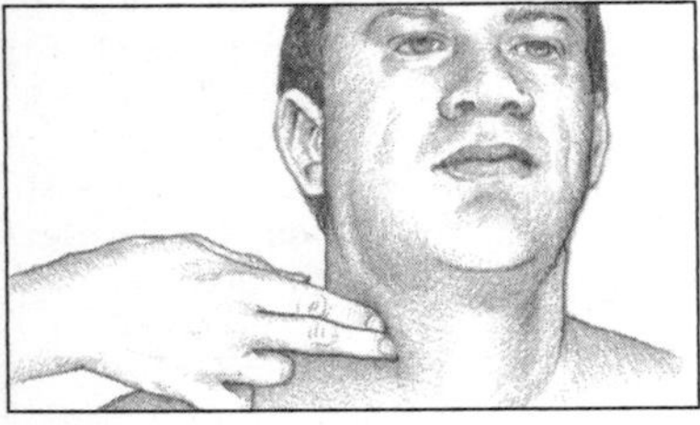

Brachial pulse
Position your fingers medial to the biceps tendon.

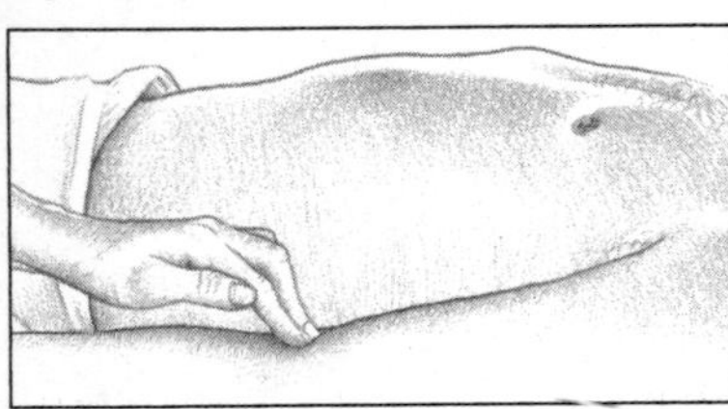

Radial pulse
Apply gentle pressure to the medial and ventral side of the wrist, just below the base of the thumb.

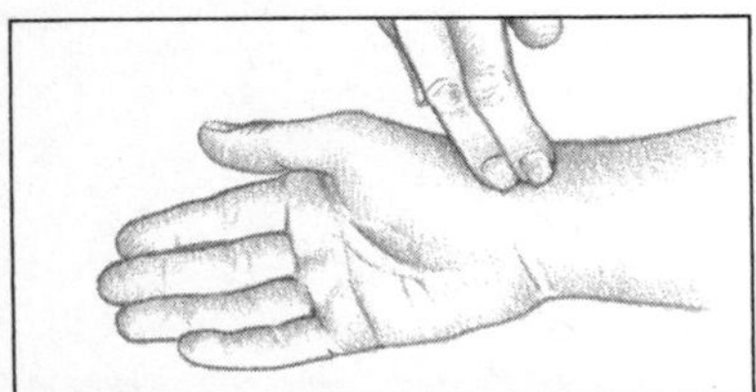

Femoral pulse
Press relatively hard at a point inferior to the inguinal ligament. For an obese patient, palpate in the crease of the groin, halfway between the pubic bone and the hip bone.

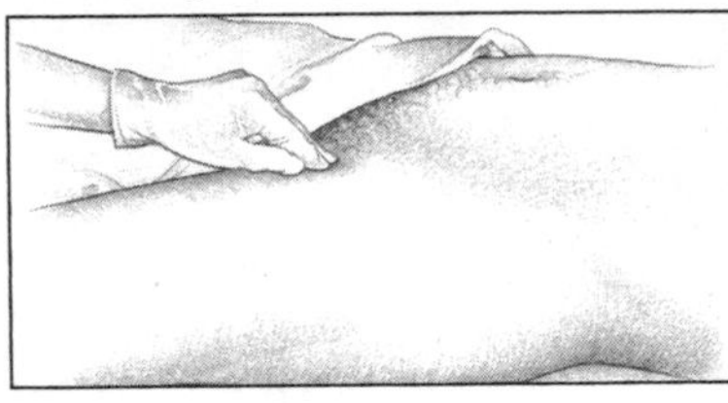

Popliteal pulse
Press firmly in the popliteal fossa at the back of the knee.

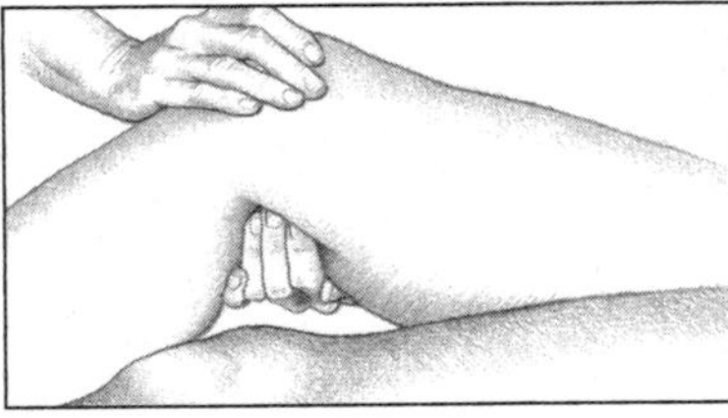

Posterior tibial pulse
Apply pressure behind and slightly below the malleolus of the ankle.

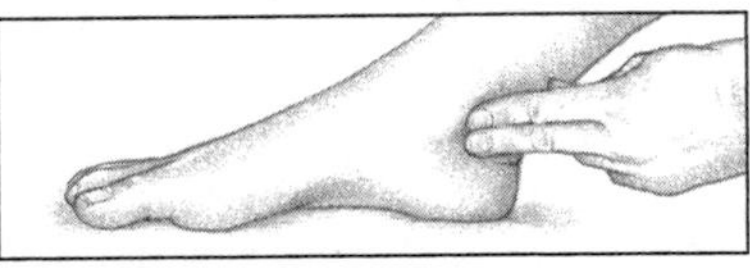

Dorsalis pedis pulse
Place your fingers on the medial dorsum of the foot while the patient points his toes down. (*Note:* The pulse is difficult to detect here and may be nonpalpable in healthy patients.)

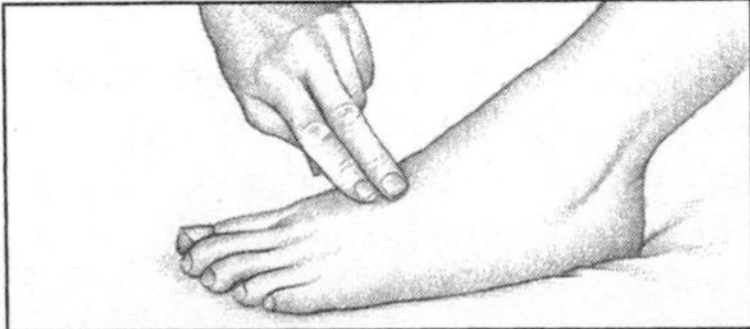

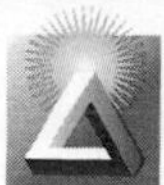

EXPERT TECHNIQUE

IDENTIFYING PULSE WAVEFORMS

To identify abnormal arterial pulses, check the waveforms below and see which one matches the patient's peripheral pulse.

Weak pulse
A weak pulse has a decreased amplitude with a slower upstroke and downstroke. Possible causes of a weak pulse include increased peripheral vascular resistance, such as happens in cold weather or severe heart failure; and decreased stroke volume, as with hypovolemia or aortic stenosis.

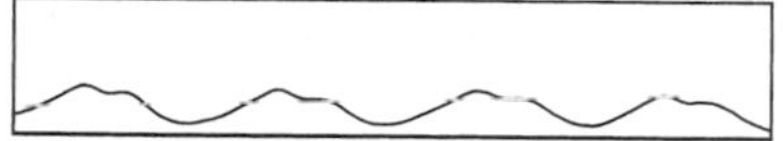

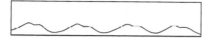

Bounding pulse
A bounding pulse has a sharp upstroke and downstroke with a pointed peak. The amplitude is elevated. Possible causes of a bounding pulse include increased stroke volume, as with aortic insufficiency; or stiffness of arterial walls, as with aging.

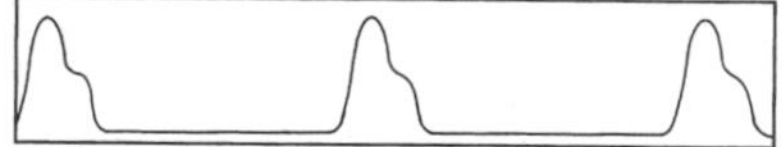

Pulsus alternans
Pulsus alternans has a regular, alternating pattern of a weak and a strong pulse. This pulse is associated with left-sided heart failure.

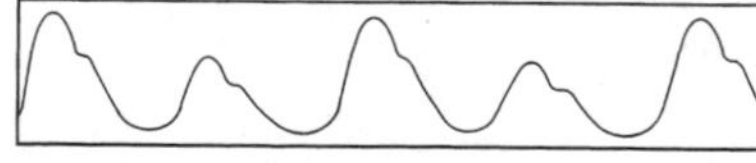

Pulsus bigeminus
Pulsus bigeminus is similar to alternating pulse but occurs at irregular intervals. This pulse is caused by premature atrial or ventricular beats.

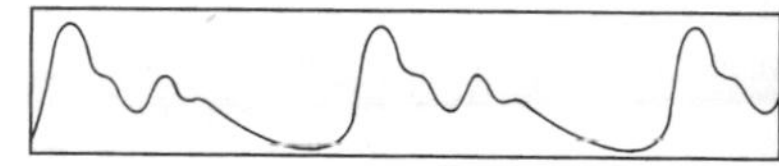

Pulsus paradoxus
Pulsus paradoxus has increases and decreases in amplitude associated with the respiratory cycle. Marked decreases occur when the patient inhales. Pulsus paradoxus is associated with pericardial tamponade, advanced heart failure, and constrictive pericarditis.

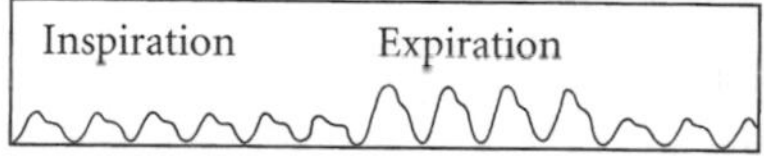

Pulsus biferiens
Pulsus biferiens shows an initial upstroke, a subsequent downstroke, and then another upstroke during systole. Pulsus biferiens is caused by aortic stenosis and aortic insufficiency.

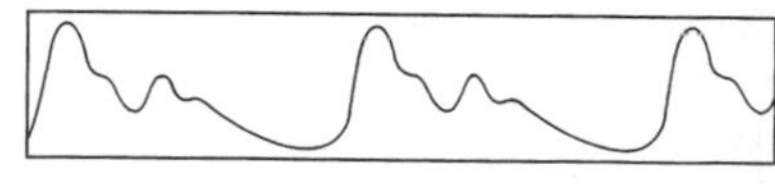

Abnormal findings

A patient's chief complaint may be due to any of the number of signs and symptoms related to the cardiovascular system. Common findings include decreased or increased blood pressure, bruits, increased capillary refill time, chest pain, fatigue, atrial or ventricular gallop, intermittent claudication, jugular vein distention, palpitations, absent or weak pulse, and peripheral edema. Cyanosis, a common finding associated with the respiratory system, also is a common finding related to the cardiovascular system. See chapter 8, Respiratory system, for further discussion of this finding. The following history, physical examination, and analysis summaries will help assess each finding quickly and accurately. After obtaining further information, begin to interpret the findings. (See *Cardiovascular system: Interpreting your findings.*)

Blood pressure, decreased

Low blood pressure refers to inadequate intravascular pressure to maintain oxygen requirements of the body's tissues.

Normal blood pressure varies considerably; what qualifies as low blood pressure for one person may be perfectly normal for another. Consequently, every blood pressure reading must be compared against the patient's baseline. Typically, a reading below 90/60 mm Hg, or a drop of 30 mm Hg from the baseline, is considered low blood pressure.

History

If the patient is conscious, ask him about associated symptoms. For example, find out if he feels unusually weak or fatigued; if he has had nausea, vomiting, or dark or bloody stools; if his vision is blurred; or if his gait is unsteady. Ask him if he has palpitations or chest or abdominal pain or difficulty breathing. Then ask if he has had episodes of dizziness or fainting. Find out if these episodes occur when he stands up suddenly. If so, take the patient's blood pressure while he's lying down, sitting, and then standing; compare readings. A drop in systolic or diastolic pressure of 10 to 20 mm Hg or more and an increase in heart rate of more than 15 beats/minute between position changes suggest orthostatic hypotension.

Physical assessment

Next, continue with a physical examination. Inspect the skin for pallor, sweating, and clamminess. Palpate peripheral pulses. Note paradoxical pulse — an accentuated fall in systolic pressure during inspiration — which suggests pericardial tamponade. Then auscultate for abnormal heart sounds, such as gallops and murmurs; heart rate, signaling bradycardia or tachycardia; and heart rhythm. Auscultate the lungs for abnormal breath sounds, such as diminished sounds, crackles, wheezing; breath rate, signaling bradypnea or tachypnea; and breath rhythm, such as agonal or Cheyne-Stokes respirations. Look for signs of hemorrhage, including visible bleeding and palpable masses, bruising, and tenderness. Assess the patient for abdominal rigidity and rebound tenderness; auscultate for abnormal bowel sounds. Carefully assess the patient for possible sources of infection such as open wounds.

Analysis

Although commonly linked to shock, decrease blood pressure may also result from a cardiovascular, respiratory, neurologic, or metabolic disorder. Hypoperfusion states especially affect the kidneys, brain, and heart, and may lead to renal failure, change in level of consciousness (LOC), or myocardial ischemia. Low blood pressure may be drug-induced or may accompany diagnostic tests — typically those using contrast media. It may stem from stress or change of position — specifically, rising abruptly from a supine or sitting position to a standing position (orthostatic hypotension). Low blood pressure can reflect an expanded intravascular space, as in severe infections, allergic reactions, or adrenal in sufficiency; reduced intravascular volume, as in dehydration and hemorrhage; or decreased cardiac output, as in impaired cardiac muscle contractility. Because the body's pressure-regulating mechanisms are complex and interrelated, a combination of these factors usually contributes to low blood pressure.

AGE ISSUE *In children, normal blood pressure is lower than that in adults. Because accidents occur frequently in children, suspect trauma or shock first as a possible cause of low blood pressure. Remember that low blood pressure typically doesn't accompany head injury in adults because intracranial hemorrhage is insufficient to cause hypovolemia. However, it does accompany head injury in infants and young children; their expandable cranial vaults allow significant blood loss into the cranial space, resulting in hypovolemia. Another common cause of low blood pressure in children is dehydration, which results from failure to thrive or from persistent diarrhea and vomiting for as little as 24 hours.*

In elderly patients, low blood pressure commonly results from the use of multiple drugs with this potential adverse effect, a problem that needs to be addressed. Orthostatic hypotension due to autonomic dysfunction is another common cause.

(Text continues on page 245.)

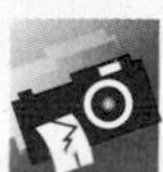

CLINICAL PICTURE

CARDIOVASCULAR SYSTEM: INTERPRETING YOUR FINDINGS

After you assess the patient, a group of findings may lead you to a particular disorder of the cardiovascular system. This chart shows some common groups of findings for major signs and symptoms related to the cardiovascular assessment, along with their probable causes.

Sign or symptom and findings	Probable cause
Blood pressure, decreased	
▪ Orthostatic hypotension ▪ Fatigue ▪ Weakness ▪ Nausea, vomiting ▪ Abdominal discomfort ▪ Weight loss ▪ Fever ▪ Tachycardia ▪ Hyperpigmentation of fingers, nails, nipples, scars, and body folds	Adrenal insufficiency, acute
▪ Fall in systolic pressure to less than 80 mm Hg or to 30 mm Hg less than baseline ▪ Tachycardia ▪ Narrowed pulse pressure ▪ Diminished Korotkoff sounds ▪ Peripheral cyanosis ▪ Pale, cool clammy skin ▪ Restlessness and anxiety	Cardiogenic shock
***Blood pressure, decreased** (continued)*	
▪ Fall in systolic pressure to less than 80 mm Hg or to 30 mm Hg less than baseline ▪ Diminished Korotkoff sounds ▪ Narrowed pulse pressure ▪ Rapid weak irregular pulse ▪ Cyanosis of extremities ▪ Pale, cool clammy skin	Hypovolemic shock
▪ Fever ▪ Chills ▪ Low blood pressure ▪ Tachycardia and tachypnea (early) ▪ Increasingly severe low blood pressure as condition progresses with narrowed pulse pressure	Septic shock
Blood pressure, elevated	
▪ Elevated diastolic pressure with orthostatic hypotension ▪ Constipation ▪ Muscle weakness ▪ Polyuria ▪ Polydipsia ▪ Personality changes	Aldosteronism, primary

(continued)

CARDIOVASCULAR SYSTEM: INTERPRETING YOUR FINDINGS *(continued)*

Sign or symptom and findings	Probable cause
Blood pressure, elevated *(continued)*	
▪ Elevated pressure with widened pulse pressure ▪ Truncal obesity ▪ Moon face	Cushing's syndrome
▪ Elevated pressure; possibly asymptomatic ▪ Suboccipital headache ▪ Light-headedness ▪ Tinnitus ▪ Fatigue	Hypertension
Bruits	
▪ Pulsatile abdominal mass ▪ Systolic bruit over aorta ▪ Rigid tender abdomen ▪ Mottled skin ▪ Diminished peripheral pulses ▪ Claudication	Aortic aneurysm, abdominal
▪ Systolic bruits over one or both carotid arteries ▪ Dizziness ▪ Vertigo ▪ Headache ▪ Syncope ▪ Aphasia ▪ Dysarthria ▪ Sudden vision loss ▪ Hemiparesis or hemiparalysis signaling transient ischemic attack	Carotid artery stenosis
Bruits *(continued)*	
▪ Bruits over femoral arteries and other arteries in the legs ▪ Diminished, absent femoral, popliteal, or pedal pulses ▪ Intermittent claudication ▪ Numbness, weakness, pain, and cramping in legs ▪ Cool, shiny skin and hair loss on affected extremity	Peripheral vascular disease
Capillary refill time, increased	
▪ Increased refill time with absent pulses distal to obstruction ▪ Affected limb cool and pale or cyanotic ▪ Intermittent claudication ▪ Moderate to severe pain, numbness, paresthesia, or paralysis of affected limb	Arterial occlusion, acute
▪ Increased refill time as a compensatory mechanism ▪ Shivering ▪ Fatigue ▪ Weakness ▪ Decreased level of consciousness ▪ Slurred speech ▪ Ataxia ▪ Muscle stiffness	Hypothermia

CARDIOVASCULAR SYSTEM: INTERPRETING YOUR FINDINGS *(continued)*

Sign or symptom and findings	Probable cause
Capillary refill time, increased *(continued)*	
▪ Refill time prolonged in fingers ▪ Blanching of fingers followed by cyanosis, then erythema before fingers return to normal	Raynaud's disease
Chest pain	
▪ A feeling of tightness or pressure in the chest described as pain or a sensation of indigestion or expansion ▪ Pain may radiate to the neck, jaw, and arms, classically to the inner aspect of the left arm ▪ Pain begins gradually, reaches a maximum, then slowly subsides ▪ Pain is provoked by exertion, emotional stress, or a heavy meal ▪ Pain typically lasts 2 to 10 minutes (usually no more than 20 minutes) ▪ Dyspnea ▪ Nausea and vomiting ▪ Tachycardia ▪ Dizziness ▪ Diaphoresis	Angina
Chest pain *(continued)*	
▪ Crushing substernal pain, unrelieved by rest or nitroglycerin ▪ Pain that may radiate to the left arm, jaw, neck, or shoulder blades ▪ Pain that lasts from 15 minutes to hours ▪ Pallor ▪ Clammy skin ▪ Dyspnea ▪ Diaphoresis ▪ Feeling of impending doom	Myocardial infarction
▪ Sharp, severe pain aggravated by inspiration, coughing, or pressure ▪ Shallow, splinted breaths ▪ Dyspnea ▪ Cough ▪ Local tenderness and edema	Rib fracture
Fatigue	
▪ Fatigue following mild activity ▪ Pallor ▪ Tachycardia ▪ Dyspnea	Anemia
▪ Persistent fatigue unrelated to exertion ▪ Headache ▪ Anorexia ▪ Constipation ▪ Sexual dysfunction ▪ Loss of concentration ▪ Irritability	Depression

(continued)

CARDIOVASCULAR SYSTEM: INTERPRETING YOUR FINDINGS *(continued)*

Sign or symptom and findings	Probable cause
***Fatigue** (continued)*	
■ Progressive fatigue ■ Cardiac murmur ■ Exertional dyspnea ■ Cough ■ Hemoptysis	Valvular heart disease
Gallop, atrial	
■ Intermittent gallop during attack, disappearing when attack is over ■ Possible paradoxical S_2 or new murmur ■ Chest tightness, pressure, or achiness that radiates	Angina
■ Atrial gallop accompanied by soft short diastolic murmur on left sternal border ■ Possible soft, short midsystolic murmur ■ Tachycardia ■ Dyspnea ■ Jugular vein distention, crackles, and possibly angina	Aortic insufficiency
■ Atrial gallop occurring early in the onset of disease ■ Possibly asymptomatic or with headache, weakness, dizziness, or fatigue ■ Epistaxis, tinnitus	Hypertension
Gallop, ventricular	
■ S_3 with atrial gallop and soft short diastolic murmur over left sternal border ■ S_2 possibly soft or absent ■ Tachycardia ■ Dyspnea ■ Jugular vein distention and crackles	Aortic insufficiency
■ Ventricular gallop accompanied by alternating pulse and altered S_1 and S_2 ■ Fatigue ■ Dyspnea ■ Orthopnea ■ Chest pain ■ Palpitations ■ Crackles ■ Peripheral edema ■ Atrial gallop	Cardiomyopathy
■ Ventricular gallop with early or holosystolic decrescendo murmur at apex ■ Atrial gallop ■ Widely split S_2 ■ Sinus tachycardia ■ Tachypnea ■ Orthopnea ■ Crackles ■ Fatigue ■ Jugular vein distention	Mitral insufficiency

CARDIOVASCULAR SYSTEM: INTERPRETING YOUR FINDINGS *(continued)*

Sign or symptom and findings	Probable cause
Intermittent claudication	
▪ Pain in lower extremities along the femoral and popliteal arteries ▪ Diminished or absent popliteal and pedal pulses ▪ Coolness of affected limb; pallor on elevation ▪ Numbness, tingling, paresthesia ▪ Ulceration and possible gangrene	Arteriosclerosis obliterans
▪ Pain in the instep ▪ Erythema along extremity blood vessels ▪ Feet becoming cold, cyanotic, and numb on exposure to cold; then becoming reddened, hot, and tingling ▪ Impaired peripheral pulses	Buerger's disease
Jugular vein distention	
▪ Distention with anxiety, restlessness ▪ Cyanosis ▪ Chest pain ▪ Dyspnea ▪ Hypotension ▪ Clammy skin ▪ Tachycardia ▪ Muffled heart sounds ▪ Pericardial friction rub ▪ Pulsus paradoxus	Cardiac tamponade
Jugular vein distention (continued)	
▪ Sudden or gradual distention ▪ Weakness and anxiety ▪ Cyanosis ▪ Dependent edema of legs and sacrum ▪ Steady weight gain ▪ Confusion ▪ Hepatomegaly ▪ Nausea and vomiting ▪ Abdominal discomfort ▪ Anorexia	Heart failure
▪ Vein distention more prominent on inspiration ▪ Chest pain ▪ Fluid retention and dependent edema ▪ Hepatomegaly ▪ Ascites ▪ Pericardial friction rub	Pericarditis, chronic constrictive
Palpitations	
▪ Paroxysmal palpitations ▪ Diaphoresis ▪ Facial flushing ▪ Trembling ▪ Impending sense of doom ▪ Hyperventilation ▪ Dizziness	Acute anxiety attack

(continued)

CARDIOVASCULAR SYSTEM: INTERPRETING YOUR FINDINGS *(continued)*

Sign or symptom and findings	Probable cause
***Palpitations** (continued)*	
▪ Paroxysmal or sustained palpitations ▪ Dizziness ▪ Weakness ▪ Fatigue ▪ Irregular, rapid, or slow pulse rate ▪ Decreased blood pressure ▪ Confusion ▪ Diaphoresis	Arrhythmias
▪ Sustained palpitations ▪ Fatigue ▪ Irritability ▪ Hunger ▪ Cold sweats ▪ Tremors ▪ Anxiety	Hypoglycemia
Peripheral edema	
▪ Headache ▪ Bilateral leg edema with pitting ankle edema ▪ Weight gain despite anorexia ▪ Nausea ▪ Chest tightness ▪ Hypotension ▪ Pallor ▪ Palpitations ▪ Inspiratory crackles	Heart failure
***Peripheral edema** (continued)*	
▪ Bilateral arm edema accompanied by facial and neck edema ▪ Edematous areas marked by dilated veins ▪ Headache ▪ Vertigo ▪ Vision disturbances	Superior vena cava syndrome
▪ Moderate to severe, unilateral or bilateral leg edema ▪ Darkened skin ▪ Stasis ulcers around the ankle	Venous insufficiency
Pulse, absent or weak	
▪ Weak or absent pulse distal to affected area ▪ Sudden tearing pain in chest and neck radiating to upper and lower back and abdomen ▪ Syncope ▪ Loss of consciousness ▪ Weakness or transient paralysis of legs or arms ▪ Diastolic murmur ▪ Systemic hypotension ▪ Mottled skin below the waist	Aortic aneurysm, dissecting

CARDIOVASCULAR SYSTEM: INTERPRETING YOUR FINDINGS *(continued)*

Sign or symptom and findings	Probable cause
Pulse, absent or weak *(continued)*	
▪ Absence of pulses distal to obstruction; usually unilaterally weak and then absent ▪ Cool, pale, cyanotic affected limb ▪ Increased capillary refill time ▪ Moderate to severe pain and paresthesia ▪ Line of color and temperature demarcating the level of obstruction	Arterial occlusion
▪ Weakening and loss of peripheral pulses ▪ Aching pain distal to occlusion that worsens with exercise and abates with rest ▪ Cool skin with decreased hair growth ▪ Possible impotence in males	Peripheral vascular disease

Blood pressure, elevated

Elevated blood pressure — an intermittent or sustained increase in blood pressure exceeding 140/90 mm Hg — strikes more men than women and twice as many Blacks as Whites. By itself, this common sign is easily ignored by the patient; because he can't see or feel it. However, its causes can be life-threatening.

Hypertension has been reported to be two to three times more common in women taking hormonal contraceptives than those not taking them. Women age 35 and older who smoke cigarettes should be strongly encouraged to stop; if they continue to smoke, they should be discouraged from using hormonal contraceptives.

History

If you detect sharply elevated blood pressure, quickly rule out possible life-threatening causes. After ruling out life-threatening causes, complete a more leisurely history and physical examination. Determine if the patient has a history of cardiovascular or cerebrovascular disease, diabetes, or renal disease. Ask about a family history of high blood pressure — a likely finding with essential hypertension, pheochromocytoma, or polycystic kidney disease. Then ask about its onset and if the high blood pressure appeared abruptly. Ask the patient's age. Sudden onset of high blood pressure in middle-aged or elderly patients suggests renovascular stenosis. Although essential hypertension may begin in childhood, it typically isn't diagnosed until near age 35.

Note headache, palpitations, blurred vision, and sweating. Ask about wine-colored urine and decreased urine output; these signs suggest glomerulonephritis, which can cause elevated blood pressure.

Obtain a drug history, including past and present prescriptions, herbal preparations, and over-the-counter drugs especially decongestants.

CRITICAL POINT *Ephedra (ma huang), ginseng, and licorice may cause high blood pressure or irregular heartbeat. St. John's wort can also raise blood pressure, especially when taken with substances that antagonize hypericin, such as amphetamines, cold and hay fever medications, nasal decongestants, pickled foods, beer, coffee, wine, and chocolate.*

If the patient is already taking an antihypertensive, determine how well he complies with the regimen. Ask about his perception of the elevated blood pressure. Find out how serious he believes it is and if he expects drug therapy will help. Explore psychosocial or environmental factors that may impact blood pressure control.

Physical assessment

Obtain vital signs and check for orthostatic hypotension. Take the patient's blood pressure with him laying down, sitting, and then standing. Normally, systolic pressure falls and diastolic pressure rises on standing. With orthostatic hypotension, both pressures fall.

Using a funduscope, check for intraocular hemorrhage, exudate, and papilledema, which characterize severe hypertension. Perform a thorough cardiovascular assessment. Check for carotid bruits and jugular vein distention. Assess skin color, temperature, and turgor. Palpate peripheral pulses. Auscultate for abnormal heart sounds, including gallops, louder S_2, murmurs; and heart rate, including bradycardia, tachycardia, or rhythm. Then auscultate for abnormal breath sounds, such as crackles or wheezing; breath rate, such as bradypnea or tachypnea; and breath rhythm.

Palpate the abdomen for tenderness, masses, or liver enlargement. Auscultate for abdominal bruits. Renal artery stenosis produces bruits over the upper abdomen or in the costovertebral angles. Easily palpable, enlarged kidneys and a large, tender liver suggest polycystic kidney disease. Obtain a urine sample to check for microscopic hematuria.

Analysis

Elevated blood pressure may develop suddenly or gradually. A sudden, severe rise in pressure (exceeding 180/110 mm Hg) may indicate life-threatening hypertensive crisis. However, even a less dramatic rise may be equally significant if it heralds a dissecting aortic aneurysm, increased intracranial pressure, myocardial infarction, eclampsia, or thyrotoxicosis.

Usually associated with essential hypertension, elevated blood pressure may also result from a renal or endocrine disorder, a treatment that affects fluid status, such as dialysis, or a drug's adverse effect. Ingestion of large amounts of certain foods, such as black licorice and cheddar cheese, may temporarily elevate blood pressure.

Sometimes elevated blood pressure may simply reflect inaccurate blood pressure measurement. However, careful measurement alone doesn't ensure a clinically useful reading. To be useful, each blood pressure reading must be compared with the patient's baseline. Also, serial readings may be necessary to establish elevated blood pressure.

The patient may experience elevated blood pressure in a health care provider's office (known as "white-coat hypertension"). In such cases, 24-hour blood pressure monitoring is indicated to confirm elevated readings in other settings. In addition, other risk factors for coronary artery disease (CAD), such as smoking and elevated cholesterol levels, need to be addressed.

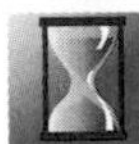

AGE ISSUE *Normally, blood pressure in children is lower than it is in adults. In children, elevated blood pressure may result from lead or mercury poisoning, essential hypertension, renovascular stenosis, chronic pyelonephritis, coarctation of aorta, patent ductus arteriosus, glomerulonephritis, adrenogenital syndrome, or neuroblastoma. In elderly patients, atherosclerosis commonly produces isolated systolic hypertension.*

Bruits

Typically an indicator of life- or limb-threatening vascular disease, bruits are swishing sounds caused by turbulent blood flow. They're characterized by location, duration, intensity, pitch, and time of onset in the cardiac cycle. Loud bruits produce in tense vibration and a palpable thrill. A thrill, however, doesn't provide any further clue to the causative disorder or to its severity.

History

If you detect a bruit, be sure to check for further vascular damage and perform a thorough cardiac assessment.

Physical assessment

If you detect bruits over the abdominal aorta, check for a pulsating mass or a bluish discoloration around the umbilicus (Cullen's sign). Either of these signs — or severe, tearing pain in the abdomen, flank, or lower back — may signal life-threatening dissection of an aortic aneurysm. Also check peripheral pulses, comparing intensity in the upper versus lower extremities.

If you detect bruits over the thyroid gland, ask the patient if he has a history of hyperthyroidism or signs and symptoms, such as nervousness, tremors, weight loss, palpitations, heat intolerance, and (in females) amenorrhea.

CRITICAL POINT *Watch for signs and symptoms of life-threatening thyroid storm, such as tremor, restlessness, diarrhea, abdominal pain, and hepatomegaly.*

If you detect carotid artery bruits, be alert for signs and symptoms of a transient ischemic attack, including dizziness, diplopia, slurred speech, flashing lights, and syncope. These findings may indicate impending stroke. Be sure to evaluate the patient frequently for changes in LOC and muscle function.

If you detect bruits over the femoral, popliteal, or subclavian artery, watch for signs and symptoms of decreased or absent peripheral circulation — edema, weakness, and paresthesia. Ask the patient if he has a history of intermittent claudication. Frequently check distal pulses and skin color and temperature. Also watch for the sudden absence of pulse, pallor, or coolness, which may indicate a threat to the affected limb.

Analysis

Bruits are most significant when heard over the abdominal aorta; the renal, carotid, femoral, popliteal, or subclavian artery; or the thyroid gland. They're also significant when heard consistently despite changes in patient position and when heard during diastole.

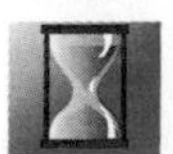

AGE ISSUE *In young children, bruits are common but are usually of little significance — for example, cranial bruits are normal until age 4. However, certain bruits may be significant. Because birthmarks commonly accompany congenital arteriovenous fistulas, carefully auscultate for bruits in a child with port-wine spots or cavernous or diffuse hemangiomas.*

Elderly people with atherosclerosis may experience bruits over several arteries. Bruits related to carotid artery stenosis are particularly important because of the high incidence of associated stroke.

Capillary refill time, increased

Capillary refill time is the duration required for color to return to the nail bed of a finger or toe after application of slight pressure, which causes blanching. This duration reflects the quality of peripheral vasomotor function. Normal capillary refill time is less than 3 seconds.

History

Capillary refill time is typically tested during a routine cardiovascular assessment. It isn't tested with suspected life-threatening disorders because other, more characteristic signs and symptoms appear earlier.

Physical examination

If you detect increased capillary refill time, take the patient's vital signs and check pulses in the affected limb. Does the limb feel cold or look cyanotic? Ask the patient about pain or any unusual sensations in his fingers or toes, especially after exposure to cold.

Take a brief medical history, especially noting previous peripheral vascular disease. Find out which medications the patient is taking.

Analysis

Increased refill time isn't diagnostic of any disorder but must be evaluated along with other signs and symptoms. However, this sign usually signals obstructive peripheral arterial disease or decreased cardiac output.

Chest pain

Chest pain can arise suddenly or gradually, and its cause may be difficult to ascertain initially. The pain can radiate to the arms, neck, jaw, or back. It can be steady or intermittent, mild or acute. It can range in character from a sharp shooting sensation to a feeling of heaviness, fullness, or even indigestion. It can be provoked or aggravated by stress, anxiety, exertion, deep breathing, or eating certain foods.

History

If the patient's chest pain isn't severe, proceed with the health history. Ask if the patient feels diffuse pain or can point to the painful area.

Sometimes a patient won't perceive the sensation he's feeling as pain, so ask whether he has any discomfort radiating to the neck, jaw, arms, or back. If he does, ask him to describe it, such as dull, aching, or pressure-like sensation; or a sharp, stabbing, knifelike pain. Find out if he feels it on the surface or deep inside.

Next, find out whether the pain is constant or intermittent. If it's intermittent, ask him how long it lasts. Ask if movement, exertion, breathing, position changes, or the eating of certain foods worsens or helps relieve the pain. Find out what in particular seems to bring on the pain.

Review the patient's history for cardiac or pulmonary disease, chest trauma, intestinal disease, or sickle cell anemia. Find out what medication he's taking, if any, and ask about recent dosage or schedule changes.

Physical assessment
When taking the patient's vital signs, note the presence of tachycardia, paradoxical pulse, and hypertension or hypotension. Also look for jugular vein distention and peripheral edema. Observe the patient's breathing pattern, and inspect his chest for asymmetrical expansion. Auscultate his lungs for pleural friction rub, crackles, rhonchi, wheezing, or diminished or absent breath sounds. Next, auscultate for murmurs, clicks, gallops, or pericardial friction rub. Palpate for lifts, heaves, thrills, gallops, tactile fremitus, and abdominal mass or tenderness.

Analysis
Chest pain usually results from disorders that affect thoracic or abdominal organs, such as the heart, pleurae, lungs, esophagus, rib cage, gallbladder, pancreas, or stomach. An important indicator of several acute and life-threatening cardiopulmonary and GI disorders, chest pain can also result from musculoskeletal and hematologic disorders, anxiety, and drug therapy.

Keep in mind that cardiac-related pain may not always occur in the chest. Pain originating in the heart is transmitted through the thoracic region via the upper five thoracic region via the upper five thoracic spinal cord segments. Thus, it maybe referred to areas served by the cervical or lower thoracic segments, such as the neck and arms. Upper thoracic segments innervated skin as well as skeletal muscles, making the origin of the pain hard to determine.

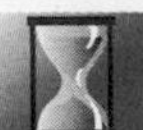

AGE ISSUE *Even children old enough to talk may have difficulty describing chest pain. Observe nonverbal clues, such as restlessness, facial grimaces, or holding of the painful area. Ask the child to point to the painful area and then to where the pain goes (to find out if it's radiating). Determine the pain's severity by asking the parents if the pain interferes with the child's normal activities and behavior. Elderly patients may have a higher risk of developing life-threatening conditions, such as a myocardial infarction (MI), angina, and aortic dissection. Carefully evaluate chest pain in this population.*

Fatigue
Fatigue is a feeling of excessive tiredness, lack of energy, or exhaustion, accompanied by a strong desire to rest or sleep. This common symptom is distinct from weakness, which involves the muscles, but may occur with it.

History
Obtain a history to identify the patient's fatigue pattern. Ask about related symptoms and any recent viral illness or stressful changes in lifestyle.

Explore nutritional habits and appetite or weight changes. Carefully review the patient's medical and psychiatric history for chronic disorders that commonly produce fatigue. Ask about a family history of such disorders.

Physical assessment
Observe the patient's general appearance for overt signs of depression or organic illness. Is he unkempt or expressionless? Does he appear tired or sickly, or have a slumped posture? If warranted, evaluate his mental status, noting especially mental clouding, attention deficits, agitation, or psychomotor retardation.

Analysis
Fatigue that worsens with activity and improves with rest generally indicates a physical disorder; the opposite pattern, a psychological disorder. Fatigue lasting longer than 4 months, constant fatigue that's unrelieved by rest, and transient exhaustion that quickly gives way to bursts of energy are other

findings associated with psychological disorders.

Fatigue is a normal and important response to physical overexertion, prolonged emotional stress, and sleep deprivation. However, it can also be a nonspecific symptoms of a psychological or physiologic disorder, especially viral infection and endocrine, cardiovascular, or neurologic disease.

Fatigue reflects hypermetabolic and hypometabolic states in which nutrients needed for cellular energy and growth are lacking because of overly rapid depletion, impaired replacement mechanisms, insufficient hormone production, or inadequate nutrient intake or metabolism. Cardiac causes include heart failure, MI, and valvular heart disease.

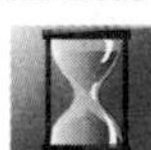

AGE ISSUE *When evaluating a child for fatigue, ask his parents if they've noticed any change in his activity level. Fatigue without an organic cause occurs normally during accelerated growth phases in preschool age and prepubescent children. However, psychological causes of fatigue must be considered—for example, a depressed child may try to escape problems at home or school by taking refuge in sleep. In the pubescent child, consider the possibility of drug abuse, particularly of hypnotics and tranquilizers. Always ask elderly patients about fatigue because this symptom may be insidious and mask more serious underlying conditions in this age-group.*

Gallop, atrial

An atrial or presystolic gallop is an extra heart sound (known as S_4) that's heard or often palpated immediately before S_1, late in diastole. This low-pitched sound is heard best with the bell of the stethoscope pressed lightly against the cardiac apex. Some clinicians say that an S_4 has the cadence of the "Ten" in Tennessee (Ten = S_4; nes = S_1; see = S_4).

History

When the patient's condition permits, ask about a history of hypertension, angina, valvular stenosis, or cardiomyopathy. If appropriate, have him describe the frequency and severity of anginal attacks.

Physical assessment

Carefully auscultate the chest for S_4. Use the bell of the stethoscope. Note any murmurs or abnormalities in the first and second heart sounds. Then listen for pulmonary crackles. Next, assess peripheral pulses, noting an alternating strong and weak pulse. Finally, palpate the liver to detect enlargement or tenderness, and assess for jugular vein distention and peripheral edema.

Analysis

S_4 gallop typically results from hypertension, conduction defects, valvular disorders, or other problems such as ischemia. Occasionally, it helps differentiate angina from other causes of chest pain. It results from abnormal forceful atrial contraction caused by augmented ventricular filling or by decreased left ventricular compliance. An atrial gallop usually originates from left atrial contraction, is heard at the apex, and doesn't vary with inspiration. A left-sided S_4 can occur in hypertensive heart disease, coronary artery disease, aortic stenosis, and cardiomyopathy. It may also originate from right atrial contraction. A right-sided S_4 is indicative of pulmonary hypertension and pulmonary stenosis. If so, it's heard best at the lower left sternal border and intensifies with inspiration.

An atrial gallop seldom occurs in normal hearts; however, it may occur in athletes with physiologic hypertrophy of the left ventricle.

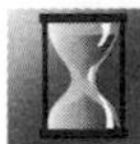

AGE ISSUE *In children, an atrial gallop may occur normally, especially after exercise. However, it may also result from congenital heart diseases, such as atrial septal defect, ventricular septal defect, patent ductus arteriosus, and severe pulmonary valvular stenosis.*

Because the absolute intensity of an atrial gallop doesn't decrease with age, as it does with an S_1, the relative intensity of S_4 increases compared with S_1. This explains the increased frequency of an audible S_4 in elderly patients and why this sound may be considered a normal finding in older patients.

Gallop, ventricular

A ventricular gallop is a heart sound known as S_3, associated with rapid ventricular filling in early diastole. Usually palpable, this low-frequency sound occurs about 0.15 second after S_2. It may originate in either the left or right ventricle. A right-sided gallop usually sounds louder on inspiration and is heard best along the lower left sternal border or over the xiphoid region. A left-sided gallop usually sounds louder on expiration and is heard best at the apex.

History

Focus the history on the cardiovascular system. Begin the history by asking the patient if he has had any chest pain. If so, have him describe its character, location, frequency, duration, and any alleviating or aggravating factors. Also ask about palpitations, dizziness, or syncope. Find out if the patient has difficulty breathing after exertion, while lying down, or at rest. Ask the patient if he has a cough. Also ask about a history of cardiac disorders. Find out if the patient is currently receiving any treatment for heart failure. If so, find out which medications he's taking.

Physical assessment

During the physical examination, carefully auscultate for murmurs or abnormalities in S_1 and S_2. Then listen for pulmonary crackles. Next, assess peripheral pulses, noting an alternating strong and weak pulse. Finally, palpate the liver to detect enlargement or tenderness, and assess for jugular vein distention and peripheral edema.

Analysis

Ventricular gallops are easily overlooked because they're usually faint. Fortunately, certain techniques make their detection more likely. These include auscultating in a quiet environment; examining the patient in the supine, left lateral, and semi-Fowler's positions; and having the patient cough or raise his legs to augment the sound.

AGE ISSUE *A physiologic ventricular gallop normally occurs in children and adults younger than age 40; however, most people lose this S_3 by age 40. This gallop may also occur during the third trimester of pregnancy. Abnormal S_3 (in adults older than age 40) can be a sign of decreased myocardial contractility, myocardial failure, and volume overload of the ventricle, as in mitral and tricuspid valve regurgitation.*

Although the physiologic S_3 has the same timing as the pathologic S_3, its intensity waxes and wanes with respiration. It's also heard more faintly if the patient is sitting or standing.

A pathologic ventricular gallop may be one of the earliest signs of ventricular failure. It may result from one of two mechanisms: rapid deceleration of blood entering a stiff, noncompliant ventricle, or rapid acceleration of blood associated with in creased flow into the ventricle. A gallop that persists despite therapy indicates a poor prognosis.

Patients with cardiomyopathy or heart failure may develop both a ventricular gallop and an atrial gallop—a condition known as a summation gallop.

Intermittent claudication

Typically occurring in the legs, intermittent claudication is cramping limb pain brought on by exercise and relieved by 1 to 2 minutes of rest. This pain may be acute or chronic. Without treatment, it may progress to pain at rest.

History

If the patient has chronic intermittent claudication, gather history data first. Ask how far he can walk before pain occurs and how long he must rest before it subsides. Find out if he can walk less further now than before, or if he needs to rest longer. Next, ask if the pain-rest pattern varies and if this symptom has affected his lifestyle.

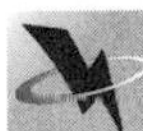

CRITICAL POINT *If the patient has sudden intermittent claudication with severe or aching leg pain at rest, check the leg's temperature and color and palpate femoral, popliteal, posterior tibial, and dorsalis pedis pulses. Ask about numbness and tingling. Suspect acute arterial occlusion if pulses are absent; if the leg feels cold and looks pale, cyanotic, or mottled; and if paresthesia and pain are present. Mark the area of pallor, cyanosis, or mottling, and reassess it frequently, noting an increase in the area.*

Obtain a history of risk factors for atherosclerosis, such as smoking, diabetes, hypertension, and hyperlipidemia. Next, ask about associated signs and symptoms, such as paresthesia in the affected limb and visible changes in the color of the fingers (white to blue to pink) when he's smoking, exposed to cold, or under stress. If the patient is male, ask if he experiences impotence.

Physical assessment

Focus the physical examination on the cardiovascular system. Palpate for femoral, popliteal, dorsalis pedis, and posterior tibial pulses. Note character, amplitude, and bilateral equality. Note any diminished or absent popliteal and pedal pulses with the femoral pulse present.

Listen for bruits over the major arteries. Note color and temperature differences between his legs or compared with his arms; also note where on his leg the changes in temperature and color occur. Elevate the affected leg for 2 minutes; if it becomes pale or white, blood flow is severely decreased. When the leg hangs down, how long does it take for color to return? (Thirty seconds or longer indicates severe disease.) If possible, check the patient's deep tendon reflexes after exercise; note if they're diminished in his lower extremities.

Examine his feet, toes, and fingers for ulceration, and inspect his hands and lower legs for small, tender nodules and erythema along blood vessels. Note the quality of his nails and the amount of hair on his fingers and toes. Physical findings include pallor on elevation, rubor on dependency (especially the toes and soles), loss of hair on the toes, and diminished arterial pulses.

If the patient has arm pain, inspect his arms for a change in color (to white) on elevation. Next, palpate for changes in temperature, muscle wasting, and a pulsating mass in the subclavian area. Palpate and compare the radial, ulnar, brachial, axillary, and subclavian pulses to identify obstructed areas.

Analysis

When acute, this pain may signal acute arterial occlusion. Intermittent claudication is most common in men ages 50 to 60 with a history of diabetes mellitus, hyperlipidemia, hypertension, or tobacco use. With chronic arterial occlusion, limb loss is uncommon because collateral circulation usually develops.

With occlusive artery disease, intermittent claudication results from an inadequate blood supply. Pain in the calf (the most common area) or foot indicates disease of the femoral or popliteal arteries; pain in the buttocks and upper thigh, disease of the aortoiliac arteries. During exercise, the pain typically results from the release of lactic acid due to anaerobic metabolism in the ischemic segment, secondary to obstruction. When exercise stops, the lactic acid clears and the pain subsides. Diminished femoral and distal pulses may indicate disease of the terminal aorta or iliac branches. Absent pedal and popliteal pulses with normal femoral pulses may suggest atherosclerotic disease of the femoral artery. Absent pedal pulses with normal femoral and popliteal pulses may indicate Buerger's disease.

Intermittent claudication may also have neurologic cause: narrowing of the vertebral column at the level of the cauda equina. This condition creates pressure on the nerve roots to the lower extremities. Walking stimulates circulation to the cauda equina, causing increased pressure on those nerves and resultant pain.

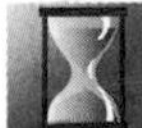

AGE ISSUE *In children, intermittent claudication rarely occurs. Although it sometimes develops in patients with coarctation of aorta, extensive compensatory collateral circulation typically prevents manifestation of this sign. Muscle cramps from exercise and growing pains may be mistaken for intermittent claudication in children.*

Jugular vein distention

Jugular vein distention is the abnormal fullness and height of the pulse waves in the internal or external jugular veins. For a patient in a supine position with his head elevated 45 degrees, a pulse wave height greater than 1¼″ to 1½″ (3 to 4 cm) above the angle of Louis indicates distention.

History

If the patient isn't in severe distress, obtain a personal history. Find out if he has recently gained weight, has difficulty putting on his shoes, and if his ankles are swollen. Ask about chest pain, shortness of breath, paroxysmal nocturnal dyspnea, anorexia, nausea or vomiting, and a history of cancer or cardiac, pulmonary, hepatic, or renal disease. Obtain a drug history noting diuretic use and dosage. Find out if the patient is taking drugs as prescribed. Ask the patient about his regular diet patterns, noting a high sodium intake.

Physical assessment
Next, perform a physical examination, beginning with vital signs. Tachycardia, tachypnea, and increased blood pressure indicate fluid overload that's stressing the heart. Inspect and palpate the patient's extremities and face for edema. Then weigh the patient and compare that weight to his baseline.

Auscultate his lungs for crackles and his heart for gallops, a pericardial friction rub, and muffled heart sounds. Inspect his abdomen for distention, and palpate and percuss for an enlarged liver. Finally, monitor urine output and note any decrease.

Analysis
Engorged, distended veins reflect increased venous pressure in the right side of the heart, which in turn, indicates an increased central venous pressure. This common sign characteristically occurs in heart failure and other cardiovascular disorders, such as constrictive pericarditis, tricuspid stenosis, and obstruction of the superior vena cava.

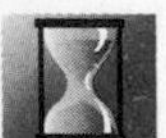

AGE ISSUE *In most infants and toddlers, jugular vein distention is difficult (sometimes impossible) to evaluate because of their short, thick necks. Even in school-age children, measurement of jugular vein distention can be unreliable because the sternal angle may not be the same distance (2" to 2¾" [5 to 7 cm] above) the right atrium as it is in adults.*

Palpitations
Defined as a conscious awareness of one's heartbeat, palpitations are usually felt over the precordium or in the throat or neck. The patient may describe them as pounding, jumping, turning, fluttering, or flopping, or as missing or skipping beats. Palpitations may be regular or irregular, fast or slow, paroxysmal or sustained.

History
If the patient isn't in distress, obtain a complete cardiac history. Ask about cardiovascular or pulmonary disorders, which may produce arrhythmias. Find out if the patient as a history of hypertension or hypoglycemia.

Obtain a drug history. Ask the patient if he has recently started cardiac glycoside therapy. In addition, ask about caffeine, tobacco, and alcohol consumption. Ask about associated symptoms, such as weakness, fatigue, and angina.

To help characterize the palpitations, ask the patient to simulate their rhythm by tapping his finger on a hard surface. An irregular "skipped beat" rhythm points to premature ventricular contractions, whereas an episodic racing rhythm that ends abruptly suggests paroxysmal atrial tachycardia.

Physical assessment
If the patient isn't in distress, perform a complete physical assessment of the cardiovascular system. Auscultate for gallops, murmurs, and abnormal breath sounds.

Analysis
Although frequently insignificant, palpitations are a common chief complaint that may result from a cardiac or metabolic disorder or from the adverse effects of certain drugs. Nonpathologic palpitations may occur with a newly implanted prosthetic valve because the valve's clicking sound heightens the patient's awareness of his heartbeat. Transient palpitations may accompany emotional stress, such as fright, anger, and anxiety, or physical stress, such as exercise and fever. They can also accompany the use of stimulants, such as tobacco and caffeine.

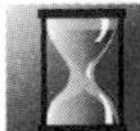

AGE ISSUE *In children, palpitations commonly result from fever and congenital heart defects, such as patent ductus arteriosus and septal defects. Because many children have difficulty describing this symptom, focus your attention on objective measurements, such as cardiac monitoring, physical examination, and laboratory test results.*

Peripheral edema
The result of excess interstitial fluid in the arms or legs, peripheral edema may be unilateral or bilateral, slight or dramatic, or pitting or nonpitting.

History
Begin by asking how long the patient has had the edema and if it developed suddenly or gradually. Find out if the edema decreases if the patient elevates his arms or legs, if it's worse in the mornings, and if it gets progressively worse during the day.

Find out if the patient recently injured the affected extremities or had surgery or an illness that may have immobilized him. Ask about a history of cardiovascular disease. Find out what medication he's taking and which drugs he has taken in the past.

Physical assessment

Begin the assessment by examining each extremity for pitting edema. In pitting edema, pressure forces fluid into the underlying tissues, causing an indentation that slowly fills. In nonpitting edema, pressure leaves no indentation in the skin, but the skin may feel unusually firm. Because edema may compromise arterial blood flow, palpate peripheral pulses to detect insufficiency. Observe the color of the extremity and look for unusual vein patterns. Then palpate for warmth, tenderness, and cords and gently squeeze the muscle against the bone to check for deep pain. Finally, note any skin thickening or ulceration in the edematous areas.

Analysis

Peripheral edema signals a localized fluid imbalance between the vascular and interstitial spaces. It may result from trauma, a venous disorder, or a bone or cardiac disorder.

Cardiovascular causes of arm edema are superior vena cava syndrome, which leads to slowly progressing arm edema accompanied by facial and neck edema with dilated veins marking these edematous areas, and thrombophlebitis, which may cause arm edema, pain, and warmth.

Leg edema is an early sign of right-sided heart failure. It can also signal thrombophlebitis and chronic venous insufficiency.

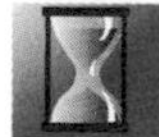

AGE ISSUE *Uncommon in children, arm edema can result from trauma. Leg edema, also uncommon, can result from osteomyelitis, leg trauma or, rarely, heart failure.*

Pulse, absent or weak

An absent or weak pulse may be generalized or affect only one extremity.

History

When time allows, obtain a complete cardiovascular history from the patient. Note any history of trauma MI, heart failure, recent cardiac surgery, infection, venous problems, or allergy.

CRITICAL POINT *If you detect an absent or weak pulse, quickly palpate the remaining arterial pulses to distinguish between localized or generalized loss or weakness. Then quickly check other vital signs, evaluate cardiopulmonary status, and obtain a brief history and intervene accordingly.*

Physical assessment

Carefully check the rate, amplitude, and symmetry of all pulses. Note any confusion or restless, hypotension, and cool pale clammy skin.

Analysis

When generalized, absent or weak pulse is an important indicator of such life-threatening conditions as shock and arrhythmia. Localized loss or weakness of a pulse that's normally present and strong may indicate acute arterial occlusion, which could require emergency surgery. However, the pressure of palpation may temporarily diminish or obliterate superficial pulses, such as the posterior tibial or the dorsal pedal. Thus, bilateral weakness or absence of these pulses doesn't necessarily indicate an underlying disorder.

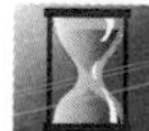

AGE ISSUE *In infants and small children, radial, dorsal pedal, and posterior tibial pulses aren't easily palpable, so be careful not to mistake these normally hard-to-find pulses for weak or absent pulses. Instead, palpate the brachial, popliteal, or femoral pulses to evaluate arterial circulation to the extremities. In children and young adults, weak or absent femoral and more distal pulses may indicate coarctation of the aorta.*

Breasts and axillae

With breast cancer becoming increasingly prevalent, more women are aware of the disease, along with its risk factors, treatments, and diagnostic measures. By staying informed and performing monthly breast self-examinations, women can take control of their health and seek medical care when they notice a change in their breasts. Additionally, it's important to assess your male patients as breast cancer can occur occasionally in this population, with signs and symptoms mimicking those found in women.

Yet, no matter how informed a woman is, she can still feel anxious during clinical breast examinations, even if she hasn't noticed any changes or problems. That's because the social and psychological significance of the female breasts go far beyond their biological function. The breast is more than just a delicate structure; it's a delicate subject. During the assessment, provide privacy and proceed carefully and professionally, helping your patient feel more at ease.

Breast anatomy

Knowledge of the basic anatomy of the breasts and axillae will help guide your assessment and give you clues to recognizing any abnormalities. The breasts, also called mammary glands in women, lie on the anterior chest wall. (See *Structures of the female breast.*)

They're located vertically between the second or third and the sixth or seventh ribs over the pectoralis major muscle and the serratus anterior muscle, and horizontally

STRUCTURES OF THE FEMALE BREAST

This illustration shows a lateral cross section of the female breast.

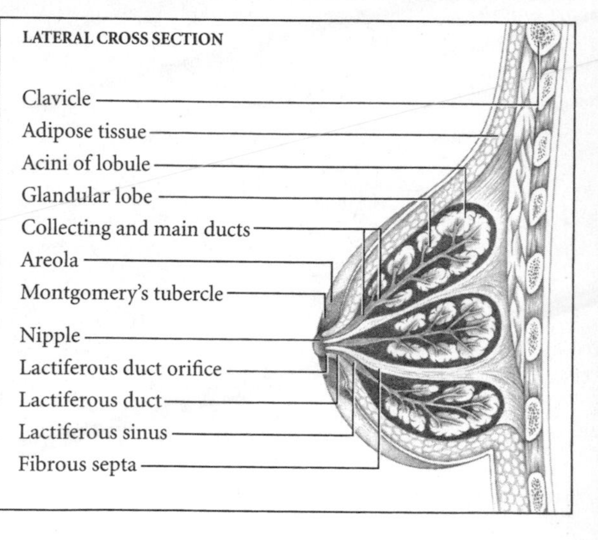

between the sternal border and the midaxillary line.

Each breast has a centrally located nipple of pigmented erectile tissue ringed by an areola that's darker than the adjacent tissue.

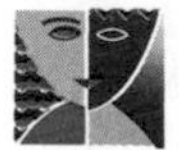

CULTURAL INSIGHT *Among different races, the pigment of the nipple and areola vary, becoming darker as skin tone darkens. Whites have light-colored nipples and areolae, usually pink or light beige. People with darker complexions, such as Blacks and Asians, have medium brown to almost black nipples and areolae.*

Sebaceous glands, also called Montgomery's tubercles, are scattered on the areola surface, along with hair follicles.

Support structures

Beneath the skin are glandular, fibrous, and fatty tissues that vary in proportion with age, weight, sex, and other factors such as pregnancy. A small triangle of tissue, called the tail of Spence, projects into the axilla. Attached to the chest-wall musculature are fibrous bands called Cooper's ligaments that support each breast.

Lobes and ducts

In women, each breast is surrounded by 12 to 25 glandular lobes containing alveoli that produce milk. The lactiferous ducts from each lobe transport milk to the nipple. In men, the breast has a nipple, an areola, and mostly flat tissue bordering the chest wall.

Lymph node chains

The breasts also hold several lymph node chains, each serving different areas. The pectoral lymph nodes drain lymph fluid from most of the breast and anterior chest. The brachial nodes drain most of the arm. The subscapular nodes drain the posterior chest wall and part of the arm. The midaxillary nodes, located near the ribs and the serratus anterior muscle high in the axilla, are the central draining nodes for the pectoral, brachial, and subscapular nodes.

In women, the internal mammary nodes drain the mammary lobes. The superficial lymphatic vessels drain the skin. In both men and women, the lymphatic system is the most common route for cancer cells to spread. (See *Lymph node chains,* page 256.)

LYMPH NODE CHAINS

This illustration shows the different lymph node chains in the breast, axilla, and upper arm.

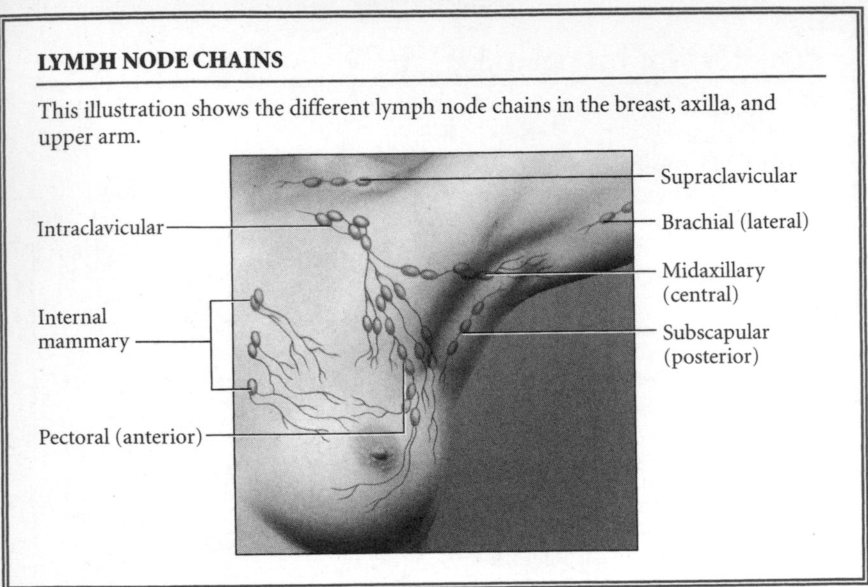

Breast physiology

A basic function of the female breast is to secrete milk that's used to nourish infants. However, a woman's breasts make many transformations throughout the life cycle. Their appearance starts changing at puberty and continues changing during the reproductive years, pregnancy, and menopause. (See *Breast changes through the life span.*)

Puberty

Breast development is an early sign of puberty in girls. It usually occurs between ages 8 and 13. *Menarche,* the start of the menstrual cycle, typically occurs about 2 years later. Development of breast tissue in girls younger than age 8 is abnormal, and the patient should be referred to a health care provider.

Breast development usually starts with the breast and nipple protruding as a single mound of flesh. The shape of the adult female breast is formed gradually. During puberty, breast development is commonly unilateral or asymmetrical.

Reproductive years

During the reproductive years, a woman's breasts may become full or tender in response to hormonal fluctuations during the menstrual cycle. During pregnancy, breast changes occur in response to hormones from the corpus luteum and the placenta.

The areola becomes deeply pigmented and increases in diameter. The nipple becomes darker, more prominent, and erect. The breasts enlarge due to the proliferation and hypertrophy of the alveolar cells and lactiferous ducts. As veins engorge, a venous pattern may become visible. Also, striae may appear as a result of stretching, and Montgomery's tubercles may become prominent.

Postmenopause

After menopause, estrogen levels decrease, causing glandular tissue to atrophy and be replaced with fatty deposits. The breasts become flabbier and smaller than they were before menopause. As the ligaments relax, the breasts hang loosely from the chest. The nipples flatten, losing some of their erectile quality. The ducts around the nipples may feel like firm strings.

Health history

In the assessment interview, establish a rapport with the patient by explaining what

BREAST CHANGES THROUGH THE LIFE SPAN

These illustrations show how a woman's breasts typically change from prepuberty through menopause.

BEFORE AGE 10

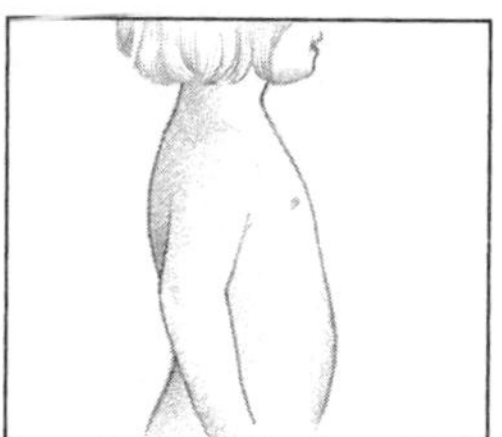

BETWEEN AGES 10 AND 14

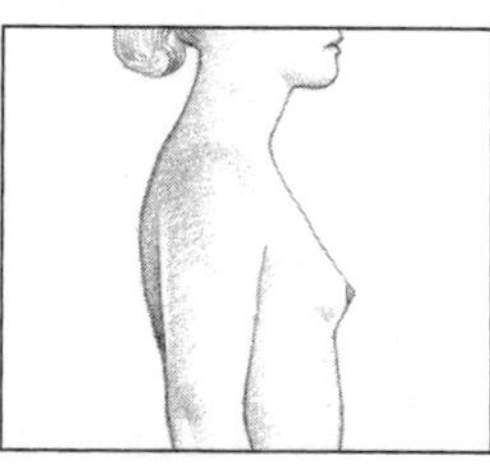

DURING ADULTHOOD (HAVING NEVER GIVEN BIRTH)

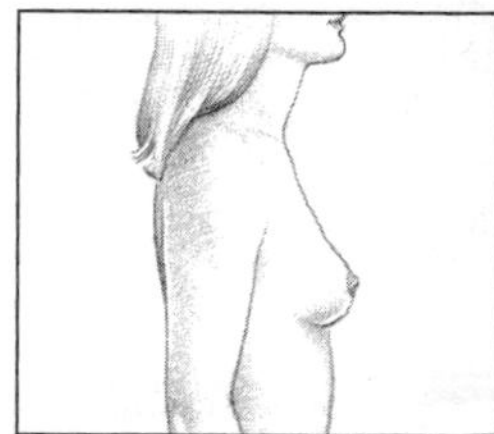

DURING PREGNANCY

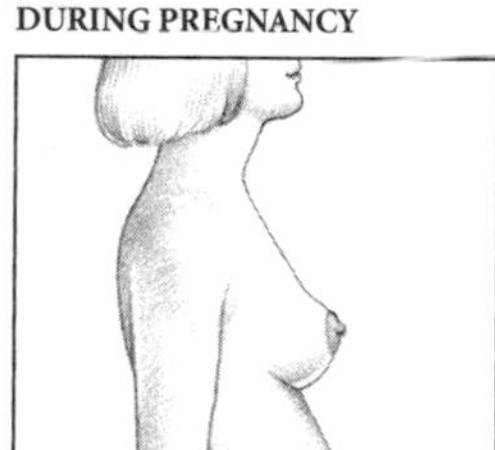

AFTER PREGNANCY

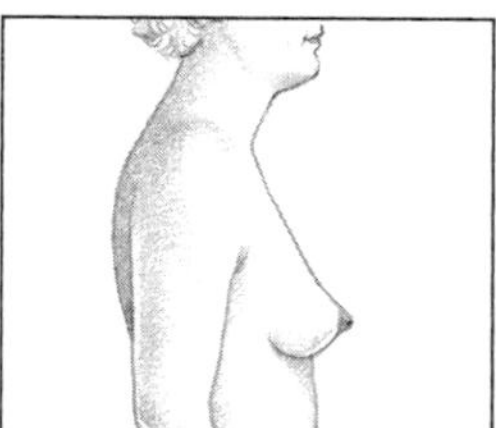

AFTER MENOPAUSE

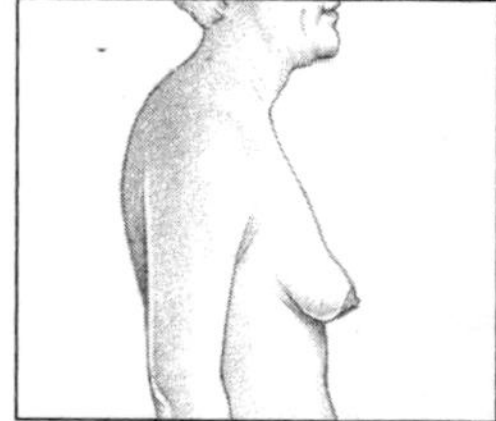

will be happening during the breast examination. The quantity and quality of the information gathered depends on your relationship with the patient. Gain the patient's trust by being sensitive to concerns and feelings. Also ask about other aspects of current health and the patient's health and family history.

Chief complaint

Common complaints about the breasts include breast pain, breast tenderness, nipple discharge and rash, nodules, masses, and other changes. Complaints such as these—whether they come from women or men—warrant further investigation.

To investigate breast complaints, ask about onset, duration, and severity. For women, find out what day of the menstrual cycle the signs or symptoms appear. Ask the patient what relieves or worsens the signs and symptoms.

Breast pain, also known as *mastalgia,* commonly results from benign breast disease. It may occur during rest or movement and may be aggravated by manipulation or palpation. It may be an indicator of breast cancer, although an unreliable one. Breast pain may be superficial, resulting from surface cuts, furuncles, contusions, and similar lesions; severe and localized, such as from nipple fissures and inflammation in the papillary ducts and areolae; tender, due to stromal distention in the breast parenchyma; or severe and constant, such as from a tumor that affects nerve endings or from inflammatory lesions that not only distend the stroma, but also irritate sensory nerve endings. In some cases, the pain may also radiate to the back, arms, and neck.

Breast tenderness refers to pain elicited by physical contact. If your patient has breast pain, ascertain whether it's unilateral or bilateral; cyclic, intermittent, or constant; and dull or sharp. In women, breast tenderness may occur before menstruation and during pregnancy. Before menstruation, breast pain or tenderness stems from increased mammary blood flow due to hormonal changes. During pregnancy, breast tenderness and throbbing, tingling, or prickling sensations may occur, also from hormonal changes. In postmenopausal women, breast pain secondary to benign breast disease is rare.

In men, breast pain may stem from gynecomastia (especially during puberty and senescence), reproductive tract anomalies, and organic disease of the liver or of the pituitary, adrenal cortex, and thyroid glands. In adolescent males, transient gynecomastia can cause breast pain during puberty.

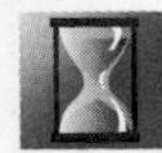

AGE ISSUE *Elderly patients may fail to report breast pain because of decreased pain perception and cognitive function. Be aware that breast pain can also be caused by trauma from falls or physical abuse.*

Breast nodules are a commonly reported gynecologic complaint that has two primary causes: benign breast disease and cancer. Benign breast disease, the leading cause of nodules, can stem from cyst formation in obstructed and dilated lactiferous ducts, hypertrophy or tumor formation in the ductal system, and inflammation or infection.

Although fewer than 20% of breast nodules are malignant, the signs of breast cancer aren't easily distinguished from those of benign breast disease. Breast cancer is a leading cause of death among women but can occur occasionally in men, with the same signs and symptoms as those found in women. Thus, make sure to always evaluate breast nodules in both sexes.

If your patient reports a breast nodule, or lump, it may be found in any part of the breast, including in the axilla. A woman familiar with the feel of her breasts and who performs monthly breast self-examinations can detect a nodule that's 5 mm or less in size — considerably smaller than the 1-cm nodule that's readily detectable by an experienced examiner. However, a woman may fail to report a nodule for fear of breast cancer. (See *Evaluating breast lumps*.)

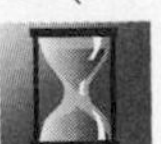

AGE ISSUE *In children and adolescent patients, most nodules reflect the normal response of breast tissue to hormonal fluctuations. For instance, the breasts of young teenage girls may normally contain cordlike nodules that become tender just before menstruation. In young boys — as well as women between ages 20 and 30 — a transient breast nodule may result from juvenile mastitis, which usually affects one breast. Signs of inflammation are present in a firm mass beneath the nipple.*

Current health history

Because certain breast changes are a normal part of aging in women, ask the patient how old she is. Ask her if she has noticed breast changes and, if so, to describe them in detail. Find out when the changes occurred. Then ask if she has breast pain, tenderness, discharge, or rash, and if she has noticed changes or problems in her underarm area.

Ask the patient which medications she takes regularly — birth control pills with estrogen, for instance. Also, ask about other hormonal methods of birth control, such as contraceptive patches or vaginal rings. Ask about her diet, especially caffeine use. Hormonal contraceptives can cause breast swelling and tenderness, and ingestion of caffeine has been linked to fibrocystic disease of the breasts.

Ask the patient if she eats a high-fat diet, is under a lot of stress, and if she smokes or drinks alcohol. Discuss the possible link between those risk factors and breast cancer.

Past health history

Ask the patient if she has ever had breast lumps, a breast biopsy, or breast surgery, including an enlargement or a reduction. If she has had breast cancer, fibroadenoma, or fibrocystic disease, ask for more information, such as when it occurred and any treatments she had.

Next, inquire about her menstrual cycle, and record the date of her last menstrual period. If the patient has been pregnant, ask about the number of pregnancies and live births that she has had. Find out how old she was each time she became pregnant, if she had complications, and if she breast-fed.

Family history

Ask the patient if any family members have had breast disorders, especially breast cancer. Also, ask about the incidence of other types of cancer. Having a close relative with breast cancer greatly increases the patient's risk of having the disease. Teach the patient how to examine her breasts and about the importance of regular clinical breast exami-

EVALUATING BREAST LUMPS

If you detect a breast lump during your assessment, evaluate it using this flowchart. Masses may be further investigated with a biopsy.

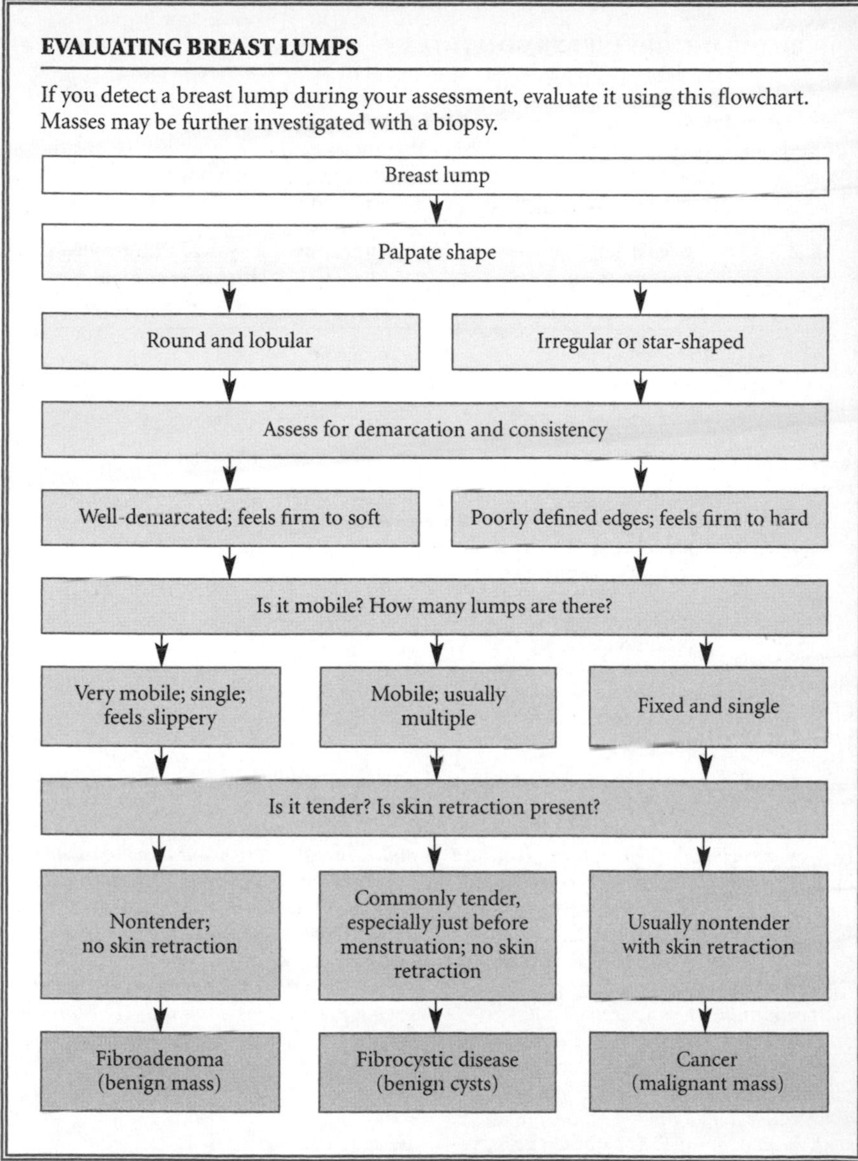

nations and mammograms. (See *Scheduling breast examinations,* page 260.)

Psychosocial history

Ask the patient about psychosocial factors as well. Ask her if she smokes, drinks alcohol, or uses any drugs. Find out what kind of support system she has, such as family and friends. Also, find out if she has young children or older adults to care for. Determine any psychosocial concerns she has and address them as needed.

Physical assessment

Breast examinations can be stressful for the female patient. To reduce the patient's anxi-

SCHEDULING BREAST EXAMINATIONS

The American Cancer Society and the American College of Radiology recommend the schedule shown below for regular breast examinations. Depending on their needs, some patients may follow a schedule that their health care provider has modified. Annual mammograms should be performed earlier for women with a family history of breast cancer or those with a genetic predisposition.

Age	Breast self-examination	Mammography	Physical examination (includes clinical breast examination)
20 to 34	Monthly, 7 to 10 days after menses begins	Not recommended	Every 3 years
35 to 39	Monthly, 7 to 10 days after menses begins	One baseline mammogram within this time span	Every 3 years
40 and older	Monthly, 7 to 10 days after menses begins (Postmenopausal women should examine their breasts on the same date each month. Have them pick a date that is significant to them so they'll remember.)	Yearly	Yearly

ety, provide privacy, take measures to ensure comfort, and explain what the examination involves.

CRITICAL POINT *Because the incidence of breast cancer in men is rising, it's important to perform breast examinations in your male patients. Men with breast disorders may feel uneasy or embarrassed about being examined because they see their condition as being unmanly. Remember that a man needs a gentle, professional manner as much as a woman does.*

Be sure to examine a man's breasts thoroughly during a complete physical assessment. Don't overlook palpation of the nipple and areola in male patients; assess for the same changes you would in a female. Breast cancer in men usually occurs in the areolar area.

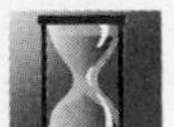

AGE ISSUE *Adolescent boys may have temporary stimulation of breast tissue due to the hormone estrogen, which is produced in males and females. Breast enlargement in boys usually stops when they begin producing adequate amounts of the male sex hormone testosterone. Older men may have gynecomastia, or breast enlargement, due to age-related hormonal alterations or as an adverse effect of certain medications. It may also be caused by cirrhosis, leukemia, thyrotoxicosis, the administration of a hormone, or a hormonal imbalance.*

Breast examination

Before examining the breasts, make sure the room is well-lit. Have the patient disrobe from the waist up and sit with her arms at her sides. Keep both breasts uncovered so you can observe them simultaneously to detect differences. Examine both breasts with the patient in supine, sitting, and forward-leaning positions.

Inspection

Observe the breast skin; it should be smooth, undimpled, and the same color as the rest of the patient's skin. Check for edema, which can accompany lymphatic obstruction and may signal cancer. Note breast size and symmetry. Asymmetry may occur normally in some adult women, with the left breast usually larger than the right.

Next, inspect the patient's breasts while she holds her arms over her head and then while she has her hands on her hips. Having the patient assume these positions will help to detect skin or nipple dimpling that might not have been obvious before.

If the patient has large or pendulous breasts, have her stand with her hands on the back of a chair and lean forward. This position helps reveal subtle breast or nipple asymmetry.

If the patient has a dimpled area on her breast, carefully inspect the area. Note if it's swollen, red, or warm to the touch. Look for any bruises or contusions. Ask the patient to tense her pectoral muscles by pressing her hips with both hands or by raising her hands over her head and note any increase in puckering. Gently pull the skin upward toward the clavicle to see if dimpling is exaggerated.

Observe if the skin moves freely over both breasts. If you can see a lump, describe its size, location, consistency, mobility, and delineation. Note what relation the lump has to breast dimpling. Gently mold the breast skin around the lump and observe if the dimpling is exaggerated. Also, examine breast and axillary lymph nodes, noting any enlargement.

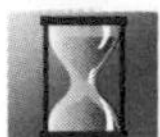

AGE ISSUE *Dimpling usually affects women older than age 40 but also occurs occasionally in men.* *(See* Dimpling and peau d'orange.*)*

Observe the breast for nipple retraction, the inward displacement of the nipple below the level of surrounding breast tissue.

CRITICAL POINT *Nipple retraction can easily be confused with nipple inversion, a common abnormality that's congenital in some patients and doesn't usually signal underlying disease. A retracted nipple appears flat and broad, whereas an inverted nipple can be pulled out from the sulcus where it hides.*

DIMPLING AND PEAU D'ORANGE

These illustrations show two abnormalities in breast tissue: dimpling and peau d'orange.

Dimpling

Dimpling usually suggests an inflammatory or malignant mass beneath the skin's surface. The illustration below shows breast dimpling and nipple inversion caused by a malignant mass above the areola.

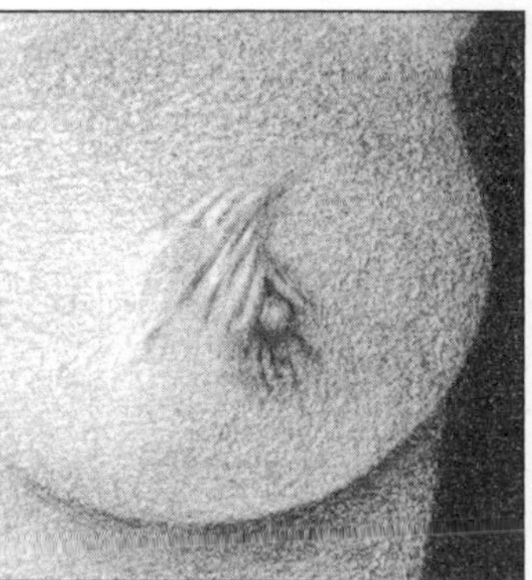

Peau d'orange

Peau d'orange, as shown below, is usually a late sign of breast cancer, but it can also occur with breast or axillary lymph node infection. The skin's orange-peel appearance comes from lymphatic edema around deepened hair follicles.

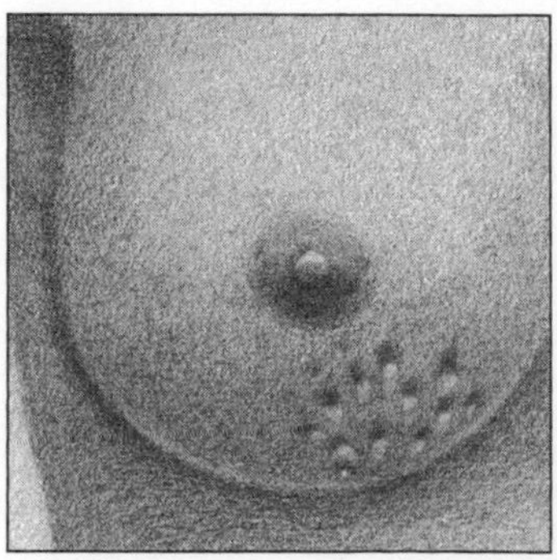

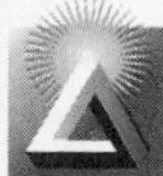

EXPERT TECHNIQUE

PALPATING THE BREASTS

Performing breast palpation
Use your three middle fingers to palpate the patient's breasts systematically. Rotating your fingers gently against the chest wall, move in concentric circles. Make sure you include the tail of Spence in your examination.

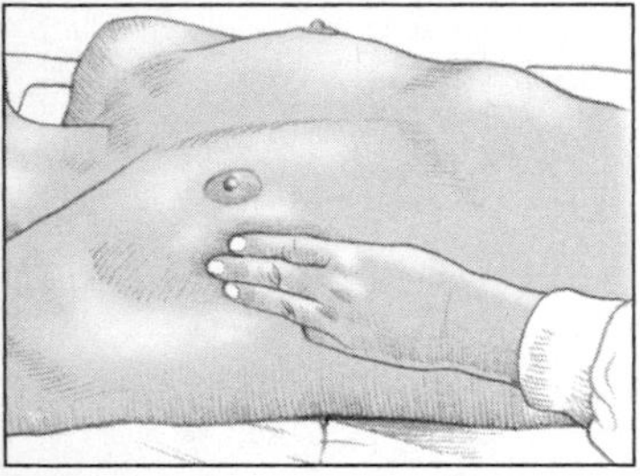

Examining the areola and nipple
After palpating the breasts, palpate the areola and nipple. Gently squeeze the nipple between your thumb and index finger to check for discharge.

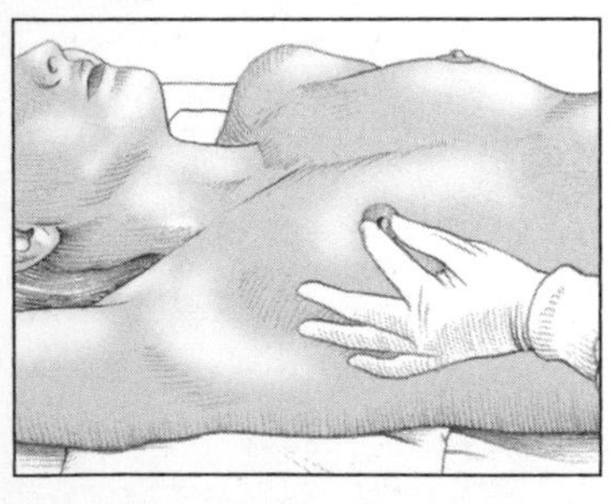

Both nipples should point in the same direction. If they're flattened or inverted, ask the patient when she first noticed the inversion. Also ask her if she has had nipple discharge. If so, ask her to describe the color and character of the discharge.

Prominent veins in the breast may indicate cancer in some patients but are normal in pregnant women due to engorgement.

Acute mastitis, or breast inflammation usually associated with lactation, causes reddening of the skin and abrasions or cracking. Fever and other signs of systemic infection may also occur.

Palpation

Before palpating the breasts, ask the patient to lie in a supine position, and place a small pillow under her shoulder on the side you're examining. This causes the breast on that side to protrude.

Have the patient put her hand behind her head on the side you're examining. This spreads the breast more evenly across the chest and makes finding nodules easier. If her breasts are small, she can leave her arm at her side.

To perform palpation, place your fingers flat on the breast and compress the tissues gently against the chest wall, palpating in concentric circles outward from the nipple. Palpate the entire breast, including the periphery, tail of Spence, and areola. For a patient with pendulous breasts, palpate down or across the breast with the patient sitting upright. (See *Palpating the breasts.*)

During palpation, note the consistency of the breast tissue. Normal consistency varies widely, depending in part on the proportions of fat and glandular tissue. Check for nodules and unusual tenderness. Remember that nodularity, fullness, and mild tenderness are normal premenstrual symptoms; so, be sure to ask the patient what stage she is in her menstrual cycle.

Tenderness may also be related to cysts and cancer.

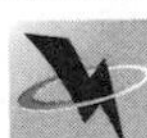

CRITICAL POINT *A lump or mass that feels different from the rest of the breast tissue may be a pathologic change and warrants further investigation. Hard, irregular, poorly circumscribed nodules that are fixed to the skin or underlying tissues, strongly suggest breast cancer. If you find what you think is an abnormality, check the patient's other breast. Keep in mind that the inframammary ridge at the lower edge of the breast is normally firm and can be mistaken for a tumor.*

If you palpate a mass, record these characteristics:

- size in centimeters
- shape — round, discoid, regular, or irregular

IDENTIFYING LOCATIONS OF BREAST LESIONS

Mentally divide the breast into four quadrants and a fifth segment, the tail of Spence. Describe your findings according to the appropriate quadrant or segment. You can also think of the breast as a clock, with the nipple as the center. Then specify locations according to the time (2 o'clock, for example). Either way, specify the location of a lesion or other findings by the distance in centimeters from the nipple.

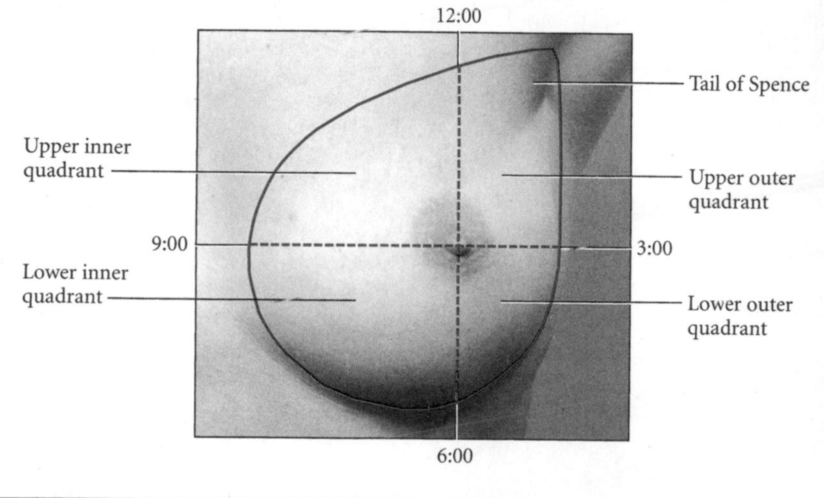

- consistency — soft, firm, or hard
- mobility
- degree of tenderness
- location, using the quadrant or clock method. (See *Identifying locations of breast lesions.*)

If the patient has fibrocystic breasts, you may palpate one or more well-defined, moveable lumps or cysts. Fibrocystic disease is a benign condition that results from excess fibrous tissue formation and hyperplasia of the linings of the mammary ducts.

If the patient has fibroadenoma, which is also a benign condition, you may palpate a small, round, painless, well-defined, mobile lump that may be soft but is usually solid, firm, and rubbery.

In a patient with a malignant breast mass, the mass may be palpated in any part of the breast, though it's usually found in the upper outer quadrant as a hard, immobile, irregular lump. Note other findings such as nipple discharge and edematous breast skin with enlarged pores, discoloration, and an orange-peel appearance.

Finally, palpate the nipple, noting its elasticity. It should be rough, elastic, and round. The nipple also typically protrudes from the breast. Compress the nipple and areola to detect discharge. If discharge is present and the patient isn't pregnant or lactating, assess the color, consistency, and quantity of the discharge. If possible, obtain a cytologic smear. To obtain a smear, put on gloves, place a glass slide over the nipple, and smear the discharge on the slide. Spray the slide with a fixative, label it with the patient's name and date, and send it to the laboratory, according to your facility's policy.

If the patient has a milky, bilateral discharge, called *galactorrhea*, this may reflect pregnancy or prolactin or other hormonal imbalance. A nonmilky, unilateral discharge suggests local breast disease.

Axillae examination

To examine the axillae, use the techniques of inspection and palpation. With the patient sitting or standing, inspect the skin of the

EXPERT TECHNIQUE

PALPATING THE AXILLAE

To palpate the axillae, have the patient sit or lie down. Make sure you wear gloves if an ulceration or discharge is present. Ask the patient to relax her arm, and support it with your nondominant hand.

Keeping the fingers of your dominant hand together, reach high into the apex of the axilla (as shown). Position your fingers so they're directly behind the pectoral muscles, pointing toward the midclavicle. Sweep your fingers downward against the ribs and serratus anterior muscle to palpate the midaxillary or central lymph nodes. Repeat palpation on the patient's other side.

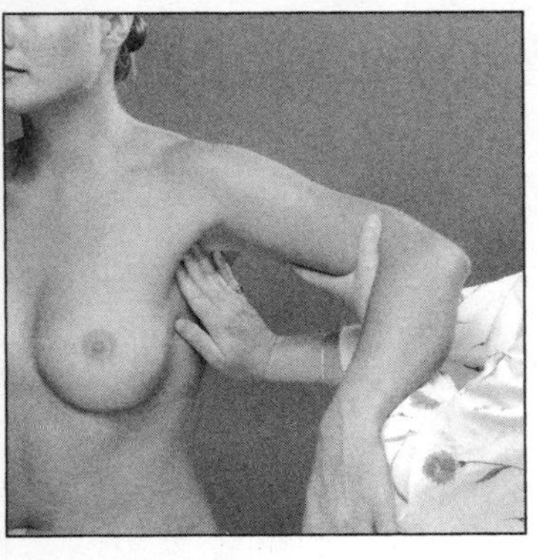

axillae for rashes, infections, or unusual pigmentation.

If the patient has a rash this could suggest a sweat gland infection. Deeply pigmented skin that feels velvety could be associated with internal malignancy.

Before palpating, ask the patient to relax her arm on the side you're examining. Support her elbow with one of your hands. Cup the fingers of your other hand, and reach high into the apex of the axilla. Place your fingers directly behind the pectoral muscles, pointing toward the midclavicle. (See *Palpating the axillae.*)

Axillary node palpation

Next, try to palpate the central nodes by pressing your fingers downward and in toward the chest wall. You can usually palpate one or more of the nodes, which should be soft, small, and nontender. If you feel a hard, large, or tender lesion, try to palpate the other groups of lymph nodes for comparison.

To palpate the pectoral and anterior nodes, grasp the anterior axillary fold between your thumb and fingers and palpate inside the borders of the pectoral muscles. Palpate the lateral nodes by pressing your fingers along the upper inner arm. Try to compress these nodes against the humerus. To palpate the subscapular or posterior nodes, stand behind the patient and press your fingers to feel the inside of the muscle of the posterior axillary fold.

Neck node palpation

If the axillary nodes appear abnormal, next you should assess the nodes in the clavicular area. To do this, have the patient relax her neck muscles by flexing her head slightly forward. Stand in front of her and hook your fingers over the clavicle beside the sternocleidomastoid muscle. Rotate your fingers deeply into this area to feel the supraclavicular nodes.

Abnormal findings

A patient's chief complaint may be for any of a number of signs and symptoms related to the breasts and axillae. Some common findings include breast dimpling, breast nodules, breast pain, breast ulcer, nipple retraction, and peau d'orange. The following history, physical examination, and analysis summaries will help you assess each one quickly and accurately. After obtaining further information, begin to interpret the findings. (See *Breasts and axillae: Interpreting your findings.*)

Breast dimpling

Breast dimpling is the puckering or retraction of skin on the breast. Dimpling usually affects women older than age 40, but also occasionally occurs in men.

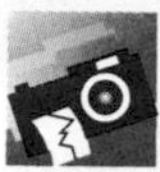

CLINICAL PICTURE

BREASTS AND AXILLAE: INTERPRETING YOUR FINDINGS

After you assess the patient, a group of findings may lead you to a particular disorder of the breasts and axillae. The chart below shows some common groups of findings for major signs and symptoms related to an assessment of the breasts and axillae, along with their probable causes.

Sign or symptom and findings	Probable cause
Breast dimpling	
■ Firm, irregular, nontender lump ■ Nipple retraction, deviation, inversion, or flattening ■ Enlarged axillary lymph nodes	Breast abscess
■ History of trauma to fatty tissue of the breast (patient may not remember such trauma) ■ Tenderness and erythema ■ Bruising ■ Hard, indurated, poorly delineated lump that's fibrotic and fixed to underlying tissue or overlying skin ■ Signs of nipple retraction	Fat necrosis
■ Heat ■ Erythema ■ Swelling ■ Pain and tenderness ■ Flulike signs and symptoms, such as fever, malaise, fatigue, and aching	Mastitis
Breast nodule	
■ Single nodule that feels firm, elastic, and round or lobular, with well-defined margins ■ Extremely mobile, "slippery" feel ■ No pain or tenderness ■ Size varies greatly from that of a pinhead to very large ■ Grows rapidly ■ Usually located around the nipple or on the lateral side of the upper outer quadrant	Fibroadenoma
■ Hard, poorly delineated nodule ■ Fixed to the skin or underlying tissue ■ Breast dimpling ■ Nipple deviation or retraction ■ Usually located in the upper outer quadrant (almost one-half) ■ Nontender ■ Serous or bloody discharge ■ Edema or peau d'orange of the skin overlying the mass ■ Axillary lymphadenopathy	Breast cancer

(continued)

BREASTS AND AXILLAE: INTERPRETING YOUR FINDINGS *(continued)*

Sign or symptom and findings	Probable cause
Breast nodule *(continued)*	
▪ Smooth, round, slightly elastic nodules ▪ Increase in size and tenderness just before menstruation ▪ Mobile ▪ Clear, watery (serous) discharge or sticky nipple ▪ Bloating ▪ Irritability ▪ Abdominal cramping	Fibrocystic breast disease
Breast pain	
▪ Tender, palpable abscesses on the periphery of the areola ▪ Fever ▪ Inflamed sebaceous Montgomery's tubercles	Areolar gland abscess
▪ Unilateral breast pain or tenderness ▪ Serous or bloody nipple discharge, usually only from one duct ▪ Small, soft, poorly delineated mass in the ducts beneath the areola	Intraductal papilloma
▪ Small, well-delineated nodule ▪ Localized erythema ▪ Induration	Infected sebaceous cyst
Breast ulcer	
▪ Ulceration that doesn't heal within 1 month ▪ Palpable breast nodule ▪ Skin dimpling ▪ Nipple retraction ▪ Bloody or serous nipple discharge ▪ Erythema ▪ Enlarged axillary lymph nodes ▪ Maceration of breast tissue	Breast cancer
▪ Bright red papular patches with scaly borders ▪ Pain and burning	*Candida albincans* infection
▪ Bright red unilateral nipple excoriation possibly extending to the areola ▪ Serous or bloody nipple discharge ▪ Extreme nipple itching	Paget's disease
Nipple retraction	
▪ Poorly defined, rubbery nodule beneath the areola with a blue-green discoloration ▪ Areolar burning, itching, swelling, tenderness, and erythema ▪ Nipple pain with a thick, sticky, grayish, multiductal discharge	Mammary duct ectasia
▪ History of breast surgery that may have caused underlying scarring	Previous surgery

BREASTS AND AXILLAE: INTERPRETING YOUR FINDINGS *(continued)*

Sign or symptom and findings	Probable cause
Peau d'orange	
▪ Pitting of breast skin, most commonly in lactating women ▪ Malaise ▪ Breast tenderness ▪ Erythema ▪ Sudden fever ▪ Possible purulent nipple discharge ▪ Induration or palpable soft mass	Breast abscess
▪ Most commonly appearing in the dependent part of the breast or areola ▪ Firm immobile mass adhering to skin above the area of pitting ▪ Changes in contour, size, or symmetry ▪ Erosion, retraction, or deviation of the nipple with thin and watery, bloody, or purulent drainage ▪ Burning or itching sensation accompanied by a feeling of warmth	Breast cancer
Peau d'orange *(continued)*	
▪ Well-demarcated erythematous elevated area with a pitting texture ▪ Pain ▪ Warmth ▪ Generalized signs and symptoms of infection including fever and malaise	Erysipelas
▪ Raised, thickened, hyperpigmented pitting areas that tend to coalesce ▪ Weight loss ▪ Palpitations ▪ Anxiety ▪ Heat intolerance ▪ Tremor ▪ Amenorrhea	Graves' disease

History

Obtain a medical and family history, noting factors that place the patient at high risk for breast cancer. In women, ask about reproductive history including pregnancy history, because women who haven't had a full-term pregnancy until after age 30 are at higher risk for developing breast cancer. Ask the patient if her mother or a sister had breast cancer. Find out if she has a previous malignancy. Ask about the patient's dietary habits because a high-fat diet predisposes women to breast cancer.

Ask the patient if she has noticed changes in the shape of the breast. Find out if she has painful or tender areas and if the pain is cyclic. If she's breast-feeding, ask her if she has recently experienced high fever, chills, malaise, muscle aches, fatigue, or other flu-like signs or symptoms. Also, find out if she remembers sustaining any trauma to her breasts.

Physical assessment

Begin the physical assessment by carefully inspecting the dimpled area of the breast. Is it swollen, red, or warm to the touch? Do you see any bruises or contusions? Ask the patient to tense her pectoral muscles by pressing her hips with both hands or by raising her hands over her head. Does puckering increase? Then, gently pull the skin upward toward the clavicle. Is dimpling exaggerated?

Next, assess the breast for nipple retraction. Do both nipples point in the same direction? Are the nipples flattened or inverted? Does the patient report nipple discharge? If so, ask her to describe the color and character of the discharge. Observe the contour of both breasts. Are they symmetrical?

With your patient in supine, sitting, and forward-leaning positions, examine both breasts. Does the skin move freely over both breasts? If you can palpate a lump, describe its size, location, consistency, mobility, and delineation. What relation does the lump have to breast dimpling? Gently mold the breast skin around the lump. Is dimpling exaggerated?

Analysis

Breast dimpling results from abnormal attachment of the skin to underlying tissue. It suggests an inflammatory or malignant mass beneath the skin surface and usually represents a late sign of breast cancer; benign lesions usually don't produce this effect.

Because breast dimpling occurs over a mass or induration, the patient usually discovers other signs before becoming aware of this one. However, a thorough breast examination may reveal dimpling and alert the patient and health care provider to a problem.

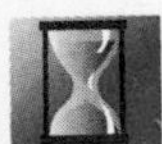

AGE ISSUE *Because breast cancer, the most likely cause of dimpling, is extremely rare in children, consider trauma a likely cause. As in adults, breast dimpling may occur in adolescents from fatty tissue necrosis caused by trauma.*

Breast nodule

A breast nodule, or lump, may be found in any part of the patient's breasts, including in the axillae.

History

If your patient reports a nodule, ask how and when she discovered it. Also ask her if the size and tenderness of the nodule varies with her menstrual cycle. Find out if it has changed since she first noticed it. Ask if she has noticed other breast signs, such as a change in breast shape, size, or contour; a discharge; or a change in the nipples.

If the patient is breast-feeding, find out if she has fever, chills, fatigue, or other flulike signs and symptoms. Ask her to describe any pain or tenderness associated with the nodule. Is the pain in one breast only? Has she sustained recent trauma to the breast?

Explore the patient's medical and family history for factors that increase her risk of breast cancer. These include eating a high-fat diet, having a mother or sister with breast cancer, or having a history of cancer, especially in the other breast. Other risk factors include nulliparity or a first pregnancy after age 30.

Physical assessment

Perform a thorough clinical breast examination. Pay close attention to the upper outer quadrant of each breast, where half the ductal tissue is located. This is the most common site of malignant breast tumors.

Carefully palpate a suspected breast nodule, noting its location, shape, size, consistency, mobility, and delineation. Note if it feels soft, rubbery, and elastic or hard. Observe if it's mobile, slipping away from your fingers as you palpate it, or firmly fixed to the adjacent tissue. Does the nodule seem to limit the mobility of the entire breast? Note the nodule's delineation. Are the borders clearly defined or indefinite? Or does the area feel more like a hardness or diffuse induration than a nodule with definite borders?

Do you feel one nodule or several small ones? Is the shape round, oval, lobular, or irregular? Inspect and palpate the skin over the nodule for warmth, redness, and edema. Palpate the lymph nodes of each breast and the axillae for enlargement.

Observe the contour of the breasts, looking for asymmetry and irregularities. Be alert for signs of retraction, such as skin dimpling and nipple deviation, retraction, or flattening. (To exaggerate dimpling, have your patient raise her arms over her head or press her hands against her hips.) Gently pull the breast skin toward the clavicle and observe for dimpling. Mold the breast skin and again observe for dimpling.

Be alert for a nipple discharge that's spontaneous, unilateral, and nonmilky (serous, bloody, or purulent). Be careful not to confuse it with the grayish discharge that can often be elicited from the nipples of a woman who has been pregnant.

Analysis

A breast nodule is a commonly reported gynecologic sign that is either caused by benign breast disease or cancer. Benign breast disease, the leading cause of nodules, can stem from cyst formation in obstructed and dilated lactiferous ducts, hypertrophy or tumor formation in the ductal system, and inflammation or infection.

Although less than 20% of breast nodules are malignant, the signs of breast cancer aren't easily distinguished from those of benign breast disease. Breast cancer is a leading cause of death among women but can occur occasionally in men. Thus, breast nodules in both sexes should always be evaluated.

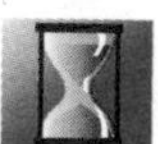

AGE ISSUE *In women age 70 and older, 75% of all breast lumps are malignant.*

Breast pain

An unreliable indicator of cancer, breast pain (also known as *mastalgia*) commonly results from benign breast disease. It may occur during rest or movement and may be aggravated by manipulation or palpation. Breast pain may be unilateral or bilateral; cyclic, intermittent, or constant; and dull or sharp.

History

Begin by asking the patient if breast pain is constant or intermittent. For either type, ask about onset and character. If intermittent, determine the relationship of pain to the phase of the menstrual cycle. Ask the patient if she's pregnant or breast-feeding. If she's not, ask about nipple discharge, and have her describe it. Or, find out if the patient has reached menopause. Ask her if she has recently experienced flulike symptoms or sustained an injury to the breast, and if she has noticed any changes in her breast shape or contour.

Next, ask your patient to describe the breast pain. She may describe it as sticking, stinging, shooting, stabbing, throbbing, or burning. Determine if the pain affects one breast or both, and ask the patient to point to the painful area.

Physical assessment

Begin the physical examination by instructing the patient to place her arms at her sides, and then inspect her breasts. Note their size, symmetry, and contour and the appearance of the skin. Remember that breast shape and size vary widely and that breasts normally change during the menstrual cycle, pregnancy, breast-feeding, and aging. Are the breasts red or edematous? Are the veins prominent?

Note the size, shape, and symmetry of the nipples and areolae. Do you detect ecchymosis, a rash, ulceration, or a discharge? Do the nipples point in the same direction? Do you see signs of retraction, such as skin dimpling or nipple inversion or flattening? Repeat your inspection, first with the patient's arms raised above her head and then with her hands pressed against her hips.

Palpate the patient's breasts, first with her seated and then with her lying down and a pillow placed under her shoulder on the side being examined. Use the pads of your fingers to compress breast tissue against the chest wall. Proceed systematically from the sternum to the midline and from the axilla to the midline, noting warmth, tenderness, nodules, masses, or irregularities. Palpate the nipple, noting tenderness and nodules, and check for discharge. Palpate axillary lymph nodes, noting any enlargement.

Analysis

Breast pain may result from surface cuts, furuncles, contusions, and similar lesions (superficial pain); nipple fissures and inflammation in the papillary ducts and areolae (severe, localized pain); stromal distention in the breast parenchyma (tenderness); a tumor that affects nerve endings (severe, constant pain); or inflammatory lesions that not only distend the stroma but also irritate sensory nerve endings (severe, constant pain). Also be aware that breast pain may radiate to the back, the arms, and sometimes the neck.

Breast tenderness in women may occur before menstruation and during pregnancy. Before menstruation, breast pain or tenderness stems from increased mammary blood flow due to hormonal changes. During pregnancy, breast tenderness and throbbing, tingling, or pricking sensations may occur, also from hormonal changes. In men, breast pain may stem from gynecomastia (especially during puberty and senescence), reproductive tract anomalies, and organic disease of the liver or of the pituitary, adrenal cortex, and thyroid glands.

AGE ISSUE *Transient gynecomastia can cause breast pain in males during puberty. In postmenopausal women, breast pain secondary to benign breast disease is rare.*

Breast ulcer

Appearing on the nipple, areola, or the breast itself, an ulcer indicates destruction of the skin and subcutaneous tissue.

History

Begin the health history by asking when the patient first noticed the ulcer and if it was preceded by other breast changes, such as nodules, edema, or nipple discharge, deviation, or retraction. Does the ulcer seem to be getting better or worse? Does it cause pain or produce drainage? Has she noticed any change in breast shape? Has she had a skin rash? If she has been treating the ulcer at home, find out how.

Review the patient's personal and family history for factors that increase the risk of breast cancer. Ask, for example, about previous cancer, especially of the breast, and mastectomy. Determine whether the patient's mother or sister has had breast cancer. Ask the patient's age at menarche and menopause because more than 30 years of menstrual activity increases the risk of breast cancer. Also ask about pregnancy because nulliparity or birth of a first child after age 30 also increases the risk of breast cancer.

If the patient recently gave birth, ask if she breast-feeds her infant or has recently weaned him. Ask if she's currently taking an oral antibiotic and if she's diabetic. All these factors predispose the patient to *Candida* infections.

Physical assessment

Inspect the patient's breast, noting any asymmetry or flattening. Look for a rash, scaling, cracking, or red excoriation on the nipples, areola, and inframammary fold. Check especially for skin changes, such as warmth, erythema, or peau d'orange. Palpate the breasts for masses, noting any induration beneath the ulcer. Then carefully palpate for tenderness or nodules around the areola and the axillary lymph nodes.

Analysis

A breast ulcer is usually a late sign of cancer, appearing well after the confirming diagnosis. However, it may be the presenting sign of breast cancer in men, who are more apt to dismiss earlier breast changes. Breast ulcers can also result from trauma, infection, or radiation.

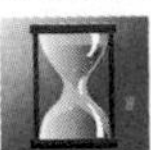

AGE ISSUE *Because of increased breast cancer risk in the elderly population, breast ulcers should be considered cancerous until proven otherwise. However, ulcers can also result from normal skin changes due to aging, such as thinning, decreased vascularity, and loss of elasticity as well as from poor skin hygiene. Breast ulcers may result from tight brassieres; traumatic ulcers, or from falls or abuse.*

Nipple retraction

Nipple retraction refers to the inward displacement of the nipple below the level of surrounding breast tissue.

History

Ask the patient when she first noticed that the nipple was retracted. Has she experienced other nipple changes, such as itching, discoloration, discharge, or excoriation? Has she noticed breast pain, lumps, redness, swelling, or warmth? Obtain a complete health history, noting risk factors of breast cancer, such as a family history or previous malignancy.

Physical assessment

Carefully examine both nipples and breasts with the patient sitting upright with her arms at her sides, with her hands pressing on her hips. Then, with her arms overhead and with the patient leaning forward so her breasts hang. Look for redness, excoriation, and discharge; nipple flattening and deviation; and breast asymmetry, dimpling, or contour differences. Note your findings.

Nipple retraction is typically confused with nipple inversion, a common abnormality that's congenital in some patients and doesn't usually signal underlying disease. A retracted nipple appears flat and broad, whereas an inverted nipple can be pulled out from the sulcus where it hides.

Try to evert the nipple by gently squeezing the areola. With the patient in a supine position, palpate both breasts for lumps, especially beneath the areola. Mold breast skin over the lump or gently pull it up toward the clavicle, looking for accentuated nipple retraction. Also, palpate axillary lymph nodes.

Analysis

Nipple retraction results from scar tissue formation within a lesion or large mammary duct. As scar tissue shortens, it pulls adjacent tissue inward, causing nipple deviation, flattening, and finally retraction. Nipple retraction may indicate an inflammatory breast lesion or cancer.

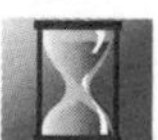

AGE ISSUE *Nipple retraction doesn't occur in prepubescent females.*

Peau d'orange

Peau d'orange, (orange peel skin) refers to the edematous thickening and pitting of breast skin.

History

Ask the patient when she first detected peau d'orange. Has she noticed any lumps, pain, or other breast changes? Does she have related signs and symptoms, such as malaise, achiness, and weight loss? Is she breastfeeding, or has she recently weaned her infant? Has she had previous axillary surgery that might have impaired lymphatic drainage of a breast?

Physical assessment

In a well-lit examining room, observe the patient's breasts. Estimate the extent of the peau d'orange and check for erythema. Assess the nipples for discharge, deviation, retraction, dimpling, and cracking. Gently palpate the area of peau d'orange, noting warmth or induration. Then palpate the entire breast, noting any fixed or mobile lumps, and the axillary lymph nodes, noting enlargement. Finally, take the patient's temperature.

Analysis

Peau d'orange is usually a late sign of breast cancer. It usually begins in the dependent part of the breast or areola. This slowly developing sign can also occur with breast or axillary lymph node infection, erysipelas, or Graves' disease. Its striking orange-peel appearance stems from lymphatic edema around deepened hair follicles. This abnormal finding also may be noted in women who are breast-feeding and develop milk stasis.

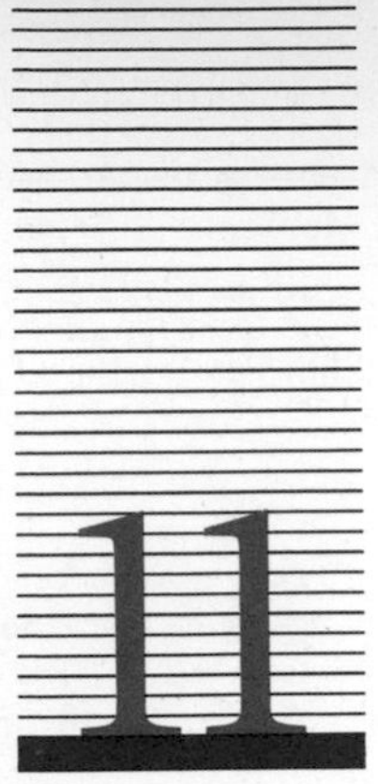

11 Gastrointestinal system

As the site of the body's digestive processes, the GI system has the critical task of supplying essential nutrients to fuel the body's brain, heart, and lungs. GI function also profoundly affects the quality of life through its impact on a person's overall health. To perform an accurate assessment of the GI system, you need a complete understanding of its anatomy and physiology and the related structures.

Anatomy and physiology

The GI system consists of two major components: the alimentary canal and the accessory GI organs. The alimentary canal, or GI tract, consists essentially of a hollow muscular tube that begins in the mouth and extends to the anus. It includes the pharynx, esophagus, stomach, small intestine, and large intestine. Accessory organs aiding GI function include the salivary glands, liver, biliary duct system (gallbladder and bile ducts), and pancreas.

Together, the GI tract and accessory organs serve two major functions:

- digestion, the breaking down of food and fluid into simple chemicals that can be absorbed into the bloodstream and transported throughout the body
- elimination of waste products from the body through excretion of stool. (See *Anatomic structures of the GI system.*)

GI tract

The GI tract is a hollow tube that begins at the mouth and ends at the anus. About 25′ (7.5 m) long, the GI tract consists of smooth muscle alternating with blood vessels and nerve tissue. Specialized circular and longitudinal fibers contract, causing

ANATOMIC STRUCTURES OF THE GI SYSTEM

This illustration shows the GI system's major anatomic structures. Understanding these structures will help you conduct an accurate physical assessment.

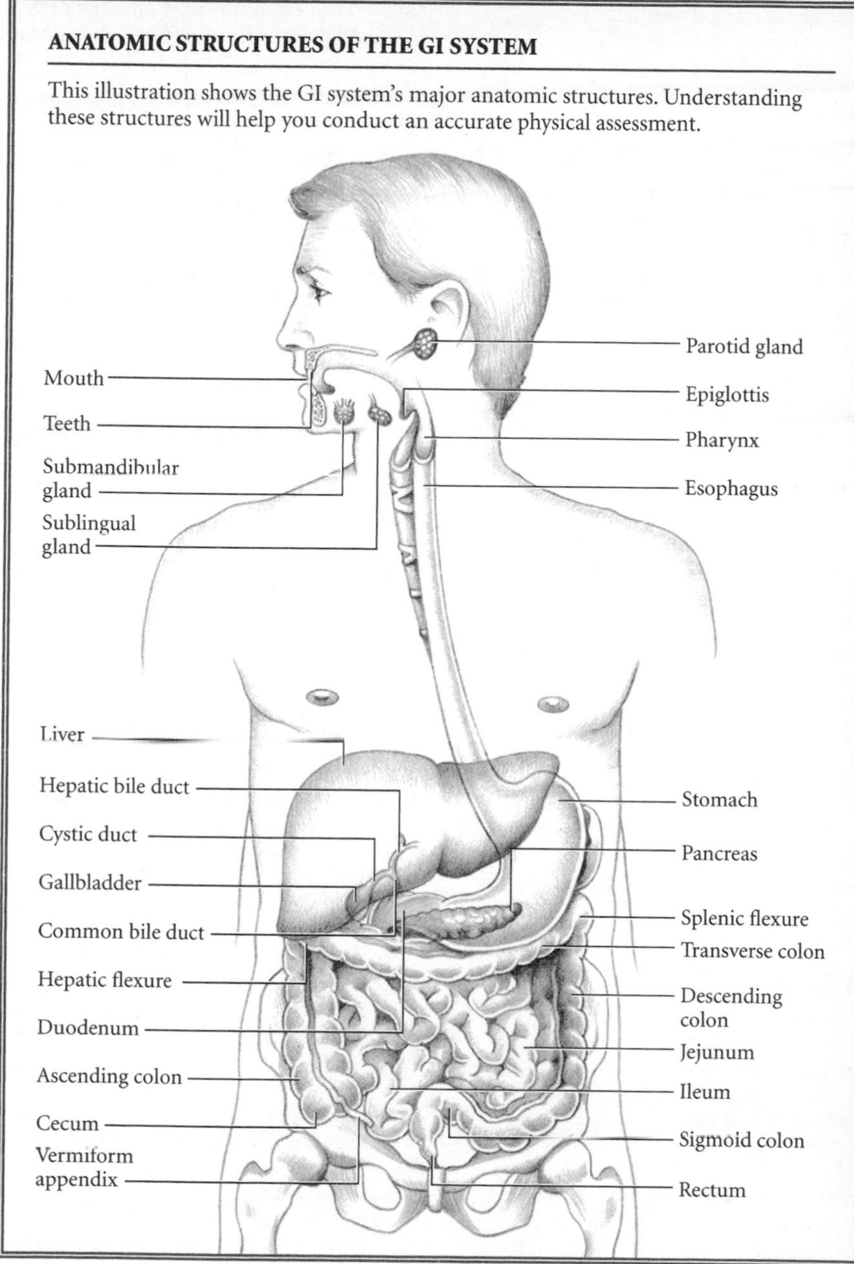

peristalsis, which aids in propelling food through the GI tract. The GI tract includes the mouth, pharynx, esophagus, stomach, small intestine, and large intestine.

Mouth

Digestive processes begin in the mouth with mastication (chewing), starch digestion (salivating), and deglutition (swallowing). The tongue provides the sense of taste. Saliva is produced by three pairs of glands that include the parotid, submandibular, and sublingual.

Pharynx

The pharynx, or throat, allows the passage of food from the mouth to the esophagus. The pharynx assists in the swallowing process and secretes mucus that aids in digestion. The epiglottis—a thin, leaf-shaped structure made of fibrocartilage—is located directly behind the root of the tongue. When food is swallowed, the epiglottis closes over the larynx, and the soft palate lifts to block the nasal cavity. These actions keep food and fluid from being aspirated into the airway.

Esophagus

The esophagus is a muscular, hollow tube about 10″ (25.5 cm) long that moves food from the pharynx to the stomach. When food is swallowed, the upper esophageal sphincter relaxes, and the food moves into the esophagus. Peristalsis then propels the food toward the stomach. The gastroesophageal sphincter at the lower end of the esophagus normally remains closed to prevent reflux of gastric contents. The sphincter opens during swallowing, belching, and vomiting. As food moves through the esophagus, glands in the esophageal mucosal layer secrete mucus, which lubricates the bolus and protects the esophageal mucosal layer from being damaged by poorly chewed foods.

Stomach

The stomach, a reservoir for food, is a dilated, saclike structure that lies obliquely in the left upper quadrant below the esophagus and diaphragm, to the right of the spleen, and partly under the liver. The stomach contains two important sphincters: the cardiac sphincter, which protects the entrance to the stomach, and the pyloric sphincter, which guards the exit.

The stomach has three major functions:

- stores food
- mixes food with gastric juices (hydrochloric acid)
- parcels food into the small intestine for further digestion and absorption.

Except for alcohol, little food absorption normally occurs in the stomach. Peristaltic contractions churn the food into tiny particles and mix it with gastric juices, forming a thick, almost liquid food bolus known as chyme. After mixing, stronger peristaltic waves move the chyme into the antrum, where it's backed up against the pyloric sphincter before being released into the duodenum, triggering the intestinal phase of digestion.

The rate of stomach emptying depends on a complex interplay of factors, including gastrin release and neural signals caused by stomach wall distention and the enterogastric reflex. In this reaction, the duodenum releases secretin and gastric-inhibiting peptide, and the jejunum secretes cholecystokinin—all of which act to decrease gastric motility.

An average meal can remain in the stomach for 3 to 4 hours. Rugae, accordion-like folds in the stomach lining, allow the stomach to expand when large amounts of food and fluid are ingested.

Small intestine

The small intestine performs most of the work of digestion and absorption. It's 20″ (6.1 m) long and named for its diameter, not its length. It has three sections: the duodenum, the jejunum, and the ileum. As food passes into the small intestine, the end products of digestion are absorbed through its thin mucous membrane lining into the bloodstream.

Carbohydrates, fats, and proteins are broken down in the small intestine. Enzymes from the pancreas, bile from the liver, and hormones from glands of the small intestine all aid digestion. These secretions mix with the food as it moves through the intestines by peristalsis.

Large intestine

The large intestine, or colon, is about 5″ (1.5 m) long and is responsible for:

- absorbing excess water and electrolytes
- storing food residue
- eliminating waste products in the form of stool.

By the time chyme passes through the small intestine and enters the ascending colon of the large intestine, it has been reduced to mostly indigestible substances.

The bolus begins its journey through the large intestine at the juncture of the ileum and cecum with the ileocecal pouch. Then the bolus moves up the ascending colon past the right abdominal cavity to the liver's lower border, crosses horizontally below the liver and stomach via the transverse colon, and descends from the left abdominal cavity to the iliac fossa through the descending colon.

From there, the bolus travels through the sigmoid colon to the lower midline of the abdominal cavity, then to the rectum, and finally to the anal canal. The anus opens to the exterior through two sphincters. The internal anal sphincter contains thick, circular smooth muscle under autonomic control. The external sphincter contains skeletal muscle under voluntary control.

Circular and longitudinal fibers of the tunica muscularis move and mix intestinal contents, and the longitudinal muscle gives the large intestine its familiar shape. These fibers gather into three narrow bands (teniae coli) down the middle of the colon and pucker the intestine into characteristic pouches (haustra coli).

The ascending and descending colons attach directly to the posterior abdominal wall for support. The transverse and sigmoid colons attach indirectly through sheets of connective tissue (mesocolon).

Although the large intestine produces no hormones or digestive enzymes, it continues the absorptive process. Through blood and lymph vessels in the submucosa, the proximal half of the intestine absorbs all but about 100 ml of the remaining water in the colon plus large amounts of sodium and chloride. The large intestine also harbors the bacteria *Escherichia coli, Enterobacter aerogenes, Clostridium welchii,* and *Lactobacillus bifidus,* which help synthesize vitamin K and break down cellulose into usable carbohydrates. Bacterial action also produces flatus, which helps propel stool toward the rectum. In addition, the mucosa produces alkaline secretions from tubular glands composed of goblet cells. This alkaline mucus lubricates the intestinal walls as food pushes through and protects the mucosa from acidic bacterial action.

In the lower colon, long and relatively sluggish contractions cause propulsive waves known as mass movements. These movements, which normally occur several times a day, propel intestinal contents into the rectum and produce the urge to defecate. Defecation normally results from the defecation reflex, a sensory and parasympathetic nerve-mediated response, along with the person's relaxation of the external anal sphincter.

Accessory GI organs

Accessory GI organs include the liver, bile ducts, gallbladder, pancreas, and vascular structures.

Liver

The liver is located in the right upper quadrant under the diaphragm. It has two major lobes, divided by the falciform ligament. The liver is the heaviest organ in the body, weighing about 3 lb (1.5 kg) in the adult.

The liver's functions include:

- metabolizing carbohydrates, fats, and proteins
- detoxifying blood
- converting ammonia to urea for excretion
- synthesizing plasma proteins, nonessential amino acids, vitamin A, and essential nutrients, such as iron and vitamins D, K, and B_{12}.

The liver also secretes bile, a greenish fluid that helps digest fats and absorb fatty acids, cholesterol, and other lipids. Bile also gives stool its color.

Bile ducts

The bile ducts provide a passageway for bile to travel from the liver to the intestines. Two hepatic ducts drain the liver and the cystic duct drains the gallbladder. These ducts converge into the common bile duct, which then empties into the duodenum.

Function of bile. A greenish liquid composed of water, cholesterol, bile salts, electrolytes, and phospholipids, bile is important in fat emulsification (breakdown) and intestinal absorption of fatty acids, cholesterol, and other lipids. When bile salts are absent from the intestinal tract, lipids are excreted and fat-soluble vitamins are absorbed poorly. Bile also aids in excretion of conjugated bilirubin (an end product of hemoglobin degradation) from the liver and thereby prevents jaundice.

The liver recycles about 80% of bile salts into bile, combining them with bile pigments (biliverdin and bilirubin — the breakdown products of red blood cells) and cholesterol. The liver produces about 500 ml of this alkaline bile in continuous secretion. Enhanced bile production can result from vagal stimulation, release of the hormone secretin, increased liver blood flow, and the presence of fat in the intestine.

The liver metabolizes digestive end products by regulating blood glucose levels. When glucose is being absorbed through the intestine (anabolic state), the liver stores glucose as glycogen. When glucose isn't being absorbed or when blood glucose levels fall (catabolic state), the liver mobilizes glucose to restore blood levels necessary for brain function.

Function of the lobules. The liver's functional unit, the lobule, consists of a plate of hepatic cells (hepatocytes) that encircle a central vein and radiate outward. The plates of hepatocytes are separated from one another by sinusoids, the liver's capillary system. Lining the sinusoids are reticuloendothelial macrophages (Kupffer's cells), which remove bacteria and toxins that have entered the blood through the intestinal capillaries.

The sinusoids carry oxygenated blood from the hepatic artery and nutrient-rich blood from the portal vein. Unoxygenated blood leaves through the central vein and flows through hepatic veins to the inferior vena cava. Bile, recycled from bile salts in the blood, leaves through bile ducts (canaliculi) that merge into the right and left hepatic ducts to form the common hepatic duct. This common duct joins the cystic duct from the gallbladder to form the common bile duct to the duodenum.

Gallbladder

The gallbladder, a 3″ to 4″ (7.5- to 10-cm) long, pear-shaped organ, is joined to the liver's ventral surface by the cystic duct. It stores and concentrates bile produced by the liver. Its 30- to 50-ml storage load increases up to 10-fold in potency. Secretion of the hormone cholecystokinin causes gallbladder contraction and relaxation of the sphincter of Oddi, releasing bile into the common bile duct for delivery to the duodenum. When the sphincter closes, bile shunts to the gallbladder for storage.

Pancreas

The pancreas, which measures about 6″ to 8″ (15 to 20.5 cm) in length, lies horizontally in the abdomen, behind the stomach. It consists of a head, tail, and body. The head of the pancreas is located in the right upper quadrant; the tail, in the left upper quadrant, attached to the duodenum. The tail of the pancreas touches the spleen.

The pancreas performs both exocrine and endocrine functions. Its exocrine function involves scattered cells that secrete more than 1,000 ml of digestive enzymes daily. Lobules and lobes of the clusters (acini) of enzyme-producing cells release their secretions into ducts that merge into the pancreatic duct. The pancreatic duct runs the length of the pancreas and joins the bile duct from the gallbladder before entering the duodenum.

Vagal stimulation and release of the hormones secretin and cholecystokinin control the rate and amount of pancreatic secretion.

The endocrine function of the pancreas involves the islets of Langerhans, which are located between the acinar cells. More than one million of these islets house two cell types: alpha cells secrete glucagon, which stimulates glycogenolysis in the liver; beta cells secrete insulin to promote carbohydrate metabolism. Both hormones flow directly into the blood, their release stimulated by blood glucose levels.

Vascular structures

The abdominal aorta also aids the GI system by supplying blood to the GI tract. It enters the abdomen, separates into the common iliac arteries, and then branches into many arteries extending the length of the GI tract.

The gastric and splenic veins drain absorbed nutrients into the portal vein of the liver. After entering the liver, the venous blood circulates and then exits the liver through the hepatic vein, emptying into the inferior vena cava.

Health history

GI signs and symptoms can have many baffling causes. For instance, if your patient is vomiting, this sign could have several implications. The patient could be pregnant, could have a viral infection or, possibly, could have a severe metabolic disorder such as hyperkalemia. Maybe the patient merely has indigestion — or maybe a cardiac crisis is building.

To help track the development of relevant signs and symptoms over time, develop a detailed patient history. The health history includes the patient's chief complaint, his current and past illnesses, a review of all body systems, and his family and psychosocial history. For best results, establish rapport with the patient by using excellent communication skills. Conduct this part of the assessment as privately as possible; many patients feel embarrassed to talk about GI functions. Speak softly so that others won't overhear the discussion.

If the patient has a hearing problem, perform the assessment in a private area or at a time when his roommate is out of the room. If the patient is in pain, help him into a comfortable position before asking questions.

ASSESSING ABDOMINAL PAIN

If your patient complains of abdominal pain, ask him to describe the type of pain he's experiencing and how and when it started. This table will help you assess the patient's pain and determine the possible causes.

Type of pain	Possible cause
Burning	Peptic ulcer, gastroesophageal reflux disease
Cramping	Biliary colic, irritable bowel syndrome, diarrhea, constipation, flatulence
Severe cramping	Appendicitis, Crohn's disease, diverticulitis
Stabbing	Pancreatitis, cholecystitis

Chief complaint

If the patient has a GI problem, he'll usually complain about pain, heartburn, nausea, vomiting, or altered bowel habits. To investigate these and other signs and symptoms, ask him about the onset, duration, location, quality, frequency, and severity of each.

Ask the patient why he's seeking care and record his words verbatim. Ask when he first noticed symptoms, keeping in mind that his answer may indicate only how long the symptoms have been intolerable, not necessarily their true duration. Clarify this point with the patient. Knowing what precipitates and relieves the patient's symptoms will provide information for a more accurate physical assessment.

Abdominal pain

One of the most common complaints associated with the GI system is abdominal pain. (See *Assessing abdominal pain.*) Abdominal pain arises from the abdominopelvic viscera, the parietal peritoneum, or the capsules of the liver, kidney, or spleen, and may be acute or chronic, diffuse, or localized.

Several types of abdominal pain exist, including:

- visceral — pain that develops slowly into a deep, dull, aching pain that's poorly localized in the epigastric, periumbilical, or hypogastric region
- somatic (parietal or peritoneal) — pain that produces sharp, more intense, and well-localized discomfort that rapidly follows the attack; movement or coughing aggravates this pain
- referred — pain that occurs from another site with the same or similar nerve supply; this sharp, well-localized, pain is felt in skin or deeper tissues and may coexist with skin hyperesthesia and muscle hyperalgesia
- inflammatory — pain that is associated with such disorders as ulcers, intestinal obstruction, appendicitis, cholecystitis, or peritonitis (For example, a duodenal ulcer can cause gnawing abdominal pain in the midepigastrium 1½ to 3 hours after eating and may even awaken the patient; antacids or food may relieve it.)
- other — pain that occurs from stretching or tension of the gut wall, traction on the peritoneum or mesentery, vigorous intestinal contraction, ischemia, and sensory nerve irritation.

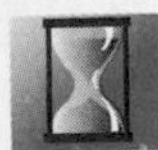

AGE ISSUE *In children, abdominal pain can signal a disorder with greater severity or different associated signs than in adults. For example, appendicitis has a higher rupture rate and mortality in children, and vomiting may be the only sign of an impending crisis. Also, acute pyelonephritis may cause abdominal pain, vomiting, and diarrhea, but not the classic urologic signs found in adults. Finally, peptic ulcer, which is becoming increasingly common in teenagers, causes nocturnal pain and colic that, unlike peptic ulcer in adults, may not be relieved by food. Other causes of abdominal pain in children include lactose intolerance, allergic-tension-fatigue syndrome, volvulus, Meckel's diverticulum, intussusception, mesenteric adenitis, diabetes mellitus, juvenile rheumatoid arthritis, heavy metal poisoning (uncommon), or an emotional need, such as a wish to avoid school or to gain adult attention.*

Nausea and vomiting

Nausea and vomiting are commonly associated with GI disorders. However, they also occur with fluid and electrolyte imbalance; infection; metabolic, endocrine, labyrinthine, and cardiac disorders; use of certain drugs; surgery; and radiation. Nausea and vomiting can be caused by existing illnesses, such as myocardial infarction, gastric and peritoneal irritation, appendicitis, bowel obstruction, cholecystitis, acute pancreatitis, and neurologic disturbances. In addition, nausea and vomiting are commonly present during the first trimester of pregnancy. They also may arise from severe pain, anxiety, alcohol intoxication, overeating, or ingestion of distasteful food or liquid.

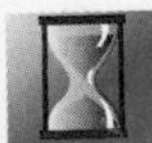

AGE ISSUE *In children, nausea — often described as stomachache — is one of the most common complaints. It can result from overeating or from any of several diverse disorders, ranging from an acute infection to a conversion reaction caused by fear. In neonates, pyloric obstruction may cause projectile vomiting, whereas Hirschsprung's disease may cause fecal vomiting. In an infant or toddler, intussusception may lead to vomiting of bile and fecal matter.*

Bowel habit changes

Ask about changes in bowel habits. Find out when the patient's last bowel movement was. Ask him if it was unusual and if he has noticed that his stools have changed in size or color or included mucus or blood.

If the patient complains about diarrhea, ask questions to elicit information about the character of the stool. Is it loose, watery, soft, formed or unformed? How often does the patient pass stool? In addition to the usual questions about onset, and duration, find out if he recently traveled abroad. Diarrhea as well as hepatitis and parasitic infections can result from ingesting contaminated food or water. Acute diarrhea may also result from acute infection, stress, fecal impaction, or use of certain drugs. Chronic diarrhea may result from chronic infection, obstructive or inflammatory bowel disease, malabsorption syndrome, an endocrine disorder, or GI surgery. Periodic diarrhea may result from food intolerance or from ingestion of spicy or high-fiber foods or caffeine.

Toxins, medications, or a GI disease, such as Crohn's disease, can cause diarrhea. Cramping, abdominal tenderness, anorexia, and hyperactive bowel sounds may accompany diarrhea. If fever occurs, the diarrhea may be caused by a toxin. One or more causes may contribute to diarrhea, and the fluid and electrolyte imbalances it produces may precipitate life-threatening arrhythmias or hypovolemic shock.

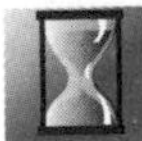

AGE ISSUE *In children, diarrhea commonly results from infection, although chronic diarrhea may be a sign of malabsorption syndrome, an anatomic defect, or allergies. Because dehydration and electrolyte imbalance occur rapidly in children, diarrhea can be life-threatening.*

If your patient complains of constipation, ascertain the characteristics of the stool. Is it hard and formed? Does the patient have to strain to pass the stool? Does the constipation alternate with diarrhea? Find out what the patient's usual bowel habits are.

Various factors such as immobility, a sedentary lifestyle, habitual laxative use, suppression of the defecation urge, acute emotional anxiety or chronic stress, and certain medications can contribute to constipation. (See *How habits and stress cause constipation.*)

The patient may complain of a dull ache in the abdomen, a full feeling, and hyperactive bowel sounds, which may be caused by irritable bowel syndrome. A patient with

HOW HABITS AND STRESS CAUSE CONSTIPATION

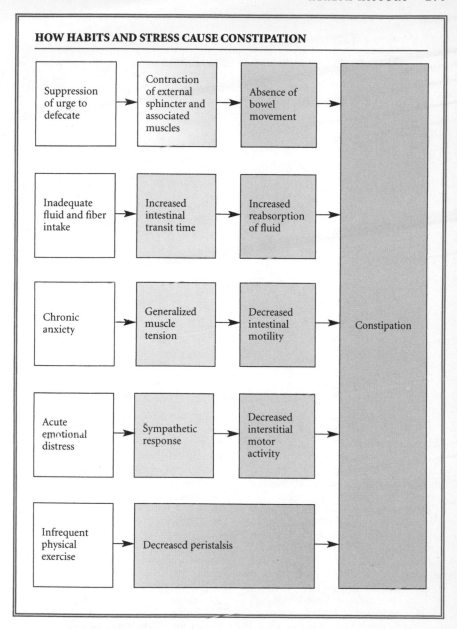

Suppression of urge to defecate →	Contraction of external sphincter and associated muscles →	Absence of bowel movement →	Constipation
Inadequate fluid and fiber intake →	Increased intestinal transit time →	Increased reabsorption of fluid →	Constipation
Chronic anxiety →	Generalized muscle tension →	Decreased intestinal motility →	Constipation
Acute emotional distress →	Sympathetic response →	Decreased interstitial motor activity →	Constipation
Infrequent physical exercise →	Decreased peristalsis →		Constipation

complete intestinal obstruction won't pass flatus or stool and won't have bowel sounds below the obstruction.

Ask the patient about any evidence of blood in the stool. Hematochezia (blood in the stool) is commonly associated with GI disorders. However, it may also result from a coagulation disorder, exposure to toxins, or a diagnostic test. Always a significant sign, hematochezia may precipitate life-threatening hypovolemia.

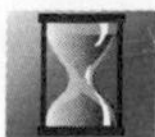

AGE ISSUE *Because elderly patients are at increased risk for colon cancer, hematochezia requires colonoscopic evaluation once perirectal lesions have been ruled out as the cause of bleeding.*

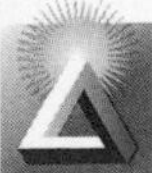

EXPERT TECHNIQUE

IDENTIFYING AREAS OF REFERRED PAIN

Pain may occur relatively near its source or distant from it. These illustrations will help to identify the areas and causes of referred pain.

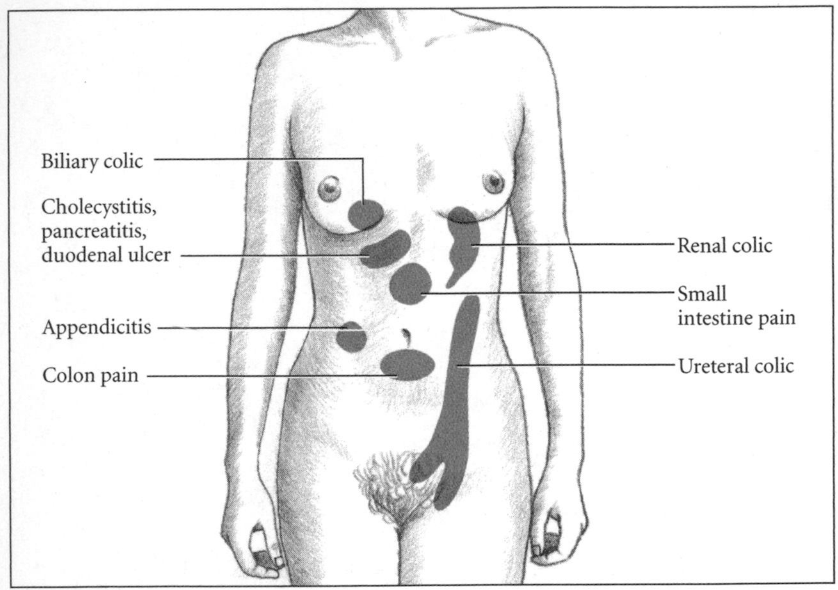

Other complaints

Ask the patient about his appetite and weight. Find out if he has lost his appetite or any weight. Ask about excessive belching or passing of gas. Find out if he has been drinking excessively. Ask him if he can eat normally and hold down foods and liquids or if he has difficulty chewing or swallowing. Dysphagia, or difficulty in swallowing, may be accompanied by weight loss. It can be caused by an obstruction, achalasia of the lower esophagogastric junction, or a neurologic disease, such as stroke or Parkinson's disease. Dysphagia can lead to aspiration and pneumonia.

Current health history

The current health history describes information relevant to the patient's chief complaint. To establish a baseline for comparison, ask the patient about his present state of health. Concentrate on:

- onset — How did the problem start? Was it gradual or sudden, with or without previous symptoms? What was the patient doing when he first noticed it?
- duration — When did the problem start? Has the patient had the problem before? If he's in pain, find out when the problem began. Is the pain continuous, intermittent, or colicky (cramplike)?
- quality — Ask the patient to describe the problem. Has he ever had it before? Was it diagnosed? If he's in pain, find out whether the pain feels sharp, dull, aching, or burning.
- severity — Ask the patient to describe how badly the problem bothers him, for example, have him rate it on a scale of 1 to 10. Does it keep him from his normal activities? Has it improved or worsened since he first noticed it? Does it wake him at night? If he's in pain, does he double over from it?
- location — Where does the patient feel the problem? Does it spread, radiate, or

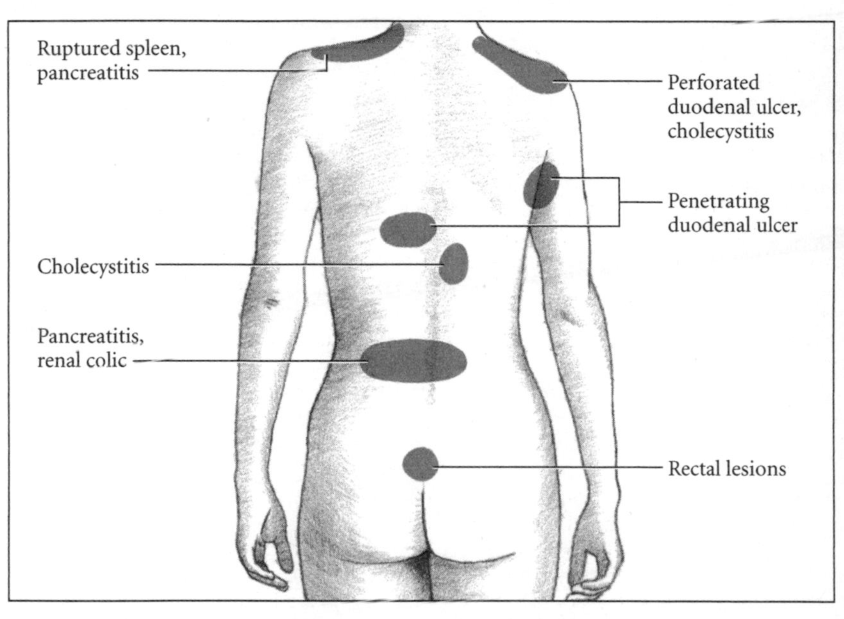

shift? Ask him to point to where he feels it most. Does he feel any pain in his shoulder, back, flank, or groin? Keep in mind pain may be referred near or far from its origin. (See *Identifying areas of referred pain.*)

Next, ask the patient to characterize his symptoms. Have him describe:

- precipitating factors — Does anything seem to bring on the problem? What makes it worse? Does it occur at the same time each day or with certain positions? Does the patient notice it after eating or drinking certain foods or after certain activities?
- alleviating factors — Does anything relieve the problem? Does the patient take any prescribed or over-the-counter (OTC) medications for relief? Has he tried anything else for relief?
- associated symptoms — What else bothers the patient when he has the problem? Has he had nausea, vomiting, and dry heaves? Has he seen blood in his vomitus (could indicate duodenal or peptic ulcer, esophageal or gastric varices, or gastritis)?

Past health history

Ask the patient whether he has had similar symptoms before and if he sought medical attention. Find out what the medical diagnosis and treatment was, if any. Ask the patient if he has had any major acute or chronic illnesses requiring hospitalization. Note the course of the illness, treatment, and any consequences. Record any surgeries in chronological order and briefly describe them. Also ask about allergies, chronic diseases, possible genetic or environmental causes, GI disorders, lifestyle, and medications.

Allergies

Ask the patient whether he's allergic to any drugs, foods, or other agents. If so, have him describe his reaction.

Chronic diseases
Find out if the patient has had cardiac or renal disease, diabetes mellitus, or cancer.

Genetic or environmental causes
Ask the patient if any of his family, friends, or coworkers have had symptoms similar to his.

GI disorders
Ask about past GI illnesses, such as an ulcer; liver, pancreas, or gallbladder disease; inflammatory bowel disease; hiatal hernia; irritable bowel syndrome; diverticulosis or diverticulitis; gastroesophageal reflux disease (GERD); hemorrhoids; cancer; or GI bleeding. Also, ask if he has had rectal or abdominal surgery or trauma.

Lifestyle
Ask whether the patient exercises. Also ask whether he drinks coffee, tea, or other caffeinated beverages such as colas. Find out if he smokes; if so, ask about how much and for how many years.

Ask the patient what he has eaten and drank in the last 24 hours and explore his usual eating habits. Some GI problems can result from certain diets or eating patterns. Ask about any late-night eating or habitually large meals. Because lack of dietary fiber (roughage) may contribute to colorectal cancer and diverticular disease, find out about the patient's fiber intake.

Medications
Record all prescribed and OTC medications the patient has taken and note their dosages and amounts, if known.

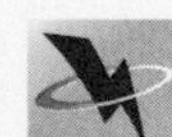

CRITICAL POINT *Several drugs — especially aspirin, nonsteroidal anti-inflammatory drugs (NSAIDs), and some antibiotics and opioids — can cause GI signs and symptoms such as nausea, vomiting, diarrhea, or constipation. If the patient has taken antibiotics in the last 30 days and has diarrhea, suspect* Clostridium difficile *infection.*

Many patients won't mention OTC preparations unless you specifically ask. However, some OTC medications, such as ibuprofen or aspirin (or those containing aspirin), herbal remedies (such as ginger and gingko biloba), and vitamins, can have GI effects. For instance, vitamins taken with iron may turn stool black.

Ask about illicit drug use and alcohol consumption. Remain tactful and nonjudgmental so the patient doesn't become defensive and give inaccurate answers.

Family history
Questioning the patient about his family may reveal environmental, genetic, or familial illnesses that may influence his current health problems and needs. Ask about the general health of his immediate relatives and spouse. If the patient's diagnosed or suspected illness has possible familial or genetic tendencies, find out whether family members have had similar problems.

GI disorders with a familial link include:

- ulcerative colitis
- colorectal cancer
- peptic ulcers
- gastric cancer
- alcoholism
- Crohn's disease.

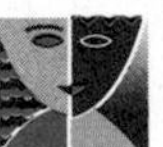

CULTURAL INSIGHT *When taking a health history, consider your patient's ethnic background. For instance, patients from Japan, Iceland, Chile, and Austria die more of gastric cancer than patients from other countries. Also, Crohn's disease is more common in Jewish patients.*

Psychosocial history
Psychological and sociologic factors as well as physical environment can profoundly affect the patient's GI health. To find out whether such factors have contributed to the patient's problem, ask about his occupation, family size, cohabitants, and home environment. Find out if the patient has been exposed to occupational or environmental hazards and whether he likes his job. Duodenal ulcers arise more commonly in individuals with marked stress or job responsibility; gastric ulcers, in laborers. Inquire about the patient's history of blood transfusions and tattoos.

Assess the patient's financial status. Inadequate resources can add to the stress of being ill and exacerbate the underlying problem.

When talking to the patient, assess his cognition and comprehension levels to help determine his health education needs. Make sure that he understands the importance of appropriate treatment.

Physical assessment

A physical assessment of the GI system should include a thorough examination of the mouth, abdomen, and rectum. To perform an abdominal assessment, always use this sequence: inspection, auscultation, percussion, and palpation. Palpating or percussing the abdomen before auscultating can change the character of the patient's bowel sounds and lead to an inaccurate assessment.

Before beginning the physical assessment, explain the techniques to be used and warn the patient that some procedures might be uncomfortable. Perform the examination in a private, quiet, warm, and well-lighted room.

Oral cavity assessment

When examining the patient's GI system, begin by assessing the oral structures. Structural problems or disorders here may affect GI functioning. Use the following information as a guide when inspecting and palpating oral structures.

Inspection

First, inspect the patient's mouth and jaw for asymmetry and swelling. Check his bite, noting malocclusion from an overbite or underbite. Inspect the inner and outer lips, teeth, gums, and oral mucosa with a penlight. Note bleeding; ulcerations; carious, loose, missing, or broken teeth; and color changes, including rashes.

Assess the sides and under the surface of the tongue checking for coating, swelling, white or reddened areas, nodules, and ulcerations. Note unusual breath odors. Examine the pharynx by pressing a tongue blade firmly down on the middle of the tongue and asking the patient to say "ah." Look for uvular deviation, tonsillar abnormalities, lesions, plaques, and exudate.

Palpation

Palpate the gums, inner lips, and cheeks for tenderness, lumps, and lesions.

Abdominal assessment

Use inspection, auscultation, percussion, and palpation to examine the abdomen. To ensure an accurate assessment, take these actions before the examination:

- Ask the patient to empty his bladder.
- Drape the genitalia and the breasts of a female patient.
- Place a small pillow under the patient's knees to help relax the abdominal muscles.
- Ask the patient to keep his arms at his sides.
- Keep the room warm. Chilling can cause abdominal muscles to become tense.
- Warm your hands and the stethoscope.
- Approach the patient slowly and avoid quick, unexpected movements.
- Speak softly, and encourage the patient to perform breathing exercises or use imagery during uncomfortable procedures. Distract the patient with conversation or questions.
- Ask the patient to point to areas of pain.
- Watch the patient's face for signs of pain such as grimacing.

CRITICAL POINT *Assess painful areas last to help prevent the patient from becoming tense.*

Inspection

Begin by mentally dividing the abdomen into four quadrants and then imagining the organs in each quadrant. (See *Abdominal quadrants,* page 284.)

To more accurately pinpoint the physical findings, remember these three terms:

- epigastric — above the umbilicus and between the costal margins
- umbilical — around the navel
- suprapubic — above the symphysis pubis.

Observe the abdomen for symmetry, checking for bumps, bulges, or masses. Also, note the patient's abdominal shape and contour. The abdomen should be flat to rounded in people of average weight. A slender patient may have a slightly concave abdomen. A bulge in the abdominal area may indicate bladder distention or hernia. A protruding abdomen may be caused by obesity, pregnancy, ascites, or abdominal distention. Gas, a tumor, or a colon filled with stool can all cause abdominal distention.

Inspect the color and integrity of the abdomen. The skin should be smooth and uniform in color. Note dilated veins. Record

ABDOMINAL QUADRANTS

To perform a systematic GI assessment, visualize the patient's abdomen by dividing it into four quadrants, as shown here.

Right upper quadrant
- Right lobe of liver
- Gallbladder
- Pylorus
- Duodenum
- Head of the pancreas
- Hepatic flexure of the colon
- Portions of the ascending and transverse colon

Right lower quadrant
- Cecum and appendix
- Portion of the ascending colon

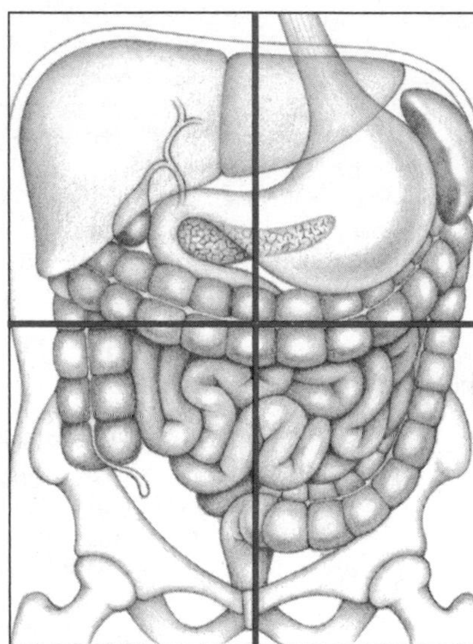

Left upper quadrant
- Left lobe of the liver
- Stomach
- Tail of the pancreas
- Splenic flexure of the colon
- Portions of the transverse and descending colon

Left lower quadrant
- Sigmoid colon
- Portion of the descending colon

the length of any surgical scars on the abdomen.

Striae, or stretch marks, can be caused by pregnancy, excessive weight gain, or ascites. New striae are pink or blue; old striae are silvery white (in patients with darker skin striae may be dark brown). Areas of abdominal redness may indicate inflammation. Bruising on the flank, or Turner's sign, indicates retroperitoneal hemorrhage. Dilated, tortuous, visible abdominal veins may indicate inferior vena cava obstruction. Cutaneous angiomas may signal liver disease.

Also observe the umbilicus, which should be located midline in the abdomen and inverted. Conditions, such as pregnancy, ascites, or an underlying mass can cause the umbilicus to protrude. Have the patient raise his head and shoulders. If his umbilicus protrudes, he may have an umbilical hernia. A bluish umbilicus, called Cullen's sign, indicates intra-abdominal hemorrhage.

Note abdominal movements and pulsations. Usually, waves of peristalsis can't be seen; if they're visible, they look like slight, wavelike motions.

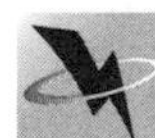

CRITICAL POINT *Visible rippling waves in the abdomen may indicate bowel obstruction and must immediately be reported.*

In thin patients, pulsation of the aorta is visible in the epigastric area. Marked pulsations may occur with hypertension, aortic insufficiency, aortic aneurysm, and other conditions causing widening pulse pressure.

Auscultation

Lightly place the stethoscope diaphragm in the right lower quadrant, slightly below and to the right of the umbilicus. Auscultate in a clockwise fashion in each of the four quadrants. Note the character and quality of bowel sounds in each quadrant. In some cases, you may need to auscultate for 5 minutes before you hear sounds. Make sure to allow enough time for listening in each quadrant before deciding that bowel sounds are absent.

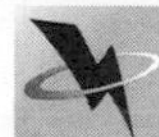

CRITICAL POINT *Before auscultating the abdomen of a patient with a nasogastric tube or another abdominal tube connected to suction, briefly clamp the tube or turn off the suction. Suction noises can obscure or mimic actual bowel sounds.*

Normal bowel sounds are high-pitched, gurgling noises caused by air mixing with fluid during peristalsis. The noises vary in frequency, pitch, and intensity and occur irregularly from 5 to 34 times per minute. They're loudest before mealtimes. Borborygmus, or stomach growling, is the loud, gurgling, splashing bowel sound heard over the large intestine as gas passes through it.

Bowel sounds are classified as normal, hypoactive, or hyperactive:

- Hyperactive bowel sounds — loud, high pitched, tinkling sounds that occur frequently — indicate increased intestinal motility and have be related to many factors, such as diarrhea, constipation, gastroenteritis, laxative use, and life-threatening intestinal obstruction.
- Hypoactive bowel sounds are heard infrequently. They're associated with ileus, bowel obstruction, or peritonitis and indicate diminished peristalsis. Recent bowel surgery or a full colon can all cause hypoactive bowel sounds. Paralytic ileus, torsion of the bowel, and the use of narcotics and other medications can decrease peristalsis. (See *Interpreting abnormal abdominal sounds,* page 286.)

Auscultate for vascular sounds with the bell of the stethoscope. Using firm pressure, listen over the aorta and renal, iliac, and femoral arteries for bruits, venous hums, and friction rubs. Friction rubs over the liver and spleen in the epigastric region may indicate splenic infarction or hepatic tumor. Abdominal bruits may be caused by aortic aneurysms or partial arterial obstruction. (See *Auscultating for vascular sounds,* page 287.)

Percussion

Direct or indirect percussion is used to detect the size and location of abdominal organs and to detect air or fluid in the abdomen, stomach, or bowel.

In direct percussion, strike the hand or finger directly against the patient's abdomen. With indirect percussion, use the middle finger of the dominant hand or a percussion hammer to strike a finger resting on the patient's abdomen. Begin percussion in the right lower quadrant and proceed clockwise, covering all four quadrants.

CRITICAL POINT *Abdominal percussion or palpation is contraindicated in patients with suspected abdominal aortic aneurysm, those who have received abdominal organ transplants, and in children with suspected Wilms' tumor. If performing abdominal percussion or palpation in patients with suspected appendicitis use extreme caution so as not to precipitate a rupture.*

During abdominal percussion, listen for two sounds: tympany and dullness. When percussing over hollow organs, such as an empty stomach or bowel, you hear a clear, hollow sound like a drum beating. This sound, tympany, predominates because air is normally present in the stomach and bowel. The degree of tympany depends on the amount of air and gastric dilation.

When percussing over solid organs — such as the liver, kidney, urine-filled bladder, or stool-filled intestines — the sound changes to dullness. Note where percussed sounds change from tympany to dullness. (See *Sites of tympany and dullness,* page 287.)

Liver percussion. Percussion of the liver can help you estimate its size. (See *Percussing and measuring the liver,* page 288.)

An enlarged liver indicates hepatomegaly. Hepatomegaly is commonly associated with patients who have hepatitis and other liver diseases. Liver borders may be obscured and difficult to assess due to effusion, fluid, or infection in the lung, or gas in the colon.

Spleen percussion. The spleen is located at about the level of the 10th rib, in the left midaxillary line. Percussion may produce a small area of dullness, generally 7″ (18 cm) or less in adults. However, the spleen usually can't be percussed because tympany from the colon masks the dullness of the spleen. It's difficult to distinguish between the dullness of the posterior flank and the dullness of the spleen.

INTERPRETING ABNORMAL ABDOMINAL SOUNDS

Sound and description	Location	Possible cause
Abnormal bowel sounds		
Hyperactive sounds (unrelated to hunger)	Any quadrant	Diarrhea, laxative use, or early intestinal obstruction
Hypoactive, then absent sounds	Any quadrant	Paralytic ileus or peritonitis
High-pitched tinkling sounds	Any quadrant	Intestinal fluid and air under tension in a dilated bowel
High-pitched rushing sounds coinciding with abdominal cramps	Any quadrant	Intestinal obstruction
Systolic bruits		
Vascular blowing sounds resembling cardiac murmurs	Over abdominal aorta	Partial arterial obstruction or turbulent blood flow
	Over renal artery	Renal artery stenosis
	Over iliac artery	Hepatomegaly
	Over femoral artery	Arterial insufficiency in the legs
Venous hum (rare)		
Continuous, medium-pitched tone with both systolic and diastolic components, created by blood flow in a large engorged vascular organ such as the liver	Epigastric and umbilical regions	Increased collateral circulation between portal and systemic venous systems such as with cirrhosis
Friction rub (rare)		
Harsh, grating sound like two pieces of sandpaper rubbing together	Over liver and spleen	Inflammation of the peritoneal surface of liver, such as from a tumor or splenic infarct (When a systolic bruit is also present, suspect liver cancer.)

To assess a patient for splenic enlargement, ask him to breathe deeply and then percuss along the 9th to 11th intercostal spaces on the left, listening for a change from tympany to dullness. Measure the area of dullness, which is called a positive splenic percussion sign.

CRITICAL POINT *During percussion, tympany produced by colonic or gastric air is heard over the spleen area. If dullness is heard, suspect splenic enlargement; if resonance is heard, suspect left kidney enlargement.*

Palpation

Abdominal palpation includes light and deep touch to help determine the size, shape, position, and tenderness of major abdominal organs, and to detect masses and fluid accumulation. Palpate all four quad-

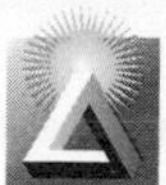

EXPERT TECHNIQUE

AUSCULTATING FOR VASCULAR SOUNDS

Use the bell of the stethoscope to auscultate for vascular sounds at the sites shown in the illustration.

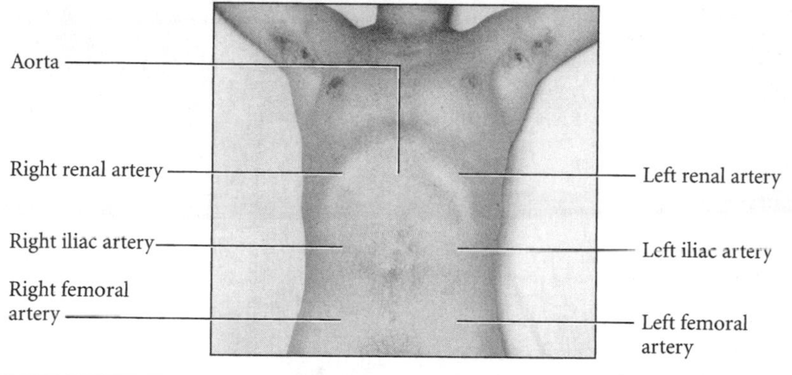

SITES OF TYMPANY AND DULLNESS

Expect to auscultate tympany and dullness in the areas shown here.

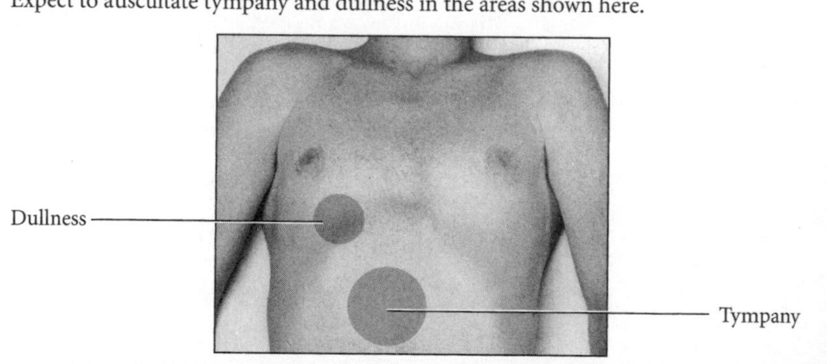

rants, leaving painful and tender areas for last. (See *Recognizing types of abdominal pain,* page 289.)

Light palpation. Light palpation helps identify muscle resistance and tenderness as well as the location of some superficial organs. To palpate, put the fingers of one hand close together, depress the skin about ½″ (1.5 cm) with your fingertips, and make gentle, rotating movements. Avoid short, quick jabs.

The abdomen should be soft and nontender. Palpate the four quadrants, noting organs, masses, and areas of tenderness or increased resistance. Determine whether resistance is due to the patient's being cold, tense, or ticklish, or whether it's due to involuntary guarding or rigidity from muscle

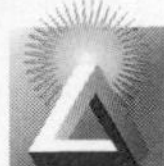

EXPERT TECHNIQUE

PERCUSSING AND MEASURING THE LIVER

To percuss and measure the liver, follow these steps:

- Identify the upper border of liver dullness. Start in the right midclavicular line in an area of lung resonance, and percuss downward toward the liver. Use a pen to mark the spot where the sound changes to dullness.
- Start in the right midclavicular line at a level below the umbilicus, and lightly percuss upward toward the liver. Mark the spot where the sound changes from tympany to dullness.
- Use a ruler to measure the vertical span between the two marked spots, as shown. In an adult, a normal liver span ranges from 2½″ to 4¾″ (6.5 to 12 cm).

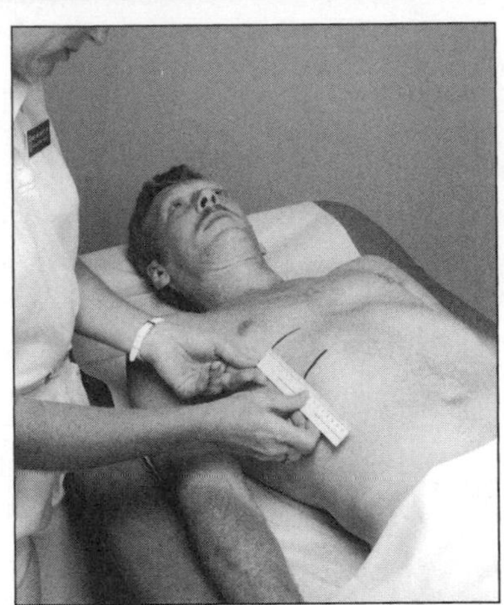

spasms or peritoneal inflammation. (See *Recognizing voluntary rigidity,* page 290.)

Help the ticklish patient relax by putting his hand over yours as you palpate. This usually decreases involuntary muscle contractions in response to touch. If he complains of abdominal tenderness even before you touch him, palpate by placing a stethoscope lightly on his abdomen.

Deep palpation. To perform deep palpation, push the abdomen down about 2″ to 3″ (5 to 7.5 cm). In an obese patient, put one hand on top of the other and push. Palpate the entire abdomen in a clockwise direction, checking for tenderness, pulsations, organ enlargement, and masses. Check for McBurney's sign. (See *Eliciting McBurney's sign,* page 290.) If you detect a mass on light or deep palpation, note its location, size, shape, consistency, type of border, degree of tenderness, presence of pulsations, and degree of mobility (fixed or mobile).

CRITICAL POINT *If the patient's abdomen is rigid, don't palpate it. He could have peritoneal inflammation, and palpation could cause pain or could rupture an inflamed organ.*

If the patient's abdomen is distended, assess its progression by taking serial measurements of abdominal girth. To do this, wrap a tape measure around the patient's abdomen at the level of the umbilicus and record the measurement. Be sure to mark the point of measurement with a felt-tip pen to ensure that subsequent readings are taken at the same point.

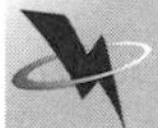

CRITICAL POINT *Don't palpate a pulsating midline mass; it may be a dissecting aneurysm, which can rupture under the pressure of palpation. Immediately report such a mass.*

LIVER PALPATION. Palpate the patient's liver to check for enlargement and tenderness. (See *Palpating the liver,* page 291.)

SPLEEN PALPATION. Unless the spleen is enlarged, it isn't palpable. (See *Palpating the spleen,* page 291.)

A markedly enlarged spleen descends into the left lower quadrant of the abdomen. A notch felt along its medial border distinguishes an enlarged spleen from an enlarged kidney.

RECOGNIZING TYPES OF ABDOMINAL PAIN

When assessing your patient with abdominal pain, use this chart to quickly identify the affected organ and the most likely source of the pain.

Affected organ	Visceral pain	Parietal pain	Referred pain
Stomach	Midepigastrium	Midepigastrium and left upper quadrant	Shoulders
Small intestine	Periumbilical area	Over affected site	Midback (rare)
Appendix	Periumbilical area	Right lower quadrant	Right lower quadrant
Proximal colon	Periumbilical area and right flank for ascending colon	Over affected site	Right lower quadrant and back (rare)
Distal colon	Hypogastrium and left flank for descending colon	Over affected site	Left lower quadrant and back (rare)
Gallbladder	Midepigastrium	Right upper quadrant	Right subscapular area
Ureters	Costovertebral angle	Over affected site	Groin; scrotum in men, labia in women (rare)
Pancreas	Midepigastrium and left upper quadrant	Midepigastrium and left upper quadrant	Back and left shoulder
Ovaries, fallopian tubes, and uterus	Hypogastrium and groin	Over affected site	Inner thighs

CRITICAL POINT *If you do feel the spleen, stop palpating immediately because compression can cause rupture.*

Specialized assessments

When assessing a patient's abdomen, it may be necessary to perform specialized assessments to check for rebound tenderness or ascites. The techniques of fluid wave, shifting dullness, and ballottement are discussed here.

Rebound tenderness

Perform the test for rebound tenderness when you suspect peritoneal inflammation. Check for rebound tenderness at the end of the examination.

Choosing a site away from the painful area, position your hand at a 90-degree angle to the abdomen. Push down slowly and deeply into the abdomen, then withdraw your hand quickly. Rapid withdrawal causes the underlying structures to rebound suddenly and results in a sharp, stabbing pain on the inflamed side. Alternatively, indirect-

EXPERT TECHNIQUE

RECOGNIZING VOLUNTARY RIGIDITY

Distinguishing voluntary from involuntary abdominal rigidity is a must for accurate assessment. Review this comparison so that you can quickly tell the two apart.

Voluntary rigidity
- Usually symmetrical
- More rigid on inspiration (expiration causes muscle relaxation)
- Eased by relaxation techniques, such as positioning the patient comfortably and talking to him in a calm, soothing manner
- Painless when the patient sits up using his abdominal muscles alone

Involuntary rigidity
- Usually asymmetrical
- Equally rigid on inspiration and expiration
- Unaffected by relaxation techniques
- Painful when the patient sits up using his abdominal muscles alone

EXPERT TECHNIQUE

ELICITING MCBURNEY'S SIGN

To elicit McBurney's sign, help the patient into a supine position, with his knees slightly flexed and his abdominal muscles relaxed. Then, palpate deeply and slowly in the right lower quadrant over McBurney's point—located about 2″ (5 cm) from the right anterior superior spine of the ilium, on a line between the spine and the umbilicus. Point pain and tenderness, a positive McBurney's sign, indicates appendicitis.

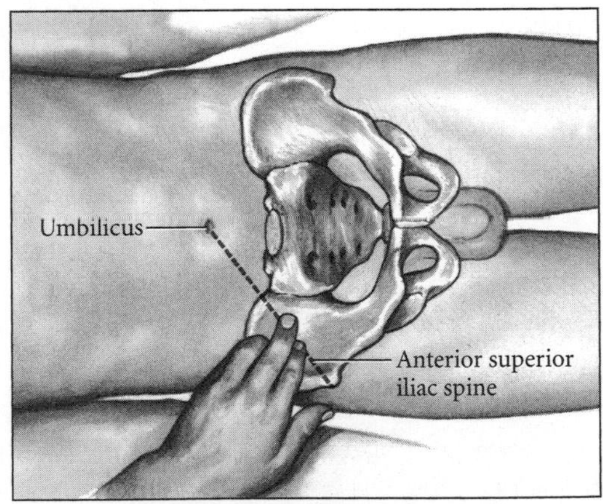

ly percuss the area lightly. (See *Eliciting rebound tenderness,* page 292.)

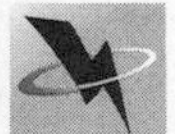

CRITICAL POINT *Peritonitis or appendicitis can cause rebound tenderness. However, not all patients have the classic right lower quadrant pain. Some older adults with appendicitis have less abdominal rigidity than younger patients. Because appendicitis may be accompanied by increased abdominal wall resistance and guarding, perform the maneuver for rebound tenderness only once—repeating the maneuver can rupture an inflamed appendix.*

Ascites

Ascites, a large accumulation of fluid in the peritoneal cavity, can be caused by advanced

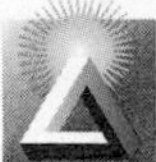

EXPERT TECHNIQUE

PALPATING THE LIVER

These illustrations demonstrate the correct hand positions for two methods of palpating the liver.

Palpating the liver

- Place the patient in the supine position. Standing at his right side, place your left hand under his back at the approximate location of the liver.
- Place your right hand slightly below the mark you made earlier at the liver's upper border. Point the fingers of your right hand toward the patient's head just under the right costal margin.
- As the patient inhales deeply, gently press in and up on the abdomen until the liver brushes under your right hand. The edge should be smooth, firm, and somewhat round. Note any tenderness.

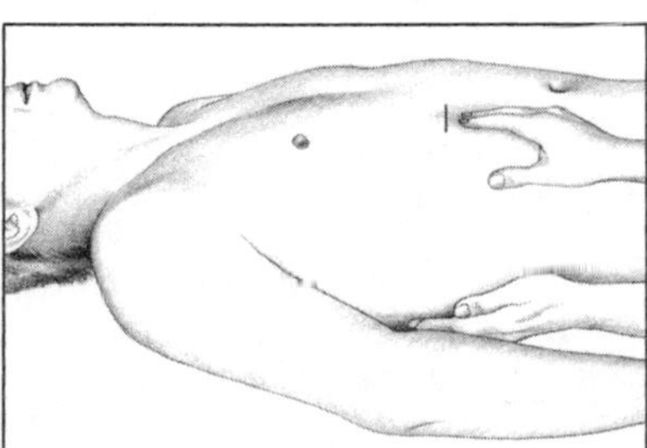

Hooking the liver

- Hooking is an alternate way of palpating the liver. To hook the liver, stand next to the patient's right shoulder, facing his feet. Place your hands side by side, and hook your fingertips over the right costal margin, below the lower mark of dullness.
- Ask the patient to take a deep breath as you push your fingertips in and up. If the liver is palpable, you may feel its edge as it slides down in the abdomen as he inhales.

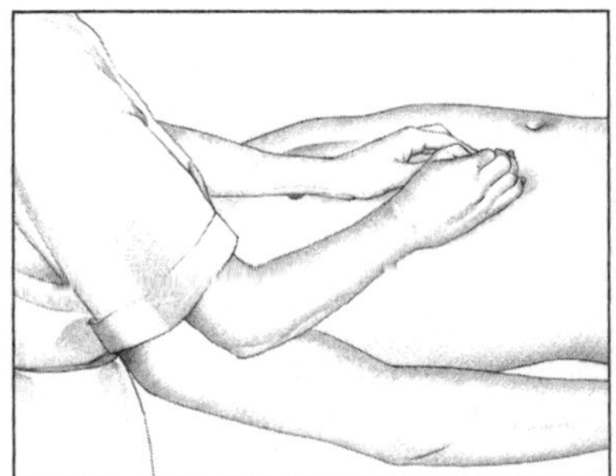

EXPERT TECHNIQUE

PALPATING THE SPLEEN

Although a normal spleen isn't palpable, an enlarged spleen is. To palpate the spleen, stand on the patient's right side. Use your left hand to support his posterior left lower rib cage. Ask him to take a deep breath. Then, with your right hand on his abdomen, press up and in toward the spleen, as shown.

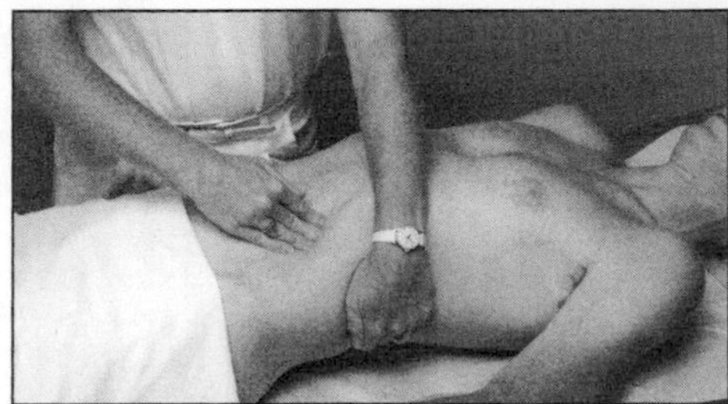

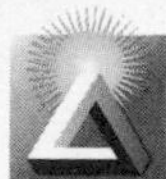

EXPERT TECHNIQUE

ELICITING REBOUND TENDERNESS

Palpating the abdomen

To elicit rebound tenderness, help the patient into a supine position, and push your fingers deeply and steadily into his abdomen (as shown). Then quickly release the pressure. Pain that results from the rebound of palpated tissue—rebound tenderness—indicates peritoneal inflammation or peritonitis.

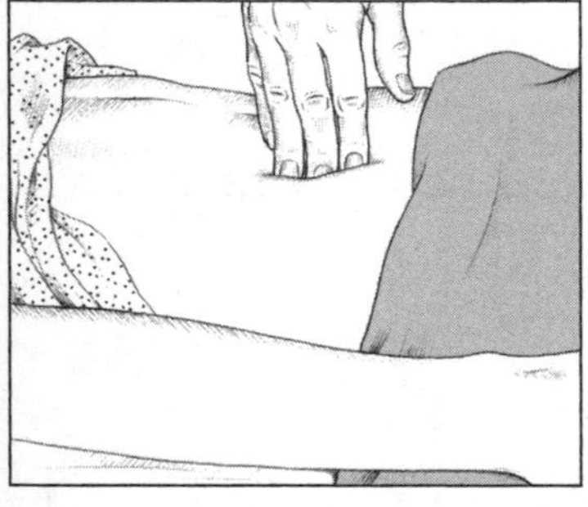

Percussing the abdomen

You can also elicit this symptom on a miniature scale by percussing the patient's abdomen lightly and indirectly (as shown). Or, simply ask the patient to cough. This allows you to elicit rebound tenderness without having to touch the patient's abdomen and may also increase his cooperation because he won't associate exacerbation of his pain with your actions.

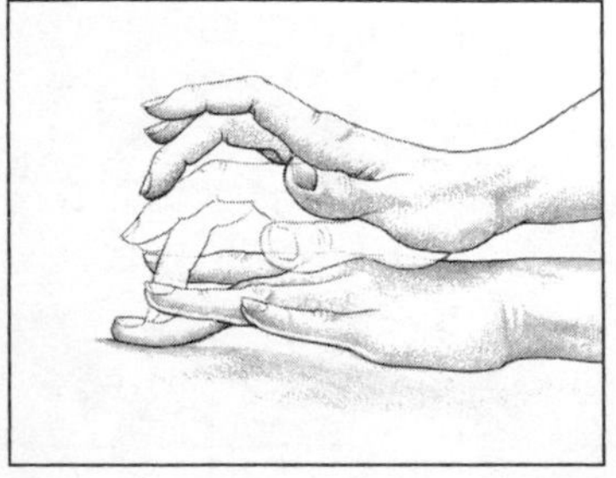

liver disease, heart failure, pancreatitis, or cancer.

If ascites is present, use a tape measure to measure the fullest part of the abdomen. Mark this point on the patient's abdomen with indelible ink to ensure consistent measurement. This measurement is important, especially if fluid removal or paracentesis is performed.

Two maneuvers are useful in checking for ascites: assessing for shifting dullness and assessing for fluid wave. (See *Detecting ascites.*)

Shifting dullness. A protuberant abdomen with bulging flanks suggests ascites. Percuss the abdomen outward from the umbilicus in several directions. Fluid sinks with gravity so if ascites is present, dependent areas of the abdomen will be dull and gas-filled bowel that floats to the top will be tympanic.

Now ask the patient to turn on his side. Percuss again. In a patient without ascites the borders between tympany and dullness will remain about the same. If ascites is present, the dullness shifts to the more dependent side and the tympany shifts to the top.

Fluid wave. Have an assistant place the ulnar edge of her hand firmly on the patient's abdomen at its midline. Then, standing and facing the patient's head, place the palm of your right hand against the patient's left flank. Give the right abdomen a firm tap with your left hand. If ascites is present, you may see and feel a "fluid wave" ripple across the abdomen.

Ballottement

Ballottement involves lightly tapping or bouncing your fingertips against the abdominal wall. This technique helps elicit abdominal muscle resistance or guarding that can be missed with deep palpation, or it may detect the movement or bounce of a freely movable mass. Your fingers should also bounce at the underlying dense liver tissue in the right upper quadrant. If the patient has ascites, you may need to use deep ballottement.

To do so, push fingertips deeply inward in a rapid motion; then quickly release the pressure, maintaining fingertip contact with the abdominal wall. You should feel the

EXPERT TECHNIQUE

DETECTING ASCITES

To differentiate ascites from other causes of abdominal distention, check for shifting dullness and fluid wave, as described here:

Shifting dullness

Step 1. With the patient in a supine position, percuss from the umbilicus outward to the flank, as shown. Draw a line on the patient's skin to mark the change from tympany to dullness.

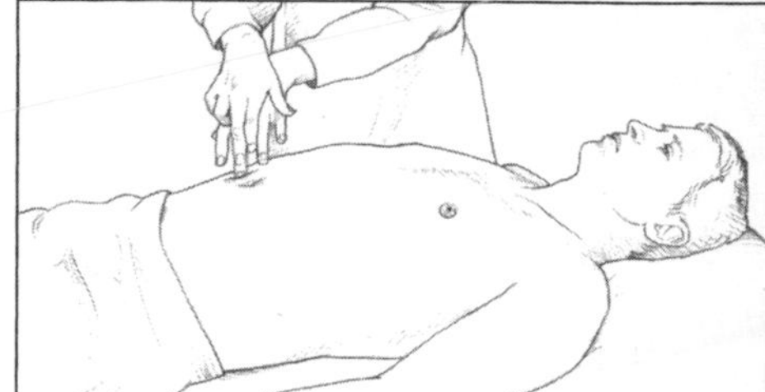

Step 2. Turn the patient onto his side. (Note that this positioning causes ascitic fluid to shift.) Percuss again and mark the change from tympany to dullness. Any difference between these lines can indicate ascites.

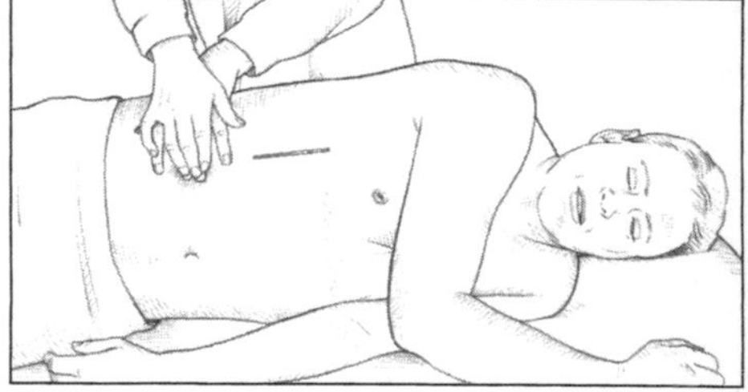

Fluid wave

Have another person press deeply into the patient's midline to prevent vibration from traveling along the abdominal wall. Place one of your palms on one of the patient's flanks, as shown. Strike the opposite flank with your other hand. If you feel the blow in the opposite palm, ascitic fluid is present.

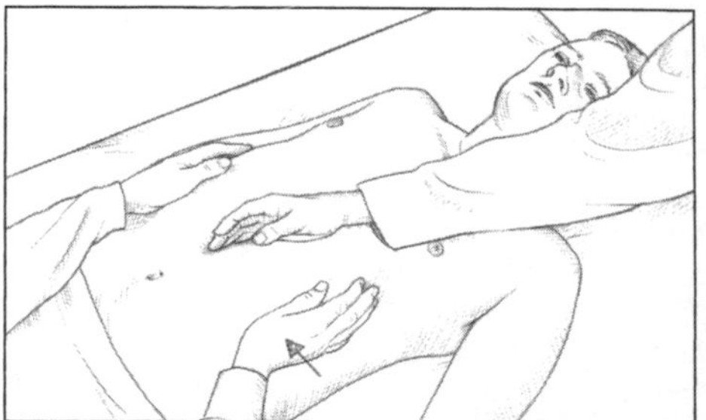

movement of an underlying organ or a movable mass toward your fingertips.

Rectal and anal assessment

If the patient is age 40 or older, perform a rectal examination as part of the GI assessment. Before performing this assessment, make sure to explain the procedure to the patient.

Inspection

First, inspect the perianal area. Put on gloves and spread the buttocks to expose the anus and surrounding tissue, checking for fissures, lesions, scars, inflammation, discharge, rectal prolapse, and external hemorrhoids. Ask the patient to strain as if he's having a bowel movement; this may reveal internal hemorrhoids, polyps, or fissures. The skin in the perianal area is normally somewhat darker than that of the surrounding area.

Palpation

Next palpate the rectum. Apply a water-soluble lubricant to a gloved index finger. Warn the patient that he'll feel some pressure. Ask the patient to strain down. As the sphincter relaxes, gently insert the finger into the rectum, toward the umbilicus. If you feel the sphincter tighten, pause and reassure the patient. Continue the examination when the sphincter relaxes again. Rotate the finger clockwise and counterclockwise to palpate all aspects of the rectal wall for nodules, tenderness, irregularities, and fecal impaction. The rectal wall should feel smooth and soft. In a female patient, try to feel the posterior side of the uterus through the anterior rectal wall. In a male patient, assess the prostate gland when palpating the anterior rectal wall; the prostate should feel firm and smooth.

With the lubricated finger fully inserted, ask the patient to bear down again; this may cause any lesions higher in the rectum to move down to a palpable level.

To assess anal sphincter competence, ask the patient to tighten the anal muscles around your finger. Finally, withdraw your finger and examine it for blood, mucus, or stool. Test fecal matter adhering to the glove for occult blood using a guaiac test.

Ongoing assessment

Whenever a patient reports a GI complaint, he'll need reassessment. Don't assume, for instance, that a previously assessed dysfunction is causing the patient's present abdominal pain. The pain's nature and location may have changed, indicating more extensive involvement or perhaps a new disorder. To avoid unduly alarming the patient, reassure him that ongoing assessment doesn't necessarily mean he has a significant health problem. Tell him that repeated evaluations aid diagnosis and treatment.

Abnormal findings

A patient may seek care for any of a number of signs and symptoms related to the GI system. Some common findings include abdominal distention, abdominal mass, abdominal pain, abdominal rigidity, abnormal bowel sounds (hyperactive or hypoactive), constipation, diarrhea, dyspepsia, hematemesis, hematochezia, melena, nausea and vomiting, pyrosis, and clay-colored stools. Dysphagia is also a common GI complaint. (See chapter 7, Ears, nose, and throat, which discusses this symptom.) The following history, physical examination, and analysis summaries will help you assess each one quickly and accurately. After obtaining further information, begin to interpret the findings. (See *GI system: Interpreting your findings.*)

Abdominal distention

Abdominal distention refers to increased abdominal girth — the result of increased intra-abdominal pressure forcing the abdominal wall outward. Distention may be mild or severe, depending on the amount of pressure. It may be localized or diffuse and may occur gradually or suddenly. Acute abdominal distention may signal life-threatening peritonitis or acute bowel obstruction.

History

If the patient's abdominal distention isn't acute, ask about its onset and duration and associated signs. A patient with localized distention may report a sensation of pressure, fullness, or tenderness in the affected area. With generalized distention, the patient may report a bloated feeling, a pounding heart, and difficulty breathing deeply or when lying flat. The patient may also feel unable to bend at his waist. Ask about abdominal pain, fever, nausea, vomiting, anorexia, altered bowel habits, and weight gain or loss.

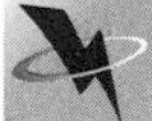

CRITICAL POINT *With abdominal distention, quickly check for signs of hypovolemia, such as pallor, diaphoresis, hypotension, rapid thready pulse, rapid shallow breathing, decreased urine output, poor capillary refill, and altered mentation. Ask the patient if he's experiencing severe abdominal pain or difficulty breathing. Find out about any recent accidents, and observe the patient for signs of trauma and peritoneal bleeding, such as Cullen's or Turner's sign. Then auscultate all abdominal quadrants, noting rapid and high-pitched, diminished, or absent bowel sounds. (If you don't*

(Text continues on page 303.)

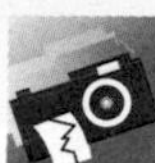

CLINICAL PICTURE

GI SYSTEM: INTERPRETING YOUR FINDINGS

After you assess the patient, a group of findings may lead you to a particular disorder of the GI system. The chart below shows some common groups of findings for major signs and symptoms related to an assessment of the GI system, along with their probable causes.

Sign or symptom and findings	Probable cause
Abdominal distention	
■ Generalized distention with ascites ■ Positive fluid wave ■ Shifting dullness ■ Umbilical eversion with dilated veins around umbilicus ■ Feeling of fullness or weight gain ■ Vague abdominal pain ■ Fever ■ Anorexia ■ Nausea and vomiting ■ Constipation or diarrhea ■ Bleeding tendencies ■ Severe pruritus ■ Spider angiomas ■ Leg edema ■ Possible splenomegaly	Cirrhosis
■ Intermittent, localized distention ■ Lower abdominal pain or cramping usually relieved by defecation or passage of flatus ■ Alternating diarrhea and constipation ■ Nausea ■ Dyspepsia ■ Straining and urgency at defecation ■ Feeling of incomplete evacuation ■ Small mucus-streaked stools	Irritable bowel syndrome
Abdominal distention *(continued)*	
■ Dramatic distention with loops of bowel possibly visible on abdomen ■ Constipation ■ Tympany ■ High-pitched bowel sounds ■ Sudden onset of colicky lower abdominal pain that becomes persistent ■ Fecal vomiting ■ Diminished peristaltic waves and bowel sounds (late)	Large bowel obstruction
■ Localized or generalized distention ■ Fluid wave and shifting dullness ■ Sudden and severe abdominal pain that worsens with movement ■ Rebound tenderness ■ Abdominal rigidity ■ Taut skin over abdomen ■ Hypoactive or absent bowel sounds ■ Fever and chills ■ Hyperalgesia ■ Nausea and vomiting	Peritonitis

(continued)

GI SYSTEM: INTERPRETING YOUR FINDINGS *(continued)*

Sign or symptom and findings	Probable cause
Abdominal mass	
▪ Pulsating abdominal mass with systolic bruit over aorta ▪ Constant upper abdominal pain or low back or dull abdominal pain; pain severe if aneurysm ruptures ▪ Mottled skin below the waist ▪ Absent femoral and pedal pulses ▪ Lower blood pressure in the legs than in the arms ▪ Mild to moderate tenderness with guarding and abdominal rigidity ▪ Possible shock	Abdominal aortic aneurysm
▪ Right lower quadrant mass ▪ Occult bleeding with anemia ▪ Abdominal aching, pressure, or dull cramps ▪ Weakness ▪ Fatigue ▪ Exertional dyspnea ▪ Vertigo ▪ Intestinal obstruction	Colon cancer, right side
▪ Smooth, round fluctuant mass resembling a distended bladder in the suprapubic region ▪ Mild pelvic discomfort ▪ Low back pain ▪ Menstrual irregularities ▪ Hirsutism	Ovarian cyst
Abdominal mass *(continued)*	
▪ Round multinodular mass in suprapubic region ▪ Menorrhagia ▪ Feeling of heaviness and pressure in abdomen ▪ Constipation ▪ Urinary frequency or urgency	Uterine fibroids
Abdominal pain	
▪ Localized abdominal pain, described as steady, gnawing, burning, aching, or hungerlike, high in the midepigastrium, slightly off center, usually on the right ▪ Pain begins 2 to 4 hours after a meal ▪ Ingestion of food or antacids brings relief ▪ Changes in bowel habits ▪ Heartburn or retrosternal burning	Duodenal ulcer
▪ Pain and tenderness in the right or left lower abdominal quadrant, may become sharp and severe on standing or stooping ▪ Abdominal distention ▪ Mild nausea and vomiting ▪ Occasional menstrual irregularities ▪ Slight fever	Ovarian cyst

GI SYSTEM: INTERPRETING YOUR FINDINGS *(continued)*

Sign or symptom and findings	Probable cause
Abdominal pain *(continued)*	
▪ Referred, severe upper abdominal pain, tenderness, and rigidity that diminish with inspiration ▪ Fever, shaking chills, achiness ▪ Blood-tinged or rusty sputum ▪ Dry, hacking cough ▪ Dyspnea	Pneumonia
Abdominal rigidity	
▪ Mild to moderate rigidity accompanied by constant upper abdominal pain possibly radiating to lower back; increased pain when lying down and possibly relieved by sitting up or leaning forward ▪ Pulsating mass in epigastrium with systolic bruit over aorta; pulsations ceasing after rupture ▪ Mottled skin below the waist ▪ Absent femoral and pedal pulses ▪ Lower blood pressure in legs than in arms ▪ Mild to moderate tenderness with guarding	Abdominal aortic aneurysm dissection
Abdominal rigidity *(continued)*	
▪ Localized or generalized rigidity ▪ Sudden and severe abdominal pain ▪ Abdominal tenderness ▪ Guarding ▪ Hyperalgesia ▪ Hypoactive or absent bowel sounds ▪ Nausea and vomiting ▪ Fever, chills ▪ Tachycardia, tachypnea ▪ Hypotension	Peritonitis
Bowel sounds, hyperactive	
▪ Insidious onset of hyperactive sounds ▪ Diarrhea ▪ Cramping abdominal pain possibly relieved by defecation ▪ Anorexia ▪ Low-grade fever ▪ Abdominal distention, tenderness ▪ Fixed mass in right lower quadrant	Crohn's disease
▪ Hyperactive sounds along with cramping abdominal pain every few minutes; bowel sounds later becoming hypoactive and then absent ▪ Nausea, vomiting ▪ Abdominal distention ▪ Constipation; bowel part distal to obstruction may continue to empty for up to 3 days	Bowel obstruction, mechanical

(continued)

GI SYSTEM: INTERPRETING YOUR FINDINGS *(continued)*

Sign or symptom and findings	Probable cause
Bowel sounds, hyperactive *(continued)*	
▪ Abrupt onset of hyperactive sounds ▪ Bloody diarrhea ▪ Anorexia ▪ Abdominal pain ▪ Nausea and vomiting ▪ Fever ▪ Tenesmus ▪ Weight loss ▪ Arthralgias ▪ Arthritis	Ulcerative colitis
Bowel sounds, hypoactive	
▪ Hypoactive after a period of hyperactivity ▪ Acute colicky abdominal pain in the quadrant of the obstruction possibly radiating to the flank or lumbar region ▪ Nausea and vomiting ▪ Constipation ▪ Abdominal distention and bloating	Bowel obstruction, mechanical
▪ Hypoactive sounds that may become absent ▪ Abdominal distention ▪ Generalized discomfort ▪ Constipation or passage of small liquid stools and flatus	Paralytic ileus
Constipation	
▪ Constipation or diarrhea with left lower quadrant pain and tenderness ▪ Possible palpable tender firm, fixed abdominal mass ▪ Mild nausea, flatulence ▪ Possible low-grade fever	Diverticulitis
▪ Constipation occurring early on and insidiously ▪ Fatigue ▪ Sensitivity to cold ▪ Anorexia with weight gain ▪ Menorrhagia ▪ Decreased memory ▪ Hearing impairment ▪ Muscle cramps ▪ Paresthesia	Hypothyroidism
▪ Chronic constipation possibly with intermittent watery diarrhea or alternating with diarrhea ▪ Nausea ▪ Abdominal distention and tenderness relieved with defecation ▪ Intense urge to defecate with feelings of incomplete bowel evacuation ▪ Scybalous stools with mucus	Irritable bowel syndrome

GI SYSTEM: INTERPRETING YOUR FINDINGS *(continued)*

Sign or symptom and findings	Probable cause
Constipation *(continued)*	
■ Constipation along with ocular disturbances such as nystagmus, blurred vision, and diplopia ■ Vertigo ■ Sensory disturbances ■ Motor weakness ■ Seizures ■ Paralysis ■ Muscle spasticity ■ Ataxia ■ Intention tremor ■ Hyperreflexia ■ Dysarthria or dysphagia	Multiple sclerosis
Diarrhea	
■ Soft, unformed stools or watery diarrhea that may be foul-smelling or grossly bloody ■ Abdominal pain, cramping, and tenderness ■ Fever	*Clostridium difficile* infection
■ Diarrhea occurs within several hours of ingesting milk or milk products ■ Abdominal pain, cramping, and bloating ■ Borborygmi ■ Flatus	Lactose intolerance
■ Recurrent bloody diarrhea with pus or mucus ■ Hyperactive bowel sounds ■ Cramping lower abdominal pain ■ Occasional nausea and vomiting	Ulcerative colitis
Dyspepsia	
■ Dyspepsia ranging from vague feeling of fullness or pressure to a boring or aching sensation in the middle or right epigastrium usually occurring 1½ to 3 hours after eating ■ Relief with food intake or antacid ingestion ■ Pain possibly awakening the patient at night with heartburn and fluid regurgitation ■ Abdominal tenderness ■ Weight gain	Duodenal ulcer
■ Dyspepsia with heartburn after eating ■ Epigastric pain ■ Possible vomiting, fullness, and abdominal distention; relief not always with food intake ■ Weight loss ■ GI bleeding	Gastric ulcer
■ Feeling of fullness usually with severe continuous or intermittent epigastric pain radiating to the back or through the abdomen ■ Anorexia ■ Nausea, vomiting ■ Jaundice ■ Dramatic weight loss ■ Hyperglycemia ■ Steatorrhea ■ Turner's or Cullen's sign	Pancreatitis, chronic

(continued)

GI SYSTEM: INTERPRETING YOUR FINDINGS *(continued)*

Sign or symptom and findings	Probable cause
Dyspepsia *(continued)*	
■ Early onset of dyspepsia ■ Anorexia ■ Nausea and vomiting ■ Bloating ■ Diarrhea ■ Abdominal cramps ■ Epigastric pain ■ Weight gain ■ Edema, pruritus, pallor, hyperpigmentation, uremic frost, ecchymoses, sexual dysfunction, poor memory, irritability, headache, drowsiness, muscle twitching, seizures, and oliguria with continued renal system deterioration	Uremia
Hematemesis	
■ Moderate to severe GI bleeding in emesis with bleeding in other body systems ■ Epistaxis ■ Ecchymosis ■ Thrombocytopenia	Coagulation disorders
■ Coffee-ground or massive, bright-red vomitus ■ Hypotension ■ Tachycardia ■ Abdominal distention ■ Melena ■ Painless hematochezia ranging from slight oozing to massive rectal hemorrhage	Esophageal varices, rupture
Hematemesis *(continued)*	
■ Hematemesis accompanied by pyrosis, flatulence, dyspepsia, and postural regurgitation aggravated by lying down or stooping ■ Dysphagia ■ Retrosternal angina-like chest pain ■ Weight loss ■ Halitosis ■ Aspiration	Gastroesophageal reflux disease (GERD)
■ Hematemesis triggered by severe vomiting, retching, or straining ■ Severe bleeding leading to shock	Mallory-Weiss syndrome
Hematochezia	
■ Moderate to severe rectal bleeding ■ Epistaxis ■ Purpura	Coagulation disorders
■ Bright-red rectal bleeding with or without pain ■ Diarrhea or ribbon-shaped stools ■ Stools may be grossly bloody ■ Weakness and fatigue ■ Abdominal aching and dull cramps	Colon cancer
■ Chronic bleeding with defecation ■ Painful defecation	Hemorrhoids

GI SYSTEM: INTERPRETING YOUR FINDINGS *(continued)*

Sign or symptom and findings	Probable cause
Melena	
▪ Melena occurring early on if mass on right side of colon; occurring late or rarely if mass on left side ▪ Abdominal aching, pressure, or cramps ▪ Weakness, fatigue ▪ Anemia ▪ Diarrhea or obstipation; pencil-like stools if mass on the left ▪ Anorexia ▪ Weight loss	Colon cancer
▪ Melena, hematochezia, and hematemesis ▪ Signs of shock such as tachycardia; tachypnea; hypotension; and cool, clammy skin ▪ Agitation and confusion signaling hepatic encephalopathy	Esophageal varices, ruptured
▪ Melena accompanied by hematemesis ▪ Mild epigastric or abdominal discomfort exacerbated by eating ▪ Belching ▪ Nausea and vomiting ▪ Malaise	Gastritis
Melena *(continued)*	
▪ Melena signaling life-threatening hemorrhage ▪ Decreased appetite ▪ Nausea and vomiting ▪ Hematemesis ▪ Hematochezia ▪ Left epigastric pain that's gnawing, burning, or sharp often described as heartburn or indigestion	Peptic ulcer
Nausea and vomiting	
▪ Nausea and vomiting follow or accompany abdominal pain ▪ Pain progressing rapidly to severe, stabbing pain in the right lower quadrant (McBurney's sign) ▪ Abdominal rigidity and tenderness ▪ Constipation or diarrhea ▪ Tachycardia	Appendicitis
▪ Nausea and vomiting of undigested food ▪ Diarrhea ▪ Abdominal cramping ▪ Hyperactive bowel sounds ▪ Fever	Gastroenteritis

(continued)

GI SYSTEM: INTERPRETING YOUR FINDINGS *(continued)*

Sign or symptom and findings	Probable cause
Nausea and vomiting *(continued)*	
▪ Nausea and vomiting ▪ Headache with severe, constant, throbbing pain ▪ Fatigue ▪ Photophobia ▪ Light flashes ▪ Increased noise sensitivity	Migraine headache
Pyrosis	
▪ Severe pyrosis that's chronic usually occurring 30 to 60 minutes after eating; possibly triggered by foods or beverages; becoming worse when lying down or bending; relieved with sitting or standing upright ▪ Postural regurgitation ▪ Dysphagia ▪ Flatulent dyspepsia ▪ Dull, retrosternal pain possibly radiating	GERD
▪ Eructation after eating and accompanied by heartburn, regurgitation of sour-tasting fluid, and abdominal distention ▪ Dull, substernal or epigastric pain possibly radiating to shoulder ▪ Dysphagia ▪ Nausea ▪ Weight loss ▪ Dyspnea, tachypnea, cough ▪ Halitosis	Hiatal hernia
Pyrosis *(continued)*	
▪ Pyrosis and indigestion signaling start of an attack ▪ Gnawing, burning pain in left epigastrium arising 2 to 3 hours after eating or when stomach is empty; relieved with intake of food or antacid	Peptic ulcer disease
Stools, clay-colored	
▪ Stools followed by unexplained pruritus that worsens at bedtime ▪ Weakness, fatigue ▪ Weight loss ▪ Vague abdominal pain ▪ Jaundice ▪ Hyperpigmentation ▪ Nocturnal diarrhea, steatorrhea ▪ Purpura ▪ Bone and back pain	Biliary cirrhosis

GI SYSTEM: INTERPRETING YOUR FINDINGS *(continued)*

Sign or symptom and findings	Probable cause
Stools, clay-colored *(continued)*	
▪ Clay-colored stools due to obstruction of common bile duct, possibly alternating with normal-colored stools if blockage is intermittent ▪ Dyspepsia ▪ Biliary colic if obstruction sudden and severe; pain in right upper quadrant possibly radiating to epigastrium or shoulder blades unrelieved by antacids ▪ Tachycardia ▪ Restlessness ▪ Nausea ▪ Intolerance of certain foods ▪ Vomiting ▪ Upper abdominal tenderness ▪ Fever ▪ Chills ▪ Jaundice	Cholelithiasis
▪ Clay-colored stools signaling start of icteric phase; followed by jaundice in 1 to 5 days ▪ Mild weight loss ▪ Dark urine ▪ Anorexia ▪ Tender hepatomegaly	Hepatitis
▪ Clay-colored stools with dark urine and jaundice ▪ Severe epigastric pain radiating to the back and aggravated by lying down ▪ Nausea and vomiting ▪ Fever ▪ Abdominal rigidity and tenderness ▪ Hypoactive bowel sounds ▪ Crackles at lung bases	Pancreatitis, acute
▪ Clay-colored stool with obstruction of common bile duct ▪ Abdominal or back pain ▪ Jaundice ▪ Pruritus ▪ Nausea and vomiting ▪ Anorexia ▪ Weight loss ▪ Fatigue, weakness ▪ Fever	Pancreatic cancer

hear bowel sounds immediately, listen for at least 5 minutes.) Gently palpate the abdomen for rigidity. Remember that deep or extensive palpation may increase pain. Begin emergency interventions if you detect abdominal distention and rigidity along with abnormal bowel sounds and patient complaints of pain.

Obtain a medical history, noting GI or biliary disorders that may cause peritonitis or ascites, such as cirrhosis, hepatitis, or inflammatory bowel disease. Also, note chronic constipation. Find out about any recent abdominal surgery, which can lead to abdominal distention. Ask about recent accidents, even minor ones, like falling off a stepladder.

Physical assessment

Perform a complete physical examination. Don't restrict the examination to the abdomen because important clues about the cause of the distention can be missed. Next, stand at the foot of the bed and observe the recumbent patient for abdominal asymmetry to determine if distention is localized or generalized. Then assess abdominal contour by stooping at his side. Inspect for tense, glistening skin and bulging flanks, which may indicate ascites. Observe the umbilicus because an everted umbilicus may indicate ascites or umbilical hernia. An inverted umbilicus also may indicate distention from gas; it's also common in obesity.

Inspect the abdomen for signs of inguinal or femoral hernia and for incisions that may point to adhesions, which lead to intestinal obstruction. Then auscultate for bowel sounds, abdominal friction rubs (indicating peritoneal inflammation), and bruits (indicating an aneurysm). Listen for succussion splash, normally heard in the stomach when the patient moves or when palpation disturbs the viscera. However, an abnormally loud splash indicates fluid accumulation, suggesting gastric dilation or obstruction.

Next, percuss and palpate the abdomen to determine if distention results from air, fluid, or both. If you hear a tympanic note in the left lower quadrant, this suggests an air-filled descending or sigmoid colon. A tympanic note throughout a generally distended abdomen suggests an air-filled peritoneal cavity. A dull percussion note throughout a generally distended abdomen suggests a fluid-filled peritoneal cavity. Shifting of dullness laterally with the patient in the decubitus position also indicates a fluid-filled abdominal cavity. A pelvic or intra-abdominal mass causes local dullness upon percussion and should be palpable. Obesity causes a large abdomen without shifting dullness, prominent tympany, or palpable bowel or other masses, with generalized rather then localized dullness.

Next, palpate the abdomen for tenderness, noting whether it's localized or generalized. Watch for peritoneal signs and symptoms, such as rebound tenderness, guarding, rigidity, or McBurney's, obturator, and psoas sign. Female patients should undergo a pelvic examination; males, a genital examination. All patients who report abdominal pain should undergo a digital rectal examination with fecal occult blood testing. Finally, measure abdominal girth for a baseline value. Mark the flanks with a felt-tipped pen as a reference for subsequent measurements.

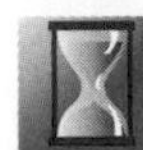

AGE ISSUE *A young child's abdomen is normally rounded so distention may be difficult to observe. However, a child's abdominal wall is less well-developed than an adult's, making palpation easier. When percussing the abdomen, remember that children normally swallow air when eating and crying, resulting in louder-than-normal tympany. Minimal tympany with abdominal distention may result from fluid accumulation or solid masses. To check for abdominal fluid, test for shifting dullness instead of for a fluid wave. (In a child, air swallowing and incomplete abdominal muscle development make the fluid wave difficult to interpret.) If the child won't cooperate with the physical examination, allow him sit in the parent's lap. Gather clues by observing the child while he's coughing, walking, or climbing. Remove all his clothing to avoid missing any diagnostic clues. Also, gently perform a rectal examination.*

Analysis

Abdominal distention may result from fat, flatus, a fetus (pregnancy or intra-abdominal mass [pregnancy]), or fluid. Fluid and gas are normally present in the GI tract but not in the peritoneal cavity. However, if fluid and gas are unable to pass freely through the GI tract, abdominal distention occurs. In the peritoneal cavity, distention may reflect acute bleeding, accumulation of ascitic fluid, or air from perforation of an abdominal organ.

Abdominal distention doesn't always signal disease. For example, in anxious patients or those with digestive distress, localized distention in the left upper quadrant can result from aerophagia — the unconscious swallowing of air. Generalized distention can result from ingestion of fruits or vegetables with large quantities of unabsorbable carbohydrates, such as legumes, or from abnormal food fermentation by microbes. Rule out pregnancy in all females with abdominal distention.

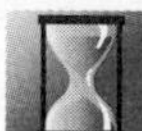
AGE ISSUE *In neonates, ascites usually results from GI or urinary perforation; in older children, from heart failure, cirrhosis, or nephrosis. Besides ascites, congenital malformations of the GI tract (such as intussusception and volvulus) may cause abdominal distention. A hernia may cause distention if it produces an intestinal obstruction. In addition, overeating and constipation can cause distention. With age, fat tends to accumulate in the lower abdomen and near the hips, even when body weight is stable. This accumulation, together with weakening abdominal muscles, commonly produces a potbelly, which some elderly patients interpret as fluid collection or evidence of disease.*

Abdominal mass

Commonly detected on routine physical examination, an abdominal mass is localized swelling in one abdominal quadrant. Distinguishing an abdominal mass from a normal structure requires skillful palpation. At times, palpation must be repeated with the patient in a different position or performed by a second health care provider to verify initial findings.

History

If the patient's abdominal mass doesn't suggest an aortic aneurysm, continue with a detailed health history. Ask the patient if the mass is painful. If so, ask if the pain is constant or if it occurs only on palpation. Observe if it's localized or generalized. Determine if the patient was already aware of the mass. If he was, find out if he noticed any change in the size or location of the mass.

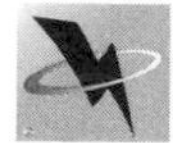
CRITICAL POINT *If the patient has a pulsating midabdominal mass and severe abdominal or back pain, suspect an aortic aneurysm.*

Next, review the patient's medical history, paying close attention to GI disorders. Ask the patient about GI symptoms, such as constipation, diarrhea, rectal bleeding, abnormally colored stools, and vomiting. Find out if he has noticed a change in appetite. Ask a female patient whether her menstrual cycles are regular and when the first day of her last menstrual period occurred.

Physical assessment

A complete physical examination should be performed. Next, auscultate for bowel sounds in each quadrant. Listen for bruits or friction rubs, and check for enlarged veins. Lightly palpate and then deeply palpate the abdomen, assessing any painful or suspicious areas last. Note the patient's pain when you locate the mass. Some masses can be detected only with the patient in a supine position; others require a side-lying position.

Estimate the size of the mass in centimeters. Determine its shape, such as if it's round or sausage-shaped. Describe its contour as smooth, rough, sharply defined, nodular, or irregular. Determine the consistency of the mass, such as if it's doughy, soft, solid, or hard. Also, percuss the mass. A dull sound indicates a fluid-filled mass; a tympanic sound, an air-filled mass.

Next, determine if the mass moves with your hand or in response to respiration. Assess whether the mass is free-floating or attached to intra-abdominal structures. To determine whether the mass is located in the abdominal wall or the abdominal cavity, ask the patient to lift his head and shoulders off the examination table, thereby contracting his abdominal muscles. While the muscles are contracted, try to palpate the mass. If you can, the mass is in the abdominal wall; if you can't, the mass is within the abdominal cavity.

After the abdominal examination is complete, perform a pelvic, genital, and rectal examination.

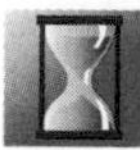
AGE ISSUE *In infants, detecting an abdominal mass can be challenging; however, make palpation easier by allowing the infant to suck on his bottle or pacifier to prevent crying, which causes abdominal rigidity and interferes with palpation. Make sure to avoid tickling him because laughter also causes abdominal rigidity. Also, reduce his apprehension by distracting him with cheerful conversation. Rest your hand on his abdomen for a few moments before palpation. If he remains sensitive, place his hand under yours as you palpate. Consider allowing the child to remain on the parent's or caregiver's lap. Finally, perform a gentle rectal examination.*

Analysis

Typically, an abdominal mass develops insidiously and may represent an enlarged organ, a neoplasm, an abscess, a vascular defect, or a fecal mass. A palpable abdominal mass is an important clinical sign and usually represents a serious and perhaps life-threatening disorder — abdominal aortic aneurysm rupture.

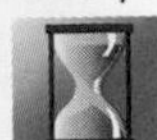

AGE ISSUE *In neonates, most abdominal masses result from renal disorders, such as polycystic kidney disease or congenital hydronephrosis. In older infants and children, abdominal masses usually are caused by enlarged organs, such as the liver and spleen. Other common causes include Wilms' tumor, neuroblastoma, intussusception, volvulus, Hirschsprung's disease (congenital megacolon), pyloric stenosis, and abdominal abscess. In thin, elderly patients, use ultrasonography to evaluate a prominent midepigastric mass.*

Abdominal pain

Abdominal pain usually results from a GI disorder, but it can be caused by a reproductive, genitourinary (GU), musculoskeletal, or vascular disorder; use of certain drugs; or exposure to toxins. At times, such pain signals life-threatening complications.

History

If the patient has no life-threatening signs or symptoms, take his health history. Ask if the pain is constant or intermittent and when it began. Constant, steady abdominal pain suggests organ perforation, ischemia, or inflammation or blood in the peritoneal cavity. Intermittent, cramping abdominal pain suggests that the patient may have obstruction of a hollow organ.

If pain is intermittent, find out the duration of a typical episode. Also, ask the patient where the pain is located and whether it radiates to other areas. Find out if movement, coughing, exertion, vomiting, eating, elimination, or walking worsens or relieves the pain. The patient may report abdominal pain as indigestion or gas, so have him describe it in detail.

Ask the patient about drug and alcohol use and history of vascular, GI, GU, or reproductive disorders. Ask female patients about the date of last menses, changes in menstrual pattern, or dyspareunia.

Next, ask the patient about appetite changes. Also ask about the onset and frequency of nausea or vomiting. Find out about any changes in bowel habits, such as constipation, diarrhea, and changes in stool consistency; and the last bowel movement. Also, find out about urinary frequency, urgency, or pain. Ask the patient if his urine is cloudy or pink.

Physical assessment

Assess skin turgor and mucous membranes. Inspect his abdomen for distention or visible peristaltic waves and, if indicated, measure abdominal girth.

Auscultate for bowel sounds, and characterize their motility. Percuss all quadrants, carefully noting the percussion sounds. Palpate the entire abdomen for masses, rigidity, and tenderness. Check specifically for costovertebral angle tenderness, abdominal tenderness with guarding, and rebound tenderness.

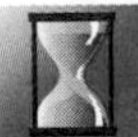

AGE ISSUE *Because many children have difficulty describing abdominal pain, pay close attention to nonverbal cues, such as wincing, lethargy, or unusual positioning (such as a side-lying position with knees flexed to the abdomen). Observing the child while he coughs, walks, or climbs may offer some diagnostic clues. Also, remember that a parent's description of the child's complaints is a subjective interpretation of what the parent believes is wrong.*

Analysis

Abdominal pain arises from the abdominopelvic viscera, the parietal peritoneum, or the capsules of the liver, kidney, or spleen, and may be acute or chronic, diffuse, or localized. Visceral pain develops slowly into a deep, dull, aching pain that's poorly localized in the epigastric, periumbilical, or hypogastric region. In contrast, somatic parietal or peritoneal pain produces a sharp, more intense, and well-localized discomfort that rapidly follows the insult. Movement or coughing aggravates this pain.

Pain may also be referred to the abdomen from another site with the same or similar nerve supply. This sharp, well-localized, referred pain is felt in skin or deeper tissues and may coexist with skin hyperesthesia and muscle hyperalgesia.

Mechanisms that produce abdominal pain include stretching or tension of the gut wall, traction on the peritoneum or mesentery, vigorous intestinal contraction, inflammation, ischemia, and sensory nerve irritation.

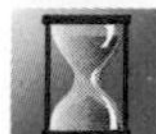

AGE ISSUE *Advanced age may decrease the symptoms of acute abdominal disease. Pain may be less severe, fever less pronounced, and signs of peritoneal inflammation diminished or absent.*

Abdominal rigidity

Abdominal rigidity (muscle spasm, involuntary guarding), refers to abnormal muscle tension or inflexibility of the abdomen. Rigidity may be voluntary or involuntary.

History

If the patient's condition allows further assessment, take a brief health history. Find out when the abdominal rigidity began and if it's associated with abdominal pain. If so, ask if the pain began at the same time. Determine whether the abdominal rigidity is localized or generalized and if it's always present. Find out if its site has changed or remained constant. Next, ask about aggravating or alleviating factors, such as position changes, coughing, vomiting, elimination, and walking. Then explore other signs and symptoms.

Physical assessment

Inspect the abdomen for peristaltic waves, which may be visible in extremely thin patients. Also, check for a visibly distended bowel loop. Next, auscultate bowel sounds. Perform light palpation to locate the rigidity and to determine its severity. Avoid deep palpation, which may exacerbate abdominal pain. Finally, check for poor skin turgor and dry mucous membranes, which indicate dehydration.

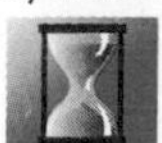

AGE ISSUE *In a child, voluntary rigidity may be difficult to distinguish from involuntary rigidity if the associated pain makes him restless, tense, or apprehensive. However, in any child with suspected involuntary rigidity, your priority is early detection of dehydration and shock, which can rapidly become life-threatening.*

Analysis

Voluntary rigidity reflects the patient's normal fear or nervousness upon palpation; involuntary rigidity reflects potentially life-threatening peritoneal irritation or inflammation. Involuntary rigidity most commonly results from GI disorders but may also result from pulmonary and vascular disorders and from the effects of insect toxins. Usually, it's accompanied by fever, nausea, vomiting, and abdominal tenderness, distention, and pain.

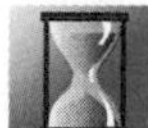

AGE ISSUE *In a child, abdominal rigidity can stem from gastric perforation, hypertrophic pyloric stenosis, duodenal obstruction, meconium ileus, intussusception, cystic fibrosis, celiac disease, and appendicitis. Advanced age and impaired cognition decrease pain perception and intensity. Weakening of abdominal muscles may decrease muscle spasms and rigidity.*

Bowel sounds, hyperactive

Sometimes audible without a stethoscope, hyperactive bowel sounds reflect increased intestinal motility (peristalsis). They're commonly characterized as rapid, rushing, gurgling waves of sounds.

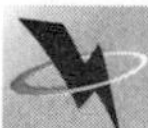

CRITICAL POINT *After detecting hyperactive bowel sounds, quickly check vital signs and ask the patient about associated symptoms, such as abdominal pain, vomiting, and diarrhea. If he reports cramping abdominal pain or vomiting, continue to auscultate for bowel sounds. If bowel sounds stop abruptly, suspect complete bowel obstruction.*

History

After ruling out life-threatening conditions, obtain a detailed medical and surgical history. Ask the patient if he has had hernia or abdominal surgery because these may cause mechanical intestinal obstruction. Find out if he has a history of inflammatory bowel disease. Also, ask about recent eruptions of gastroenteritis among family members, friends, or coworkers. If the patient has traveled recently, even within the United States, ask him if he was aware of any endemic illnesses.

In addition, determine whether stress may have contributed to the patient's problem. Ask about food allergies and recent ingestion of unusual foods or fluids. Check for fever, which suggests infection.

Physical assessment
First, begin the physical examination by auscultating the abdomen in all four quadrants. Then gently inspect, percuss, and palpate the abdomen.

Analysis
Hyperactive bowel sounds may stem from life-threatening bowel obstruction or GI hemorrhage, or from GI infection, inflammatory bowel disease (which usually follows a chronic course), food allergies, or stress.

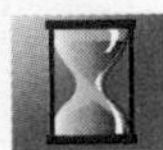

AGE ISSUE *In children, hyperactive bowel sounds usually result from gastroenteritis, erratic eating habits, excessive ingestion of certain foods such as unripened fruit, or food allergy.*

Bowel sounds, hypoactive
Hypoactive bowel sounds, detected by auscultation, are diminished in regularity, time, and loudness from normal bowel sounds. In themselves, hypoactive bowel sounds don't signal an emergency; in fact, they're considered normal during sleep. However, they may indicate absent bowel sounds, which can indicate a life-threatening disorder.

History
Look for related symptoms and ask the patient about the location, onset, duration, frequency, and severity of any pain. Cramping or colicky abdominal pain usually indicates a mechanical bowel obstruction, whereas diffuse abdominal pain usually indicates intestinal distention related to paralytic ileus.

Ask the patient about any recent vomiting, when it began, how often it occurs, and if it's bloody. Also, ask about any changes in bowel habits, such as a history of constipation and the last time he had a bowel movement or expelled gas.

Obtain a detailed medical and surgical history of any conditions that may cause mechanical bowel obstruction, such as an abdominal tumor or hernia. Find out if the patient has a history of severe pain; trauma; conditions that can cause paralytic ileus such as pancreatitis; bowel inflammation or gynecologic infection, which may produce peritonitis; or toxic conditions such as uremia. Ask him if he has recently had radiation therapy or abdominal surgery, or ingested an opiate, which can decrease peristalsis and cause hypoactive bowel sounds.

Physical assessment
After the health history is complete, perform a careful physical examination. Inspect the abdomen for distention, noting surgical incisions and obvious masses. Gently percuss and palpate the abdomen for masses, gas, fluid, tenderness, and rigidity. Measure abdominal girth to detect any subsequent increase in distention. Also check for poor skin turgor, hypotension, narrowed pulse pressure, and other signs of dehydration and electrolyte imbalance, which may result from paralytic ileus.

Analysis
Hypoactive bowel sounds result from decreased peristalsis, which, in turn, can result from a developing bowel obstruction. The obstruction may be mechanical as from a hernia, tumor, or twisting; vascular as from an embolism or thrombosis; or neurogenic as from mechanical, ischemic, or toxic impairment of bowel innervation.

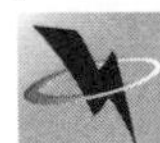

CRITICAL POINT *Severe pain, abdominal rigidity, guarding, and fever, accompanied by hypoactive bowel sounds, may indicate paralytic ileus from peritonitis. Immediately prepare for emergency interventions if these signs and symptoms occur.*

Hypoactive bowel sounds can result from the use of certain drugs, such as opiates or anticholinergics, abdominal surgery, and radiation therapy.

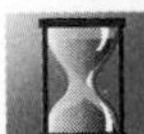

AGE ISSUE *In children, hypoactive bowel sounds may simply be due to bowel distention from excessive swallowing of air while eating or crying. However, be sure to observe children for further signs and symptoms of illness. As with adults, sluggish bowel sounds in children may signal the onset of paralytic ileus or peritonitis.*

Constipation
Constipation is defined as small, infrequent, or difficult bowel movements. Because normal bowel movements can vary in frequency and from individual to individual, consti-

pation must be determined in relation to the patient's normal elimination pattern.

Constipation usually occurs when the urge to defecate is suppressed and the muscles associated with bowel movements remain contracted. Because the autonomic nervous system controls bowel movements — by sensing rectal distention from fecal contents and by stimulating the external sphincter — any factor that influences this system may cause bowel dysfunction.

History

Ask the patient to describe the frequency of his bowel movements and the size and consistency of his stools. Find out how long he has been constipated. Acute constipation usually has an organic cause, such as an anal or rectal disorder. In a patient over age 45, a recent onset of constipation may be an early sign of colorectal cancer. Conversely, chronic constipation typically has a functional cause and may be related to stress.

Ask the patient if he has pain related to constipation. If so, find out when he first noticed the pain, and where it's located. Cramping, abdominal pain, and distention suggest obstipation — extreme, persistent constipation due to intestinal tract obstruction. Ask the patient if defecation worsens or helps relieve the pain. Defecation usually worsens pain, but with disorders such as irritable bowel syndrome, it may relieve it. Ask the patient to describe a typical day's menu; estimate his daily fiber and fluid intake. Ask him, too, about any changes in eating habits, medication or alcohol use, or physical activity. Find out about recent emotional distress. Ask if his constipation has affected his family life or social contacts. Also, ask about his job. A sedentary or stressful job can contribute to constipation.

Find out whether the patient has a history of GI, rectoanal, neurologic, or metabolic disorders; abdominal surgery; or radiation therapy. Then ask about the medications he's taking, including over-the-counter preparations, such as laxatives, mineral oil, stool softeners, and enemas.

Physical assessment

Inspect the abdomen for distention or scars from previous surgery. Then auscultate for bowel sounds, and characterize their motility. Percuss all four abdominal quadrants, and gently palpate for abdominal tenderness, a palpable mass, and hepatomegaly. Next, examine the patient's rectum. Spread his buttocks to expose the anus, and inspect for inflammation, lesions, scars, fissures, and external hemorrhoids. Use a disposable glove and lubricant to palpate the anal sphincter for laxity or stricture. Also, palpate for rectal masses and fecal impaction. Finally, obtain a stool sample and test it for occult blood.

Analysis

Constipation may be a minor annoyance or, uncommonly, a sign of a life-threatening disorder such as acute intestinal obstruction. Untreated, constipation can lead to headache, anorexia, and abdominal discomfort and can adversely affect the patient's lifestyle and well-being.

Constipation may be caused by a GI disorder, but it also may result from endocrine, metabolic or neurologic disorders, such as diabetic neuropathy or hypothyroidism, hypercalcemia or cirrhosis, or multiple sclerosis or a spinal cord lesion, respectively. It can result from rectoanal surgery, which may traumatize nerves, and abdominal irradiation, which may cause intestinal stricture. Constipation can result from several life-threatening disorders, such as acute intestinal obstruction and mesenteric artery ischemia, but it doesn't signal these conditions.

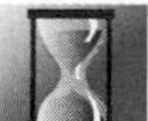

AGE ISSUE *In bottle-fed infants, the high content of casein and calcium in cow's milk can produce hard stools and possible constipation. Other causes of constipation in infants include inadequate fluid intake, Hirschsprung's disease, and anal fissures. In older children, constipation usually results from inadequate fiber intake and excessive intake of milk; it can also result from bowel spasm, mechanical obstruction, hypothyroidism, reluctance to stop playing for bathroom breaks, and the lack of privacy in some school bathrooms. In elderly patients, acute constipation is usually associated with underlying structural abnormalities. Chronic constipation, however, is chiefly caused by lifelong bowel and dietary habits and laxative use.*

Diarrhea

Usually a chief sign of an intestinal disorder, diarrhea is an increase in the volume, frequency, and liquidity of stools compared with the patient's normal bowel habits. It varies in severity and may be acute or chronic.

History

Begin by exploring signs and symptoms associated with the patient's diarrhea. Ask the patient if he has abdominal pain and cramps, difficulty breathing, and weakness or fatigue. Find out his drug history and if he has had GI surgery or radiation therapy recently.

Ask the patient to briefly describe his diet and if he has any known food allergies. Last, find out if he's under unusual stress.

Physical assessment

If the patient isn't in shock, proceed with a brief physical examination. Evaluate hydration, check skin turgor, and take blood pressure with the patient lying, sitting, and standing. Inspect the abdomen for distention, and palpate for tenderness. Auscultate bowel sounds. Take the patient's temperature, and note any chills. Also, look for a rash. Conduct a rectal examination and a pelvic examination if indicated.

Analysis

Acute diarrhea may result from acute infection, stress, fecal impaction, or use of certain drugs. Chronic diarrhea may result from chronic infection, obstructive and inflammatory bowel disease, malabsorption syndrome, an endocrine disorder, or GI surgery. Periodic diarrhea may result from food intolerance or from ingestion of spicy or high-fiber foods or caffeine. One or more causes may contribute to diarrhea. Certain fluid and electrolyte imbalances may precipitate life-threatening arrhythmias or hypovolemic shock.

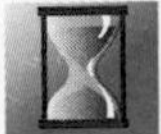

AGE ISSUE *In children, diarrhea commonly results from infection, although chronic diarrhea may result from malabsorption syndrome, an anatomic defect, or allergies. Because dehydration and electrolyte imbalance occur rapidly in children, diarrhea can be life-threatening. Diligent monitoring and immediate fluid replacement are crucial. In the elderly patient with new-onset segmental colitis, always consider ischemia before diagnosing the patient with Crohn's disease.*

Dyspepsia

Dyspepsia refers to an uncomfortable fullness after meals that's associated with nausea, belching, heartburn and, possibly, cramping and abdominal distention. Frequently aggravated by spicy, fatty, or high-fiber foods and by excess caffeine intake, dyspepsia without other diseases involved indicates impaired digestive function.

History

If the patient complains of dyspepsia, begin by asking him to describe it in detail. Ask him how often and when it occurs, specifically in relation to meals. Find out if any drugs or activities relieve or aggravate it. Ask if he has had nausea, vomiting, melena, hematemesis, cough, or chest pain, and if he's taking any prescription drugs or has recently had surgery. Find out if the patient has a history of renal, cardiovascular, or pulmonary disease.

Ask if the patient has noticed any change in the amount or color of his urine.

If the patient's experiencing an unusual or overwhelming amount of emotional stress, determine his coping mechanisms and their effectiveness.

Physical assessment

Focus the physical examination on the abdomen. Inspect for distention, ascites, scars, obvious hernias, jaundice, uremic frost, and bruising. Then auscultate for bowel sounds and characterize their motility. Palpate and percuss the abdomen, noting any tenderness, pain, organ enlargement, or tympany. Finally, examine other body systems. Ask about behavior changes, and evaluate level of consciousness. Auscultate for gallops and crackles. Percuss the lungs to detect consolidation. Note peripheral edema and any swelling of lymph nodes.

Analysis

Dyspepsia is caused by GI disorders and, to a lesser extent, by cardiac, pulmonary, and renal disorders and the effects of drugs. This abnormal finding apparently results when altered gastric secretions lead to excess stomach acidity. Dyspepsia may also result from emotional upset and overly rapid eating or improper chewing. It usually occurs a few hours after eating and lasts for a variable period of time. Its severity depends on the amount and type of food eaten and on GI motility. Additional food or an antacid may relieve the discomfort.

Drugs, such as NSAIDs, especially aspirin, commonly cause dyspepsia. Diuretics, antibiotics, antihypertensives, corticosteroids, and many other drugs can cause dyspepsia, depending on the patient's tolerance of the dosage.

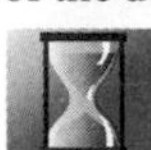

AGE ISSUE *In adolescents, dyspepsia may occur with peptic ulcer disease, but it isn't relieved by food. It may also occur in congenital pyloric stenosis, but projectile vomiting after meals is a more characteristic sign. It may also result from lactose intolerance.*

Hematemesis

Hematemesis, the vomiting of blood, usually indicates GI bleeding above the ligament of Treitz, which suspends the duodenum at its junction with the jejunum. Bright-red or blood-streaked vomitus indicates fresh or recent bleeding. Dark-red, brown, or black vomitus (the color and consistency of coffee grounds) indicates that blood has been retained in the stomach and partially digested.

History

If the patient's hematemesis isn't immediately life-threatening, begin by taking a thorough health history. First, have the patient describe the amount, color, and consistency of the vomitus. Find out when he first noticed this sign and if he has ever had hematemesis. Also ask if he has had bloody or black, tarry stools. Note whether hematemesis is usually preceded by nausea, flatulence, diarrhea, or weakness. Ask about recent bouts of retching with or without vomiting.

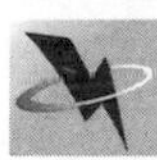

CRITICAL POINT *Hematemesis is always an abnormal finding and its severity depends on the amount, source, and rapidity of the bleeding. Massive hematemesis (500 to 1,000 ml of blood) may be life-threatening. If the patient has massive hematemesis, check his vital signs. If you detect signs of shock—such as tachypnea, hypotension, and tachycardia—place the patient in a supine position, and elevate his feet 20 to 30 degrees. Institute emergency interventions, such as starting a large-bore I.V. line for emergency fluid replacement, obtaining a blood sample for typing and cross-matching and other laboratory studies, and administering oxygen.*

Next, ask about a history of ulcers or liver or coagulation disorders. Find out how much alcohol the patient drinks, if any. Ask if he regularly takes aspirin or other NSAIDs, such as phenylbutazone or indomethacin. These drugs may cause erosive gastritis or ulcers.

Physical assessment

Begin the physical examination by checking for orthostatic hypotension, an early warning sign of hypovolemia. Take blood pressure and pulse with the patient in supine, sitting, and standing positions. A decrease of 10 mm Hg or more in systolic pressure or an increase of 10 beats/minute or more in pulse rate indicates volume depletion. After obtaining other vital signs, inspect the mucous membranes, nasopharynx, and skin for any signs of bleeding or other abnormalities. Finally, palpate the abdomen for tenderness, pain, or masses. Note lymphadenopathy.

Analysis

Although hematemesis usually results from a GI disorder, it may stem from a coagulation disorder or from a treatment that irritates the GI tract. Esophageal varices may also cause hematemesis. Swallowed blood from epistaxis or oropharyngeal erosion may also cause bloody vomitus. Hematemesis may be precipitated by straining, emotional stress, and the use of NSAIDs or alcohol. In a patient with esophageal varices, hematemesis may be a result of trauma from swallowing hard or partially chewed food.

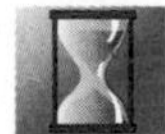

AGE ISSUE *In children, hematemesis is much less common than in adults and may be related to foreign-body ingestion. Occasionally, neonates develop hematemesis after swallowing maternal blood during delivery or breast-feeding from a cracked nipple. Hemorrhagic disease of the neonate and esophageal erosion may also cause hematemesis in infants; such cases require immediate fluid replacement. In elderly patients, hematemesis may be caused by a vascular anomaly, an aortoenteric fistula, or*

upper GI cancer. In addition, chronic obstructive pulmonary disease, chronic liver or renal failure, and chronic NSAID use all predispose elderly people to hemorrhage secondary to coexisting ulcerative disorders.

Hematochezia

Hematochezia refers to the passage of bloody stools. It ranges from formed, blood-streaked stools to liquid, bloody stools that may be bright-red, dark mahogany, or maroon in color. This abnormal finding usually develops abruptly and is heralded by abdominal pain.

Hematochezia usually indicates and may be the first sign of GI bleeding below the ligament of Treitz. Usually preceded by hematemesis, hematochezia may also accompany rapid hemorrhage of 1 L or more from the upper GI tract.

History

If the hematochezia isn't immediately life-threatening, ask the patient to fully describe the amount, color, and consistency of bloody stools. If possible, also inspect and characterize the stools yourself.

Ask the patient about the stools and how long they've been bloody. Find out if they always look the same or if the amount of blood varies. Ask about associated symptoms. Explore the patient's medical history, focusing on GI and coagulation disorders. Ask about use of GI irritants, such as alcohol, aspirin, and other NSAIDs.

Physical assessment

Begin the physical examination by checking for orthostatic hypotension, an early sign of shock. Take the patient's blood pressure and pulse while he's lying down, sitting, and standing. If systolic pressure decreases by 10 mm Hg or more or if pulse rate increases by 10 beats/minute or more when he changes position, suspect volume depletion and impending shock.

Examine the skin for petechiae or spider angiomas. Palpate the abdomen for tenderness, pain, or masses. Also, note lymphadenopathy. Finally, perform a digital rectal examination to rule out any rectal masses.

Analysis

Although hematochezia is commonly associated with GI disorders, it may also result from a coagulation disorder, exposure to toxins, or a diagnostic test. Always a significant abnormal finding, hematochezia may precipitate life-threatening hypovolemia.

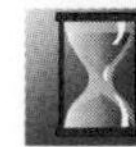

AGE ISSUE *In children, hematochezia is much less common than in adults; however, when it does occur it may result from a structural disorder, such as intussusception or Meckel's diverticulum, or from inflammatory disorders, such as peptic ulcer disease or ulcerative colitis. In children, ulcerative colitis typically produces chronic, rather than acute, signs and symptoms and may also cause slow growth and maturation related to malnutrition. Suspect sexual abuse in all cases of rectal bleeding in children.*

Melena

A common sign of upper GI bleeding, melena is the passage of black, tarry stools containing digested blood. Characteristic color results from bacterial degradation and hydrochloric acid acting on the blood as it travels through the GI tract. At least 60 ml of blood is needed to produce this abnormal finding.

History

If the patient's condition permits, ask when he discovered his stools were black and tarry. Ask about the frequency and quantity of bowel movements. Find out if he has had melena before. Ask about other signs and symptoms, notably hematemesis or hematochezia, and about use of NSAIDs, alcohol, or other GI irritants. Also, find out if he has a history of GI lesions. Ask if the patient takes iron supplements, which can also cause black stools. Obtain a drug history, noting the use of warfarin or other anticoagulants.

Physical assessment

First, inspect the patient's mouth and nasopharynx for evidence of bleeding. Then, perform an abdominal examination that includes auscultation, palpation, and percussion.

Analysis

Severe melena can signal acute bleeding and life-threatening hypovolemic shock. Usually, melena indicates bleeding from the esophagus, stomach, or duodenum, although it can also indicate bleeding from the jejunum, ileum, or ascending colon. This abnormal finding can also result from swallowing blood, as in epistaxis; from taking certain drugs; or from ingesting alcohol. Because false melena may be caused by ingestion of lead, iron, bismuth, or licorice (which produces black stools without the presence of blood), all black stools should be tested for occult blood.

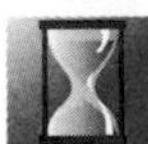

AGE ISSUE *Neonates may experience melena neonatorum due to extravasation of blood into the alimentary canal. In older children, melena usually results from peptic ulcer, gastritis, or Meckel's diverticulum.*

Nausea and vomiting

Nausea is a sensation of profound revulsion to food or of impending vomiting. Typically accompanied by autonomic signs such as hypersalivation, diaphoresis, tachycardia, pallor, and tachypnea — it's closely associated with vomiting.

Vomiting is the forceful expulsion of gastric contents through the mouth. Characteristically preceded by nausea, vomiting results from a coordinated sequence of abdominal muscle contractions and reverse esophageal peristalsis.

History

Begin by obtaining a complete medical history, focusing on GI, endocrine, and metabolic disorders, recent infections, and cancer, along with its treatment.

Ask your patient to describe the onset, duration, and intensity of nausea and vomiting. Find out what started it, what makes it subside, and if he experiences nausea and vomiting together.

Explore related complaints, particularly abdominal pain, anorexia and weight loss, changes in bowel habits or stools, excessive belching or flatus, and bloating or fullness. If possible, collect, measure, and inspect the character of the vomitus, or have the patient describe it to you. Ask the female patient if she is or could be pregnant.

Physical assessment

First, inspect the skin for jaundice, bruises, and spider hemangiomas, and assess skin turgor. Inspect the abdomen for distention, and auscultate for bowel sounds and bruits. Palpate for rigidity and tenderness, and test for rebound tenderness. Next, palpate and percuss the liver for enlargement. Assess other body systems as appropriate.

Analysis

Nausea and vomiting, common indications of a GI disorder, also occur with fluid and electrolyte imbalance; infection; metabolic, endocrine, labyrinthine, and cardiac disorders; use of certain drugs; surgery; and radiation.

Often present during the first trimester of pregnancy, nausea and vomiting may also arise from severe pain, anxiety, alcohol intoxication, overeating, or ingestion of distasteful food or liquids.

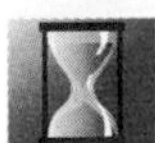

AGE ISSUE *Elderly patients have increased dental caries; tooth loss; decreased salivary gland function, which causes mouth dryness; decreased gastric acid output and motility; and decreased sense of taste and smell. All of these can contribute to nonpathologic nausea. However, intestinal ischemia, which is common in this age-group, should always be ruled out as a potential cause.*

Pyrosis

Caused by reflux of gastric contents into the esophagus, pyrosis (heartburn) is a substernal burning sensation that rises in the chest and may radiate to the neck or throat. It's commonly accompanied by regurgitation, which also results from gastric reflux.

History

Ask the patient if he has had heartburn before. Find out what foods or beverages trigger it. Ask him if stress or fatigue aggravate his discomfort. Find out if movement, a certain body position, or ingestion of very hot or cold liquids worsens or helps relieve the heartburn. Ask where the pain is located and whether it radiates to other areas. Also, find out if the patient regurgitates sour- or bitter-tasting fluids. Ask about any associated signs and symptoms.

Physical assessment

Focus the physical examination on the abdomen. Inspect for distention, ascites, scars, obvious hernias, jaundice, and bruising. Then auscultate for bowel sounds and characterize their motility. Palpate and percuss the abdomen, noting any tenderness, pain, organ enlargement, or tympany.

Analysis

Serving as a barrier to reflux, the lower esophageal sphincter (LES) normally relaxes only to allow food to pass from the esophagus into the stomach. However, hormonal fluctuations, mechanical stress, and the effects of certain foods and drugs can lower LES pressure. When LES pressure falls and intra-abdominal or intragastric pressure rises, the normally contracted LES relaxes inappropriately and allows reflux of gastric acid or bile secretions into the lower esophagus. There, the acids or secretions irritate and inflame the esophageal mucosa, producing pyrosis. Persistent inflammation can cause LES pressure to decrease even more and may trigger a recurrent cycle of reflux and pyrosis.

Because increased intra-abdominal pressure contributes to reflux, pyrosis commonly occurs with pregnancy, ascites, or obesity. It also accompanies various GI disorders, connective tissue diseases, and the use of numerous drugs. Pyrosis usually develops after meals or when the patient lies down (especially on his right side), bends over, lifts heavy objects, or exercises vigorously. It typically worsens with swallowing and improves when the patient sits upright or takes an antacid.

CRITICAL POINT *A patient experiencing a myocardial infarction (MI) may mistake chest pain for pyrosis. However, he'll probably develop other signs and symptoms—such as dyspnea, tachycardia, palpitations, nausea, and vomiting—that will help distinguish an MI from pyrosis. And, obviously, his chest pain won't be relieved by an antacid.*

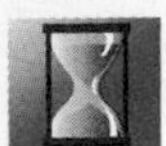

AGE ISSUE *A child may have difficulty distinguishing esophageal pain from pyrosis. To gain information, help him describe the sensation. Elderly patients with peptic ulcer disease commonly present with nonspecific abdominal discomfort or weight loss. Elderly patients are also at greater risk for complications from NSAIDs, and many of them develop pyrosis due to intolerance to spicy foods.*

Stools, clay-colored

Normally, bile pigments give the stool its characteristic brown color. However, interference with the formation or release of these pigments into the intestine leads to clay-colored stools. These stools are commonly associated with jaundice and dark "cola-colored" urine.

History

After documenting when the patient first noticed clay-colored stools, explore associated signs and symptoms, such as abdominal pain, nausea and vomiting, fatigue, anorexia, weight loss, and dark urine. Find out if the patient has trouble digesting fatty foods or heavy meals. Ask him if he bruises easily.

Next, review the patient's medical history for gallbladder, hepatic, or pancreatic disorders. Find out if he has ever had biliary surgery or recently undergone barium studies (barium lightens stool color for several days.) Also, ask about antacid use because large amounts may lighten stool color. Note a history of alcoholism or exposure to other hepatotoxic substances.

Physical assessment

Assess the patient's general appearance, take his vital signs, and check his skin and eyes for jaundice. Then examine the abdomen; inspect for distention, ascites, and auscultate for hypoactive bowel sounds. Percuss and palpate for masses and rebound tenderness. Finally, obtain urine and stool specimens for laboratory analysis.

Analysis

Pale, putty-colored stools usually result from hepatic, gallbladder, or pancreatic disorders. Hepatocellular degeneration or biliary obstruction may interfere with the formation or release of the bile pigments that give the stools their characteristic color. Biliary surgery that causes bile duct stricture may lead to clay colored stools.

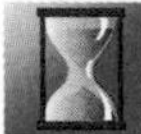

AGE ISSUE *In infants with biliary atresia, clay-colored stools may occur. Because elderly patients with cholelithiasis have a greater risk of developing complications if the condition isn't treated, surgery should be considered early on for treatment of persistent symptoms.*

Endocrine system

The endocrine system functions primarily as the regulatory system for the entire body. It consists of eight glands that produce hormones — powerful chemicals that profoundly affect a person's life. Hormones influence a person's growth and development, physical appearance, body functions, and emotional status. A disorder or imbalance of the endocrine system, therefore, affects not only a person's body functions but also his physical and emotional well-being.

Anatomy and physiology

A basic understanding of the anatomy and physiology of the three major components of the endocrine system will help guide your assessment. They include the:

- glands — specialized cell clusters or organs
- hormones — chemical substances secreted by glands in response to stimulation
- receptors — protein molecules that trigger specific physiologic changes in a target cell in response to hormonal stimulation.

Knowing how to assess the endocrine system properly aids in identifying subtle abnormalities that can signal a patient's problems with this system.

Endocrine glands

The endocrine glands are one of two major groups of glands in the body. The digestive and salivary glands compose the larger group, called exocrine glands because they discharge their secretions directly onto an epithelial surface through an excretory duct (*exo* means outward). Conversely, the endocrine glands (*endo* means within) discharge their secretions — six hormones —

STRUCTURES OF THE ENDOCRINE SYSTEM

Endocrine glands secrete hormones directly into the bloodstream to regulate body function. This illustration shows the location of the major endocrine glands, except the gonads.

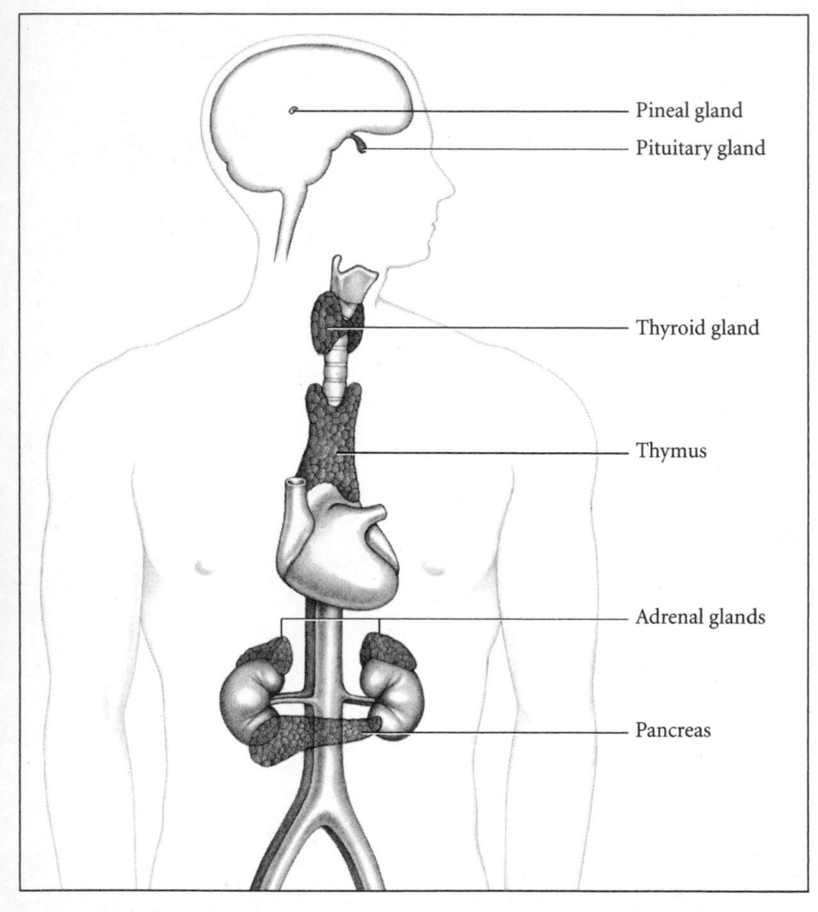

directly into the bloodstream to regulate body functions.

Negative feedback controls hormonal secretion. Once a hormone achieves its physiologic effect on the target organ, the information travels back to the producing gland to inhibit further secretion. When an inadequate amount of hormone is secreted, negative feedback causes the producing gland to release more.

The endocrine system includes the pituitary, thyroid, parathyroid, and adrenal glands; the islet cells of the pancreas, thymus, pineal gland, and the gonads (ovaries or testes). (See *Structures of the endocrine system.*)

Remember that endocrine glands aren't the only sites of hormone production; specialized cells in other organs also secrete hormones. The kidneys, for example, produce erythropoietin, and the cells of the gastric and duodenal mucosa produce gastrin. However, these hormone-producing cells aren't part of the endocrine system.

Pituitary gland

The pituitary—a small, pea-shaped gland located at the base of the brain—connects with the hypothalamus via the infundibulum, from which it receives chemical and nervous stimulation. (See *Understanding the effects of the hypothalamus.*) The gland sits in a small depression within the sphenoid bone, called the sella turcica, or pituitary fossa. Located near the pituitary is the optic chiasm, where nerve fibers from both eyes cross as they convey impulses to the brain.

The pituitary consists of an anterior lobe, a posterior lobe, and a small, rudimentary intermediate lobe that's actually part of the anterior lobe. The anterior and the posterior lobes differ not only in their embryologic origin but also in their structure and the way they interact with the hypothalamus.

Anterior pituitary. The anterior pituitary, also know as the *adenohypophysis,* consists of cords of epithelial cells, including eosinophils, basophils, and chromophobes. Many of these cells contain granules of stored hormone. The hypothalamus communicates with the anterior lobe through a specialized network of blood vessels called the portal system. Capillaries around the hypothalamus merge into larger vessels that travel down the pituitary stalk and eventually become capillaries again around the cells of the anterior lobe. Through this vascular pathway, releasing hormones from the hypothalamus reach the anterior pituitary cells, stimulating them to secrete hormones. Each anterior pituitary hormone has a releasing hormone in the hypothalamus. Only some of these hormones have corresponding hypothalamic inhibitory hormones.

The anterior pituitary, the larger region, produces at least six hormones:

- growth hormone (GH), or somatotropin, which functions for general tissue growth
- thyroid-stimulating hormone (TSH), or thyrotropin, which triggers the secretion of thyroid hormone
- corticotropin (ACTH), which stimulates the adrenal glands to produce and secrete adrenocortical hormones, mainly affecting the glucocorticoids responsible for controlling carbohydrate, fat, and protein metabolism
- follicle-stimulating hormone (FSH), known as a gonadotropic hormone, which along with luteinizing hormone (LH), regulate the growth and maturation of germ cells and control sex hormone production by the gonads
- LH, also known as a *gonadotropic hormone*
- prolactin, which maintains the corpus luteum and secretion of progesterone and promotes breast milk secretion provided that the breast has been stimulated previously by estrogen and progesterone.

Posterior pituitary. The posterior pituitary, made up of nerve fibers and specialized cells

UNDERSTANDING THE EFFECTS OF THE HYPOTHALAMUS

The hypothalamus is the integrative center of the endocrine and autonomic nervous systems. It helps control some endocrine glands through neural and hormonal stimulation.

Stimulating the posterior pituitary
Neural pathways connect the hypothalamus to the posterior pituitary gland. These hypothalamic neurons stimulate the posterior pituitary gland to secrete two effector hormones—antidiuretic hormone (ADH) and oxytocin—which are stored in the posterior pituitary. When ADH is secreted, the body retains water. Oxytocin stimulates uterine contractions during labor and milk secretion in lactating women.

Regulating the anterior pituitary
The hypothalamus also produces many other inhibiting and stimulating hormones and other factors, which it uses to regulate functions of the anterior pituitary.

that resemble nerve cells, connects more directly to the hypothalamus than does the anterior lobe. Nerve cell bodies in the hypothalamus send their axons down the pituitary stalk to establish direct contact with the cells in the posterior lobe. Hormones produced by the hypothalamus travel down the nerve axons to the posterior lobe; here they're stored and released, as needed, in response to nerve impulses from the hypothalamus. Thus, the posterior pituitary, unlike the anterior lobe, stores—but doesn't actually produce—the hormones it releases.

The posterior pituitary makes up about 25% of the gland. It serves as a storage area for antidiuretic hormone (ADH), or vasopressin, and oxytocin, which are produced by the hypothalamus. ADH affects the permeability of the renal collecting tubules, causing them to absorb more water so that a more concentrated urine is excreted. Oxytocin stimulates uterine contractions and contributes to milk release from lactating breasts.

Thyroid gland

The thyroid gland consists of two lateral lobes, each measuring about 1½″ (4 cm) from top to bottom and ¾″ (2 cm) in width. An isthmus connects the two lobes in the middle. The thyroid is located in the lower part of the neck and overlies the trachea with the isthmus below the cricoid cartilage and the lateral lobes along the lower margins of the thyroid cartilage. A fibrous capsule surrounds the gland, and loose connective tissue fixes it to the trachea. Consequently, the thyroid moves with the larynx and the trachea during swallowing. The lower portions of the sternocleidomastoid muscles partially cover the lateral lobes.

Histologically, the thyroid gland consists of minute, spherical vesicles called thyroid follicles. These follicles synthesize the two thyroid hormones—triiodothyronine (T_3) and thyroxine (T_4) collectively referred to as thyroid hormone. T_3 and T_4 control the rate of the body's metabolic processes and influence growth and development. Thyroid hormone regulates metabolism by speeding cellular respiration. The thyroid also contains small groups of slightly larger cells, located adjacent to the follicles. These parafollicular cells secrete a hormone called calcitonin, which maintains blood calcium levels. It does this by inhibiting the release of calcium from the bone. Secretion of calcitonin is controlled by the calcium concentration of the fluid surrounding the thyroid cells.

Parathyroid glands

The parathyroids are four small glands, only a few millimeters in diameter, located on the posterior surface of the thyroid gland's lateral lobes, one in each corner.

The parathyroid glands working together as one unit secrete parathyroid hormone (PTH). This hormone regulates the ionized calcium and phosphate levels in the blood by controlling calcium and phosphate release from bone, calcium and phosphate absorption from the intestine, and the rate of calcium and phosphate excretion from the kidneys. PTH causes loss of phosphate in the urine at the same time as it causes increased renal tubular reabsorption of calcium. Control of PTH secretion is by a feedback mechanism involving the extracellular fluid concentration of calcium ions. If calcium levels fall, the parathyroids secrete more PTH than usual; if calcium levels rise, PTH secretion decreases. Calcitonin, which has the opposite effect of PTH on calcium metabolism, plays only a minor role in the regulation of blood calcium levels.

Adrenal glands

The adrenals are paired, triangular glands that sit atop the kidneys. Each gland weighs only a few grams, measures about 1½″ (4 cm) in diameter, and consists of two separate structures—the adrenal cortex and the adrenal medulla.

Adrenal cortex. The adrenal cortex, the major part of the gland, is the outer layer and forms the major bulk of the adrenal gland. It has three zones, or cell layers:

- zona glomerulosa, the outermost zone, which produces mineralocorticoids, primarily aldosterone
- zona fasciculata, the middle and largest zone, which produces the glucocorticoids cortisol (hydrocortisone), cortisone, and corticosterone as well as small amounts of the sex hormones androgen and estrogen
- zona reticularis, the innermost zone, which produces mainly glucocorticoids and some sex hormones.

Adrenal medulla. The adrenal medulla, or inner layer of the adrenal gland, functions as part of the sympathetic nervous system and produces two catecholamines: epinephrine and norepinephrine. Because catecholamines play an important role in the autonomic nervous system (ANS), the adrenal medulla is considered a neuroendocrine structure.

Pancreas

The pancreas functions primarily as an exocrine gland. As an exocrine gland, acinar cells make up most of the gland and regulate pancreatic exocrine function. As an endocrine gland, it's involved in secretion of vital hormones. The endocrine part of the pancreas consists of more than a million tiny clusters of alpha, beta, and delta cells, known collectively as the *islets of Langerhans. Alpha cells,* which make up about 20% of the total, secrete glucagon, a hormone that raises blood glucose levels. *Beta cells,* the most numerous type (about 75% of the total), secrete insulin, which lowers blood glucose levels. As the chief hormone secreted by the islets, insulin regulates carbohydrate metabolism and influences protein and fat metabolism. It acts mainly on liver cells, muscle, and adipose tissue. Insulin promotes entry of glucose into the cells and favors utilization of glucose as a source of energy. It also promotes storage of glucose as glycogen in liver and muscle cells and favors both conversion of glucose to fat and fat storage in adipose tissue. The remaining 5% of the islet cells—*delta cells*—secrete somatostatin, a hormone that inhibits the release of GH, corticotrophin, and certain other hormones.

Thymus

The thymus is located below the sternum and contains lymphatic tissue. It reaches maximal size at puberty and then starts to atrophy.

Because the thymus produces T cells, which are important in cell-mediated immunity, its major role seems to be related to the immune system. However, the thymus also produces the peptide hormones thymosin and thymopoietin. These hormones promote growth of peripheral lymphoid tissue.

Pineal gland

The pineal gland lies at the back of the third ventricle of the brain. It produces the hormone melatonin, which may play a role in the neuroendocrine reproductive axis as well as other widespread actions.

Gonads

The gonads include the ovaries (in females) and the testes (in males).

Ovaries. The ovaries are paired, oval glands that are situated on either side of the uterus. They produce ova and the steroidal hormones estrogen and progesterone. These hormones have four functions:

- They promote development and maintenance of female sex characteristics.
- They regulate the menstrual cycle.
- They maintain the uterus for pregnancy.
- Along with other hormones, they prepare the mammary glands for lactation.

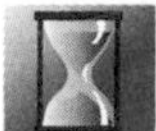

AGE ISSUE *During menopause, a normal part of the aging process in women, ovarian senescence causes permanent cessation of menstrual activity. Changes in endocrine function during menopause vary from woman to woman but normally estrogen levels diminish and follicle-stimulating hormone production increases.*

Testes. The testes are paired structures that lie in the scrotum (an extra-abdominal pouch) in the male. They produce spermatozoa and the male sex hormone testosterone. Testosterone stimulates and maintains male sex characteristics.

Hormones

Hormones are complex chemical substances that trigger or regulate the activity of an organ or a group of cells. Hormones are classified by their molecular structure as polypeptides, steroids, or amines.

Polypeptides

Polypeptides are protein compounds made of many amino acids that are connected by peptide bonds. They include:

- anterior pituitary hormones (GH, TSH, FSH, LH, and prolactin)
- posterior pituitary hormones (ADH and oxytocin)
- PTH

■ pancreatic hormones (insulin and glucagon).

Steroids

Steroids are derived from cholesterol. They include:

■ adrenocortical hormones secreted by the adrenal cortex (aldosterone and cortisol)

■ sex hormones secreted by the gonads (estrogen and progesterone in females and testosterone in males).

Amines

Amines are derived from tyrosine, an essential amino acid found in most proteins. They include:

■ thyroid hormones (T_4 and T_3)

■ catecholamines (epinephrine, norepinephrine, and dopamine).

Hormone release and transport

Although all hormone release results from endocrine gland stimulation, release patterns of hormones vary greatly. For example:

■ corticotropin (secreted by the anterior pituitary) and cortisol (secreted by the adrenal cortex) are released in spurts in response to body rhythm cycles. Levels of these hormones peak in the morning.

■ Secretion of PTH (by the parathyroid gland) and prolactin (by the anterior pituitary) occurs fairly evenly throughout the day.

■ Secretion of insulin by the pancreas has both steady and sporadic release patterns.

Receptors

When a hormone reaches its target site, it binds to a specific receptor on the cell membrane or within the cell. Polypeptides and some amines bind to membrane receptor sites. The smaller, more lipid-soluble steroids and thyroid hormones diffuse through the cell membrane and bind to intracellular receptors.

After binding occurs, each hormone produces unique physiologic changes, depending on its target site and its specific action at that site. A particular hormone may have different effects at different target sites.

Hormonal regulation

To maintain the body's delicate equilibrium, a feedback mechanism regulates hormone production and secretion. The mechanism involves hormones, blood chemicals and metabolites, and the nervous system. This system may be simple or complex. (See *Regulating the endocrine system.*)

For normal function, each gland must contain enough appropriately programmed secretory cells to release active hormone on demand. Secretory cells need supervision. A secretory cell can't sense on its own when to release the hormone or how much to release. It gets this information from sensing and signaling systems that integrate many messages. Together, stimulatory and inhibitory signals actively control the rate and duration of hormone release. When released, the hormone travels to target cells, where a receptor molecule recognizes it and binds to it. (See *Target cells,* page 322.)

Hormone release

Four basic mechanisms control hormone release:

■ the pituitary-target gland axis

■ the hypothalamic-pituitary-target gland axis

■ chemical regulation

■ nervous system regulation.

Pituitary-target gland axis. The pituitary gland regulates other endocrine glands — and their hormones — through secretion of trophic hormones — releasing and inhibiting hormones. These hormones include:

■ corticotropin, which regulates adrenocortical hormones

■ TSH, which regulates T_4 and T_3

■ LH, which regulates gonadal hormones.

The pituitary gets feedback about target glands by continuously monitoring levels of hormones produced by these glands. If a change occurs, the pituitary corrects it in one of two ways:

■ by increasing the trophic hormones, which stimulate the target gland to increase production of target gland hormones

■ by decreasing the trophic hormones, thereby decreasing target gland stimulation and target gland hormone levels.

Hypothalamic-pituitary-target gland axis. The hypothalamus also produces trophic hormones that regulate anterior pituitary hormones. By controlling anterior pituitary hormones, which regulate the target gland

REGULATING THE ENDOCRINE SYSTEM

This diagram shows the negative feedback mechanism that regulates the endocrine system.

Simple feedback

Simple feedback occurs when the level of one substance regulates the secretion of hormones. For example, a low serum calcium level stimulates the parathyroid gland to release parathyroid hormone (PTH). PTH, in turn, promotes resorption of calcium. A high serum calcium level inhibits PTH secretion.

Complex feedback

When the hypothalamus receives negative feedback from target glands, the mechanism is more complicated. Complex feedback occurs through an axis established between the hypothalamus, pituitary gland, and target organ. For example, secretion of corticotropin-releasing hormone from the hypothalamus stimulates release of corticotropin by the pituitary, which in turn stimulates cortisol secretion by the adrenal gland (the target organ). A rise in serum cortisol levels inhibits corticotropin secretion by decreasing corticotropin-releasing hormone.

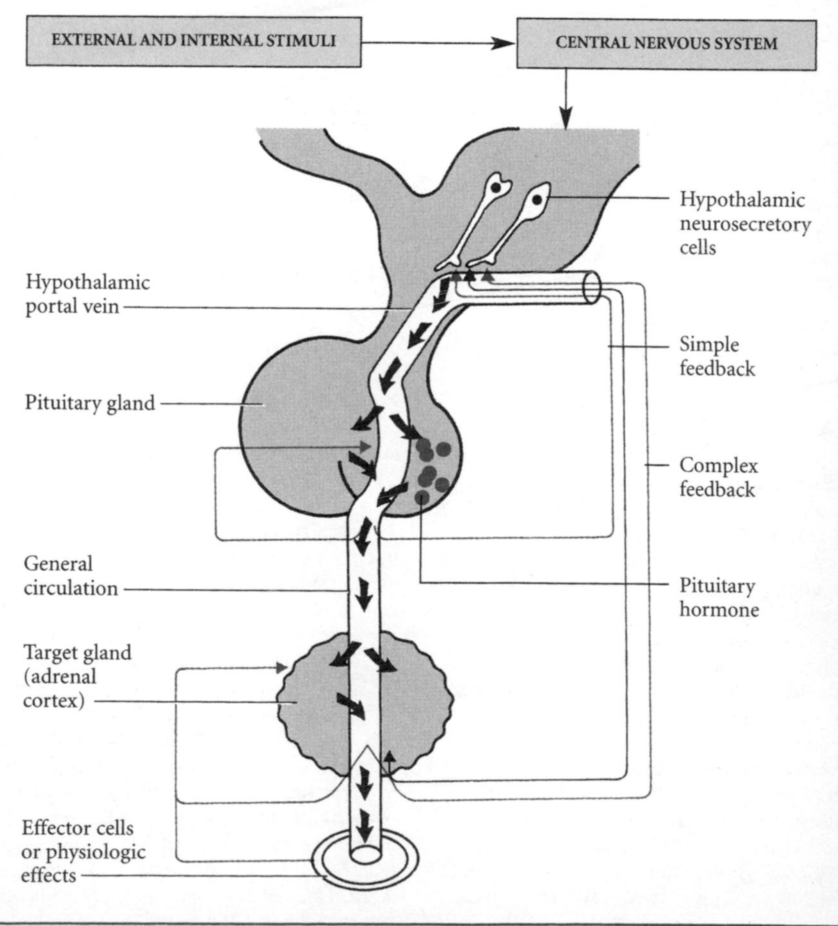

TARGET CELLS

Hormones act only on cells that have receptors specific to that hormone. The sensitivity of a target cell depends on how many receptors it has for a particular hormone; the more receptor sites, the more sensitive the target cell.

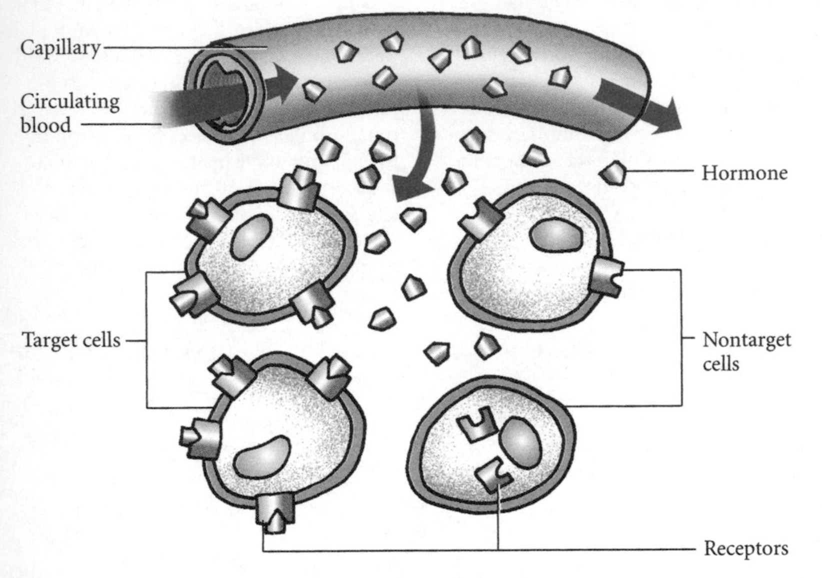

hormones, the hypothalamus affects target glands as well.

Chemical regulation. Endocrine glands not controlled by the pituitary gland may be controlled by specific substances that trigger gland secretions. For example, blood glucose level is a major regulator of glucagon and insulin release. When the blood glucose level rises, the pancreas is stimulated to increase insulin secretion and suppress glucagon secretion. A depressed level of blood glucose, on the other hand, triggers increased glucagon secretion and suppresses insulin secretion.

Nervous system regulation. The central nervous system (CNS) helps to regulate hormone secretion in several ways. The hypothalamus controls pituitary hormones. Because hypothalamic nerve cells stimulate the posterior pituitary to produce ADH and oxytocin, these hormones are controlled directly by the CNS.

Nervous system stimuli — such as hypoxia (oxygen deficiency), nausea, pain, stress, and certain drugs — also affect ADH levels.

The ANS controls catecholamine secretion by the adrenal medulla.

The nervous system also affects other endocrine hormones. For example, stress, which leads to sympathetic stimulation, causes the pituitary to release corticotropin.

AGE ISSUE *Elderly patients experience a decreased ability to tolerate stress. The most obvious and serious indication of this diminished stress response occurs in glucose metabolism. Normally, fasting blood sugar levels aren't significantly different in young and older adults. But when stress stimulates an older person's pancreas, the blood sugar concentration increase is greater and lasts longer than in a younger adult. This decreased glucose tolerance occurs as a normal part of aging.*

Health history

When assessing a patient's endocrine system, remember that it affects many, if not all, of the other body systems. In fact, make sure you evaluate the endocrine system when you assess any of a patient's body systems, because, for instance, an endocrine disorder may cause cardiovascular, reproductive, or nervous system signs and symptoms.

Ask the patient's age and ethnic background to help determine if variations specifically related to growth, pubertal development, or hair distribution are within normal limits.

Chief complaint

Because of the endocrine's interrelationship with other body systems, the patient's chief complaints can be wide-ranging and numerous. Attempt to focus questions on the complaints that are causing the patient the most difficulty. Some of the most common chief complaints regarding endocrine disorders include fatigue and weakness, weight changes, abnormalities of sexual maturity or function, mental status changes, and polyuria and polydipsia.

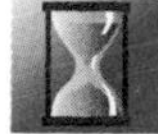

AGE ISSUE *In children, the most common signs and symptoms of endocrine abnormalities are growth and developmental disturbances. However, these disturbances are typically so subtle that only a thorough physical examination will reveal them. Parents may want their child examined because he's restless or doing poorly in school.*

Current health history

To initiate the history, ask the patient some general questions that address all body systems. Ask if he has noticed any changes in his skin such as bruising or in the amount or distribution of his body hair. Find out if his eyes burn or feel gritty when he closes them. Also, ask him how his sense of smell is.

Then ask the patient to elaborate on his chief complaint. Focus the discussion on the onset, duration, quality, severity, location, precipitating factors, alleviating factors, and associated symptoms. Ask such questions as:

- What causes it? What makes it better? Worse?
- How does it feel, look, or sound and how much of it is there?
- Where is it? Does it spread?
- Does it interfere with activities? If so, ask the patient to rate the interference on a scale of 1 to 10.
- When did it begin? How often does it occur? Is it sudden or gradual?

Remember that these chief complaints may be related to an endocrine disturbance or they may be psychogenic. Careful questioning helps to differentiate between the two. Then depending on the complaint, explore the history of his present illness, such as fatigue and weakness, changes in weight, abnormalities of sexual maturation or function, mental status changes, and conditions, such as polyuria and polydipsia.

Fatigue and weakness

Ask the patient about fatigue and if it's constant or intermittent. If it's intermittent, ask him when it occurs, for instance, when he wakes up in the morning or at the end of the day. Find out if the patient feels more tired after strenuous exercise and if rest makes him feel better. Fatigue is a nonspecific complaint that occurs in both organic and psychological illnesses.

Fatigue from organic causes is intermittent—worse at the end of the day and after exercise, better in the morning and after rest. Find out if your patient's feeling of weakness is generalized or localized. In many cases, generalized weakness indicates systemic illness, such as an endocrine disorder; localized weakness may suggest a neurologic disorder. Ask if he feels numbness or tingling in his arms or legs. These sensations may indicate peripheral neuropathy, which occurs in some endocrine disorders.

Weight changes

Ask the patient how much he usually weighs. Find out the least and most he has ever weighed and use these figures as baselines. Ask him how long he was gaining (or losing) weight, if he's still gaining (or losing) weight, and if his weight gain (or loss) was intentional. Answers to these questions should help to determine if the patient's weight changes are from an organic disorder or from overeating (or strict dieting).

Ask the patient about his nutrition. Find out what his daily food intake is, including alcoholic beverages. Ask him if his appetite has increased or decreased. If it has decreased, ask him whether the decrease is constant or whether he's intermittently hungry. Persistent loss of appetite suggests an organic cause; intermittent loss of appetite may indicate a psychogenic problem, such as depression. Finally, ask the patient if he's eating more but still losing weight. This condition may result from an endocrine disorder.

Sexual maturation or function abnormalities

Ask your female patient at what age she began to menstruate. Have her describe the volume of her normal flow, asking for instance, if it's heavy and how many days it lasts. Find out when she had her last normal period. Ask about missed periods and if she could be pregnant. Find out if the patient is under a great deal of stress, because severe stress can cause amenorrhea. If your patient has children, ask if her periods resumed normally after childbirth. Unless the patient is breast-feeding her child, nonresumption of menstruation may indicate an endocrine disorder.

Ask both male and female patients if their sexual desire has increased or decreased and when this change occurred. Find out how often your patient normally experiences sexual desire. Ask female patients if their breast size has changed. Endocrine disorders can cause breast enlargement, especially in men. Make sure such enlargement isn't from weight gain. Also find out if the patient's breasts have been secreting milk. Lactation from an endocrine disorder can occur in both men and women. (See chapter 14, Female genitourinary system and chapter 15, Male genitourinary system, for more information on assessing these systems.)

Mental status changes

Ask your patient if he has difficulty coping with his problems. Find out if he's nervous; if so, ask him how often. Ask the patient if he has difficulty sitting still. Find out if these feelings are triggered by specific events. Endocrine disorders can cause nervous behavior or emotional lability. Ask the patient if he has been feeling confused recently and, if so, how long he has felt this way. Find out if the onset was quick or gradual and if the confusion is constant or intermittent. Ask about previous episodes. Confusion caused by endocrine disorders has a quick onset and is usually intermittent. Next, ask the patient about his sleeping patterns, such as if he has difficulty sleeping. Ask whether he has difficulty falling asleep or staying asleep, and how long he has been having difficulty sleeping. Find out how many hours he sleeps and if that's different from his usual pattern. Ask the patient if he feels he has to sleep during the day, if he's sleepy all day, and how long he has felt this way. Also ask him if he wakes up refreshed. Changes in sleep patterns may result from endocrine disorders. Certain endocrine disorders may produce hallucinations and delusions, so note any reference to thought disorders during your conversation with the patient.

Polyuria and polydipsia

Ask the patient how long he has been passing large quantities of urine and if the onset was sudden or gradual. Find out how many times per day he urinates. Ask if he passes large quantities of urine every time he urinates or only sometimes. Varying amounts suggest dysuria, not polyuria. Ask the patient if he wakes up at night to urinate. This may suggest a urinary tract disorder instead of an endocrine disorder.

Ask the patient if his thirst is insatiable and if it's constant or variable. Find out if he prefers ice-cold fluids. A preference for ice-cold fluids may suggest an endocrine disorder; no preference may indicate psychogenic polydipsia. Find out how much fluid the patient drinks at present and how much he used to drink. Also, ask the patient if he urinates less frequently when he's deprived of fluid. Answers to these questions help you distinguish the compulsive drinker from a patient with polydipsia, which is caused by an endocrine condition.

Past health history

When recording your patient's past history for assessment of a suspected endocrine condition, focus on these key areas:

- *Trauma.* Repeated fractures may indicate adrenal or parathyroid problems; fracture at the base of the skull may cause midbrain injury, resulting in pituitary and hypothalamus dysfunction. Fright, stress, or trauma may precipitate diabetes insipidus.

- *Surgical procedures.* Bilateral oophorectomy results in decreased estrogen and progesterone production, leading to signs and symptoms of the climacteric, such as amenorrhea. Neck surgery may cause thyroid function abnormalities. Partial or total adrenalectomy may result in adrenal crisis. Hypophysectomy impairs regulation of fluid volume by antidiuretic hormone. Also, the stress from any surgery can precipitate endocrine disorders, such as pheochromocytoma.
- *Obstetric history.* Gestational diabetes mellitus may suggest possible impaired blood glucose control predisposing the patient to diabetes mellitus, as may giving birth to an infant weighing more than 10 lb (4.5 kg).
- *Drugs.* Prescription and over-the-counter medications and herbal remedies including those for sleep problems, diet, or anxiety, may mask or simulate symptoms of endocrine disorders
- *General.* Unexplained neuromuscular disorders and such nonspecific symptoms as nervousness, fatigue, and weakness may indicate underlying hyperthyroidism. Thyroid test results may reveal previous thyroid problems. Long-standing obesity contributes to the development of diabetes mellitus. Irradiation can cause glandular atrophy. Meningitis or encephalitis can cause hypothalamic disturbances.

Family history

Because certain endocrine disorders are inherited and others have strong familial tendencies, a thorough family history is essential. Ask your patient if anyone in his family is (or was) obese, or has had diabetes mellitus, thyroid disease, or hypertension. Diabetes mellitus has an especially strong familial tendency. Thyroid conditions, such as goiter, also show familial tendencies. Pheochromocytoma may result from an autosomal dominant trait. Delayed puberty recurs in certain families; in women, this condition causes primary amenorrhea.

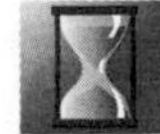

AGE ISSUE *When assessing a child, obtaining a thorough family history from one or both parents is essential because endocrine disorders may be hereditary or demonstrate a familial tendency. An older child or adolescent can probably give you a more accurate history of his physical growth and sexual development than his parents can, so interview the child, too, when this is possible.*

Psychosocial history

A key aspect of the patient's psychosocial history is environment. Although rare, iodine deficiency in local water and food may cause thyroid enlargement.

Inquire about the patient's activities of daily living. Ask about his diet. Specifically, determine whether he has any unusual eating habits. For instance, does your patient routinely follow a strict, limited, or fad-food diet? Adolescent girls typically diet unnecessarily and may develop severe nutritional deficiencies and extreme weight loss, which can cause amenorrhea.

Also, determine whether your patient uses recreational drugs or drinks alcohol regularly; if he does, ask how much and how often. Intoxication or withdrawal from drugs or alcohol can produce signs and symptoms that mimic endocrine disorders.

Review of systems

When completing the health history, ask the patient specific questions related to all body systems. First, review the patient's overall general health status, including the frequency of infections. Then focus questions on these systems:

- *Integumentary system.* Changes in skin, including hair growth and pattern may occur. For example, hirsutism occurs with ovarian and adrenocortical disorders that result in increased androgen production. Excessive hair loss may be an autoimmune response. Loss of axillary and pubic hair may result from a pituitary disorder. Episodes of flushing and diaphoresis may occur in association with abnormal heat intolerance, a classic complaint of patients with hyperthyroidism. Abnormal cold intolerance may indicate hypothyroidism.
- *Eyes.* Exophthalmos is present in endocrine disorders involving the thyroid. Partial loss of vision may indicate a pituitary tumor.
- *Mouth and throat.* Hoarseness can indicate laryngeal nerve compression from a tumor or, in women, excessive androgen production. Difficulty swallowing may be the

result of compression or displacement of the esophagus by an enlarged thyroid gland.

- *Cardiovascular system.* Orthostatic hypotension occurs in adrenal disorders. Palpitations with sweating and flushing may result from the hormonal imbalances of an endocrine disorder, such as hyperthyroidism, or possibly from an adrenal tumor that increases epinephrine production. Leg swelling from heart failure or myxedema occurs in patients with thyroid disorders.
- *Nervous system.* Tremors during periods of sustained posture, for instance, when a patient holds his arm out in front of his body for a period of time, may occur in patients with thyroid disorders. Paresthesia may result from peripheral neuropathies associated with certain endocrine disorders.
- *Musculoskeletal system.* Arthralgia, bone pain, and extremity enlargement may result from disorders of the growth process.
- *Respiratory system.* Stridor or dyspnea may occur in the patient with an enlarged thyroid gland that compresses his trachea.
- *GI system.* Frequent loose bowel movements may accompany hyperthyroidism; constipation may accompany hypothyroidism.

Physical assessment

Due to the endocrine system's interrelationship with all other body systems, physical assessment of a patient's endocrine function consists of a complete evaluation of his body. Make sure the lighting in the examining room is adequate, because the assessment depends primarily on inspection. Palpation and auscultation also will be used to assess a patient's thyroid gland.

General assessment

Begin your assessment of the endocrine system by focusing on the patient's general physical appearance and emotional status. Observe the patient's apparent state of health, and note any signs of distress. Assess general body development including height and weight, body build and posture, and proportion of body parts. Also, note the distribution of body fat. In men, fat tissue should be distributed evenly over the entire body. In women, fat tissue normally concentrates in the shoulders, breasts, buttocks, inner thighs, and pubic symphysis. In men and women who are obese, excessive fat accumulates in these same areas.

CRITICAL POINT *When assessing the endocrine system, distinguish between the fat distribution of obesity and that of Cushing's syndrome: In a patient with Cushing's syndrome, fat is concentrated on the face, neck, interscapular area, trunk, and pelvic girdle.*

While you talk with your patient, observe his activity level. Look to see if he moves briskly or are his movements extremely slow. The former may indicate hyperthyroidism; the latter, hypothyroidism. Note his speech — its coherence, quality, and speed. The patient with hyperthyroidism can't get his words out fast enough; the patient with myxedema sounds hoarse and slurs his words.

Next, assess your patient's vital signs. Take his blood pressure in both arms while lying, sitting, and standing. Compare the findings with normal expected values and the patient's baseline measurements, if available.

CRITICAL POINT *Hypertension occurs in many endocrine disorders, particularly pheochromocytoma and Cushing's syndrome. Hyperthyroidism causes systolic blood pressure elevations. Arrhythmias may accompany metabolic disturbances.*

When taking a patient's apical pulse, note its quality and character. In an adult, a heart rate below 60 or above 100 beats/minute may suggest thyroid disease. Deep, rapid respirations (Kussmaul's respirations) may indicate diabetic ketoacidosis.

Inspection

Systematically inspect the patient's overall appearance and examine all areas of the body

Skin assessment

Focus first on skin color. Observe for hyperpigmentation, both generalized and localized, on the patient's exposed areas and at pressure points. Remember, hyperpigmentation can range from tan to brown.

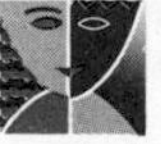

CULTURAL INSIGHT *When assessing skin pigmentation, consider racial and ethnic variations. For example, hyperpigmented gums are normal in*

Blacks but may indicate Addison's disease in Whites. Use the sclera, conjunctiva, mouth, nail beds, and palms to obtain the most accurate information.

Also, observe the patient for areas of hypopigmentation (vitiligo), which may be associated with Addison's disease, thyroid disorders, or diabetes mellitus. Inspect the patient's sclerae to help distinguish yellow pigmentation caused by myxedema from jaundice. Jaundice causes yellowing of the sclerae; myxedema doesn't.

Next, examine the patient's skin for hydration and texture. Dry, rough skin may be a sign of hypothyroidism or dehydration; smooth, flushed skin can accompany hyperthyroidism. Observe for areas of lipoatrophy and wasting, which may appear at injection sites in patients with diabetes mellitus. Easy bruising may be associated with the tissue breakdown of Cushing's syndrome. Skin lesions and ulcerations commonly appear in patients with diabetes mellitus. Also look for poor wound healing, which is associated with the peripheral circulation problems characteristic of some endocrine disorders, such as diabetes mellitus.

Hair and nail assessment

Observe your patient's nails, noting color, shape, and quality. Thick, brittle nails may suggest hypothyroidism; thin, brittle nails may result from hyperthyroidism. Also note the attachment of the nail to the nail bed. Separation of the nail from the bed, beginning at the nail edge, may suggest a thyroid disorder. Increased nail pigmentation occurs in Addison's disease.

Inspect the patient's hair for abnormalities. Note the amount of scalp and body hair. Check for abnormal patterns of hair loss or hair growth; if your patient is a woman, note any excessive facial, chest, or abdominal hair (hirsutism). Remember to consider racial and ethnic variations in texture and distribution of hair. Observe for hair thinning or loss on the outer eyebrows, axillae, and genitalia in both men and women.

Note the texture of the patient's hair by inspecting and touching it. Fine, soft, silky hair is characteristic of hyperthyroidism, in contrast to the coarse, dry, brittle hair you'll find in patients with hypothyroidism.

Face and neck assessment

Carefully inspect your patient's face. First, study his expression. Does he stare and look alarmed? Or, is his expression dull and apathetic? Note any coarsening of facial features, such as his nose, lips, and ears, and check for a prominent forehead and protruding lower jaw. These are possible signs of a growth abnormality. "Moon face" is a sign of Cushing's syndrome. Also observe for facial edema, especially around the patient's eyes. With your index finger, apply firm pressure to this area and watch for pitting. Nonpitting facial edema, especially if accompanied by periorbital edema, may indicate hypothyroidism.

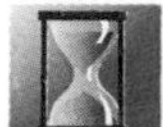

AGE ISSUE *Always inspect the child's face to determine if his facial appearance correlates with his age. In cretinism, for example, a child retains his infantile facial appearance.*

Eyes. After observing your patient's entire face, carefully inspect his eyes. Observe their position and alignment. Be especially alert for abnormal protrusion of the eyeball with obvious lid retraction (exophthalmos), which may indicate increased thyroid function.

Test extraocular movements through the six cardinal positions of gaze (see chapter 6, Eyes). Note any evidence of extraocular muscle paralysis or reduced function, which can develop secondary to diabetic neuropathy or thyroid dysfunction. Test for eye convergence, which is usually poor in a patient with hypothyroidism. Inspect the relation of the upper eyelids to the eyeballs as the patient moves his eyes to gaze upward and then down. "Lid lag" — a margin of white sclera between the upper lid and the iris as the patient's gaze moves down — may indicate hyperthyroidism.

Test the patient's visual acuity and then test his visual fields. Some endocrine disorders, such as pituitary tumors, may cause visual field defects and reduced visual acuity.

Using an oblique light source, inspect for opacities in the cornea and the lens of the patient's eye. Premature cataracts may appear in a patient with diabetes or hypoparathyroidism. When performing a funduscopic examination, be alert for microaneurysms (tiny red spots), hemorrhages (large, slightly irregular red spots), and exudates (yellow spots), which are characteristic of diabetic retinopathy. Watch for arteriolar narrowing, which may be present in a patient with long-term hypertension associated with pheochromocytoma and Cushing's syndrome.

Mouth. Next, examine the patient's mouth. Inspect the buccal mucosa for color and condition. Look for patchy, brown pigmentation of the gums, a possible sign of Addison's disease. Have the patient extend his tongue and inspect it color, size, lesions, positioning, and tremors or unusual movements. An enlarged tongue is associated with myxedema. Also note the patient's breath odor. If it smells fruity, like acetone, he may be in diabetic ketoacidosis.

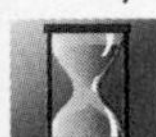

AGE ISSUE *When inspecting a child's mouth, check if the number of teeth corresponds with normal expectations for the child's age. Delayed eruption of teeth occurs in hypothyroidism and hypopituitarism.*

Neck. Carefully inspect the patient's neck. First, move any hair and clothing away from his neck to check contour and symmetry with the patient's neck held straight. Then, inspect his slightly extended neck for symmetry and midline positioning and for symmetry of the trachea.

Use tangential lighting directed downward from the patient's chin to see the thyroid gland. Observe for any visible signs of thyroid enlargement or asymmetry. An enlarged thyroid gland may be diffuse and asymmetrical. Note how the thyroid gland moves when the patient swallows. Ask him if he has difficulty swallowing, and if he has any hoarseness or neck pain.

Chest assessment

Evaluate the overall size, shape, and symmetry of the patient's chest, noting any deformities. In females, assess the breasts for size, shape, symmetry, pigmentation (especially on the nipples and in skin creases), and nipple discharge (galactorrhea). In males, observe for bilateral or unilateral breast enlargement (gynecomastia) and nipple discharge.

Abdomen assessment

Inspect the patient's abdomen for shape, contour, and fat distribution. Abnormalities in these areas are associated with endocrine disorders. Look carefully at the skin, noting any purple-red striae. Observe your female patients for abdominal hair distribution.

External genitalia assessment

Inspect the patient's external genitalia for sexual maturation, particularly the size of the testes or clitoris. Small testes may indicate hypogonadism; an enlarged clitoris suggests virilization. Also note the amount and distribution of pubic hair.

Musculoskeletal assessment

Inspect the size and proportions of your patient's body. Extremely short stature suggests dwarfism; disproportionate body parts, such as enlarged hands or feet, may be caused by excessive amounts of growth hormone, as in acromegaly.

Next, inspect the patient's vertebral column for such deformities as an enlarged disk or kyphosis, which may appear in acromegaly and hyperparathyroidism. Observe the joints for enlargement and deformity, and use range-of-motion tests to check for stiffness and pain. All these signs and symptoms can result from hypothyroidism.

Inspect the patient's muscles of the arms and legs for tremors. To do so, have the patient hold both arms outstretched in front with the palms down and fingers separated. Place a sheet of paper on the outstretched fingers and watch for trembling.

Note any muscle wasting or atrophy, especially in the upper arms. Have the patient grasp your hands to assess strength and symmetry of his grip.

Inspect the legs for muscle development, symmetry, color, and hair distribution. Examine the feet for size and note lesions, corns, calluses or marks from socks or shoes. Inspect the toes and the spaces between them for maceration and fissures.

Neurologic assessment

Assess the patient's level of consciousness. Assess your patient's sensitivity to pain, touch, and vibration, and his position sense. Sensory loss may occur in diabetic neuropathy; paresthesias can result from hypothy-

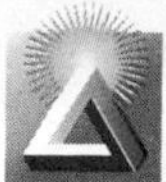

EXPERT TECHNIQUE

PALPATING THE THYROID

Palpation steps

- First, stand in front of the patient and place your index and middle fingers below the cricoid cartilage on both sides of the trachea.
- Next, palpate for the thyroid isthmus as he swallows.
- Then ask the patient to flex his neck toward the side being examined as you gently palpate each lobe.

In most cases, only the isthmus connecting the two lobes is palpable. However, if the patient has a thin neck, you may feel the whole gland. If he has a short, stocky neck, you may have trouble palpating even an enlarged thyroid.

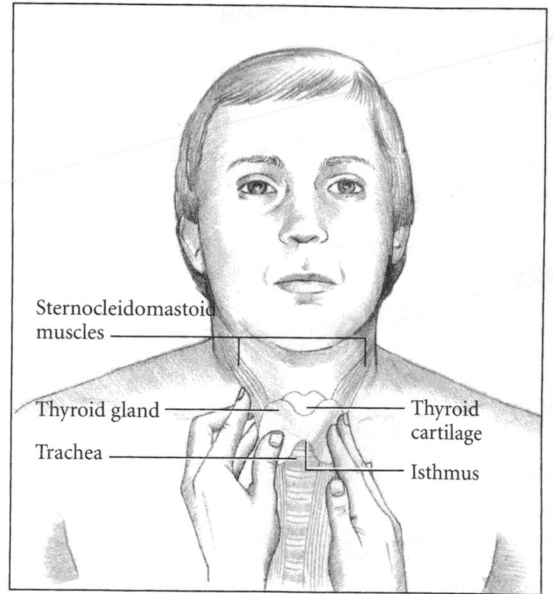

Locating the right and left lobe

- First, use your right hand to displace the thyroid cartilage slightly to your left.
- Next, hook your left index and middle fingers around the sternocleidomastoid muscle, as shown above, to palpate for thyroid enlargement.
- Then examine the left lobe by using your left hand to displace the thyroid cartilage and your right hand to palpate the lobe.

roidism, diabetes, and acromegaly. Note any loss of motor function. Wristdrop or ankledrop may signal extreme diabetic neuropathy.

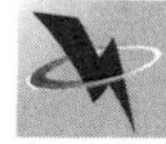

CRITICAL POINT *Alterations in consciousness may occur in a patient with uncontrolled diabetes or myxedema.*

Assess deep tendon reflexes in your patient, noting any evidence of hyperreflexia with delayed relaxation associated with hyperthyroidism and hypoparathyroidism. Hyporeflexia, especially with ankle jerk reflex, may occur in a patient with hypothyroidism or diabetic neuropathy.

Palpation

When assessing a patient's endocrine system, palpation is primarily completed for the thyroid gland. If inspection of other body systems reveals abnormalities, then other body systems can be palpated as well.

Thyroid palpation

To examine the thyroid, stand facing the patient or behind him, and ask him to lower his chin, which relaxes the neck muscles and makes the examination easier. (See *Palpating the thyroid.*)

Palpate the thyroid gland for size, shape, symmetry, tenderness, and nodules. When palpating from the front, use your index and middle fingers to feel for the thyroid isthmus, below the cricoid cartilage, as the patient swallows. Swallowing raises the larynx, the trachea, and the thyroid gland—but not the lymph nodes and other structures.

Palpate one lobe at a time. Ask the patient to flex his neck slightly to the side you're examining. To palpate the right lobe, use your right hand to move the thyroid cartilage slightly to the right. Then, grasp the sternocleidomastoid muscle with your left hand (tips of index and middle fingers behind the muscle, thumb in front), and try to palpate for the right lobe of the thyroid between your fingers.

To palpate the left lobe, use your left hand to move the thyroid cartilage and your right hand to palpate. To palpate the thyroid from behind the patient, gently place the fingers of both hands on either side of the trachea, just below the thyroid cartilage. Try to feel the thyroid isthmus as your patient swallows. While you're palpating one lobe at a time, ask the patient to flex his neck to the side being examined. To feel for the right lobe, use your left hand to move the thyroid cartilage to the right. Grasp the sternocleidomastoid muscle with your right hand, while placing your middle fingers deep into and in front of the muscle. For the left lobe, use your right hand to move the cartilage to the left and your left hand to palpate.

In most patients, you won't feel the thyroid gland, but you may feel the isthmus. You may see or feel a normal thyroid in a patient with a thin neck.

CRITICAL POINT *When you do palpate a large mass, don't confuse thick neck musculature with an enlarged thyroid or goiter. An enlarged thyroid may feel finely lobulated, like a well-defined organ. Thyroid nodules feel like a knot, protuberance, or swelling. A firm, fixed nodule may be a tumor.*

When you detect an enlarged thyroid, perform Kocher's test to determine if it's compressing the patient's trachea. Ask your patient to inspire deeply as you apply slight pressure on the gland's lateral lobes. If the enlarged gland is causing tracheal compression, the pressure you apply will produce stridor on deep inspiration. When you elicit a positive response to Kocher's test, observe your patient for dyspnea.

Testing for hypocalcemia. Determine if the patient is experiencing hypocalcemic tetany (a rapid drop in serum calcium levels from deficient or ineffective PTH secretion from hypoparathyroidism or surgical removal of the parathyroid gland) by testing for Chvostek's sign and Trousseau's sign. (See *Assessing for hypocalcemia.*)

Test for Chvostek's sign by tapping one finger in front of the patient's ear at the angle of the jaw, over the facial nerve. If contracture of the lateral facial muscles results, Chvostek's sign is positive.

To check for Trousseau's sign, apply a blood pressure cuff to the patient's arm just above the antecubital area. Inflate the cuff until you've occluded the blood supply to his arm. If this procedure precipitates carpal spasm displayed by finger contractions and inability to open the hand, Trousseau's sign is positive.

Auscultation

If you palpate an enlarged thyroid, auscultate the gland for systolic bruits. Place the bell of the stethoscope over one of the thyroid's lateral lobes. Then listen carefully for a bruit—a low, soft, rushing sound. This occurs in hyperthyroidism because accelerated blood flow through the thyroid arteries produces vibrations. If necessary, ask the patient to hold his breath and avoid swallowing, so tracheal sounds don't interfere with auscultation.

To distinguish a bruit from a venous hum, listen for the rushing sound, then gently occlude the jugular vein with your fingers on the side you're auscultating and listen again. A venous hum, produced by jugular blood flow, disappears during venous compression; however, a bruit doesn't disappear.

Abnormal findings

A patient's chief complaint may be for any of a number of signs and symptoms related to the endocrine system. The most significant findings include cold intolerance, fatigue, heat intolerance, hirsutism, moon face, polydipsia, polyuria, thyroid enlarge-

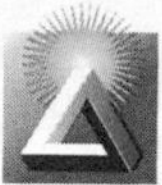

EXPERT TECHNIQUE

ASSESSING FOR HYPOCALCEMIA

In patients with tetany associated with hypocalcemia, there are two signs that indicate this condition: Chvostek's and Trousseau's signs. To elicit these signs, follow the procedures described here. Immediately notify the health care provider if you detect them.

While conducting these tests, watch the patient for laryngospasm, monitor his cardiac status, and have resuscitation equipment nearby. Keep in mind the discomfort these tests typically cause.

Chvostek's sign

To elicit Chvostek's sign, tap the patient's facial nerve just in front of the earlobe and below the zygomatic arch or between the zygomatic arch and the corner of the mouth, as shown.

A positive response, indicating latent tetany, ranges from simple mouth-corner twitching to twitching of all facial muscles on the side tested. Simple twitching may be normal in some patients. However, a more pronounced response usually confirms Chvostek's sign.

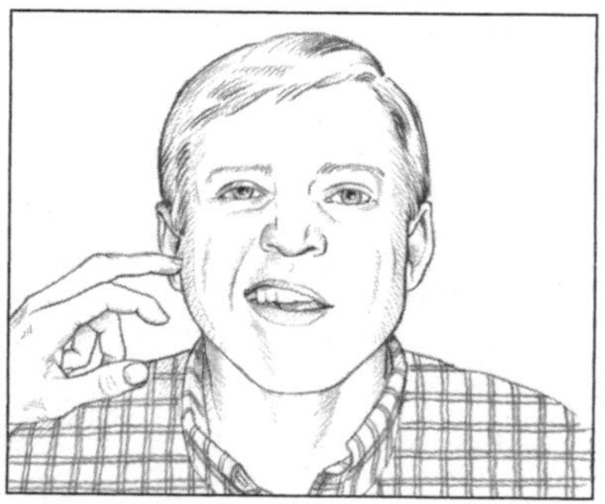

Trousseau's sign

To test for Trousseau's sign, occlude the brachial artery by inflating a blood pressure cuff on the patient's upper arm to a level between diastolic and systolic blood pressure. Maintain this inflation for 3 minutes while observing the patient for Trousseau's sign, or carpal spasm, as shown.

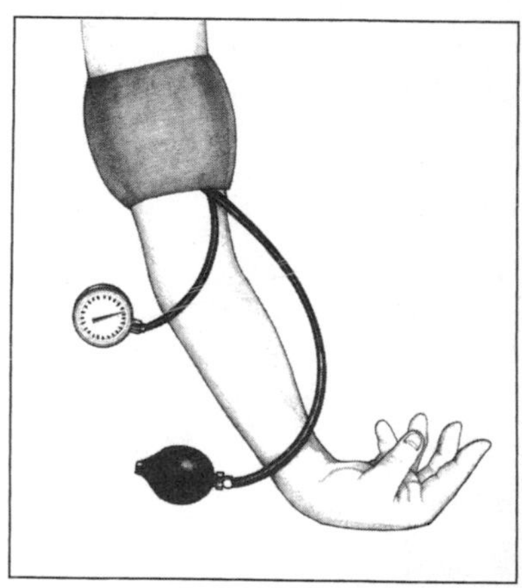

ment, and tremors. The following history, physical examination, and analysis summaries will help you assess each one quickly and accurately. After obtaining further information, begin to interpret the findings. (See *Endocrine system: Interpreting your findings,* pages 332 to 336.)

Cold intolerance

Usually developing gradually, this increased sensitivity to cold temperatures reflects damage to the body's temperature-regulating mechanism, based on interactions between the hypothalamus and the thyroid gland.

History

Find out when the patient first noticed cold intolerance. For instance, ask him when he began to use more blankets or wear heavier clothing. Ask about associated signs and symptoms, such as changes in vision or in the texture or amount of body hair. Ask the female patient about changes in her normal menstrual pattern.

(Text continues on page 336.)

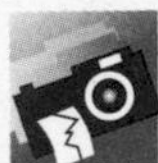

CLINICAL PICTURE

ENDOCRINE SYSTEM: INTERPRETING YOUR FINDINGS

After you assess the patient, a group of findings may lead you to a particular disorder of the endocrine system. The chart below shows some common groups of findings for major signs and symptoms related to an assessment of the endocrine system, along with their probable causes.

Sign or symptom and findings	Probable cause
Cold intolerance	
▪ Gradual onset of cold intolerance with shivering ▪ Cold dry thin skin with waxy pallor ▪ Fine wrinkles around the mouth ▪ Fatigue, lethargy ▪ Menstrual disturbances ▪ Impotence ▪ Decreased libido ▪ Nervousness ▪ Irritability	Hypopituitarism
▪ Early onset of cold intolerance that progressively worsens ▪ Fatigue ▪ Anorexia with weight gain ▪ Constipation ▪ Menorrhagia ▪ Loss of libido ▪ Slowed mental processes	Hypothyroidism
Fatigue	
▪ Mild fatigue after exertion and stress becoming more severe and persistent ▪ Weakness ▪ Weight loss with GI disturbances such as nausea, vomiting, abdominal pain, and chronic diarrhea ▪ Hyperpigmentation ▪ Orthostatic hypotension ▪ Weak irregular pulse	Adrenal insufficiency
▪ Insidious or abrupt onset fatigue ▪ Weight loss ▪ Blurred vision ▪ Polyuria ▪ Polydipsia ▪ Polyphagia	Diabetes mellitus
▪ Fatigue accompanied by lethargy and weakness occurring slowly ▪ Irritability ▪ Anorexia ▪ Amenorrhea or impotence ▪ Decreased libido ▪ Hypotension ▪ Dizziness ▪ Headache ▪ Cold intolerance	Hypopituitarism

ENDOCRINE SYSTEM: INTERPRETING YOUR FINDINGS *(continued)*

Sign or symptom and findings	Probable cause
Heat intolerance	
▪ Dramatic fluctuations in body temperature with alternating heat and cold intolerances ▪ Amenorrhea ▪ Disturbed sleep patterns ▪ Increased thirst and urination ▪ Increased appetite and weight gain ▪ Impaired visual acuity ▪ Headache ▪ Personality changes	Hypothalamic disease
▪ Heat intolerance accompanied by enlarged thyroid, nervousness ▪ Weight loss despite increased appetite ▪ Diaphoresis ▪ Diarrhea ▪ Tremor ▪ Palpitations	Thyrotoxicosis
Hirsutism	
▪ Hirsutism with enlarged hands and feet ▪ Coarsened facial features ▪ Prognathism ▪ Increased diaphoresis and need for sleep ▪ Oily skin ▪ Fatigue ▪ Weight gain ▪ Heat intolerance ▪ Lethargy	Acromegaly
***Hirsutism** (continued)*	
▪ Rapidly progressive hirsutism ▪ Truncal obesity ▪ Buffalo hump ▪ Moon face ▪ Oligomenorrhea ▪ Amenorrhea ▪ Muscle wasting ▪ Thin skin with purple striae	Adrenocortical carcinoma
▪ Increased hair growth on the face, abdomen, breasts, chest, or upper thighs ▪ Truncal obesity ▪ Moon face ▪ Thin skin ▪ Purple striae ▪ Ecchymoses ▪ Petechiae ▪ Muscle wasting ▪ Poor wound healing ▪ Hypertension ▪ Weakness and fatigue ▪ Excessive diaphoresis ▪ Hyperpigmentation ▪ Menstrual irregularities ▪ Personality changes	Cushing's syndrome

(continued)

ENDOCRINE SYSTEM: INTERPRETING YOUR FINDINGS *(continued)*

Sign or symptom and findings	Probable cause
Moon face	
▪ Moon face of varying severity ▪ Buffalo hump ▪ Truncal obesity with slender arms and legs ▪ Thin transparent skin with purple striae and ecchymoses ▪ Acne ▪ Diaphoresis ▪ Muscle wasting ▪ Elevated blood pressure ▪ Personality changes ▪ Hirsutism and menstrual irregularities (in females) ▪ Gynecomastia and impotence (in males)	Hypercortisolism
Polydipsia	
▪ Polydipsia, polyuria, and polyphagia ▪ Nocturia ▪ Weakness ▪ Fatigue ▪ Weight loss ▪ Dehydration	Diabetes mellitus
▪ Polydipsia, polyuria, and nocturia ▪ Fatigue ▪ Failure to lactate ▪ Decreased pubic and axillary hair growth ▪ Reduced libido	Sheehan's syndrome
Polyphagia	
▪ Polyphagia with weight loss ▪ Polydipsia and polyuria ▪ Nocturia ▪ Fatigue ▪ Weakness ▪ Signs of dehydration	Diabetes mellitus
▪ Polyphagia with appetite changes and cravings ▪ Abdominal bloating ▪ Behavioral changes ▪ Headache ▪ Paresthesia ▪ Diarrhea or constipation ▪ Edema ▪ Temporary weight gain ▪ Breast swelling and tenderness	Premenstrual syndrome
▪ Constant polyphagia accompanied by weight loss ▪ Weakness ▪ Nervousness ▪ Diarrhea ▪ Tremors ▪ Diaphoresis ▪ Dyspnea ▪ Thin, brittle hair and nails ▪ Enlarged thyroid	Thyrotoxicosis

ENDOCRINE SYSTEM: INTERPRETING YOUR FINDINGS *(continued)*

Sign or symptom and findings	Probable cause
Polyuria	
▪ Polyuria of approximately 5 L/day with a urine specific gravity of 1.005 or less ▪ Polydipsia ▪ Nocturia ▪ Fatigue ▪ Signs of dehydration	Diabetes insipidus
▪ Polyuria usually less than 5 L/day with a urine specific gravity over 1.020 ▪ Polydipsia, polyphagia ▪ Weight loss ▪ Weakness ▪ Frequent urinary tract infections and yeast vaginitis	Diabetes mellitus
Thyroid enlargement	
▪ Gland enlargement ▪ Weight gain despite anorexia ▪ Fatigue ▪ Cold intolerance ▪ Constipation ▪ Menorrhagia ▪ Slowed intellectual and motor activity ▪ Dry pale cool skin ▪ Dry sparse hair ▪ Thick brittle nails ▪ Dull expression with periorbital edema (eventually)	Hypothyroidism
Thyroid enlargement *(continued)*	
▪ Fever and gland enlargement with tenderness if due to infection ▪ Asymptomatic except for gland enlargement due to autoimmune reaction	Thyroiditis
▪ Gland enlargement ▪ Nervousness ▪ Heat intolerance ▪ Fatigue ▪ Weight loss despite increased appetite ▪ Diarrhea ▪ Sweating ▪ Palpitations ▪ Tremors ▪ Smooth warm flushed skin ▪ Fine soft hair ▪ Exophthalmos ▪ Nausea and vomiting	Thyrotoxicosis
Tremors	
▪ Fine tremors of the hand ▪ Nervousness ▪ Weight loss ▪ Fatigue ▪ Palpitations ▪ Dyspnea ▪ Increased heat intolerance ▪ Enlarged thyroid gland ▪ Exophthalmos	Graves' disease

(continued)

ENDOCRINE SYSTEM: INTERPRETING YOUR FINDINGS *(continued)*

Sign or symptom and findings	Probable cause
Tremors *(continued)*	
■ Rapid fine intention tremor accompanied by confusion, weakness, tachycardia, diaphoresis, and cold, clammy skin ■ Mild generalized headache early on ■ Profound hunger ■ Nervousness ■ Blurred or double vision	Hypoglycemia
■ Contralateral ataxic tremors and other abnormal movements ■ Oculomotor palsy with contralateral hemiplegia ■ Paralysis of vertical gaze ■ Stupor or coma	Thalamic syndrome

Sign or symptom and findings	Probable cause
Tremors *(continued)*	
■ Rapid fine intention tremor of hands and tongue ■ Clonus ■ Hyperreflexia ■ Babinski's reflex ■ Tachycardia, cardiac arrhythmias ■ Palpitations ■ Anxiety ■ Dyspnea ■ Diaphoresis ■ Heat intolerance ■ Weight loss despite increased appetite ■ Diarrhea ■ Enlarged thyroid gland ■ Possible exophthalmos	Thyrotoxicosis

Also find out if the patient has recently moved from a different climate.

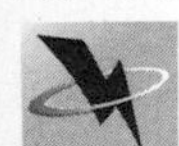

CRITICAL POINT *A person may suffer transitory cold intolerance when moving from a tropical to a temperate climate.*

Obtain a brief health history. Ask the patient if he has a history of hypothyroidism or hypothalamic disease. Find out what medications he's taking and if he's complying with the prescribed schedule and dosage. Ask him if the regimen been changed recently.

Physical assessment

Begin the physical examination by taking the patient's vital signs and checking for hypothermia, dry skin, and hair loss. Then ask the patient to straighten and extend his arms. Observe if his hands are shaking. During the examination, note if the patient shivers or complains of chills. Provide a blanket if necessary.

Typically, the cold intolerance results from tumors involving the hypothalamus or a hormonal deficiency.

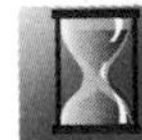

AGE ISSUE *In infants, some degree of cold intolerance is normal because fat distribution is decreased and the temperature-regulating mechanism is immature at birth. An infant with cold intolerance due to hypothyroidism may have subtle, nonspecific signs of the underlying disorder, or none at all. Typically, the infant shivers and has a subnormal temperature, below 86° F (30° C); cold, mottled skin, especially on the extremities; and blue lips. Cold intolerance is common in older people because of metabolic changes associated with aging, thus reflecting a normal age-related change.*

Fatigue

Fatigue is a feeling of excessive tiredness, lack of energy, or exhaustion accompanied by a strong desire to rest or sleep. This common symptom is distinct from weakness, which involves the muscles, but may occur with it.

History

Obtain a careful history to identify the patient's fatigue pattern. Fatigue that worsens with activity and improves with rest generally indicates a physical disorder; the opposite pattern, a psychological disorder.

Fatigue lasting longer than 4 months, constant fatigue that's unrelieved by rest, and transient exhaustion that quickly gives way to bursts of energy are other findings associated with psychological disorders.

Ask about related symptoms and any recent viral or bacterial illness or stressful changes in lifestyle. Explore nutritional habits and any appetite or weight changes. Carefully review the patient's medical and psychiatric history for any chronic disorders that commonly produce fatigue. Ask about a family history of such disorders.

Obtain a thorough drug history, noting use of any narcotic or drug with fatigue as an adverse effect. Ask about alcohol and drug use patterns. Determine the patient's risk for carbon monoxide poisoning, and inquire as to whether the patient has a carbon monoxide detector.

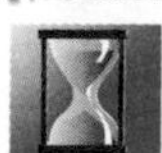

AGE ISSUE *Always ask older patients about fatigue because this symptom may be insidious and mask more serious underlying conditions. When evaluating a child for fatigue, ask his parents if they've noticed any change in his activity level. Fatigue without an organic cause occurs normally during accelerated growth phases in preschool-age and prepubescent children. However, psychological causes of fatigue must be considered—for example, a depressed child may try to escape problems at home or school by taking refuge in sleep. In the pubescent child, consider the possibility of drug abuse, particularly of hypnotics and tranquilizers.*

Physical assessment

Observe the patient's general appearance for overt signs of depression or organic illness. Note if he is unkempt or expressionless or he appears tired or sickly, or has a slumped posture. If warranted, evaluate his mental status, noting especially mental clouding, attention deficits, agitation, or psychomotor retardation.

Analysis

Fatigue is a normal and important response to physical overexertion, prolonged emotional stress, and sleep deprivation. However, it can also be a nonspecific symptom of a psychological or physiologic disorder—especially viral or bacterial infection and endocrine, cardiovascular, or neurologic disease.

Fatigue reflects both hypermetabolic and hypometabolic states in which nutrients needed for cellular energy and growth are lacking because of overly rapid depletion, impaired replacement mechanisms, insufficient hormone production, or inadequate nutrient intake or metabolism.

Heat intolerance

Heat intolerance refers to the inability to withstand high temperatures or to maintain a comfortable body temperature. This symptom produces a continuous feeling of overheated and, at times, profuse diuresis. It usually develops gradually and is chronic.

History

Ask the patient when he first noticed his heat intolerance. Find out if he gradually used fewer blankets at night. Ask the patient if he has to turn up the air conditioning to keep cool. Ask if it's difficult for him to adjust to warm weather and if he sweats while in a hot environment. Find out if his appetite or weight has changed. Also, ask about unusual nervousness or other personality changes. Then take a drug history, especially noting use of amphetamines or amphetamine-like drugs. Ask the patient if he takes a thyroid drug; if so, find out the daily dose and when he last took it.

Physical assessment

When beginning the physical assessment, notice how much clothing the patient is wearing. After taking vital signs, inspect the patient's skin for flushing and diaphoresis. Also, note tremors and lid lag.

Analysis

Most cases of heat intolerance result in thyrotoxicosis. With this disorder, excess thyroid hormone stimulates peripheral tissues, increasing basal metabolism and producing excess heat. Although rare, hypothalamic disease may also cause intolerance to heat and cold.

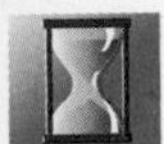

AGE ISSUE *Rarely, maternal thyrotoxicosis may be passed to the neonate, resulting in heat intolerance. More commonly, acquired thyrotoxicosis appears in children between ages 12 and 14, although this too is infrequent. Dehydration may also make a child sensitive to heat.*

Hirsutism

Hirsutism is the excessive growth of coarse body hair in females. In mild hirsutism, fine and pigmented hair appears on the sides of the face and the chin (but doesn't form a complete beard) and on the extremities, chest, abdomen, and perineum. In moderate hirsutism, coarse and pigmented hair appears on the same areas. In severe hirsutism, coarse hair also covers the whole beard area, the proximal interphalangeal joints, and the ears and nose.

History

Begin by asking the patient where on her body she first noticed excessive hair and at what age. Find out where and how quickly other hirsute areas developed. Ask her if she uses any hair removal technique; if so, find out how often she uses it and when she last used it.

Next, obtain a menstrual history, including the patient's age at menarche, the duration of her periods, the usual amount of blood flow, and the number of days between periods.

Also ask about medications. If the patient is taking a drug containing an androgen or progestin compound, or another drug that can cause hirsutism, find out its name, dosage, schedule, and therapeutic aim. Ask her if she misses doses or takes extra ones.

Physical assessment

Next, examine the hirsute areas. Observe for excessive hair appearing on the upper lip and other body parts as well. Note if the hair is fine but pigmented, or dense and coarse. Also note if the patient is obese. Observe the patient for signs of virilization, such as deepening of the voice, breast atrophy, temporal hair recession, muscle hypertrophy, loss of female body contour, and clitoral enlargement.

Analysis

Excessive androgen (male hormone) production stimulates hair growth on the pubic region, axillae, chin, upper lip, cheeks, anterior neck, sternum, linea alba, forearms, abdomen, back, and upper arms. Hirsutism may also occur with normal levels of androgens when there's an increased sensitivity of the skin to the hormones.

Depending on the degree of excess androgen production, hirsutism may be associated with acne and increased skin oiliness, increased libido, and menstrual irregularities (including anovulation and amenorrhea). Extremely high androgen levels cause further virilization, including such signs as breast atrophy, loss of female body contour, frontal balding, and deepening of the voice.

Hirsutism may result from endocrine abnormalities and idiopathic causes. It may also occur in pregnancy from transient androgen production by the placenta or corpus luteum, and in menopause from increased androgen and decreased estrogen production.

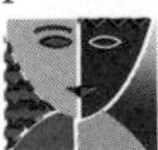

CULTURAL INSIGHT *Some patients have a strong familial predisposition to hirsutism, which may be considered normal in the context of their genetic background, culture, and race. Although hirsutism is a female characteristic, excessive hair growth may be present in female and male family members.*

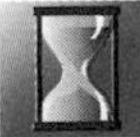

AGE ISSUE *Childhood hirsutism can stem from congenital adrenal hyperplasia. It's usually detected at birth because affected infants have ambiguous genitalia. Rarely, a mild form becomes apparent after puberty when hirsutism, irregular bleeding or amenorrhea, and signs of virilization appear. Hirsutism that occurs at or after puberty commonly results from polycystic ovary disease. Hirsutism can occur after menopause if peripheral conversion of estrogen is poor.*

Moon face

Moon face is a distinctive facial adiposity. Its typical characteristics include marked facial roundness and puffiness, a double chin, a prominent upper lip, and full supraclavicular fossae.

History

Ask the patient when he first noticed his facial adiposity, and try to obtain a pre-onset photograph to help evaluate the extent of the change.

Ask about weight gain and any personal or family history of endocrine disorders, obesity, or cancer. Find out if the patient has noticed any fatigue, irritability, depression, or confusion. Ask female patients of child bearing age to determine the date of her last menses and whether she has experienced any menstrual irregularities.

Ask about medications such as a glucocorticoid. Find out the name of the drug, dosage and schedule, route of administration, and reason for therapy. Also ask if the dosage has ever been modified and, if so, when and why.

Physical assessment

Take the patient's vital signs, weight, and height. Assess the patient's overall appearance for other characteristic signs of hypercortisolism, including virilism in a female or gynecomastia in a male. Also assess for purple striae on the skin, muscle weakness due to loss of muscle mass from increased catabolism, and skeletal growth retardation in children.

Analysis

Moon face usually indicates hypercortisolism resulting from ectopic or excessive pituitary production of corticotropin, adrenal adenoma or carcinoma, or long-term glucocorticoid therapy. Although the presence of moon face doesn't help differentiate causes of hypercortisolism, it does indicate a need for diagnostic testing.

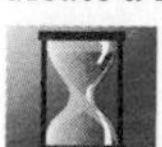

AGE ISSUE *Moon face is rare in children. In an infant or a young child, it usually indicates adrenal adenoma or carcinoma or, rarely, cri du chat syndrome. After age 7, it usually indicates abnormal pituitary secretion of corticotropin in bilateral adrenal hyperplasia.*

Polydipsia

Polydipsia refers to excessive thirst. It's a common symptom associated with endocrine disorders.

History

Obtain the patient's health history. Find out how much fluid the patient drinks each day. Ask him how often and how much he typically urinates. Find out if the need to urinate awakens him at night. Determine if he or anyone in his family has diabetes or kidney disease. Find out what medications he uses. Ask him if his lifestyle has recently changed, and if so, have the changes upset him.

Physical assessment

If the patient has polydipsia, take his blood pressure and pulse when he's in supine and standing positions. A decrease of 10 mm Hg in systolic pressure and a pulse rate increase of 10 beats/minute from the supine to the sitting or standing position may indicate hypovolemia. If you detect these changes, ask the patient about recent weight loss. Check for signs of dehydration, such as dry mucous membranes and decreased skin turgor. I.V. replacement fluids may be needed.

Analysis

Polydipsia is a common symptom associated with endocrine disorders and certain drugs. It may reflect decreased fluid intake, increased urine output, or excessive loss of water and salt.

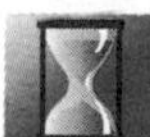

AGE ISSUE *In children, polydipsia usually stems from diabetes insipidus or diabetes mellitus. Rare causes include pheochromocytoma, neuroblastoma, and Prader-Willi syndrome. However, some children develop habitual polydipsia that's unrelated to any disease.*

Polyphagia

Polyphagia refers to voracious or excessive eating. Depending on the underlying cause, polyphagia may cause weight gain.

History

Begin the assessment by asking the patient what he has eaten and drank within the last 24 hours. If he easily recalls this information, ask about his intake for the 2 previous days, for a broader view of his dietary habits. Note the frequency of meals and the amount and types of food eaten. Find out if the patient's eating habits have changed recently. Ask if he has always had a large appetite. Also ask if his overeating alternates with periods of anorexia. Ask about conditions that may trigger overeating, such as stress, depression, or menstruation. Determine if the patient actually feels hungry, or if he's eating simply because food is available. Find out if he ever vomits or has a headache after overeating.

Explore related signs and symptoms. Ask the patient if he recently gained or lost weight. Find out if he feels tired, nervous, or excitable. Ask if he has experienced heat intolerance, dizziness, palpitations, diarrhea, or increased thirst or urination. Obtain a complete drug history, including the use of laxatives or enemas.

Physical assessment

During the physical examination, weigh the patient. Tell him his current weight, and watch for any expression of disbelief or anger. Inspect the skin to detect dryness or poor turgor. Palpate the thyroid for enlargement.

Analysis

Polyphagia is a common symptom can be persistent or intermittent. It commonly results from endocrine and psychological disorders as well as the use of certain drugs.

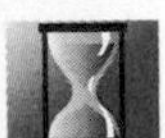

AGE ISSUE *In children, polyphagia commonly results from type 1 diabetes. In infants ages 6 to 18 months, it can result from a malabsorptive disorder such as celiac disease. However, polyphagia may occur normally in a child who is experiencing a sudden growth spurt.*

Polyuria

A relatively common sign, polyuria is the daily production and excretion of more than 3 L of urine. It's usually reported by the patient as increased urination, especially when it occurs at night.

History

If the patient doesn't display signs of hypovolemia, explore the frequency and pattern of the polyuria. Find out when it began, how long it's lasted, and if it was precipitated by a certain event. Ask the patient to describe the pattern and amount of his daily fluid intake. Check for a history of visual deficits, headaches, or head trauma, which may precede diabetes insipidus. Also check for a history of urinary tract obstruction, diabetes mellitus, renal disorder, chronic hypokalemia or hypercalcemia, or psychiatric disorder (both past and present). Find out the schedule and dosage of any drugs the patient is taking.

CRITICAL POINT *The patient with polyuria is at risk for developing hypovolemia. Evaluate fluid status first. Take vital signs, noting increased body temperature, tachycardia, and orthostatic hypotension (10 mm Hg decrease in systolic blood pressure upon standing and 10 beats per minute increase in heart rate upon standing). Inspect for dry skin and mucous membranes, decreased skin turgor and elasticity, and reduced perspiration. Ask the patient if he's unusually tired or thirsty. Find out if he has recently lost more than 5% of his body weight. If the patient is hypovolemic, fluid replacement therapy is needed.*

Physical assessment

In addition to assessing the patient's overall status and body systems, pay particular attention to a neurologic examination, noting especially any change in the patient's level of consciousness. Then palpate the bladder and inspect the urethral meatus. Obtain a urine specimen and check its specific gravity.

Analysis

Polyuria is aggravated by overhydration, consumption of caffeine or alcohol, and excessive ingestion of salt, glucose, or other hyperosmolar substances.

Polyuria usually results from the use of certain drugs, such as a diuretic, or from a psychological, neurologic, or renal disorder. It can reflect central nervous system dysfunction that diminishes or suppresses secretion of antidiuretic hormone (ADH), which regulates fluid balance. Or, when ADH levels are normal, it can reflect renal impairment. In both of these pathophysiologic mechanisms, the renal tubules fail to reabsorb sufficient water, causing polyuria.

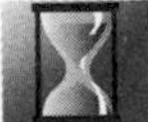

AGE ISSUE *In children, the major causes of polyuria are congenital nephrogenic diabetes insipidus, medullary cystic disease, polycystic renal dis-*

ease, and distal renal tubular acidosis. Because a child's fluid balance is more delicate than an adult's, urine specific gravity must be checked at each voiding. The child also must be assessed for signs of dehydration, including a decrease in body weight; decreased skin turgor; pale, mottled, or gray skin; dry mucous membranes; decreased urine output; and absence of tears when crying.

Thyroid enlargement

An enlarged thyroid gland can result in hyperfunction or hypofunction of the gland with resulting excess or deficiency, respectively, of the hormone thyroxine. An enlarged thyroid that causes visible swelling in the front of the neck is called a *goiter.*

History

Review the patient's history for possible cause of thyroid enlargement. Important data includes a family history of thyroid disease, when the thyroid enlargement began, any previous irradiation of the thyroid or the neck, recent infections, and the use of thyroid replacement drugs.

Physical assessment

Begin the physical examination by inspecting the patient's trachea for midline deviation. Although you can usually see the enlarged gland, you should always palpate it. To palpate the thyroid gland, you'll need to stand behind the patient. Give the patient a cup of water, and have him extend his neck slightly. Place the fingers of both hands on the patient's neck, just below the cricoid cartilage and just lateral to the trachea. Tell the patient to take a sip of water and swallow. The thyroid gland should rise as he swallows. Use your fingers to palpate laterally and downward to feel the whole thyroid gland. Palpate over the midline to feel the isthmus of the thyroid.

During palpation, be sure to note the size, shape, and consistency of the gland, and the presence or absence of nodules. Using the bell of a stethoscope, listen over the lateral lobes for a bruit. The bruit is typically continuous.

Analysis

An enlarged thyroid gland can result from inflammation, physiologic changes, iodine deficiency, and thyroid tumors. If no infection is present, enlargement is usually slow and progressive.

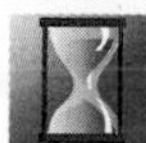

AGE ISSUE *Congenital goiter, a syndrome of infantile myxedema or cretinism, is characterized by mental retardation, growth failure, and other signs and symptoms of hypothyroidism. Early treatment can prevent mental retardation.*

Tremors

The most common type of involuntary muscle movement, tremors are regular rhythmic oscillations that result from alternating contraction of opposing muscle groups. Tremors can be characterized by their location, amplitude, and frequency. They're classified as resting, intention, or postural. Resting tremors occur when an extremity is at rest and subside with movement. They include the classic pill-rolling tremor of Parkinson's disease. Conversely, intention tremors occur only with movement and subside with rest. Postural (or action) tremors appear when an extremity or the trunk is actively held in a particular posture or position. A common type of postural tremor is called an essential tremor.

History

Begin the patient history by asking the patient about the tremor's onset (sudden or gradual) and about its duration, progression, and any aggravating or alleviating factors. Find out if the tremor interferes with the patient's normal activities. Ask if he has other symptoms. Find out if he has noticed any behavioral changes or memory loss (the patient's family or friends may provide more accurate information on this).

Explore the patient's personal and family medical history for a neurologic (especially seizures), endocrine, or metabolic disorder. Obtain a complete drug history, noting especially the use of phenothiazines. Also, ask about alcohol use.

Physical assessment

Assess the patient's overall appearance and demeanor, noting mental status. Test range of motion and strength in all major muscle groups while observing for chorea, athetosis, dystonia, and other involuntary movements. Check deep tendon reflexes and, if possible, observe the patient's gait.

Analysis

Tremors are typical signs of extrapyramidal or cerebellar disorders. However, they can also result from certain drugs. Tremorlike movements may also be elicited, such as asterixis — the characteristic flapping tremor seen in hepatic failure. Stress or emotional upset tends to aggravate a tremor. Alcohol commonly diminishes postural tremors.

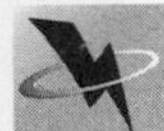

CRITICAL POINT *Herbal products, such as ephedra (ma huang), have been known to cause serious adverse reactions, which may include tremors. An early sign of manganese toxicity is a resting tremor.*

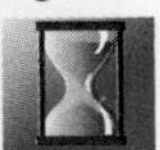

AGE ISSUE *A normal neonate may display coarse tremors with stiffening — an exaggerated hypocalcemic startle reflex — in response to noises and chills. Pediatric-specific causes of pathologic tremors include cerebral palsy, fetal alcohol syndrome, and maternal drug addiction.*

13 Hematologic and immune systems

Most systems of the body are composed of groups of organs. In contrast, the hematologic or blood-forming system consists of bone marrow and blood cells. The immune system consists primarily of billions of cells that circulate throughout the cardiovascular system as well as other structures, such as lymph nodes, distributed throughout the body.

The hematologic and immune systems directly affect — and are affected by — every organ system. The two systems are distinct, yet closely related. Their cells share a common origin in the bone marrow, and the immune system uses the bloodstream to transport defensive components to the site of an invasion. Although some hematologic and immune disorders cause hallmark signs and symptoms (for example, the butterfly rash of systemic lupus erythematosus (SLE) or the plethora of polycythemia), detecting other problems in these systems can be extremely challenging. Therefore, a careful and thorough history and physical assessment is crucial to identify nonspecific symptoms that can appear in any body system but reflect a hematologic or immune dysfunction.

Hematologic system

The hematologic system consists of the blood and bone marrow. Blood delivers oxygen and nutrients to all tissues, removes wastes, and transports gases, blood cells, immune cells, and hormones throughout the body.

The hematologic system manufactures new blood cells through a process called *hematopoiesis.* Multipotential stem cells in bone marrow give rise to distinct cell types,

TRACING BLOOD CELL FORMATION

New blood cells form and develop in the bone marrow by a process called *hematopoiesis.* This chart follows the process from the formation of five unipotential stem cells from multipotential stem cells until they differentiate to form erythrocytes, granulocytes, agranulocytes, or platelets.

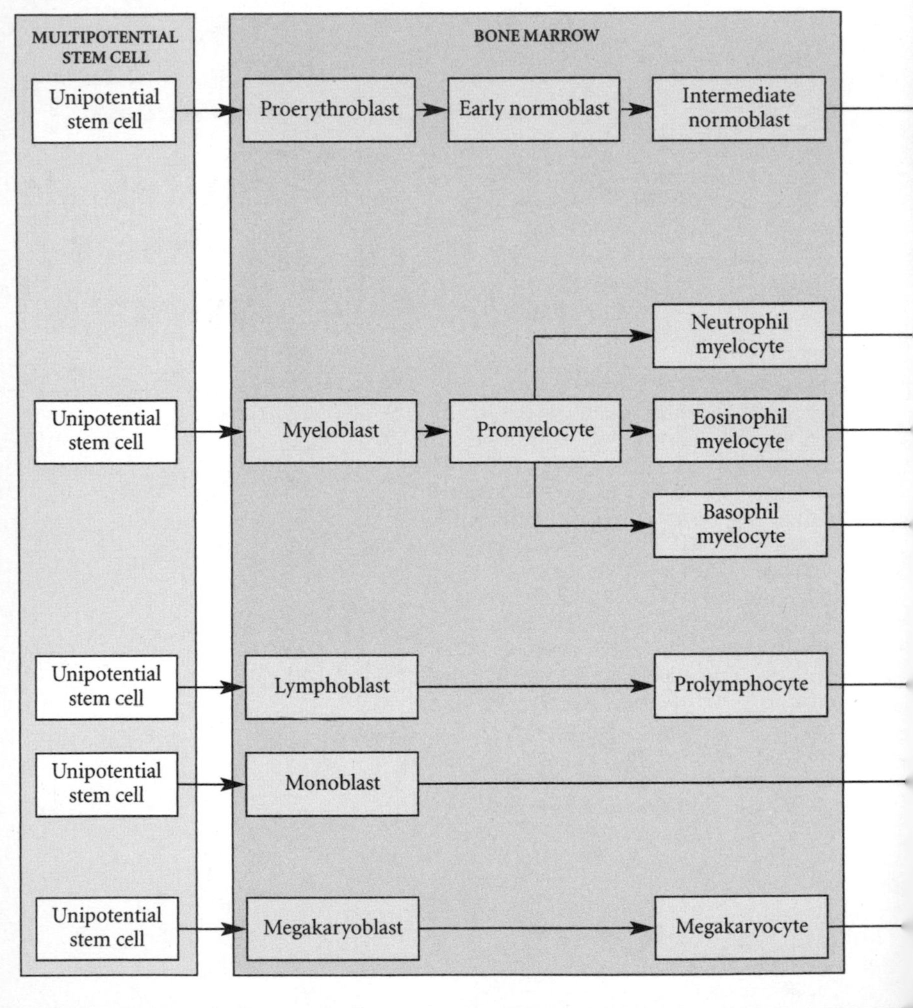

called *unipotential* stem cells. Unipotential cells differentiate into precursors of erythrocytes (red blood cells [RBCs]), leukocytes (white blood cells [WBCs], including granulocytes and agranulocytes), or thrombocytes (platelets). (See *Tracing blood cell formation.*)

RBCs and platelets function entirely within blood vessels. WBCs act mainly in the tissues outside the blood vessels.

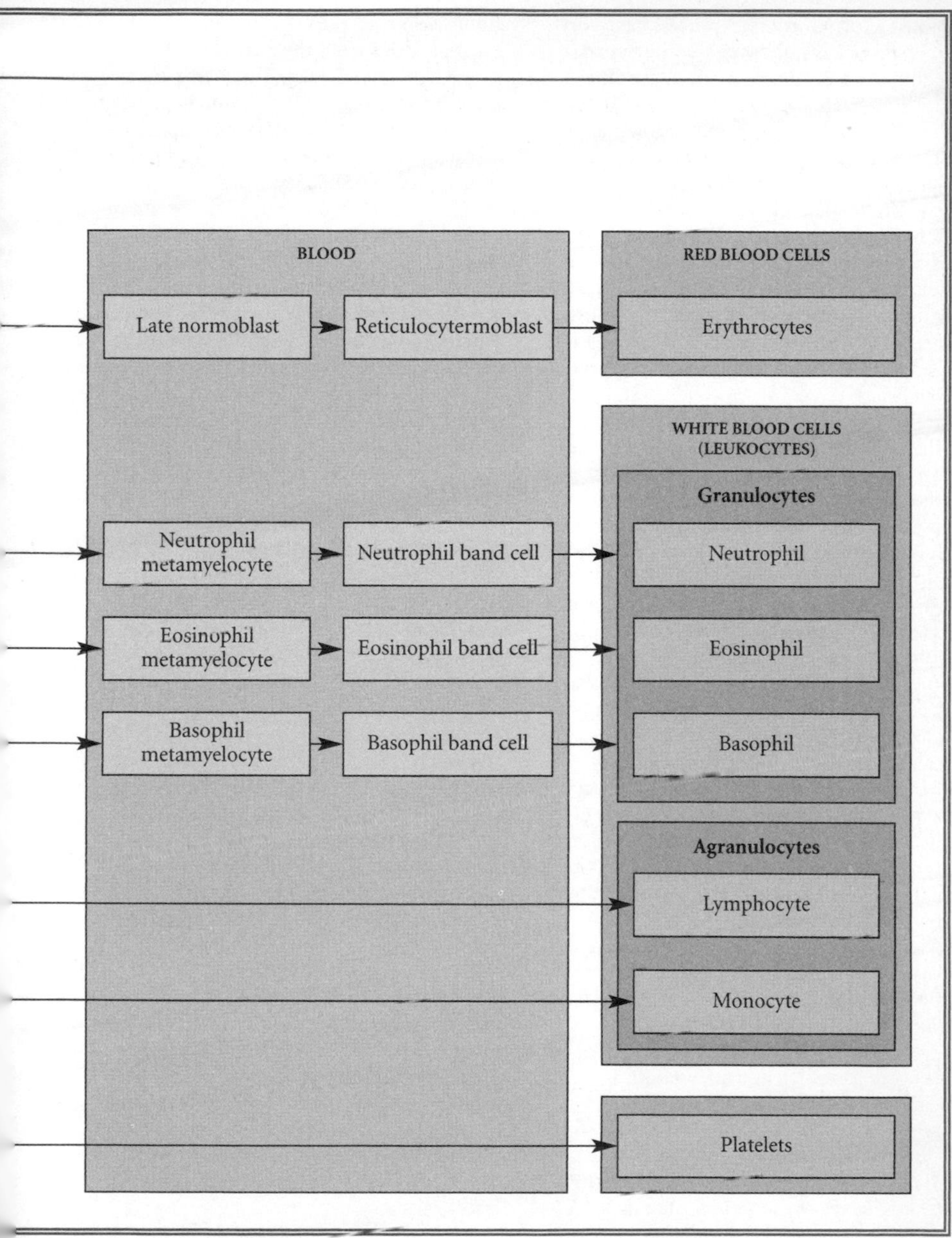

Blood components

Blood consists of various formed elements suspended in a fluid called *plasma*, which is the liquid protein of the blood.

Red blood cells

RBCs transport oxygen and carbon dioxide to and from body tissues. They contain hemoglobin, the oxygen-carrying substance that gives blood its red color. The RBC surface carries antigens, which determine a person's blood type.

RBCs form through a process called *erythropoiesis.* Lack of oxygen in the tissues stimulates RBC production. In the fetus, erythropoiesis starts in the yolk sac at about the third week. This process is gradually taken over by the liver and spleen and, after the 20th week of gestation, the red bone marrow. In an adult, erythrocyte production takes place only in the marrow of the ribs, sternum, iliac crest, cranium and, to a lesser extent, vertebral bodies. However, the rest of the bone marrow retains its ability to form erythrocytes and will produce them in extremely stressful conditions such as blood dyscrasias.

The genesis of an erythrocyte occurs when the stem cell produces a daughter cell that differentiates into an erythroblast, which eventually synthesizes hemoglobin. As the hemoglobin concentration increases, the immature cell nucleus grows smaller and is eventually pushed out of the cell. The cell continues to develop into an erythrocyte, which enters the capillaries from the bone marrow.

The mature erythrocyte is a biconcave disk about 7.7 microns in diameter and has an average life span of 120 days. The spleen isolates old, worn-out RBCs, removing them from circulation. The rate of reticulocyte release usually equals the rate of old RBC removal. When RBC depletion occurs (for example, with hemorrhage), the bone marrow increases reticulocyte production to maintain the normal RBC count.

Erythropoiesis keeps the erythrocyte count high enough for adequate oxygen supply and low enough for unimpaired blood flow. This steady production of mature erythrocytes requires various nutritional substances, such as iron, vitamin B_{12}, folic acid, and amino acids.

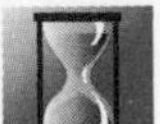

AGE ISSUE *As a person ages, fatty bone marrow replaces some active blood-forming marrow — first in the long bones and later in the flat bones. The altered bone marrow can't increase erythrocyte production as readily as before in response to such stimuli as hormones, anoxia, hemorrhage, and hemolysis. With age, vitamin B absorption may also diminish, resulting in reduced erythrocyte mass and decreased hemoglobin and hematocrit.*

The primary function of erythrocytes is to carry hemoglobin, which transports oxygen from the lungs to body tissues. Hemoglobin also transports carbon dioxide and hydrogen ions from the cells to the lungs where they are released. The erythrocytes act as an acid-base buffer. Hemoglobin and the erythrocytes are buffering compounds that help keep the pH of blood within the appropriate range, 7.35 to 7.45.

When an erythrocyte reaches the end of its life span, reticuloendothelial cells break down its hemoglobin into iron, globin, and the bile pigment bilirubin. Most of the iron is returned to the bone marrow for new hemoglobin formation. Iron in excess of the need for new RBCs is stored as either hemoglobin or hemosiderin in the cells of the reticuloendothelial system. The globin's amino acids are used in protein synthesis, and the bilirubin is excreted, primarily in bile.

White blood cells

Leukocytes or WBCs are nucleated cells derived from stem cells. Unlike erythrocytes, leukocytes contain no hemoglobin. Leukocytes are a functional part of the immune system and fall into two categories: granulocytes and agranulocytes.

Granulocytes. Granulocytes include neutrophils, eosinophils, and basophils — collectively known as *polymorphonuclear leukocytes.* All granulocytes contain a single multilobular nucleus and granules in the cytoplasm. Each cell type exhibits different properties and each is activated by different stimuli.

NEUTROPHILS. Neutrophils, the most numerous granulocytes, account for 47.6% to 76.8% of circulating WBCs. These phagocytic cells engulf, ingest, and digest foreign materials. Through a process called *diapedesis,* they leave the bloodstream by passing through the capillary walls into the tissues, then migrate to and accumulate at infection sites.

Worn-out neutrophils form the main component of pus. Bone marrow produces their replacements, immature neutrophils called *bands.* In response to infection, bone marrow must produce many immature cells and release them into circulation, elevating the band count.

EOSINOPHILS. Eosinophils account for 0.3% to 7% of circulating WBCs. These gran-

COMPARING GRANULOCYTES AND AGRANULOCYTES

White blood cells (WBCs) fight off foreign organisms. Through diapedesis, each type of WBC migrates from the bloodstream to fight different organisms.

Granulocytes

Polymorphonuclear leukocytes are the group of WBCs that include basophils, neutrophils, and eosinophils. These WBCs are the first to respond to infection, allergic reactions, and inflammatory and immune stimuli.

BASOPHILS SECRETE HISTAMINE IN RESPONSE TO INFLAMMATORY AND IMMUNE STIMULI.

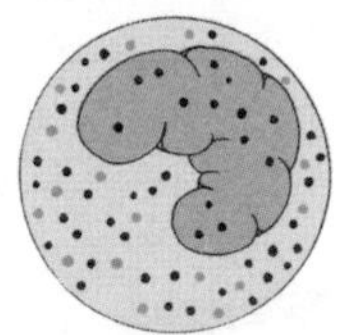

NEUTROPHILS ENGULF, INGEST, AND DIGEST FOREIGN BODIES.

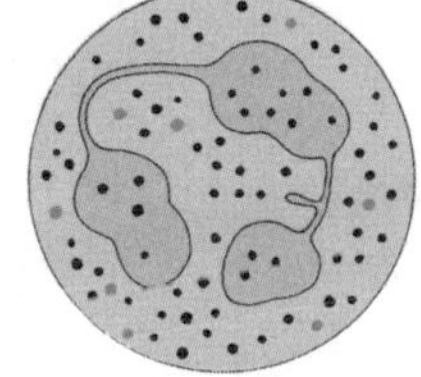

EOSINOPHILS INGEST ANTIGENS AND ANTIBODIES.

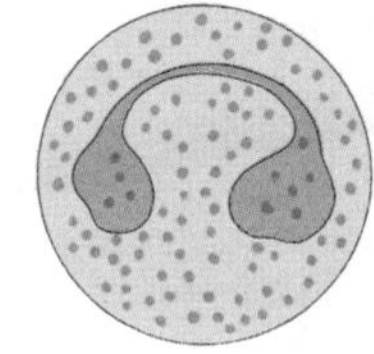

Agranulocytes

Agranulocytes, with groups of lymphocytes and monocytes, may roam freely in the body when stimulated by inflammation. However, they mainly concentrate at structures that filter large amounts of fluid, such as the liver, and defend against invading organisms. Plasma cells develop from lymphoblasts and reside in the tissue.

LYMPHOCYTES ATTACK INFECTED CELLS OR PRODUCE ANTIBODIES.

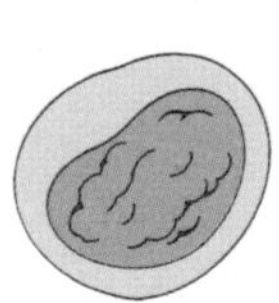

MONOCYTES INGEST BACTERIA, CELLULAR DEBRIS, AND NECROTIC TISSUE.

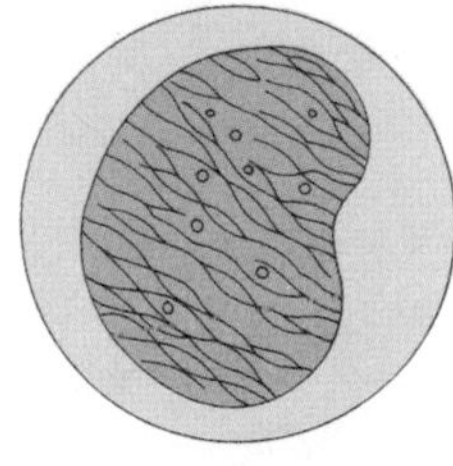

PLASMA CELLS DEVELOP FROM LYMPHOBLASTS, RESIDE IN THE TISSUE, AND PRODUCE ANTIBODIES.

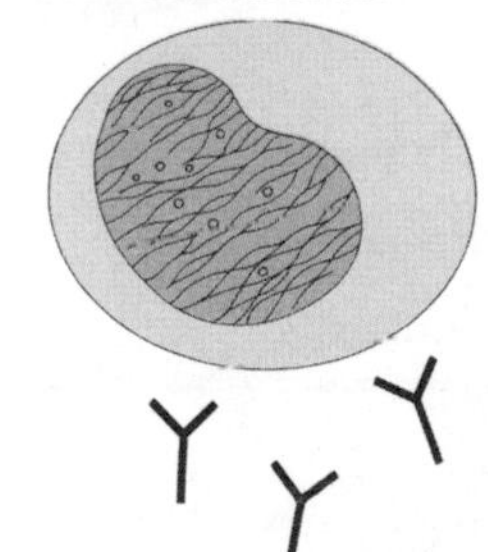

ulocytes also migrate from the bloodstream by diapedesis but do so as a response to an allergic reaction. Eosinophils accumulate in loose connective tissue, where they become involved in the ingestion of antigen-antibody complexes.

BASOPHILS. Basophils usually constitute fewer than 2% of circulating WBCs and possess minimal or no phagocytic ability. Their cytoplasmic granules secrete heparin and histamine in response to certain inflammatory and immune stimuli. Histamine makes the blood vessels more permeable and eases the passage of fluids from the capillaries into body tissues.

Agranulocytes. WBCs in the agranulocyte category — monocytes, lymphocytes, and plasma cells — lack specific cytoplasmic granules and have nuclei without lobes. (See *Comparing granulocytes and agranulocytes.*)

HOW BLOOD COAGULATES

When a blood vessel is severed or injured, three interrelated processes occur. The flowchart at right illustrates these processes.

Constriction and aggregation
Immediately after an injury occurs the affected blood vessels constrict, reducing blood flow. In addition, platelets, stimulated by the exposed collagen of the damaged cells, begin to aggregate. Aggregation provides a temporary seal and a site for clotting to take place. The platelets release a number of substances that enhance constriction and aggregation.

Coagulation pathways
Coagulation, the transformation of blood from a liquid to a solid, may be initiated through two different pathways, the intrinsic pathway or the extrinsic pathway. The intrinsic pathway is activated when plasma comes in contact with damaged vessel surfaces. The extrinsic pathway is activated when tissue factor— a substance released by damaged endothelial cells—comes into contact with one of the clotting factors.

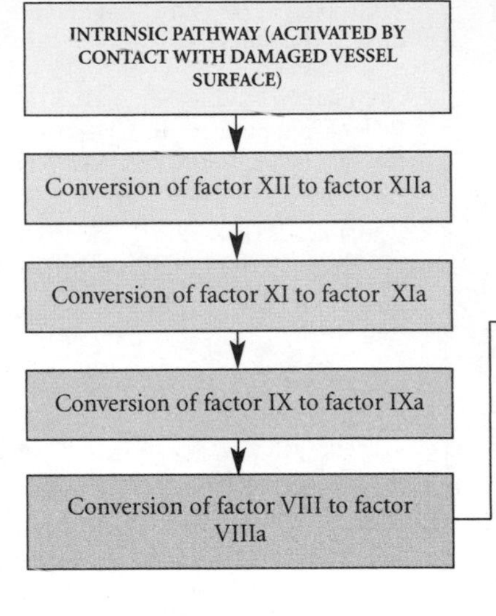

MONOCYTES. Monocytes, the largest of the WBCs, constitute only 0.6% to 9.6% of WBCs in circulation. Like neutrophils, monocytes are phagocytic and enter the tissues by diapedesis. Outside the bloodstream, monocytes enlarge and mature, becoming tissue macrophages, also called *histiocytes.*

As macrophages, monocytes may roam freely through the body when stimulated by inflammation. Usually, they remain immobile, populating most organs and tissues. Collectively, they serve as components of the reticuloendothelial system, which defends the body against infection and disposes of cell breakdown products.

Macrophages concentrate in structures that filter large amounts of body fluid, such as the liver, spleen, and lymph nodes, where they defend against invading organisms. Macrophages are efficient phagocytes that ingest microorganisms; cellular debris, including worn-out neutrophils; and necrotic tissue. When mobilized at an infection site, they phagocytize cellular remnants and promote wound healing.

COMMON PATHWAY (INITIATED IN EITHER CASE AND BEGINS CLOTTING)

EXTRINSIC PATHWAY (ACTIVATED BY DAMAGED TISSUE)

Calcium ions (Ca^{++})

Conversion of factor X to factor Xa, byproducts of intrinsic and extrinsic pathways

Tissue factor (factor III) and factor VII activated in presence of Ca++ and platelet phospholipids

Conversion of factor V to factor Va

Platelet phospholipid

Prothrombin

Thrombin

Fibrinogen

Fibrin

Factor XIII

Stabilized fibrin clot

LYMPHOCYTES. Lymphocytes, the smallest of the WBCs and the second most numerous constituting 16.2% to 43%, derive from stem cells in the bone marrow. There are two types of lymphocytes:

- T lymphocytes directly attack an infected cell.
- B lymphocytes produce antibodies against specific antigens.

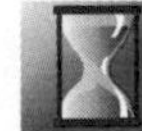

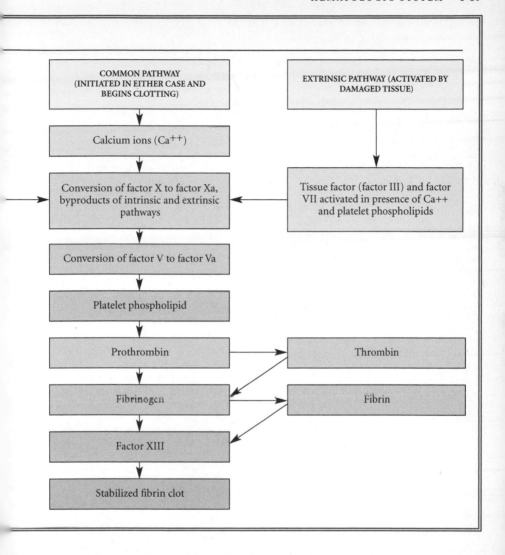

AGE ISSUE *Some persons over age 65 may exhibit a slight decrease in the range of a normal leukocyte count. When this happens, the number of B cells and total lymphocytes decreases, and T cells decrease in number and become less effective.*

PLASMA CELLS. Plasma cells develop from lymphoblasts. The plasma cells reside in the tissue and produce antibodies.

Platelets

Platelets are small, colorless, disk-shaped cytoplasmic fragments split from cells in bone marrow called *megakaryocytes.* These fragments, which have a life span of approximately 10 days, perform three vital functions, including initiating the contraction of damaged blood vessels to minimize blood loss, forming hemostatic plugs in injured blood vessels and, with plasma, providing materials that accelerate blood coagulation.

Hemostasis

Hemostasis, or blood clotting, is the complex process by which platelets, plasma, and coagulation factors interact to control bleeding . This process is called the *coagulation cascade.*

Extrinsic pathway

Initially, when a blood vessel ruptures, local vasoconstriction that's caused by a decrease in the caliber of blood vessels and platelet aggregation at the site of the injury helps to prevent hemorrhage. This activation, called the *extrinsic pathway of coagulation,* requires the release of tissue thromboplastin from the damaged cells.

Intrinsic pathway

However, formation of a more stable clot requires initiation of the complex clotting mechanisms known as the *intrinsic pathway of coagulation.* This coagulation system is activated by a protein called factor X, one of 13 substances that are necessary for coagulation and derived from plasma and tissue.

The result of the intrinsic pathway of coagulation is a *fibrin clot,* an accumulation of a fibrous, insoluble protein at the site of the injury. (See *How blood coagulates,* pages 348 and 349.)

Coagulation factors

The materials that platelets and plasma provide work with coagulation factors to serve as precursor compounds in the coagulation of blood.

Designated by name and Roman numeral, these coagulation factors are activated in a chain reaction, each one in turn activating the next factor in the chain:

- Factor I, fibrinogen, is a high-molecular-weight protein synthesized in the liver and converted to fibrin during the coagulation pathway.
- Factor II, prothrombin, is a protein synthesized in the liver in the presence of vitamin K and converted to thrombin during coagulation.
- Factor III, tissue thromboplastin, is released from damaged tissue; it's required to initiate the second phase, the extrinsic pathway of coagulation.
- Factor IV, consisting of calcium ions, is required throughout the entire clotting sequence.
- Factor V, or labile factor (proaccelerin), is a protein that's synthesized in the liver and functions during the combined pathway phase of the coagulation system.
- Factor VII, serum prothrombin conversion accelerator or stable factor (proconvertin), is a protein synthesized in the liver in the presence of vitamin K; it's activated by factor III in the extrinsic pathway of coagulation.
- Factor VIII, antihemophilic factor (antihemophilic globulin), is a protein synthesized in the liver and required during the intrinsic pathway of coagulation.
- Factor IX, plasma thromboplastin component, a protein synthesized in the liver in the presence of vitamin K, is required in the intrinsic pathway of coagulation.
- Factor X, Stuart factor (Stuart-Prower factor), is a protein synthesized in the liver in the presence of vitamin K; it's required in the combined pathway of coagulation.
- Factor XI, plasma thromboplastin antecedent, is a protein synthesized in the liver and required in the intrinsic pathway of coagulation.
- Factor XII, Hageman factor, is a protein required in the intrinsic pathway of coagulation.
- Factor XIII, fibrin stabilizing factor, is a protein required to stabilize the fibrin strands in the combined pathway of coagulation.

Blood groups

Blood groups are determined by the presence or absence of genetically determined antigens or agglutinogens (glycoproteins) on the surface of RBCs. A, B, and Rh are the most clinically significant blood antigens.

ABO groups

Testing for the presence of A and B antigens on RBCs is the most important system for classifying blood:

- Type A blood has A antigen on its surface.
- Type B blood has B antigen.
- Type AB blood has both A and B antigens.

REVIEWING BLOOD TYPE COMPATIBILITY

Precise blood typing and crossmatching can prevent the transfusion of incompatible blood, which can be fatal. Usually, typing the recipient's blood and crossmatching it with available donor blood takes less than 1 hour.

ABO compatibility

Agglutinogen, an antigen in red blood cells (RBCs), and agglutinin, an antibody in plasma, distinguish the four ABO blood groups. This chart shows ABO compatibility from the perspectives of the recipient and the donor.

Blood group	Antibodies in plasma	Compatible RBCs	Compatible plasma
Recipient			
O	Anti-A and anti-B	O	O, A, B, AB
A	Anti-B	A, O	A, AB
B	Anti-A	B, O	B, AB
AB	Neither Anti-A nor anti-B	AB, A, B, O	AB
Donor			
O	Anti-A and anti-B	O, A, B, AB	O
A	Anti-B	A, AB	A, O
B	Anti-A	B, AB	B, O
AB	Neither anti-A nor anti-B	AB	AB, A, B, O

- Type O blood has neither A nor B antigen.

Plasma may contain antibodies that interact with these antigens, causing the cells to agglutinate, or combine into a mass. However, plasma can't contain antibodies to its own cell antigen or it would destroy itself. Thus, type A blood has A antigen but no A antibodies; however, it does have B antibodies.

Precise blood-typing and crossmatching, which involves the mixing and observing for agglutination of donor cells, are essential, especially for blood transfusions. A donor's blood must be compatible with a recipient's or the result can be fatal. These blood groups are compatible:

- type A with type A or O
- type B with type B or O
- type AB with type AB, A, B, or O
- type O with type O only. (See *Reviewing blood type compatibility*.)

Rh typing

Rh typing determines whether the Rh factor is present or absent in the blood. Of the eight types of Rh antigens, only C, D, and E are common.

Typically, blood contains the Rh antigen. Blood with the Rh antigen is Rh-positive; blood without the Rh antigen is Rh-negative. Anti-Rh antibodies can appear only in a person who has become sensitized. Anti-Rh antibodies can appear in the blood of an Rh-negative person after the entry of Rh-positive RBCs in the bloodstream — for example, from a transfusion of Rh-positive blood. An Rh-negative female who carries an Rh-positive fetus may also acquire anti-Rh antibodies.

STRUCTURES OF THE IMMUNE SYSTEM

The structures of the immune system include organs and tissues in which lymphocytes predominate as well as cells that circulate in the blood. This illustration shows central, peripheral, and accessory lymphoid organs and tissues.

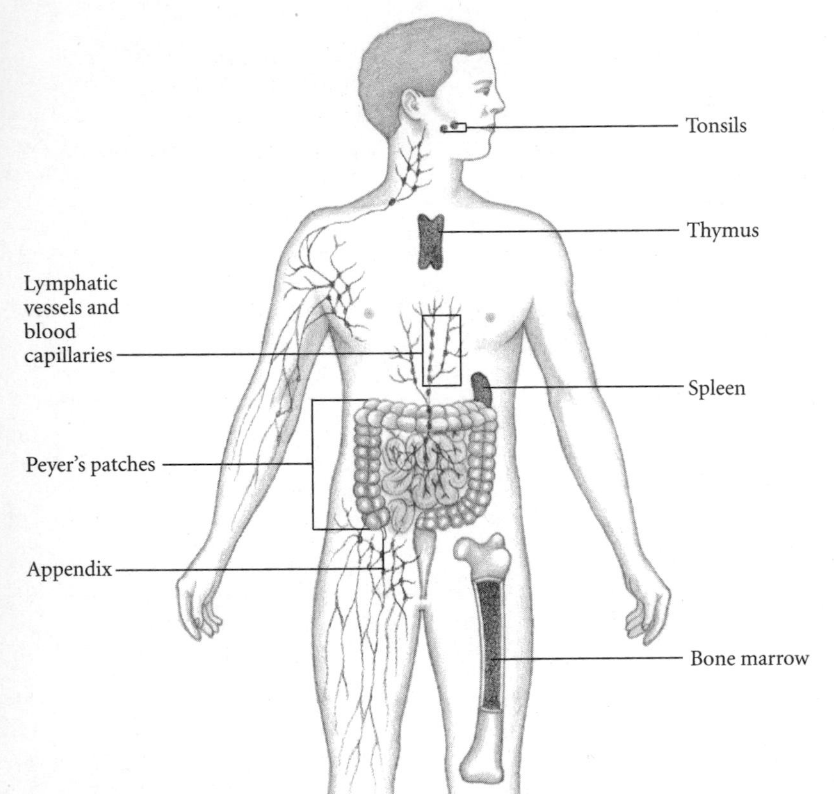

Immune system

The immune system consists of specialized cells, tissues, and organs found throughout the body. It defends the body against invasion by harmful organisms and chemical toxins. Blood plays an important part in this protective system.

Organs and tissues of the immune system are referred to as *lymphoid* because they're all involved with the growth, development, and dissemination of lymphocytes, one type of WBC. The immune system has three major divisions including the central lymphoid organs and tissues, peripheral lymphoid organs and tissues, and accessory lymphoid organs and tissues. (See *Structures of the immune system.*)

Central lymphoid organs and tissues

The bone marrow and thymus play roles in developing B cells and T cells, which are the two major types of lymphocytes.

Bone marrow

The bone marrow contains stem cells, which are multipotential that may develop into several different cell types. The immune system and blood cells develop from stem cells in a process called *hematopoiesis.*

Soon after differentiation from the stem cells, some of the cells become part of the immune system and sources of lymphocytes; others develop into phagocytes, which ingest microorganisms and cellular debris. The lymphocytes further differentiate into either B cells that mature in the bone marrow or T cells that travel to the thymus and mature. B cells and T cells are distributed throughout the lymphoid organs, especially the lymph nodes and spleen.

B cells don't attack pathogens themselves but instead produce antibodies, which attack pathogens or direct other cells, such as phagocytes, to attack them. This is known as the *humoral immune response* or *antibody-mediated response.* The response to attack foreign substances is regulated by T cells and their products, lymphokines, which, in turn, determine the immunoglobulin class that a B cell will manufacture. This is known as the *cell-mediated response.*

Thymus

In a fetus or an infant, the thymus is a two-lobed mass of lymphoid tissue located over the base of the heart in the mediastinum. The thymus forms T lymphocytes for several months after birth and gradually atrophies until only a remnant persists in adults.

In the thymus, T cells undergo a process called *T-cell education,* in which the cells learn to recognize other cells from the same body (known as *self cells*) and distinguish them from all other cells (known as *nonself cells*). There are five types of T cells with specific functions:

- *memory cells,* which are sensitized cells that remain dormant until second exposure to an antigen, also known as secondary immune response
- *lymphokine-producing cells,* which are involved in delayed hypersensitivity reactions
- *cytotoxic T cells,* which direct destruction of an antigen or the cells carrying the antigen
- *helper T cells,* also known as T4 cells, which facilitate the humoral and cell-mediated responses
- *suppressor T cells,* also known as T8 cells, which inhibit humoral and cell-mediated responses.

Peripheral lymphoid organs and tissues

The peripheral lymphoid structures include lymph and the lymphatic vessels, lymph nodes, and spleen.

Lymph

Lymph is a clear fluid that bathes body tissues. It contains a liquid portion that resembles blood plasma.

Lymphatic vessels

The lymphatic vessels form a network of thin-walled channels that drain lymph from body tissues. Lymph seeps into the lymphatic vessels through their thin walls. (See *Lymphatic vessels and lymph nodes,* page 354.)

Lymphatic capillaries are located throughout most of the body. They're wider than blood capillaries and permit interstitial fluid to flow into them but not out.

Lymph nodes

Lymph nodes are small, oval-shaped structures along the lymphatic vessels. They're most abundant in the head, neck, axillae, abdomen, pelvis, and groin. Lymph nodes remove and destroy antigens circulating in the blood and lymph.

Afferent lymphatic vessels, which resemble veins, carry lymph into the lymph nodes; the lymph slowly filters through the node and is collected into efferent lymphatic vessels.

Lymph usually travels through more than one lymph node because numerous nodes line the lymphatic vessels that drain a region. For example, axillary nodes filter drainage from the arms and femoral nodes filter drainage from the legs. This prevents organisms that enter peripheral areas from entering central areas.

Spleen

A person's spleen is in the left upper abdominal quadrant beneath the diaphragm. This dark red, oval structure is about the size of a fist. Bands of connective tissue form the dense fibrous capsule surrounding the spleen and extend into the spleen's interior. The interior spleen, called the splenic pulp, contains white and red pulp. White pulp contains compact masses of lymphocytes surrounding branches of the splenic artery. Red pulp is a network of blood-filled

LYMPHATIC VESSELS AND LYMPH NODES

Lymphatic tissues are connected by a network of thin-walled drainage channels called *lymphatic vessels.* Resembling veins, the afferent lymphatic vessels carry lymph into lymph nodes; lymph slowly filters through the node and is collected into efferent lymphatic vessels.

Lymphatic capillaries are located throughout most of the body. Wider than blood capillaries, they permit interstitial fluid to flow into them but not out. The illustrations here show the structures of the lymphatic vessels and lymph nodes.

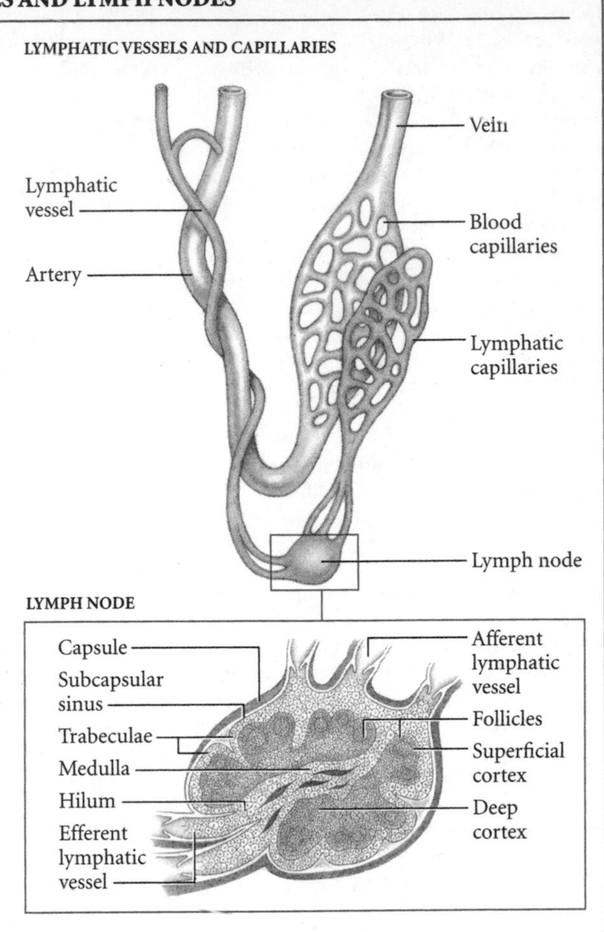

sinusoids supported by a framework of reticular fibers and mononuclear phagocytes, along with some lymphocytes, plasma cells, and monocytes.

The spleen has several functions:

- Its phagocytes engulf and break down worn out RBCs, causing the release of hemoglobin, which then breaks down into its components. These phagocytes also selectively retain and destroy damaged or abnormal RBCs and cells with large amounts of abnormal fibers.
- It filters and removes bacteria and other foreign substances that enter the bloodstream; these substances are promptly removed by splenic phagocytes.
- Splenic phagocytes interact with lymphocytes to initiate an immune response.
- It stores blood and 20% to 30% of platelets.

Accessory lymphoid organs and tissues

The tonsils, adenoids, appendix, and Peyer's patches are the accessory lymphoid organs and tissues. They remove foreign debris similar to lymph nodes. They're located in areas where microbial access is more likely to occur.

Immunity

Immunity is the body's capacity to resist invading organisms and toxins, thereby preventing tissue and organ damage.

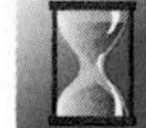

AGE ISSUE *A neonate's immune system depends on passive immunity acquired from the mother transplacentally. Development of immunity begins during the first few months after birth, when bone marrow and the reticuloendothelial system mature.*

The cells and organs of the immune system recognize, respond to, and eliminate antigens or foreign substances, such as bacteria, fungi, viruses, and parasites. They also preserve the body's internal environment by scavenging dead or damaged cells.

The immune system has three basic defensive functions that include protective surface phenomena, general host defense, and specific immune responses.

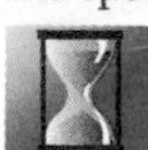

AGE ISSUE *The decline of immune system function begins at sexual maturity and continues with age. As an elderly person's immune system begins to lose its ability to differentiate between self and nonself, the incidence of autoimmune disease increases. The immune system also begins losing its ability to recognize and destroy mutant cells. In elderly people, susceptibility to infection is more likely due to decreased antibody response.*

Protective surface phenomena

Protective surface phenomena are physical, chemical, and mechanical barriers that prevent organisms from entering the body. Such phenomena include organs, structures, and processes of many body systems, including integumentary, respiratory, GI, and urinary.

Integumentary defenses. Intact and healing skin and mucous membranes physically defend against microbial invasion by preventing attachment of microorganisms. Skin desquamation, or normal cell turnover, and low pH further impede bacterial colonization.

Antibacterial substances, such as the enzyme lysozyme that's found in tears, saliva, and nasal secretions, chemically protect seromucous surfaces, such as the conjunctiva of the eye and oral mucous membranes.

Respiratory defenses. In the respiratory system, turbulent airflow through the nostrils and nasal hairs filters foreign materials. Nasal secretions contain an immunoglobulin that discourages microbe adherence, and the mucous layer lining the respiratory tract is continually sloughed off and replaced.

GI defenses. Bacteria that enter the GI system are mechanically removed through salivation, swallowing, peristalsis, and defecation. In addition, the low pH of gastric secretions is bactericidal, making the stomach virtually free from live bacteria. In addition, resident bacteria in the intestines prevent colonization by other microorganisms, protecting the rest of the GI system through a process called *colonization resistance.*

Urinary defenses. The urinary system is sterile except for the distal end of the urethra and the urinary meatus. Urine flow, low urine pH, immunoglobulin, and the bactericidal effects of prostatic fluid impede bacterial colonization. A series of sphincters also inhibits upward bacterial migration into the urinary tract.

General host defense

When an antigen does penetrate the skin or mucous membrane, the immune system launches a nonspecific cellular response to identify and remove the invader.

The first nonspecific response against an antigen, the inflammatory response, involves vascular and cellular changes that eliminate dead tissue, microorganisms, toxins, and inert foreign matter. (See *Understanding inflammation,* page 356.)

Phagocytosis occurs after inflammation or during chronic infection. In this nonspecific response, neutrophils and macrophages engulf, digest, and dispose of the antigen.

Specific immune responses

All foreign substances elicit the same general host defenses. In addition, particular microorganisms or molecules activate specific immune responses produced by lymphocytes — B cells and T cells — and can initially involve specialized sets of immune cells. Such specific responses are classified as either humoral immunity or cell-mediated immunity.

UNDERSTANDING INFLAMMATION

The inflammatory response to an antigen involves vascular and cellular changes that eliminate dead tissue, microorganisms, toxins, and inert foreign matter. This nonspecific immune response aids tissue repair in a stepwise fashion, depicted here by this flowchart.

Immediately after microorganisms invade damaged tissue, basophils release heparin, histamine, and kinins.

↓

These substances promote vasodilation and increase capillary permeability.

↓

Blood flow increases to the affected tissues, and fluid collects in them.

↓

Granulocytes — predominantly neutrophils — promptly migrate to the invasion site.

↓

At the invasion site, these cells engulf and destroy the microorganism, foreign materials, and debris from dying cells.

↓

Tissue repair results.

Humoral immunity. In humoral immunity, an invading antigen causes B cells to divide and differentiate into plasma cells. Each plasma cell then produces and secretes a large amount of antigen-specific immunoglobulin, also called *antibodies*, into the bloodstream. The humoral response is also known as an *antibody-mediated response.*

IMMUNOGLOBULINS. Immunoglobulins have a special molecular structure that creates a Y shape. The upper fork of the Y is designed to attach to a particular antigen; the lower stem enables the immunoglobulin to link with other structures in the immune system. Depending on the antigen, immunoglobulins can work in one of several ways:

- They can disable certain bacteria by linking with toxins that the bacteria produce; these immunoglobulins are called *antitoxins.*
- They can opsonize or coat bacteria, making them targets for scavenging by phagocytosis. (See *Understanding phagocytosis.*)
- Most commonly, they can link to antigens, causing the immune system to produce and circulate enzymes called *complement.*

Each of the five types of immunoglobulins (IgA, IgD, IgE, IgG, and IgM) has a specific function:

- IgA, IgG, and IgM guard against viral and bacterial invasion.
- IgD is an antigen receptor of B cells.
- IgE causes an allergic response.

After initial exposure to an antigen, a time lag occurs during which minimal or no antibody levels can be detected in the body. During this time, the B cell recognizes the antigen, and the antigen-antibody complex forms. The complex has several functions:

- A macrophage processes the antigen and presents it to antigen-specific B cells.
- The antibody activates the complement system, causing an enzymatic cascade that destroys the antigen.
- The activated complement system, which bridges humoral and cell-mediated immunity, attracts phagocytic neutrophils and macrophages to the antigen site.

COMPLEMENT SYSTEM. The complement system consists of about 25 enzymes that complement the work of antibodies by aiding phagocytosis or destroying bacteria by puncturing their cell membranes.

UNDERSTANDING PHAGOCYTOSIS

Microorganisms and other antigens that invade the skin and mucous membranes are removed by phagocytosis, a defense mechanism carried out by macrophages (mononuclear leukocytes) and neutrophils (polymorphonuclear leukocytes). These illustrations demonstrate how macrophages are an integral part of the process of phagocytosis.

Chemotaxis
Chemotactic factors attract macrophages to the antigen site.

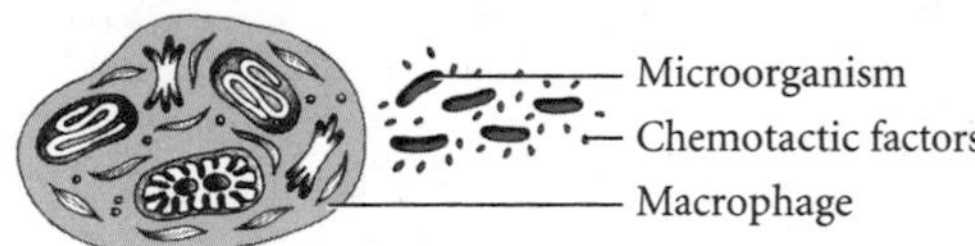

Opsonization
Antibody (immunoglobulin G) or complement fragment coats the microorganism, enhancing macrophage binding to the antigen, now called an *opsinogen.*

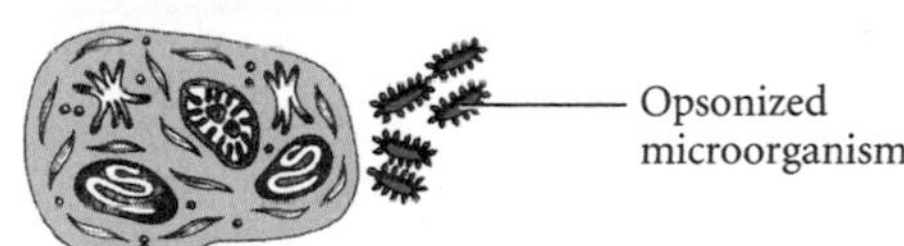

Ingestion
The macrophage extends its membrane around the opsonized microorganism, engulfing it within a vacuole (phagosome).

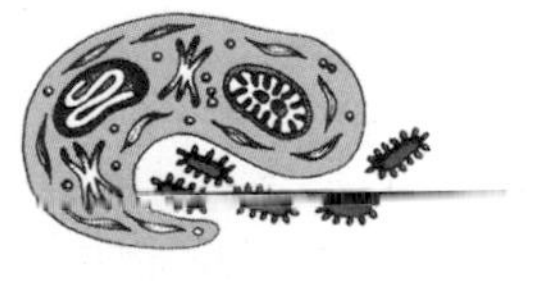

Digestion
As the phagosome shifts away from the cell periphery, it merges with lysosomes, forming a phagolysosome, where antigen destruction occurs.

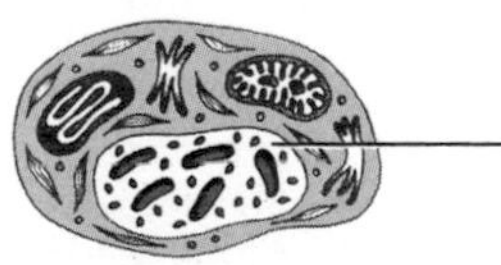

Release
When digestion is complete, the macrophage expels digestive debris, including lysosomes, prostaglandins, complement components, and interferon, which continue to mediate the immune response.

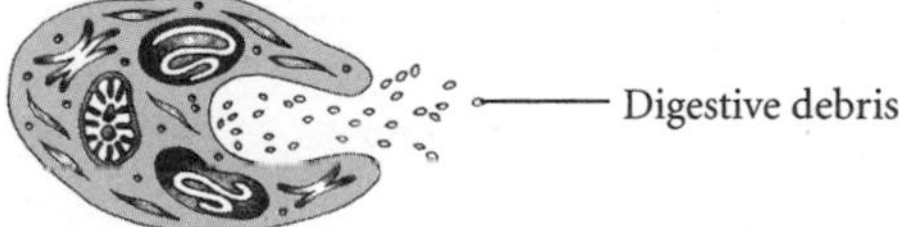

Complement proteins travel in the bloodstream in an inactive form. When the first complement substance is triggered by an antibody interlocked with an antigen, it sets in motion a ripple effect. As each component is activated in turn, it acts on the next component in a controlled sequence called the *complement cascade.*

The complement cascade leads to formation of the membrane attack complex, which enters the membrane of a target cell and creates a channel through which fluids and molecules flow in and out. The target cell then swells and eventually bursts.

Effects of the complement cascade also include the inflammatory response, resulting from the release of the contents of mast cells and basophils; stimulation and attraction of neutrophils, which participate in phagocytosis; the coating of target cells by C3b — an inactivated fragment of the complement protein C3 — making them attractive to phagocytes; viral neutralization; and lysis of cells and bacteria.

Cell-mediated immunity. Cell-mediated immunity protects the body from bacterial, viral, and fungal infections and provides resistance against transplanted cells and tumor cells.

In cell-mediated immunity, a macrophage processes the antigen, which is then presented to T cells. Some T cells become sensitized and destroy the antigen; others release lymphokines, which activate macrophages that destroy the antigen. Sensitized T cells then travel through the blood and lymphatic systems, providing ongoing surveillance for specific antigens.

Health history

Many signs and symptoms of hematologic disorders are nonspecific and difficult to assess. Others are more specific; use these to focus on possible disorders. Assess the hematologic system if the patient reports any of these specific signs or symptoms, including abnormal bleeding, bone and joint pain, exertional dyspnea, ecchymoses, fatigue and weakness, fever, lymphadenopathy, pallor, petechiae, shortness of breath, and tachycardia.

Accurately assessing a patient's immune system can likewise be challenging. Immune disorders sometimes produce characteristic signs — such as butterfly rash in SLE — but they usually cause vague symptoms, such as fatigue or dyspnea, which initially seem related to other body systems. For this reason, assess the immune system whenever a patient reports such symptoms as malaise, fatigue, frequent or recurrent infections, slow wound healing, and weight loss or decreased appetite.

Start your assessment by taking a thorough patient history. Gather information about the patient's current and previous illnesses. Also ask about the patient's family and social histories.

Obtain biographical information, particularly age, sex, race, and ethnicity, because some hematologic and immune disorders occur more frequently in certain groups of people than in others.

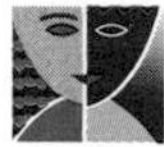

CULTURAL INSIGHT *Certain autoimmune diseases appear more often in women — especially young women — than in men. Sickle cell anemia occurs primarily in Blacks and less frequently in Mediterranean, Middle Eastern, and Asian people. Pernicious anemia occurs most frequently in Northern Europeans.*

Chief complaint

The most common chief complaints of the hematologic and immune systems include such dysfunctions as bleeding, lymphadenopathy, fatigue and weakness, fever, and joint pain. Ask the patient to elaborate on his chief complaint and document it in the patient's own words.

Current health history

Ask the patient how long he has had the problem, when it began, and if it was sudden or gradual. Ask if it occurs continuously or intermittently. If intermittently, find out how frequent and how long each episode occurs.

Next, determine the location and character of the problem and precipitating conditions. Ask what actions or measures make the problem better or worse. Also ask about other signs and symptoms that occur at the same time as the primary ones.

Abnormal bleeding

To assess for abnormal bleeding, ask if the patient has experienced any unusual blood loss. To gain additional information, begin by asking the patient if he has passed black stool, had blood in his urine or, for a female patient, if she has had unusually heavy menses. Excessive blood loss may result in anemia. Next, find out if he has frequent nosebleeds. Ask about any bruises he has noticed on his skin, especially ones for which he can't recall the cause. A platelet or clotting mechanism deficiency can result in bruises from minimal pressure or slight bumps. Ask if he bleeds for a long time when he cuts his finger or has his teeth cleaned. Such excessive bleeding suggests a defective clotting mechanism. Find out if he starts bleeding for no apparent reason and if bleeding after an injury starts slowly and lasts a long time.

All these signs and symptoms are indicative of vascular, platelet, or coagulation disorders.

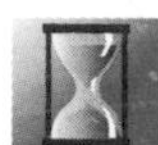

AGE ISSUE *When recording the health history of a child with a suspected hematologic disorder, check for anemia by asking the parents about these common signs and symptoms: pallor, fatigue, failure to gain weight, malaise, and lethargy. If you suspect a clotting disorder, also ask if there's a family history of abnormal bleeding tendencies.*

Lymphadenopathy

For the patient who reports swelling in the lymph nodes, ask if he has swelling in his neck, armpit, or groin. Check these areas for soreness, hardness, or redness. Ask him when he first noticed the swelling and if it's on one side, or both.

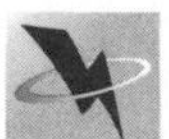

CRITICAL POINT *Enlarged lymph nodes may indicate an inflammatory process, an infection, or the elevated lymphocyte production characteristic of certain leukemias.*

Enlargement from a primary lymphatic tumor usually isn't painful. Hodgkin's disease, however, may be accompanied by red, tender, enlarged lymph nodes. A large mass may indicate a lymphoma. Ask if a biopsy has ever been done on one of these lymph nodes, which could indicate a previously diagnosed malignancy.

Fatigue and weakness

Next, ask the patient if he feels tired all the time or only during exertion. Find out if he naps during the day and how many hours he sleeps at night. Ask the patient if he's experiencing weakness and, if so, if it's more noticeable on one side or adjacent to joints. Find out if the weakness developed gradually and if it occurs persistently. Also, find out if the patient was ever told he was anemic. Fatigue and weakness on exertion can suggest moderate anemia; extreme or constant fatigue and weakness can occur in a patient with severe anemia or with neuropathy from an autoimmune disease.

Fever

If your patient reports a fever, find out how long he has had it and if his temperature ever drops to normal during the day. Intermittent fevers occur with lymphomas. Ask about periods of fever alternating with periods of normal temperature. Recurrent fever occurs in Hodgkin's disease. Find out about frequent fevers. Fever from frequent infections may suggest a poorly functioning immune system. It may also suggest rapid cell proliferation. Ask the patient if he perspires excessively with the fever or appears flushed in the face. These symptoms usually accompany an infection.

Joint pain

Finally, ask your patient if he has joint pain. Find out which joints are affected and if the joint pain occurs in several joints at the same time or if it affects additional joints. Ask about swelling, redness, or warmth appearing with the joint pain. Find out if the patient's joints are painful when he's resting or if he has early-morning stiffness. Pain in the knees, wrists, or hands may indicate an autoimmune process or hemarthrosis from a blood disorder.

Find out if the patient's bones ache. Aching bones may result from the pressure of expanding bone marrow. Ask what he does to relieve the pain. Heat application or salicylates relieve pain from an inflammatory process.

Past health history

Examine the patient's past health history for additional clues to his present condition. Look for information about allergies, immunizations, previously diagnosed illnesses in childhood and adulthood, past hospitalizations and surgeries, and current medications he uses, both prescription and over-the-counter.

Look at the patient's health history for information about such past disorders as acute leukemia, Hodgkin's disease, sarcoma, and rheumatoid arthritis that required aggressive immunosuppressant or radiation therapies. Such treatment can diminish blood cell production. Find out if the patient has received any blood products. If so, note when and how often blood product transfusions were used to assess the patient's risk of harboring a blood-borne infection.

Focus on these relevant areas when reviewing the patient's past health history:

- *Allergies* — Ask the patient about known allergies to foods, drugs, insects, or environmental pollutants. Multiple allergies are common.
- *Asthma* — A history of asthma may indicate immunopathology.
- *Autoimmune diseases* — The presence of one autoimmune disease can predispose a person to others.
- *Blood donation refusals* — A patient rejected as a blood donor may have longstanding anemia or a history of hepatitis or jaundice with an undetermined cause.
- *Blood transfusions* — A history of blood transfusions may suggest anemia. Try to determine the reason for the transfusions, how many units were given, and the patient's reaction, if any.
- *GI problems* — A patient's history of peptic ulcer with excessive bleeding may indicate the presence of anemia.
- *Immunizations* — A history of the patient's immunizations is essential. Determine if the patient has developed appropriate antibody responses to titers to the immunizations.
- *Medications* — A history of taking prescribed medications may indicate previous immune and hematologic disorders. Also, note that certain drugs, such as anticonvulsants (for example, carbamazepine and phenytoin) and antineoplastics (for example, cyclophosphamide and vincristine) can produce adverse effects in the hematologic and immune systems.
- *Radiation therapy* — Radiation therapy can cause decreased blood cell production.
- *Sore throats* — Frequent sore throats may indicate poor resistance to infection.
- *Surgery* — Gastric surgery decreases the level of intrinsic factor needed for vitamin B absorption. Bilateral nephrectomy may produce a diminished erythropoietin level. Hepatic surgery may reduce the formation of coagulation factors.

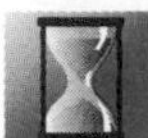

AGE ISSUE *For a child, ask the patient's mother about obstetric bleeding complications, and note any history of Rh incompatibility.*

Family history

Some hematologic and immune disorders demonstrate familial tendencies while others are hereditary. Always be sure to determine if your patient's family has a history of anemias, cancer, abnormal bleeding problems (particularly in male relatives), or immune disorders, including allergies. Note any inheritable hematologic or immune disorders and create a family genogram to determine the patient's inheritance risk.

Psychosocial history

The patient may be reluctant to discuss certain habits or lifestyles. Take steps to develop trust between you and the patient to increase cooperation. Inquire about alcohol intake, diet, sexual habits, and possible drug and tobacco abuse, which can impair hematologic or immune function.

Make sure you gather a comprehensive occupational and military service history. Exposure to certain hazardous substances can cause bone marrow dysfunction, especially leukemia. Exposure to chemicals — such as industrial cleaning fluids, glues used in some hobbies, or insecticides used in gardening or farming — may cause blood disorders.

Increased stress may reduce a patient's resistance to infection and can trigger an autoimmune disease.

Determine the patient's activities of daily living (ADLs), focusing on his diet. Specifically, evaluate his typical daily diet and inquire about idiosyncratic, religious, or cultural dietary restrictions. Also ask about recent significant dietary changes and weight loss. Inquire about specific herbal food sources that may be interfering with the absorption of medications.

Poor nutrition can greatly affect a person's immune system. For example, a severely protein-deficient diet can result in lymphoid tissue atrophy, diminished antibody response, fewer circulating T cells, and impaired cell-mediated immunity. Although infection increases the need for nutrients and caloric intake, it may paradoxically cause anorexia. Also ask about the patent's alcohol consumption. If it's excessive, he may have nutritional deficits. Ask too, about exercise and rest patterns. Problems associated with these ADLs may provide clues to an underlying hematologic or immune disorder.

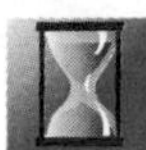

AGE ISSUE *When assessing the elderly patient's diet, ask if he lives alone and cooks for himself. Because of limited income and resources and decreased mobility, elderly patients may have diets deficient in protein, calcium, and iron — nutrients essential to the blood-forming process. Even with an adequate diet, nutrients may not be absorbed due to excessive laxative use or metabolized due to fewer enzymes. In those over age 60, about 40% have iron deficiency anemia.*

Review of systems

When obtaining the health history, be sure to question the patient about complaints or problems associated with the various body systems. For example, ask the patient about changes in his nails, such as brittleness, ridges, or flattening, which could suggest anemia. Inquire about complaints of headache, irritability, or depression. These complaints may suggest central nervous system complications associated with SLE, an autoimmune disorder.

Physical assessment

During the physical assessment, the patient will alternate between sitting and lying down. Adjust the examination table to an appropriate height for both positions. Ensure proper lighting for skin inspection — a key part of assessing the hematologic and immune systems.

CRITICAL POINT *Lighting that produces a glare may interfere with detecting subtle color changes.*

Before starting the examination, allow the patient the opportunity to urinate because deep abdominal palpation will be performed. Explain the purpose of the examination to the patient, and tell him what will be done before starting each procedure. Have the necessary equipment ready — stethoscope, sphygmomanometer, ophthalmoscope, scale, and measuring tape.

CRITICAL POINT *Note that in your physical assessment the typical order of inspection, palpation, percussion, and auscultation will be reversed. Specific structures of the hematologic and immune system (such as the spleen) differ from other body systems in that they require auscultation, percussion, and palpation, in that order, due to their sensitivity.*

General assessment

Because signs and symptoms of hematologic and immune disorders are often nonspecific, a thorough observation of your patient's general physical status is essential. Inspect his general appearance and note if he looks acutely ill. Observe his face for flushing, profuse perspiration, or grimacing as if he's in pain. Then observe for indications of chronic illness, including dehydration, pallor, emaciation, and listlessness.

Determine if the patient looks his stated age. Chronic disease and nutritional deficiencies associated with hematologic and immune disorders may make a patient look older than he is.

Next, weigh the patient and measure his height. Compare his weight to the ideal for his height, bone structure, and build. Weight loss may result from anorexia and GI problems associated with hematologic or immune conditions. If your patient appears undernourished or cachectic, assess him for chronic disease.

Next, inspect your patient for abnormal body posture, movements, or gait; these can indicate joint, spinal, or neurologic changes.

Finally, record your patient's vital signs. Start by taking his temperature. Frequent fevers can indicate a poorly functioning immune system.

CRITICAL POINT *Subnormal temperature in a patient usually accompanies a gram-negative infection.*

Note the patient's heart rate. The heart may pump harder or faster to compensate for a decreased oxygen supply resulting from anemia or decreased blood volume from bleeding. This problem can cause tachycardia, palpitations, or arrhythmias.

Measure the patient's blood pressure while he's lying, sitting, and standing. Check for orthostatic hypotension, which may be caused by septicemia or hypovolemia.

Check the patient's breathing. If he's having difficulty meeting the body's oxygen needs, he may have pronounced tachypnea.

Observe your patient's behavior to assess his mood. A chronically ill patient, regardless of the nature of his disorder, may be depressed or angry. However, irritability, confusion, hallucinations, or other symptoms of psychosis such as paranoid thinking may occur with immune disorders, particularly SLE. Forgetfulness and sleeplessness may occur with anemia. Slowed responses or a poor attention span can result from either hematologic or immune disorders.

Inspection

A key component of the physical assessment of the hematologic and immune systems is inspection. Inspection of these systems focuses on the skin, hair and nails, eyes, and the mouth, including its mucous membranes. In addition, immune system inspection also focuses on the nose and lymph nodes as well as the cardiac, respiratory, GI (including the abdomen), and genitourinary (GU) systems.

Skin inspection

Inspect your patient's skin color, noting any pallor, cyanosis, or jaundice. Pallor can result from decreased hemoglobin content. Cyanosis suggests excessive deoxygenated hemoglobin in cutaneous blood vessels caused by hypoxia, which appears in some anemias. In a patient's fingers or toes, cyanosis or pallor may result from Raynaud's phenomenon, which is seen in some autoimmune diseases.

Examine the patient's face, conjunctivae, hands, and feet for ruddy cyanosis or plethora (red, florid complexion), which appear in polycythemia. Clubbing of the digits due to thrombosis in smaller vessels may also occur. Also inspect for erythema, a possible sign of local inflammation or fever.

Look for jaundice in the patient's sclerae, mucous membranes, and skin.

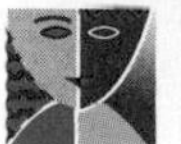

CULTURAL INSIGHT *For dark-skinned patients, also inspect the buccal mucosa, palms, and soles.*

For an edematous patient, examine the inner forearm for jaundice. An elevated bilirubin level may be secondary to increased erythrocyte hemolysis — a problem that may be hereditary or acquired.

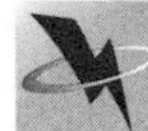

CRITICAL POINT *Excessive intake of carrots or yellow vegetables may cause yellow skin in a patient, but will not cause color change in the sclerae or mucous membranes.*

If a clotting abnormality is suspected, inspect the patient's skin for purpuric lesions, which result most commonly from thrombocytopenia. These lesions can vary in size. In adults, large blood-filled blisters may be seen in the mouth.

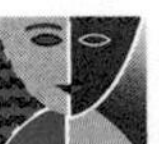

CULTURAL INSIGHT *For dark-skinned patients, assess the oral mucosa or conjunctivae for petechiae or ecchymoses. As blood is reabsorbed, the skin color changes from yellow to yellow-green. These two skin changes are difficult to detect in dark-skinned patients.*

Also inspect for such abnormalities as telangiectasias, and note their location.

Assess skin integrity, noting if the patient has signs of infection, such as abnormal temperature, wound drainage, poor wound healing, or ulceration. Evaluate the patient's skin for dryness or coarseness, which may indicate iron deficiency anemia. Check for rashes; among many possible causes, a rash can indicate autoimmune disease. Certain autoimmune diseases have uniquely characteristic rashes, such as the butterfly rash of SLE or the heliotrope rash of dermatomyositis. Note the rash's distribution.

Hair and nail inspection

Inspect the patient's hair growth patterns, noting alopecia on the arms, legs, or head.

CRITICAL POINT *Alopecia patches may occur in patients with SLE.*

Inspect the patient's nails and note any abnormalities. Specifically, note any longitudinal striation, which is associated with anemia, or koilonychia (also called *spoon nail*), which is characteristic of iron deficiency anemia. Look for platyonychia, characterized by abnormally broad or flat nails, which may precede the development of koilonychia, and for onycholysis or loosening of the nails. Then, inspect for nail clubbing, indicative of chronic hypoxia—which can result from a hematologic or immune disorder.

Eye inspection

Inspect your patient's eyelids for signs of infection or inflammation, such as edema, redness, or lesions. Note the eyes' position and alignment, and check the conjunctivae for engorged or enlarged vessels. Keratoconjunctivitis, as well as iritis and scleritis, may accompany rheumatoid arthritis. Perform an ophthalmoscopic examination to examine the patient's retinas. Vessel tortuosity may result from sickle cell anemia; hemorrhage or infiltration may suggest, among other possibilities, hemorrhagic leukemia, vasculitis, or thrombocytopenia.

CRITICAL POINT *Retinal hemorrhages and exudates suggest severe anemia and thrombocytopenia.*

Mouth inspection

Inspect the patient's buccal mucosa, lips, gums, teeth, tongue, and palate. White patches scattered throughout the mouth may indicate candidiasis, and lacy white plaques on the buccal mucosa may be associated with acquired immunodeficiency syndrome. Such lesions can occur in a patient with an immunosuppressive disorder or in one who receives chemotherapy. Red mucous membranes may result from polycythemia; an enlarged tongue from multiple myeloma, among other possible disorders; absence of papillae from pernicious anemia; and purpuras and telangiectasias from bleeding disorders. Inspect the tonsils, noting hypertrophy. Tonsillar hypertrophy appears in lymphomas; gingival hypertrophy that makes teeth look sunken may result from myelogenous leukemia. These changes occur in chronic, not acute, neoplastic diseases. Oral nasopharyngeal ulcers may accompany SLE.

Lymph node inspection

Inspect the lymph node areas where the patient reports swollen glands or lumps for color abnormalities and visible lymph node enlargement. Then inspect all other nodal regions. Proceed from head to toe to avoid missing any region. Normally, lymph nodes can't be seen. Visibly enlarged nodes suggest a current or previous inflammation. Nodes covered with red-streaked skin suggest acute lymphadenitis.

Cardiac and respiratory inspection

Inspect the patient's chest area carefully. Note signs of respiratory distress, especially dyspnea, coughing, or cyanosis. Assess the patient's peripheral circulation for Raynaud's phenomenon, which causes the intermittent arteriolar vasospasm of the fingers or toes and sometimes of the ears and nose. This phenomenon may be caused by SLE or scleroderma.

Gastrointestinal inspection

Inspect the patient's abdominal area for enlargement, distention, and asymmetry, possibly indicating a tumor. Hepatomegaly and splenomegaly may result from:

- congestion caused by cell overproduction, as in polycythemia or leukemia
- excessive cell destruction, as in hemolytic anemia.

Genitourinary inspection

Because immune dysfunction can affect the GU system, obtain a urine specimen and evaluate its color, clarity, and odor. Cloudy, malodorous urine may result from a urinary tract infection.

Inspect the urinary meatus. In a patient with WBC deficiency or immunodeficiency, the external genitalia may be focal points for inflammation, which is commonly accompanied by discharge or bleeding related to infection.

Auscultation

Auscultate the patient's precordium for heart murmurs. Ventricular enlargement and apical systolic murmurs may result from severe anemia. Mitral, aortic, and pulmonic murmurs can occur in sickle cell anemia. Tachycardia may also occur in some anemias. Heart failure or pericardial effusions may develop in a patient with SLE or rheumatoid arthritis.

Auscultate the patient's lungs, noting abnormal breath sounds. Auscultation may detect wheezing—a possible sign of allergy or asthma. Evidence of a pleural effusion, as noted by decreased or absent breath sounds on one side, may suggest rheumatoid arthritis or SLE.

With the patient lying down, auscultate the abdomen before palpation and percussion to avoid altering bowel sounds. Listen for a loud, high-pitched, tinkling sound, which heralds the early stages of intestinal obstruction. Lymphoma is a hematologic cause of such obstruction.

Next, auscultate the liver and spleen. Listen carefully over both organs for friction rubs, which are grating sounds that fluctuate with respirations. These sounds usually indicate inflammation of the organ's peritoneal covering. Splenic friction rubs also suggest infarction and inflammation.

Percussion

Percuss the patient's chest for resonance. Dullness or flatness on percussion may suggest a pleural effusion, associated with rheumatoid arthritis or SLE.

To determine liver and spleen size and, possibly, detect tumors, percuss all four abdominal quadrants and compare your findings.

The normal liver sounds dull. Establish the organ's approximate size by percussing for its upper and lower borders at the midclavicular line. To determine medial extension, percuss to the midsternal landmark.

The normal spleen also sounds dull. Percuss it from the midaxillary line toward the midline. The average-sized spleen lies near the eighth, ninth, or tenth intercostal space. Mark the liver and spleen borders with a pen for later reference.

Palpation

When assessing the hematologic and immune systems, palpation focuses on the lymph nodes, liver, and spleen. Before palpating these areas, position and drape the patient appropriately, making sure to keep the patient warm. Warm your hands, then palpate using gentle to moderate pressure.

Lymph node palpation

Palpate the patient's neck, axillary, epitrochlear, and inguinal lymph nodes as you examine the areas of the body. Use your finger pads to move skin over the area. When palpating the nodes in the patient's neck, he should be sitting. To palpate axillary nodes, the patient should remain sitting or be supine, with his arms relaxed. Use your nondominant hand to support his right arm and put your other hand as high in his right axilla as possible. Palpate against the chest wall for the lateral, anterior, posterior, central, and subclavian nodes. Use the same procedure for the patient's left axilla. For the epitrochlear nodes, palpate the medial area of his elbow. For the inguinal nodes, palpate below the inguinal ligament and along the upper saphenous vein. When palpating all nodes, note their size, consistency (hard or soft), and whether they're fixed or movable, tender or painless. (See *Palpating the lymph nodes.*)

Red streaks in the skin, palpable nodes, and lymphedema may indicate a lymphatic disorder. Enlarged palpable nodes suggest current or previous inflammation. Nodes covered by red-streaked skin suggest acute lymphadenitis and reveal an obvious infection site. Hard nodes may suggest a tumor. General lymphadenopathy can indicate an inflammatory or neoplastic process.

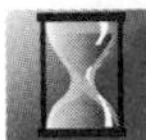

AGE ISSUE *In a child under age 12, normal lymph nodes are commonly palpable. You may feel normal cervical and inguinal nodes ranging in size from about 1/8" (3 mm) across to as much as 3/8" (1 cm) across. Moderate numbers of nodes that are cool, firm, movable, and painless indicate past infection. Palpable cervical nodes of this description, for example, can suggest a past respiratory infection.*

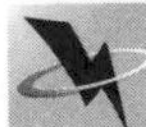

CRITICAL POINT *When palpating the patient's nodes, you may discover sternal tenderness. This problem occurs with cell packing in the marrow from anemia, leukemia, and immunoproliferative disorders.*

Liver and spleen palpation

Accurate liver palpation is difficult and can depend on the patient's size and comfort level and possible fluid accumulation. Lightly palpate all four abdominal quadrants to distinguish tender sites and muscle guard-

EXPERT TECHNIQUE

PALPATING THE LYMPH NODES

When assessing your patient for signs of an immune disorder, palpate the superficial lymph nodes of the head and neck and of the axillary, epitrochlear, inguinal, and popliteal areas, using the pads of your index and middle fingers. Always palpate gently, beginning with light pressure and gradually increasing the pressure.

Head and neck nodes

Head and neck nodes are best palpated with the patient in a sitting position.

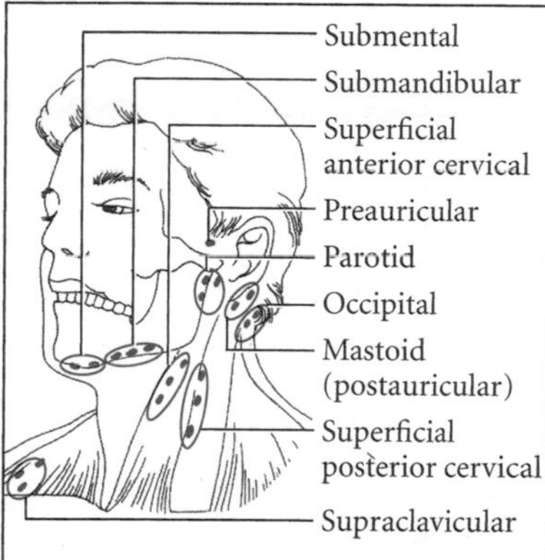

Axillary and epitrochlear nodes

Palpate the axillary and epitrochlear nodes with the patient in a sitting position. You can also palpate the axillary nodes with the patient lying in a supine position.

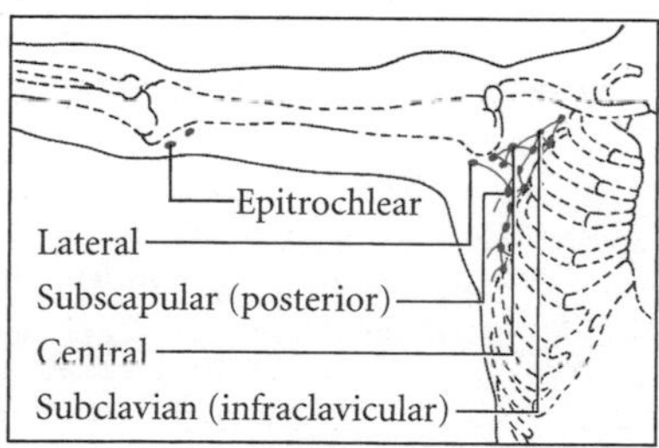

Inguinal and popliteal nodes

Palpate the inguinal and popliteal nodes with the patient lying in a supine position. You can also palpate the popliteal nodes with the patient sitting or standing.

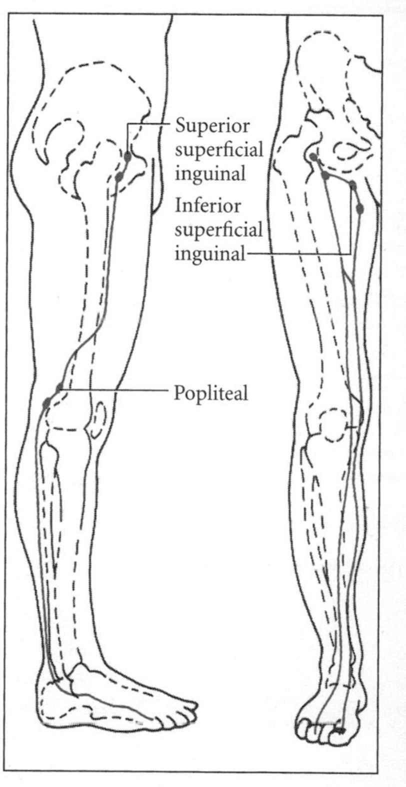

ing. Use deeper palpation to delineate abdominal organs and masses. (See chapter 11, Gastrointestinal system, for more information on liver palpation.)

If necessary, repeat the procedure, checking hand position and the pressure exerted.

CRITICAL POINT *Always palpate tender areas such as the spleen last.*

Palpate the spleen to detect tenderness and confirm splenomegaly. The spleen must be enlarged about three times its normal size to be palpable. (See *Percussing and palpating the spleen,* page 366.)

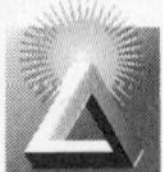

EXPERT TECHNIQUE

PERCUSSING AND PALPATING THE SPLEEN

To assess the spleen, use percussion to estimate its size and palpation to detect tenderness and enlargement. Splenic tenderness may result from infections, which are common in a patient with an immunodeficiency disorder. Splenomegaly may occur with immune disorders that cause congestion by cell overproduction or by excessive demand for cell destruction.

Percussion

To percuss the spleen, first percuss the lowest intercostal space in the left anterior axillary line as shown; percussion notes should be tympanic.

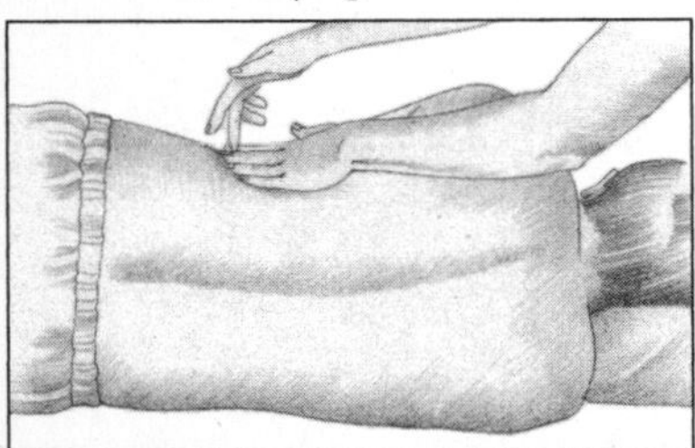

Second, ask the patient to take a deep breath, then percuss this area again. If the spleen is normal in size, the area will remain tympanic. If the tympanic percussion note changes on inspiration to dullness, the spleen is probably enlarged.

Last, to estimate spleen size, outline the spleen's edges by percussing in several directions from areas of tympany to areas of dullness.

Palpation

To palpate the spleen, first, with the patient in a supine position and you at his right side, reach across him to support the posterior lower left rib cage with your left hand. Place your right hand below the left costal margin and press inward as shown.

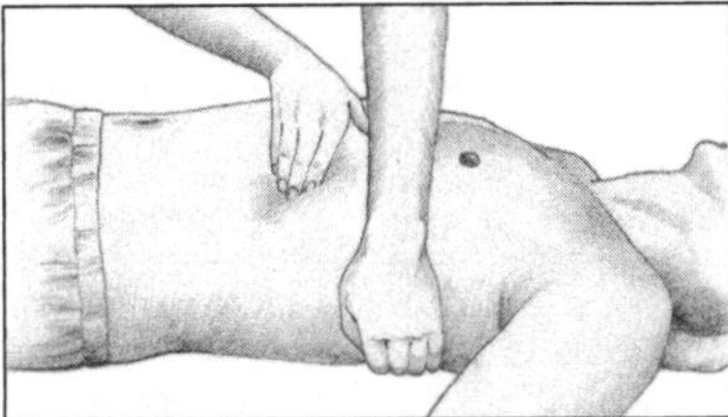

Second, instruct him to take a deep breath. The spleen normally shouldn't descend on deep inspiration below the ninth or tenth intercostal space in the posterior midaxillary line. If the spleen is enlarged, you'll feel its rigid border.

Never over-palpate the spleen; an enlarged spleen can easily rupture.

Hepatomegaly and splenomegaly may result from congestion caused by cell overproduction, as in polycythemia or leukemia, or from excessive demand for defective cell destruction, as in hemolytic anemias.

Abnormal findings

A patient's chief complaint may reveal a number of signs and symptoms related to the hematologic and immune systems. The most significant findings include dizziness, dyspnea, edema of the face, erythema, fever, lymphadenopathy, pallor, purpura, and splenomegaly. Butterfly rash, a common finding associated with SLE is described in chapter 5, Integumentary system. The following history, physical assessment, and analysis summaries will help you assess each finding quickly and accurately. After obtaining further information, begin to interpret the findings. (See *Hematologic and immune systems: Interpreting your findings.*)

Dizziness

A common symptom, dizziness is a sensation of imbalance or faintness, sometimes associated with giddiness, weakness, confusion, and blurred or double vision. Episodes

(Text continues on page 371.)

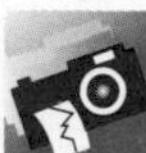

CLINICAL PICTURE

HEMATOLOGIC AND IMMUNE SYSTEMS: INTERPRETING YOUR FINDINGS

After you assess the patient, a group of findings may lead you to suspect a particular hematologic or immune disorder. The chart below shows you some common groups of findings for major signs and symptoms related to the hematologic and immune systems, along with their probable causes.

Sign or symptom and findings	Probable cause
Dizziness	
▪ Dizziness aggravated by postural changes or exertion ▪ Pallor ▪ Dyspnea ▪ Fatigue ▪ Tachycardia ▪ Bounding pulse ▪ Increased capillary refill time	Anemia
▪ Dizziness in conjunction with other signs of fluid volume deficit, such as dry mucous membranes, hypotension, or tachycardia	Hypovolemia
Dyspnea	
▪ Gradual onset of dyspnea ▪ Fatigue ▪ Weakness ▪ Syncope ▪ Tachycardia, tachypnea, restlessness, anxiety, and thirst (if severe)	Anemia
***Dyspnea** (continued)*	
▪ Acute dyspneic attacks ▪ Audible wheezing ▪ Dry cough ▪ Accessory muscle use ▪ Nasal flaring ▪ Retractions ▪ Tachypnea ▪ Tachycardia ▪ Diaphoresis ▪ Prolonged expiration ▪ Flushing or cyanosis ▪ Apprehension	Asthma
▪ Dyspnea accompanied by fever ▪ Headache ▪ Malaise ▪ Dry nonproductive cough ▪ Possible progression to respiratory failure	Severe acute respiratory syndrome
Edema of the face	
▪ Unilateral facial edema ▪ Severe throat pain ▪ Neck swelling ▪ Drooling ▪ Cervical adenopathy ▪ Fever ▪ Chills ▪ Malaise	Abscess, peritonsillar

(continued)

HEMATOLOGIC AND IMMUNE SYSTEMS: INTERPRETING YOUR FINDINGS *(continued)*

Sign or symptom and findings	Probable cause
Edema of the face *(continued)*	
▪ Facial edema, angioneurotic edema with urticaria, erythema, and flushing ▪ Hoarseness, stridor, and bronchospasms due to airway edema ▪ Hypotension ▪ Cool clammy skin	Allergic reaction
▪ Edema of the eyelids accompanied by redness ▪ Paroxysmal sneezing ▪ Itchy nose and eyes ▪ Profuse watery rhinorrhea	Rhinitis, allergic
Erythema	
▪ Reddened skin with hivelike eruptions and edema ▪ Sudden urticaria, flushing, facial edema, diaphoresis, weakness, sneezing, bronchospasm with dyspnea and tachycardia, and anaphylactic shock	Allergic reaction
▪ Acute onset of erythema as a butterfly rash ranging from a blush with swelling to a scaly, sharply demarcated, macular rash with plaques that may spread to the forehead, chin, ears, chest, and other sun-exposed areas	Systemic lupus erythematosus
Erythema *(continued)*	
▪ Erythema with telangiectasia ▪ Hyperpigmentation ▪ Ear and nose deformity ▪ Mouth, tongue, and eyelid lesions	Discoid lupus erythematosus
Fever	
▪ Low fever with possible mild elevations; remittent, intermittent, or sustained ▪ Erythema multiforme ▪ Fatigue, anorexia, and weight loss as prodromal complaints ▪ Nocturnal diaphoresis ▪ Diarrhea ▪ Persistent cough	Immune complex dysfunction
▪ Fever ranging from low to extremely high depending on causative organism ▪ Remittent, sustained, or relapsing ▪ Abrupt or insidious onset	Infectious and inflammatory disorders
Lymphadenopathy	
▪ Enlarged lymph nodes with a history of fatigue, night sweats, afternoon fevers, diarrhea, weight loss, and cough ▪ Concurrent infections beginning afterward	Acquired immunodeficiency syndrome

HEMATOLOGIC AND IMMUNE SYSTEMS: INTERPRETING YOUR FINDINGS *(continued)*

Sign or symptom and findings	Probable cause
Lymphadenopathy *(continued)*	
▪ Single to multiple enlarged lymph nodes depending on stage of disease ▪ Pruritus ▪ Fatigue ▪ Weakness ▪ Night sweats ▪ Malaise ▪ Weight loss ▪ Unexplained fever ▪ Tracheal and esophageal pressure if mediastinal lymph nodes involved	Hodgkin's disease
▪ Generalized lymphadenopathy ▪ Fatigue ▪ Malaise ▪ Pallor ▪ Low fever ▪ Prolonged bleeding time ▪ Swollen gums ▪ Weight loss ▪ Bone or joint pain ▪ Hepatosplenomegaly	Leukemia, acute lymphocytic
▪ Painless enlargement of one or more peripheral nodes ▪ Dyspnea ▪ Cough ▪ Hepatosplenomegaly ▪ Fever ▪ Night sweats ▪ Fatigue ▪ Malaise ▪ Weight loss	Non-Hodgkin's lymphoma
▪ Lymphadenopathy associated with fatigue, malaise, continuous low fever, weight loss, and vague arthralgias ▪ Joint tenderness, swelling, and warmth occurring later ▪ Joint stiffness after inactivity ▪ Subcutaneous nodules on elbows	Arthritis, rheumatoid
Pallor	
▪ Gradual development of pallor, possibly appearing sallow or grayish ▪ Fatigue ▪ Dyspnea ▪ Tachycardia ▪ Bounding pulse ▪ Atrial gallop ▪ Systolic bruit over carotid arteries ▪ Crackles and bleeding tendencies possible	Anemia
▪ Abrupt onset of pallor on arising from a recumbent position to a sitting or standing position ▪ Precipitous drop in blood pressure ▪ Increased heart rate ▪ Dizziness	Orthostatic hypotension

(continued)

HEMATOLOGIC AND IMMUNE SYSTEMS: INTERPRETING YOUR FINDINGS *(continued)*

Sign or symptom and findings	Probable cause
Purpura	
▪ Varying degrees of purpura depending on severity and underlying cause ▪ Acrocyanosis ▪ Nausea ▪ Dyspnea ▪ Seizures ▪ Severe muscle, back, and abdominal pain ▪ Oliguria due to acute tubular necrosis	Disseminated intravascular coagulation
▪ Insidious onset of purpura with scattered petechiae on distal arms and legs ▪ Epistaxis ▪ Bruising that easily occurs ▪ Hematuria ▪ Hematemesis ▪ Menorrhagia	Idiopathic thrombocytopenia purpura, chronic
▪ Erythematous patches with some scaling becoming interspersed with nodules ▪ Pruritus ▪ Discomfort ▪ Tumors and ulcerations and nontender lymphadenopathy later in the course of the disease	Hodgkin's disease
***Purpura** (continued)*	
▪ Widespread petechiae on skin, mucous membranes, retina, and serosal surfaces persisting throughout course of the disease ▪ Confluent ecchymoses uncommon ▪ Swollen and bleeding gums ▪ Epistaxis ▪ Lymphadenopathy ▪ Splenomegaly	Leukemia
▪ Scaling dermatitis with pruritus beginning on the legs and then affecting entire body ▪ Small pink to brown nodules and diffuse pigmentation ▪ Painless peripheral lymphadenopathy, usually affecting cervical nodes first	Non-Hodgkin's lymphoma
Splenomegaly	
▪ Splenomegaly with pancytopenia; anemia, neutropenia, or thrombocytopenia ▪ Weakness ▪ Fatigue ▪ Malaise ▪ Pallor ▪ Bacterial infections ▪ Bruising that easily occurs or spontaneous bleeding ▪ Left-sided abdominal pain ▪ Feeling of fullness after eating	Hypersplenism, primary

HEMATOLOGIC AND IMMUNE SYSTEMS: INTERPRETING YOUR FINDINGS *(continued)*

Sign or symptom and findings	Probable cause
Splenomegaly *(continued)*	
■ Moderate to severe splenomegaly, sometimes painful in chronic granulocytic form ■ Hepatomegaly ■ Lymphadenopathy ■ Fatigue ■ Pallor ■ Fever ■ Gum swelling ■ Bleeding tendencies ■ Weight loss ■ Anorexia ■ Abdominal, bone, and joint pain	Leukemia
■ Moderate to massive splenomegaly occurring as a late sign ■ Hepatomegaly ■ Painless lymphadenopathy ■ Scaly dermatitis with pruritus ■ Fever ■ Fatigue ■ Weight loss ■ Malaise	Lymphoma
■ Marked enlargement of the spleen late in the disorder ■ Early satiety ■ Abdominal fullness ■ Left upper quadrant or pleuritic chest pain ■ Purplish red oral mucous membranes ■ Headache ■ Dyspnea ■ Dizziness ■ Vertigo ■ Weakness ■ Fatigue ■ Finger and toe paresthesia ■ Impaired mentation ■ Tinnitus ■ Blurred or double vision ■ Scotoma ■ Increased blood pressure ■ Intermittent claudication ■ Pruritus ■ Urticaria ■ Ruddy cyanosis ■ Epigastric distress ■ Weight loss ■ Hepatomegaly ■ Bleeding tendencies	Polycythemia vera

of dizziness are usually brief; they may be mild or severe with abrupt or gradual onset. Dizziness may be aggravated by standing up quickly and alleviated by lying down and by rest.

History

If the patient isn't in acute distress, ask about a history of diabetes and cardiovascular disease. Find out if the patient is taking drugs prescribed for high blood pressure and, if so, when he took his last dose.

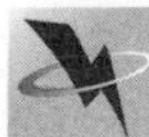

CRITICAL POINT *If the patient complains of dizziness, first ensure his safety by preventing falls. Then determine the severity and onset of the dizziness. Ask the patient to describe it, for example if it's associated with headache or blurred*

vision. Next, take the patient's blood pressure while he's lying, sitting, and standing to check for orthostatic hypotension. Ask about a history of high blood pressure. Determine if the patient is at risk for hypoglycemia. Tell the patient to lie down, and recheck his vital signs every 15 minutes. Start an I.V. line, and prepare to administer medications as ordered.

If the patient's blood pressure is normal, obtain a more complete history. Ask about myocardial infarction, heart failure, kidney disease, or atherosclerosis, which may predispose the patient to cardiac arrhythmias, hypertension, and transient ischemic attack. Find out if he has a history of anemia, chronic obstructive pulmonary disease, anxiety disorders, or head injury. Obtain a complete drug history.

Next, explore the patient's dizziness. Ask when it began, how often it occurs, and how long each episode lasts. Find out if the dizziness abates spontaneously, leads to loss of consciousness, and if it's triggered by sitting or standing up suddenly or stooping over. Ask the patient if being in a crowd makes him feel dizzy. Also, ask about emotional stress and if he has been irritable or anxious lately. Find out about insomnia or difficulty concentrating. Observe the patient for fidgeting, eyelid twitching, and if he startles easily. Ask the patient if he has palpitations, chest pain, diaphoresis, shortness of breath, or a chronic cough.

Physical assessment

Perform a physical examination. Begin with a quick neurocheck, assessing the patient's level of consciousness, motor and sensory functions, and reflexes. Then inspect for poor skin turgor and dry mucous membranes, signs of dehydration. Auscultate the patient's heart rate and rhythm. Inspect for barrel chest, clubbing, cyanosis, and use of accessory muscles. Also auscultate his breath sounds. Take the patient's blood pressure while he's lying, sitting, and standing to check for orthostatic hypotension. Test capillary refill time in the extremities, and palpate for edema.

Analysis

Dizziness typically results from inadequate blood flow and oxygen supply to the cerebrum and spinal cord. It may occur with anxiety; hematologic, respiratory, and cardiovascular disorders; and postconcussion syndrome. It's a key symptom in certain serious disorders, such as hypertension and vertebrobasilar artery insufficiency. Drugs such as anxiolytics, central nervous system depressants, narcotics, decongestants, antihistamines, antihypertensives, and vasodilators may cause dizziness.

Dizziness is commonly confused with vertigo — a sensation of revolving in space or of surroundings revolving about oneself. However, unlike dizziness, vertigo is commonly accompanied by nausea, vomiting, nystagmus, staggering gait, and tinnitus or hearing loss. Dizziness and vertigo may occur together, as in postconcussion syndrome.

AGE ISSUE *In children, dizziness is less common than in adults. Many children have difficulty describing this symptom and instead complain of tiredness, stomachache, or feeling sick. If you suspect dizziness, assess the patient for vertigo as well. A more common symptom in children, vertigo may result from a vision disorder, an ear infection, or antibiotic therapy.*

Dyspnea

Dyspnea is the sensation of difficult or uncomfortable breathing. It's usually reported as shortness of breath. Its severity varies greatly and is usually unrelated to the severity of the underlying cause. Dyspnea may arise suddenly or slowly and may subside rapidly or persist for years.

History

If a patient complains of shortness of breath, quickly look for signs of respiratory distress, such as tachypnea, cyanosis, restlessness, and accessory muscle use. Prepare to institute emergency measures including oxygen administration, I.V. fluid therapy, and monitoring.

If the patient can answer questions without increasing his distress, take a complete history. Ask if the shortness of breath began suddenly or gradually. Ask if it occurs constantly or intermittently. Find out if it occurs only during activity or also while at rest. If the patient has had dyspneic attacks before, ask if they're increasing in severity. Ask him if he can he identify what aggravates or alleviates these attacks. Also find out if he has a productive or nonproductive cough or chest pain. Ask about recent trauma, and note a history of upper respiratory tract infection, deep vein thrombophlebitis, or other disorders. Ask the patient if he smokes or is exposed to occupational toxic fumes or irritants. Find out if he also has orthopnea, paroxysmal nocturnal dyspnea, or progressive fatigue.

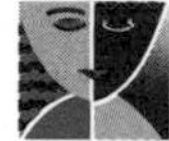

CULTURAL INSIGHT *Because dyspnea is subjective and exacerbated by anxiety, patients from cultures that are highly emotional may complain of shortness of breath sooner than those who are more stoic about symptoms of illness.*

Physical assessment

During the physical examination, look for signs of chronic dyspnea such as accessory muscle hypertrophy, especially in the shoulders and neck. Also look for pursed-lip exhalation, clubbing, peripheral edema, barrel chest, diaphoresis, and jugular vein distention.

Check the patient's blood pressure and auscultate for crackles, abnormal heart sounds or rhythms, egophony, bronchophony, and whispered pectoriloquy. Finally, palpate the abdomen for hepatomegaly, and assess the patient for edema.

Analysis

Most people normally experience dyspnea when they exert themselves, and its severity depends on their physical condition. In a healthy person, dyspnea is quickly relieved by rest.

Typically, dyspnea is a symptom of cardiopulmonary dysfunction. Pathologic causes of dyspnea include pulmonary, cardiac, neuromuscular, and allergic disorders. It may also be caused by anxiety.

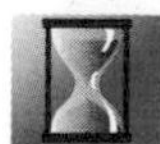

AGE ISSUE *Normally, an infant's respirations are abdominal, gradually changing to costal by age 7. Suspect dyspnea in an infant who breathes costally, in an older child who breathes abdominally, or in any child who uses his neck or shoulder muscles to help him breathe. Acute epiglottiditis and laryngotracheobronchitis (croup) can also cause severe dyspnea in a child and may even lead to respiratory or cardiovascular collapse. Older patients with dyspnea related to chronic illness may not be aware initially of a significant change in their breathing pattern. The child may hyperextend his neck, sit up, and lean forward with his mouth open to relieve the distress. His nostrils may be flared and his tongue may protrude.*

Edema of the face

Facial edema refers to either localized swelling — around the eyes, for example — or more generalized facial swelling that may extend to the neck and upper arms. Occasionally painful, this sign may develop gradually or abruptly. In some cases, it precedes the onset of peripheral or generalized edema. Mild edema may be difficult to detect; the patient or someone who's familiar with his appearance may report it before it's noticed during assessment.

History

If the patient isn't in severe distress, take his health history. Ask if facial edema developed suddenly or gradually. Find out if it's more prominent in the early morning or if it worsens throughout the day. Ask the patient if he has gained weight and, if so, how much and over what length of time. Find out if he has had a change in his appetite. Also ask if he has noticed a change in his urine color or output. Take a drug history and ask about recent facial trauma.

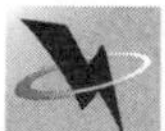

CRITICAL POINT *If the patient has facial edema and reports recent exposure to an allergen, quickly evaluate his respiratory status. Edema may also affect his upper airway, causing life-threatening obstruction. If audible wheezing, inspiratory stridor, or other signs of respiratory distress are noted, institute emergency measures including epinephrine and oxygen administration; if the patient's distress is severe, tracheal intubation, cricothyroidotomy, or tracheotomy may be required.*

Physical assessment

Begin the physical examination by characterizing the edema. Observe if it's localized to one part of the face or if it affects the entire face and other parts of the body. Determine if the edema is pitting or nonpitting, and grade its severity. Next, take vital signs, and assess neurologic status. Examine the oral cavity to evaluate dental hygiene and look for signs of infection. Visualize the oropharynx and look for soft-tissue swelling.

Analysis

Facial edema results from disruption of the hydrostatic and osmotic pressures that govern fluid movement between the arteries, veins, and lymphatics. It may result from venous, inflammatory, and certain systemic disorders; trauma; allergy; malnutrition; or the effects of certain drugs, tests, and treatments.

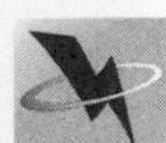

CRITICAL POINT *Long-term use of glucocorticoids may produce facial edema. Any drug that causes an allergic reaction, such as aspirin, antipyretics, penicillin, and sulfa preparations, may have the same effect. Ingestion of the fruit pulp of ginkgo biloba can cause severe erythema and edema and the rapid formation of vesicles. Feverfew and chrysanthemum parthenium can cause swelling of the lips, irritation of the tongue, and mouth ulcers. Licorice may cause facial edema and water retention or bloating, especially if used before menses.*

Erythema

Dilated or congested blood vessels produce red skin, or erythema, the most common sign of skin inflammation or irritation. Erythema may be localized or generalized and may occur suddenly or gradually. Skin color can range from bright red in patients with acute conditions to pale violet or brown in those with chronic problems. Erythema must be differentiated from purpura, which causes redness from bleeding into the skin. When pressure is applied directly to the skin, erythema blanches momentarily but purpura doesn't.

History

If erythema isn't associated with anaphylaxis, obtain a detailed health history. Find out how long the patient has had the erythema and where it first began. Find out if he has had any associated pain or itching. Ask about recent fever, upper respiratory tract infection, or joint pain. Find out if there's a history of skin disease or other illness and if he or anyone in his family has allergies, asthma, or eczema. Ask if he has been exposed to someone who has had a similar rash or who's now ill or if he recently fell or injured the area of erythema.

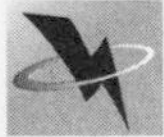

CRITICAL POINT *If your patient has sudden progressive erythema with rapid pulse, dyspnea, hoarseness, and agitation, the patient may be experiencing anaphylactic shock. Provide emergency respiratory support and give epinephrine.*

Obtain a complete drug history, including recent immunizations. Ask about food intake, use of herbal remedies, and exposure to chemicals.

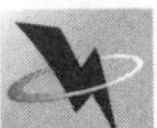

CRITICAL POINT *Ingestion of the fruit pulp of ginkgo biloba can cause severe erythema and edema of the mouth and rapid formation of vesicles. St. John's wort can cause heightened sun sensitivity, resulting in erythema or sunburn.*

Physical assessment

Begin the physical examination by assessing the extent, distribution, and intensity of erythema. Look for edema and other skin lesions, such as hives, scales, papules, and purpura. Examine the affected area for warmth, and gently palpate it to check for tenderness or crepitus.

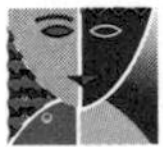

CULTURAL INSIGHT *Dark-skinned patients may have difficulty recognizing erythema; as a result, they may present with associated diseases in a more advanced state.*

Analysis

Erythema usually results from changes in the arteries, veins, and small vessels that lead to increased small-vessel perfusion. Drugs and neurogenic mechanisms can allow extra blood to enter the small vessels. Erythema can also result from trauma and tissue damage; changes in supporting tissues, which increase vessel visibility; and a number of rare disorders.

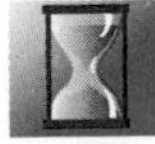

AGE ISSUE *Normally, erythema toxicum neonatorum (neonatal rash), a pink papular rash, develops during the first 4 days after birth and spontaneously disappears by day 10. Neonates and infants can also develop erythema from infections and other disorders. For example, candidiasis can produce thick white lesions over an erythematous base on the oral mucosa as well as diaper rash with beefy red erythema. Roseola, rubeola, scarlet fever, granuloma annulare, and cutis marmorata also cause erythema in children. Elderly patients commonly have well-demarcated purple macules or patches, usually on the back of the hands and on the forearms. Known as* actinic purpura, *this condition results from blood leaking through fragile capillaries. The lesions disappear spontaneously.*

Fever

Fever is a common sign that can arise from any one of several disorders. It can be classified as low (oral reading of 99° F to 100.4° F [37.2° C to 38° C]), moderate (100.5° to 104° F [38.1°C to 40° C]), or high (above 104° F). Fever over 106° F (41.1° C) causes unconsciousness and, if sustained, leads to permanent brain damage.

Fever may also be classified as remittent, intermittent, sustained, relapsing, or undulant. Remittent fever, the most common type, is characterized by daily temperature fluctuations above the normal range. Intermittent fever is marked by a daily temperature drop into the normal range and then a rise back to above normal. An intermittent fever that fluctuates widely, typically producing chills and sweating, is called hectic, or septic, fever. Sustained fever involves persistent temperature elevation with minimal fluctuation. Relapsing fever consists of alternating feverish and afebrile periods. Undulant fever refers to a gradual increase in temperature that stays high for a few days and then decreases gradually.

Further classification involves duration — either brief, less than 3 weeks, or prolonged. Prolonged fevers include fever of unknown origin, a classification used when careful examination fails to detect an underlying cause.

History

If the patient's fever is only mild to moderate, ask him when it began and how high his temperature reached. Find out if the fever disappeared, only to reappear later. Also ask if he experienced any other symptoms, such as chills, fatigue, or pain.

Obtain a complete health history, especially noting immunosuppressive treatments or disorders, infection, trauma, surgery, diagnostic testing, and the use of anesthesia or other medications. Ask about recent travel because certain diseases are endemic.

Physical assessment

Let the health history findings direct the physical examination. Because fever can accompany diverse disorders, the examination may range from a brief evaluation of one body system to a comprehensive review of all systems.

Analysis

Because these disorders can affect virtually any body system, fever in the absence of other signs and symptoms usually has little diagnostic significance. A persistent high fever, though, represents an emergency. Fever and rash commonly result from hypersensitivity to drugs such as antifungals, sulfonamides, penicillins, cephalosporins, tetracyclines, barbiturates, phenytoin, and some antitoxins. Fever can accompany chemotherapy, especially with bleomycin, vincristine, and asparaginase. It can result from drugs that impair sweating, such as anticholinergics, Phenothiazines, and monoamine oxidase inhibitors. A drug-induced fever typically disappears after the involved drug is discontinued. Fever can also stem from toxic doses of salicylates, amphetamines, and tricyclic antidepressants.

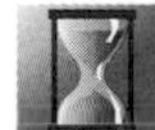

AGE ISSUE *Infants and young children experience higher and more prolonged fevers, more rapid temperature increases, and greater temperature fluctuations than older children and adults. Seizures commonly accompany extremely high fever. Aspirin use should always be avoided in children with varicella or flulike symptoms because of the risk of precipitating Reye's syndrome. Common pediatric causes of fever include varicella, croup syndrome, dehydration, meningitis, mumps, otitis media, pertussis, roseola infantum, rubella, rubeola, and tonsillitis. Fever can also occur as a reaction to immunizations and antibiotics. Elderly people may have an altered sweating mechanism that predisposes them to heatstroke when exposed to high temperatures; they may also have an impaired thermoregulatory mechanism, making temperature change a much less reliable measure of disease severity.*

Lymphadenopathy

Lymphadenopathy — enlargement of one or more lymph nodes — may result from increased production of lymphocytes or reticuloendothelial cells or from infiltration of cells that aren't normally present. This sign may be generalized, involving three or more node groups, or localized.

History
Ask the patient when he first noticed the swelling, and whether it's located on one side of his body or both. Find out if the areas are swollen, sore, hard, or red. Ask the patient if he has recently had an infection or other health problem. Also ask if a biopsy has ever been done on any node because this may indicate a previously diagnosed cancer. Find out if the patient has a family history of cancer.

Physical assessment
Palpate the entire lymph node system to determine the extent of lymphadenopathy and to detect other areas of local enlargement. Use the pads of your index and middle fingers to move the skin over underlying tissues at the nodal area. If you detect enlarged nodes, note their size in centimeters and whether they're fixed or mobile, tender or nontender, and erythematous or not. Note their texture and if the node is discrete or if it feels matted. If you detect tender, erythematous lymph nodes, check the area drained by that part of the lymph system for signs of infection, such as erythema and swelling. Also palpate for and percuss the spleen.

Analysis
Generalized lymphadenopathy may be caused by an inflammatory process, such as bacterial or viral infection, connective tissue disease, an endocrine disorder, or neoplasm. Localized lymphadenopathy most commonly results from infection or trauma affecting a specific area.

Normally, lymph nodes are discrete, mobile, soft, nontender and, except in children, nonpalpable. However, palpable nodes may also be normal in adults. Nodes that are more than 3/8″ (1 cm) in diameter are cause for concern. They may be tender and the skin overlying the lymph node may be erythematous, suggesting a draining lesion. Alternatively, they may be hard and fixed and tender or nontender, suggesting a malignant tumor.

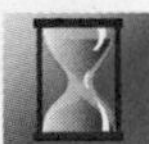

AGE ISSUE *In children, infection is the most common cause of lymphadenopathy. The condition is commonly associated with otitis media and pharyngitis.*

Pallor
Pallor is abnormal paleness or loss of skin color, which may develop suddenly or gradually. Although generalized pallor affects the entire body, it's most apparent on the face, conjunctiva, oral mucosa, and nail beds. Localized pallor commonly affects a single limb.

How easily pallor is detected varies with skin color and the thickness and vascularity of underlying subcutaneous tissue. At times, it's merely a subtle lightening of skin color that may be difficult to detect in dark-skinned persons; sometimes it's evident only on the conjunctiva and oral mucosa.

History
If the patient's condition permits, take a complete health history. Find out if the patient or anyone in his family has a history of anemia, a chronic disorder that might lead to other disorders, such as renal failure, heart failure, or diabetes. Ask about the patient's diet, particularly his intake of green vegetables.

Then explore the pallor more fully. Find out when the patient first noticed it. Ask if it occurs constantly or intermittently or when he's exposed to the cold or when he's under emotional stress. Explore associated signs and symptoms, such as fainting, orthostasis, weakness and fatigue on exertion, dyspnea, chest palpitations, menstrual irregularities, or loss of libido. If the pallor is confined to one or both legs, ask the patient if walking is painful. Ask him if his legs feel cold or numb. If pallor is confined to his fingers, ask about tingling and numbness.

Physical assessment
Start the physical examination by taking the patient's vital signs. Be sure to check for orthostatic hypotension. Auscultate the heart for gallops and murmurs and the chest for crackles. Check the patient's skin temperature — cold extremities commonly occur with vasoconstriction or arterial occlusion. Also note skin ulceration.

Examine the abdomen for splenomegaly. Finally, palpate peripheral pulses. An absent pulse in a pale extremity may indicate arterial occlusion, whereas a weak pulse may indicate low cardiac output.

Analysis

Pallor may result from decreased peripheral oxyhemoglobin or decreased total oxyhemoglobin. Decreased peripheral oxyhemoglobin reflects diminished peripheral blood flow associated with peripheral vasoconstriction, arterial occlusion, or low cardiac output. Transient peripheral vasoconstriction may occur with exposure to cold, causing nonpathologic pallor. Decreased total oxyhemoglobin usually results from anemia, the chief cause of pallor.

Purpura

Purpura is the extravasation of RBCs from the blood vessels into the skin, subcutaneous tissue, or mucous membranes. It's characterized by discoloration that's easily visible through the epidermis, usually purplish or brownish red. Purpuric lesions include petechiae, ecchymoses, and hematomas. Purpura differs from erythema in that it doesn't blanch with pressure because it involves blood in the tissues, not just dilated vessels.

History

Ask the patient when he first noticed the lesion and whether he has noticed other lesions on his body. Find out if he or his family has a history of a bleeding disorder or if he bruises easily. Find out what medications he's taking, and ask him to describe his diet. Ask about recent trauma or transfusions and the development of associated signs, such as epistaxis, bleeding gums, hematuria, and hematochezia. Also ask about systemic complaints such as fever that may suggest infection. Ask female patients about heavy menstrual flow.

Physical assessment

Inspect the patient's entire skin surface to determine the type, size, location, distribution, and severity of purpuric lesions. Also inspect the mucous membranes.

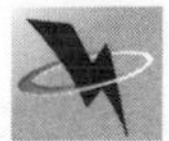

CRITICAL POINT *The same mechanisms that cause purpura can also cause internal hemorrhage, although purpura isn't a cardinal indicator of this condition.*

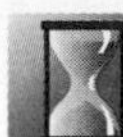

AGE ISSUE *When you assess a child with purpura, be alert for signs of possible child abuse. Signs include bruises in different stages of resolution, from repeated beatings; bruise patterns resembling a familiar object, such as a belt, hand, or thumb and finger; and bruises on the face, buttocks, or genitalia that are areas unlikely to be injured accidentally.*

Analysis

Purpura results from damage to the endothelium of small blood vessels, a coagulation defect, ineffective perivascular support, capillary fragility and permeability, or a combination of these factors. These faulty hemostatic factors, in turn, can result from thrombocytopenia or another hematologic disorder, an invasive procedure, or the use of an anticoagulant.

Additional causes are nonpathologic.

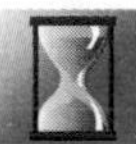

AGE ISSUE *Purpura can be a consequence of aging, when loss of collagen decreases connective tissue support of upper skin blood vessels. In an elderly or cachectic person, skin atrophy and inelasticity and loss of subcutaneous fat increase susceptibility to minor trauma, causing purpura to appear along the veins of the forearms, hands, legs, and feet.*

Prolonged coughing or vomiting can produce crops of petechiae in loose face and neck tissue. Violent muscle contraction, as occurs in seizures or weight lifting, sometimes results in localized ecchymoses from increased intraluminal pressure and rupture. High fever, which increases capillary fragility, can also produce purpura.

The anticoagulants heparin and warfarin can produce purpura. Administration of warfarin can result in painful areas of erythema that become purpuric then necrotic with an adherent black eschar. The lesions develop between the 3rd and 10th day of drug administration.

Additional causes are nonpathologic.

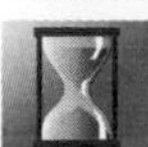

AGE ISSUE *Neonates commonly exhibit petechiae, particularly on the head, neck, and shoulders, after vertex deliveries. Thought to result from the trauma of birth, these petechiae disappear within a few days. Other causes in infants include thrombocytopenia, vitamin K deficiency, and infantile scurvy. The most common type of purpura in children is allergic purpu-*

ra. Other causes in children include trauma, hemophilia, autoimmune hemolytic anemia, Gaucher's disease, thrombasthenia, congenital factor deficiencies, Wiskott-Aldrich syndrome, acute idiopathic thrombocytopenia, von Willebrand's disease, and the rare, life-threatening purpura fulminans, which usually follows bacterial or viral infection.

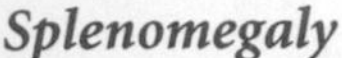

Splenomegaly

Because it occurs with various disorders and in up to 5% of normal adults, splenomegaly — an enlarged spleen — isn't a diagnostic sign by itself. However, it usually points to infection, trauma, or a hepatic, autoimmune, neoplastic, or hematologic disorder.

History

If you detect splenomegaly during a routine physical examination, begin by exploring associated signs and symptoms. Ask the patient if he has been unusually tired lately. Find out if he has frequent colds, sore throats, or other infections and if he bruises easily. Ask about left-upper-quadrant pain, abdominal fullness, and early satiety.

Physical assessment

Perform a complete assessment of all body systems. Examine the patient's skin for pallor and ecchymoses, and palpate his axillae, groin, and neck for lymphadenopathy.

Analysis

Because the spleen functions as the body's largest lymph node, splenomegaly can result from any process that triggers lymphadenopathy. For example, it may reflect reactive hyperplasia, which is a response to infection or inflammation; proliferation or infiltration of neoplastic cells; extramedullary hemopoiesis; phagocytic cell proliferation; increased blood cell destruction; or vascular congestion associated with portal hypertension.

Splenomegaly may be detected by light palpation under the left costal margin. However, because this technique isn't always advisable or effective, splenomegaly may need to be confirmed by a computed tomography or radionuclide scan.

Additional causes are nonpathologic.

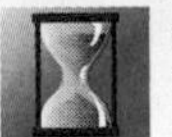

AGE ISSUE *In immunocompromised children, splenic abscess is the most common cause of splenomegaly.*

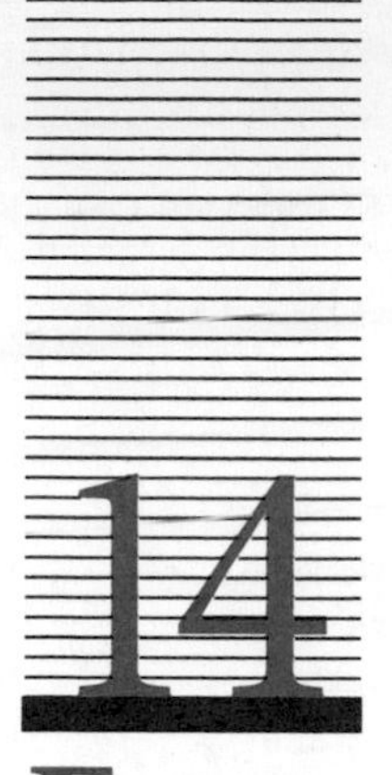

14 Female genitourinary system

The female genitourinary (GU) system encompasses the urinary tract and the reproductive organs and structures. Disorders of this system can have wide-ranging effects on other body systems. For example, ovarian dysfunction can alter endocrine balance and kidney dysfunction can affect the production of the hormone erythropoietin, which regulates the production of red blood cells.

Assessing the female GU system can be a challenging task. Many patients with urinary disorders don't realize they're ill because they only have mild signs and symptoms; therefore, it's easy to overlook underlying problems.

More women seek health care for reproductive disorders than for any other problem. Assessing those problems can be difficult because the reproductive system is complex and its functions have far-reaching psychosocial implications.

Anatomy and physiology of the urinary system

To perform an accurate assessment of the urinary system, you'll need to understand the anatomy and physiology of the kidneys, ureters, bladder, and urethra. Working together, these structures remove wastes from the body, regulate acid-base balance by retaining or excreting hydrogen ions, and regulate fluid and electrolyte balance. (See *Structures of the urinary system,* page 380.)

Kidneys

The essential functions of the urinary system — such as forming urine and maintaining homeostasis — take place in the highly vascular kidneys. These bean-shaped organs are 4½" to 5" (11.5 to 12.5 cm) long and

STRUCTURES OF THE URINARY SYSTEM

This illustration shows the main structures of the urinary system.

2½″ (6.5 cm) wide. Located retroperitoneally on either side of the lumbar vertebrae, the kidneys lie behind the abdominal organs and in front of the muscles attached to the vertebral column. The peritoneal fat layer protects them.

Crowded by the liver, the right kidney extends slightly lower than the left. Atop each kidney (suprarenal) lies an adrenal gland. At the hilus — an indentation in the kidney's medial aspect — the renal artery, renal vein, lymphatic vessels, and nerves enter the kidney. The renal pelvis, a funnel-shaped ureter extension, also enters here.

A cross section of the kidney reveals the outer renal cortex, central renal medulla, internal calyces, and renal pelvis. At the microscopic level, the nephron serves as the kidney's functional unit.

Each of the body's systems depends on the kidneys to maintain homeostasis. In turn, the kidneys depend on other body systems for the same purpose. For example, the cardiovascular system must deliver blood to the kidneys at a pressure adequate for filtration. The kidneys reciprocate by regulating fluid balance that maintains circulating blood volume and electrolyte balance necessary for proper cardiac function.

Ureters

The ureters act as ducts to allow urine to pass from the kidneys to the bladder. They measure about 10″ to 12″ (25.5 to 30.5 cm) in adults and have a diameter varying from ⅛″ to ⅜″ (2 to 8 mm), with the narrowest portion being at the ureteropelvic junction. The left kidney is higher than the right one, so the left ureter typically is slightly longer than the right one. Originating in the ureteropelvic junction of the kidneys, the ureters travel obliquely to the bladder, channeling urine via peristaltic waves that occur about one to five times per minute.

Bladder

The bladder is a hollow, spherical, muscular organ in the pelvis that serves to store urine. It lies anterior and inferior to the pelvic cavity and posterior to the symphysis pubis. Bladder capacity ranges from 500 to 600 ml in a normal adult. If the amount of stored urine exceeds bladder capacity, the bladder distends above the symphysis pubis.

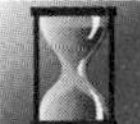

AGE ISSUE *Children and elderly patients have bladders with a lower capacity.*

The base of the bladder contains three openings that form a triangular area called the *trigone.* Two ureteral orifices act as the posterior boundary of the trigone; one urethral orifice forms its anterior boundary.

Urination results from involuntary, as by reflex, and voluntary, as learned or intentional, processes. When urine distends the bladder, the involuntary process begins. The parasympathetic nervous system fibers transmit impulses that make the bladder contract and the internal sphincter, which is located at the internal urethral orifice, relax. Then the cerebrum stimulates voluntary relaxation and contraction of the external sphincter that's located about ½″ (1.5 cm) beyond the internal sphincter.

Urethra

The urethra is a small duct that channels urine outside the body from the bladder. It has an exterior opening known as the *urinary* or *urethral meatus.* In the female, the urethra ranges from 1″ to 2″ (2.5 to 5 cm) long, with the urethral meatus located anterior to the vaginal opening.

Urine formation

Three processes—glomerular filtration, tubular reabsorption, and tubular secretion—take place in the nephrons, ultimately leading to urine formation.

The kidneys can vary the amount of substances reabsorbed and secreted in the nephrons, changing the composition of excreted urine. Normal urine constituents include sodium, chloride, potassium, calcium, magnesium, sulfates, phosphates, bicarbonates, uric acid, ammonium ions, creatinine, and urobilinogen. A few leukocytes and red blood cells (RBCs) may enter into the urine as it passes from the kidneys to the ureteral orifice. Urine may also contain drugs if the patient is taking drugs that undergo urinary excretion.

Varying with fluid intake and climate, total daily urine output averages 720 to 2,400 ml. For example, after a patient drinks a large volume of fluid, urine output increases as the body rapidly excretes excess water. If a patient restricts water intake or has an excessive intake of such solutes as sodium, urine output declines as the body retains water to restore normal fluid concentration.

Hormones

Hormones help regulate tubular reabsorption and secretion. For example, antidiuretic hormone (ADH) acts in the distal tubule and collecting ducts to increase water reabsorption and urine concentration. ADH deficiency decreases water reabsorption, causing dilute urine. Aldosterone affects tubular reabsorption by regulating sodium retention and helping to control potassium secretion by tubular epithelial cells.

By secreting the enzyme renin, the kidneys play a crucial role in blood pressure and fluid volume regulation. The distal tubules of the kidneys regulate potassium excretion. Responding to an elevated serum potassium level, the adrenal cortex increases aldosterone secretion. Through a poorly understood mechanism, aldosterone also affects the potassium-secreting capacity of distal tubular cells.

Other hormonal functions of the kidneys include secretion of the hormone erythropoietin and regulation of calcium and phosphorus balance. In response to low arterial oxygen tension, the kidneys produce erythropoietin, which travels to the bone marrow, then stimulates RBC production. To help regulate calcium and phosphorus balance, the kidneys filter and reabsorb about half of unbound serum calcium and activate vitamin D, a compound that promotes intestinal calcium absorption and regulates phosphate excretion.

Anatomy and physiology of the reproductive system

To perform an accurate assessment of the female reproductive system, you'll need to understand the anatomy and physiology of the external and internal genitalia.

External genitalia

The external genitalia, collectively called the *vulva,* consist of the mons pubis; labia majora; labia minora; clitoris, vestibule, and urethral opening; vaginal opening and perineum; and Skene's and Bartholin's glands. (See *Structures of the external genitalia,* page 382.)

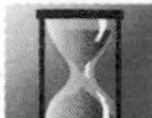

AGE ISSUE *With age, the vulva atrophies. Other changes include pubic hair loss and a flattening of the labia majora. Vulval tissue shrinks, exposing the sensitive area around the urethra and vagina to abrasions and irritation—from undergarments, for example. The introitus also constricts, tissues lose their elasticity, and the epidermis thins.*

STRUCTURES OF THE EXTERNAL GENITALIA

This illustration shows the external structures of the female genitalia.

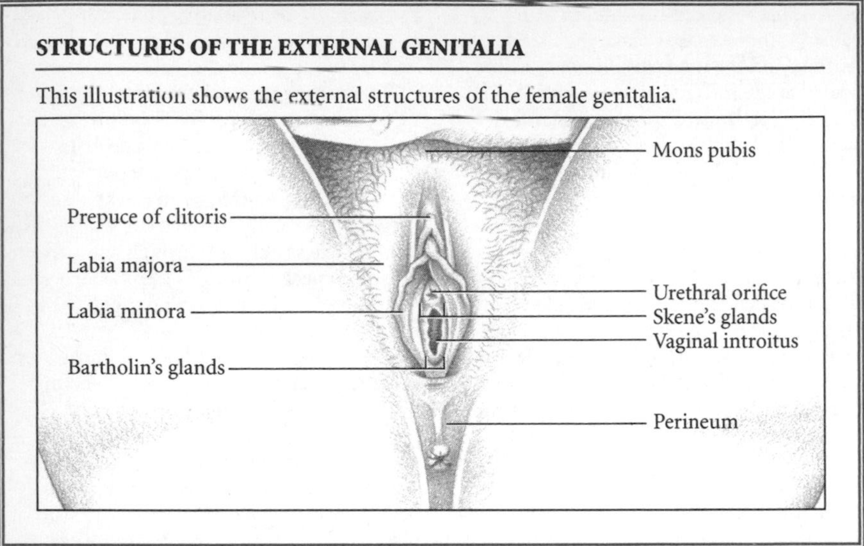

Mons pubis

The mons pubis is a mound of adipose tissue overlying the symphysis pubis and is covered with pubic hair in the adult. Pubic hair typically appears around age 10½. It may become sparse after menopause due to hormonal changes.

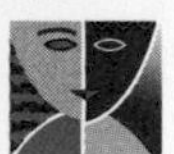

CULTURAL INSIGHT *Native Americans and Asians usually have less pubic hair than people of other races.*

Labia majora

The outer vulval lips, or *labia majora,* are two rounded folds of adipose tissue that extend from the mons pubis to the perineum. The labia majora are covered with hair.

Labia minora

The inner vulval lips are called the *labia minora.* The anterolateral and medial parts join to form the prepuce or hood, the folds of skin that cover the clitoris. The posterior union of the labia minora is called the *fourchette* or *frenulum.*

Clitoris, vestibule, and urethral opening

The clitoris is the small, protuberant organ located just beneath the arch of the mons pubis. The clitoris contains erectile tissue, venous cavernous spaces, and specialized sensory corpuscles that are stimulated during coitus. The clitoris lies between the labia minora at the top of the vestibule, which contains the urethral and vaginal openings. The urethral opening is a slit below the clitoris.

Vaginal opening and perineum

The vaginal opening, or introitus, is posterior to the urethral orifice. This opening is a thin vertical slit in women with intact hymens and a large opening with irregular edges in women whose hymens have been perforated. The hymen is a thin membranous fold that may cover the vaginal orifice or may be absent. The perineum is the area bordered anteriorly by the top of the labial fold and posteriorly by the anus.

Skene's and Bartholin's glands

Two kinds of glands have ducts that open into the vulva. Skene's glands are tiny structures just below the urethra, each containing 6 to 31 ducts. Bartholin's glands are found posterior to the vaginal opening. Neither of these glands can be seen, but they can be palpated if enlarged.

Skene's and Bartholin's glands produce fluids important for the reproductive process. They can become infected, usually with organisms known to cause sexually transmitted diseases (STDs).

STRUCTURES OF THE INTERNAL GENITALIA

These illustrations show the internal structures of the female reproductive system.

LATERAL VIEW OF INTERNAL GENITALIA

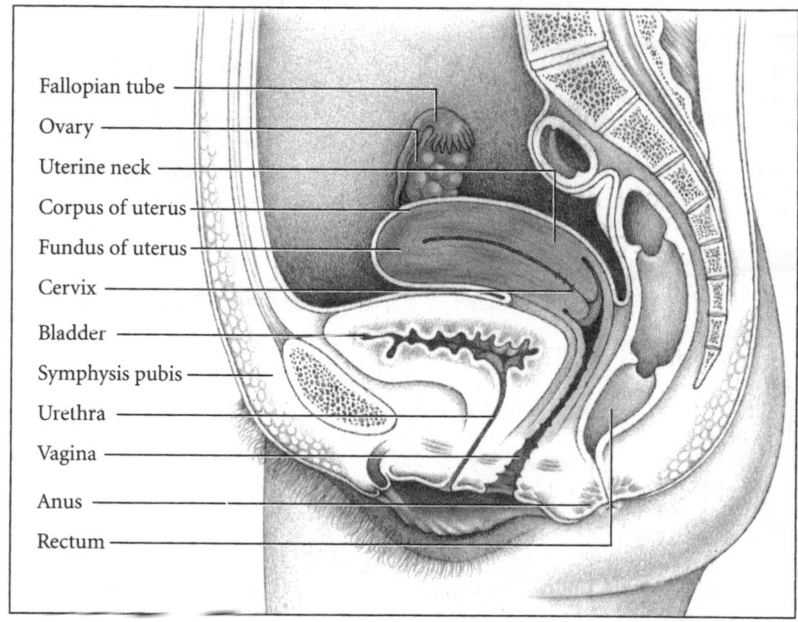

ANTERIOR CROSS-SECTIONAL VIEW OF INTERNAL GENITALIA

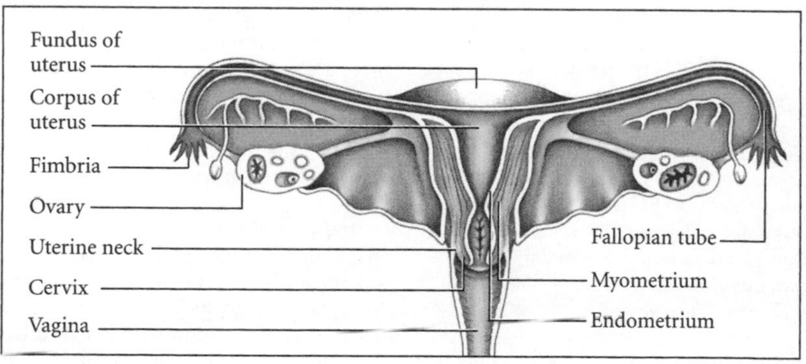

Internal genitalia

The internal genitalia include the vagina, uterus, ovaries, and fallopian tubes. (See *Structures of the internal genitalia.*)

Vagina

The vagina, a highly elastic muscular tube, is located between the urethra and the rectum. Measuring 2½″ to 2¾″ (6.5 to 7 cm) long anteriorly and 3½″ (9 cm) long posteriorly, the vagina lies at a 45-degree angle to the long axis of the body. A pink, hollow, collapsed tube that extends up and back from the vulva to the uterus, the vagina is the route of passage for childbirth and menstruation.

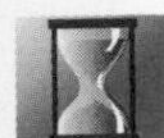

AGE ISSUE *In older women, atrophy causes the vagina to shorten and the mucus lining to be come thin, dry, less elastic, and pale because of decreased vascularity. In this state, the vaginal mucosa is highly susceptible to abrasion.*

Uterus

The uterus, a small, firm, pear-shaped, muscular organ, rests between the bladder and the rectum and usually lies at almost a 90-degree angle to the vagina. However, the position of the uterus in the pelvic cavity may vary, depending on bladder fullness. The uterus may also tip in different directions.

The mucous membrane lining the uterus is called the *endometrium;* the muscular layer, the *myometrium.* In pregnancy, the elastic, upper uterine portion, also known as the fundus, accommodates most of the growing fetus until term. The uterine neck, or isthmus, joins the fundus to the cervix, the uterine part extending into the vagina. The fundus and the isthmus make up the corpus, the main uterine body. The cervix contains mucus-secreting glands that help in reproduction and protect the uterus from pathogens. The function of the uterus is to nurture and then expel the fetus.

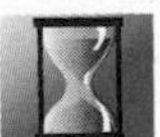

AGE ISSUE *During a woman's lifetime, the size of the uterine corpus and cervix changes, as does the percentage of space these parts occupy. For example, in a premenarchal female, the uterine corpus may occupy one-third of the uterus and the cervix may occupy two-thirds. However, in an adult multiparous female the distribution may be reversed.*

Ovaries

A pair of oval organs about 1¼″ (3 cm) long, the ovaries are usually found near the lateral pelvic wall at the height of the anterosuperior iliac spine. They produce ova and release the hormones estrogen and progesterone. The ovaries become fully developed after puberty and shrink after menopause.

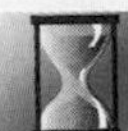

AGE ISSUE *In the adult female, ovulation usually stops 1 to 2 years before menopause. As the ovaries reach the end of their productive cycle, they become unresponsive to gonadotropic stimulation.*

Fallopian tubes

Two fallopian tubes attach to the uterus at the upper angles of the fundus. Usually nonpalpable, these 2¾″ to 5½″ (7- to 14-cm) long, narrow tubes of muscle fibers have fingerlike projections, called *fimbriae,* on the free ends that partially surround the ovaries, which help guide the ova to the uterus after expulsion from the ovaries. Fertilization of the ovum usually occurs in the outer third of the fallopian tube.

Health history

Because the urinary and reproductive systems are located so close together in women, you and your patient may have trouble differentiating signs and symptoms. Even if the patient's complaint seems minor, investigate it. Ask about its onset, duration, and severity, and about measures taken to treat it. The information you gain will help in formulating an appropriate care plan.

Urinary system history

The most common complaints of the urinary system include output changes, such as polyuria, oliguria, and anuria; voiding pattern changes, such as hesitancy, frequency, urgency, nocturia, and incontinence; urine color changes; and pain.

Chief complaint

Begin by asking the patient what her chief complaint is and, if she mentions several complaints, ask which bothers her most. Document her responses in her own words.

When gathering information, remain objective. Don't let the patient's opinions about her condition distract you from a thorough investigation. For example, a patient with a history of abdominal aneurysm who's experiencing flank pain may assume that the aneurysm is to blame. Further investigation, however, could reveal renal calculi. You can usually detect renal dysfunction by assessing other related body symptoms.

Current health history

Find out how the patient's symptoms developed and progressed. Ask how long she has had the problem, how it affects her daily routine, when and how it began, and how often it occurs. Also ask about related signs and symptoms, such as nausea and vomiting.

If she has had pain, ask about its location, radiation, intensity, and duration. Find out what precipitates, exacerbates, or relieves it. Ask her about self-help remedies and over-the-counter (OTC) medications she has used.

Also, ask the patient if she has diabetes or hypertension. Review the patient's chief complaint and obtain detailed information about it.

Output changes. To gather additional information about the complaint of output changes, ask the patient if she has noticed a change in the amount of excreted urine and how often this occurs. Find out if it occurs only if she drinks excessive fluids.

Always compare the patient's intake and output before concluding that the output is abnormal.

Voiding pattern changes. If the patient reports changes in voiding patterns, ask her how many times a day she usually urinates. Find out how many times a day she has been urinating recently. Ask her if she has noticed a change in the size of her urine stream and if her bladder still feels full after she has urinated. Then ask if she urinates small amounts frequently and if she wakes up during the night to urinate. Find out if she's unable to wait to urinate or if she has a problem controlling her urine.

Most voiding pattern changes suggest bladder dysfunction or an infectious process. In a patient with edema on bed rest, nocturia may result from rapid fluid reabsorption.

When evaluating urinary patterns, remember to distinguish between urinary frequency (frequent urination) and polyuria (excessive urination). Frequency can occur throughout the day or only at night. When frequency occurs both day and night, possible causes include infection, calculi, pregnancy, bladder hypertrophy, urethral stricture, and bladder cancer.

CRITICAL POINT *Urine retention is a urologic emergency that can result from numerous physical causes, such as urethral stricture, neurogenic disease, drug effect, or pain. In some patients, psychological factors play a part. If left untreated, it can lead to kidney damage and failure as fluid backs up and creates pressure inside the kidneys. Because retained urine provides an ideal medium for bacterial growth, pyelonephritis or sepsis may develop.*

Urine color changes. Ask the patient about the color of her urine and find out how long it has been this color. A dark amber color may indicate concentrated urine, usually associated with diminished volume or resulting from fluid losses due to diarrhea or vomiting. A clear, watery appearance may indicate dilute urine, associated with increased volume. Pale, dilute urine may suggest diabetes insipidus, increased fluid intake, or diuretic therapy. Brown or bright-red urine may contain blood. Green-brown urine suggests bile duct obstruction. Other color variations may result from taking certain medications. For example, rifampin may turn the urine orange-red or orange-brown. Methylene blue causes the urine to appear blue-green.

Pain. Ask the patient if she ever experiences pain when trying to urinate. Find out if she ever feels a burning sensation when urinating and, if so, how often. Painful spasms during urination suggest calculi. Dysuria described as a burning sensation usually indicates a disorder of the lower urinary tract.

Ask the patient if her abdomen ever feels distended and painful. Find out if she has pain over the pubic area or in her lower back and, if so, if the pain is dull or sharp. Find out if repositioning relieves suprapubic or flank pain. Position changes don't relieve pain from renal colic; however, lying down does reduce inflammatory pain.

It can be difficult to distinguish urinary pain from that of other disorders, such as appendicitis and biliary disease. To accurately assess the patient's pain, first ask her to point to the painful area. Determine the character of the pain—for example, if it's sharp or dull. Also, determine if it's constant or intermittent and if it radiates.

Different types of pain may include:

- bladder pain — typically occurring just above the pubic bone, whereas pain from renal disease typically occurs in the lumbus under the costovertebral margin, lateral to the spine, or anteriorly near the tip of the ninth rib
- dull ache in kidney area — periodically radiating to the genital area or leg on the affected side may indicate renal calculus
- ureteral pain — usually occurring between the costal margin and the pubic bone
- continuous, nonradiating pain — indicating inflammation or a tumor
- shifting pain — indicating appendicitis; whereas renal, bladder, and ureteral pain remain fixed
- colicky pain — resulting from peristaltic waves moving from the kidney to a ureteral obstruction such as renal disease
- dysuria — pain associated with urination, originating in the perineum, bladder, or urethra and occurring before, during, or after urination; if accompanied by pyuria and urinary frequency it may also suggest a lower urinary tract infection (UTI) or obstruction.

Past health history

Past illnesses and preexisting conditions can affect a patient's urinary tract health. For example, find out if the patient has ever had a UTI, kidney trauma, or renal calculus.

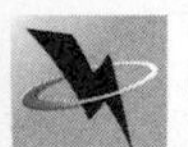

CRITICAL POINT *Patients with diabetes have an increased risk of UTIs. In addition, hypertension can contribute to renal failure and nephropathy.*

Renal calculi or trauma can alter the structure and function of the kidneys and bladder. Find out if she has problems with urinary incontinence or frequency. Ask if she has difficulty controlling her urine or if she notices that she leaks urine when she sneezes, laughs, coughs, or bears down.

For clues to the patient's present condition, it's important to explore past medical problems, including those she experienced as a child. If she has ever had a serious condition, such as kidney disease or a tumor, find out what treatment she received and its outcome. Ask similar questions about traumatic injuries, surgery, and conditions that required hospitalization.

Focus your questions to the patient on these areas:

- *Kidney or bladder problems.* Kidney and bladder stones tend to recur.
- *Systemic diseases.* Signs and symptoms of diabetic nephropathy — hypertension, edema, and azotemia — may appear 10 to 15 years after the onset of diabetes mellitus. Urinary symptoms of systemic lupus erythematosus (SLE), such as nephritis, may appear at onset or later. SLE may also produce recurrent swelling that's characteristic of nephrotic syndrome. Tuberculosis may reach the urinary tract; disseminated intravascular coagulation can lead to severe renal perfusion problems; and hepatic disease can occur with renal failure.
- *Nerve damage.* In multiple sclerosis, demyelination can affect bladder musculature, causing urinary hesitancy and chronic UTIs.
- *Sexually transmitted disease.* Gonorrhea causes urinary tract problems including discharge, dysuria, urgency, and frequency that may be the first indications of the disease.
- *Streptococcal infection.* A recent episode of streptococcal infection increases a patient's risk of glomerulonephritis.
- *Urinary tract surgery.* Make sure to ask your patient whether she has ever had surgery for a urinary disorder. If so, ask when it was performed.

Next, obtain an immunization and allergy history, including a history of medication reactions.

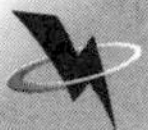

CRITICAL POINT *Allergic reactions can cause tubular damage. A severe anaphylactic reaction can cause temporary renal failure and permanent tubular necrosis.*

Also, inquire about current prescription and OTC medications, herbal remedies, alcohol use, smoking habits, and illicit drug use. Make a list of all medications and herbal preparations the patient takes. Some drugs can affect the appearance of urine; nephrotoxic drugs can alter urinary function.

Family history

For clues to risk factors, ask the patient if any blood relatives have ever been treated for renal or cardiovascular disorders, diabetes, cancer, or any other chronic illness.

Obtain information about:

- *Noninherited renal disorders.* Although they aren't hereditary, such disorders as UTIs, congenital anomalies, and urinary calculi recur in some families.
- *Hereditary renal diseases.* Polycystic kidney disease and all types of hereditary nephritis, such as Alport's syndrome, are genetically transmitted conditions that can progress to end-stage renal disease.
- *Inheritable systemic diseases.* Hypertension and diabetes mellitus can eventually cause nephropathies.

Psychosocial history

Investigate psychosocial factors that may affect the way the patient deals with her condition. Marital problems, poor living conditions, job insecurity, and other stresses can strongly affect how she feels.

Also, find out how the patient views herself. A disfiguring genital lesion or an STD can alter self-image. Try to determine what concerns she has about her condition. For example, ask her if she fears that the disease or therapy will affect her sex life. If she can express her fears and concerns, you can develop appropriate nursing interventions more easily.

Sexual history

A complete sexual history helps you identify your patient's knowledge deficits and expectations. This information may suggest a need for psychological or sexual therapy. It can also guide treatment decisions. For example, pain or discomfort associated with intercourse or diminished sexual desire may reflect disease progression or depression.

Activities of daily living

When questioning your patient about her daily activities, focus questions on her diet and sleeping patterns. Learning about your patient's diet may provide valuable information. As the patient describes her usual diet, determine if she takes in an adequate amount of fluid, salt, and protein. Ask if she's on a special diet and, if so, whether a physician prescribed it. Prolonged reducing diets involving liquid protein are associated with kidney dysfunction. Special diets for patients with renal disease include sodium, potassium, protein, and fluid restrictions.

Ask the patient about her sleep patterns. Waking up to void at night can interfere with a sound sleep. Disturbed sleep from nocturnal muscle cramps of the calves and thighs is common in early renal failure. A reversal in sleep patterns, such as staying awake at night and sleeping during the day, is also a symptom of renal failure.

Reproductive system history

Conduct your reproductive system history in a comfortable environment that protects the patient's privacy. Avoid rushing her so you don't overlook important details. Use terms that the patient understands and explain technical terms.

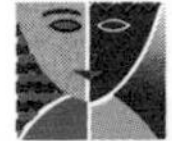

CULTURAL INSIGHT *Remember that in some cultures, discussing female physiologic function or problems is taboo.*

Ideally, the patient should be allowed to remain seated and dressed until the physical assessment. Always ask health history questions before the patient is in the lithotomy position. Commonly, the patient is asked to undress, get on the examination table, and wait for the health care provider to come in and begin the examination and interview. Some women find this demeaning as well as stressful.

Although you'll focus your questions on the reproductive system, maintain a holistic approach by inquiring about other physical and psychological concerns. Keep in mind that reproductive system problems may affect other aspects of the patient's life, including self-image and overall wellness.

Chief complaint

The most common reproductive system complaints are pain, vaginal discharge, abnormal uterine bleeding, pruritus, and infertility. To obtain the most complete data about those problems, focus on the patient's current complaints, and then explore her menstrual and contraceptive, reproductive, menopausal, family, and psychosocial history. Ask her to describe her symptoms in her own words, encouraging her to speak freely. Use open-ended questions.

Many patients feel uncomfortable answering questions about their sexual health or reproductive system. Start with the less personal questions and establish a rapport.

Menstrual and contraceptive history

When assessing the patient's menstrual history, first find out how old she was when she began menstruating. Typically, menses starts by age 14. If it hasn't, and if no secondary sex characteristics have developed, the patient should be evaluated by a specialist. Next, find out when the first day of her last menses was and how it compared with her previous periods. Then ask her when the first day of her previous menses was. Ask how often her periods occur. The normal cycle for menstruation is one menses every 21 to 38 days. Find out how long they last. The normal duration is 2 to 8 days. Ask her to describe her menstrual flow and how many pads or tampons she uses on each day of her period. Find out if she experiences pain during menstruation.

Affecting over 50% of menstruating women, dysmenorrhea (or painful menstruation) can involve sharp, intermittent pain or dull, aching pain. It's usually characterized by mild to severe cramping or colicky pain in the pelvis or lower abdomen that may radiate to the thighs and lower sacrum. This pain may precede menses by several days or accompany it and gradually subside as bleeding tapers off.

Ask the patient if she ever bleeds between periods and, if so, how much and for how long. Spotting between periods, or metrorrhagia, may be normal in patients using low-dose hormonal contraceptives or progesterone; otherwise, spotting may indicate infection or cancer. Find out if she has ever had vaginal bleeding after intercourse.

Ask the patient if she has had any uncomfortable signs and symptoms before or during her periods. Find out if the signs or symptoms involve infection, such as discharge, itching, painful intercourse, sores or lesions, fever, chills, or swelling of the vagina or vulva. Ask how often she visits the gynecologist.

To elicit information about the patient's contraceptive history, first find out if she's sexually active and, if so, are her sexual practices bisexual, homosexual, or heterosexual. Ask if she uses a hormonal contraceptive and, if so, what she uses and for how long she has used it. If she doesn't use a hormonal contraceptive, find out what method of contraception she does use, how long she has used it, and its condition, if it's a device.

Ask the patient if she smokes. If so, find out how much she smokes, how long she has smoked, and if she has ever tried a smoking-cessation program. Smoking in conjunction with the use of oral contraceptives increases the woman's risk for adverse effects.

In addition, find out about any prescription, OTC, and alternative medications that the patient takes, including the reason for taking them and the dosage. Also ask if she has ever taken drugs for recreational purposes. Many drugs affect the female reproductive system, specifically the menstrual cycle. For example, androgens, antihypertensives, antipsychotics, cytotoxics, estrogens, progestins, and steroids can cause amenorrhea. Antidepressants and thyroid hormones can cause other menstrual irregularities.

Additionally, inquire about the patient's use of alcohol and alcohol consumption. Find out how much alcohol she drinks and how long she has been drinking.

Reproductive history

When collecting data about the patient's reproductive history, first ask her if anyone has ever told her that something is wrong with her uterus or associated organs. Find out if she has ever had a positive Papanicolaou (Pap) test and when her last Pap test was. Ask if she has ever had an STD or other genital or reproductive system infection. Find out about any surgeries for a reproductive system problem. Ask the patient if she ever uses feminine hygiene products, such as douches or sprays and, if so, for what reason she uses them. Find out which products she uses and how frequently she uses them.

Next, ask the patient if she has ever been pregnant and, if so, how many times. Ask how many times she has given birth. Find out if the deliveries were vaginal or cesarean. Also find out if she has ever had problems conceiving or had treatment for infertility. Last, ask if she ever had an abortion or miscarriage.

Menopausal history

If your patient is experiencing menopause, find out more about the menopausal signs and symptoms she may be experiencing.

Ask her if she has an abnormal vaginal discharge. Ask her about external lesions or itching. Find out if she experiences pain with intercourse. If she douches, find out how often. Ask the patient when her last Pap test was and what the results were.

Ask for the date of her last menses. Ask if she's having hot flashes, mood swings, or flushing. Ask about vaginal dryness, itching, and the use of hormone replacement therapy or herbal or soy products to control symptoms. Also, ask her about bleeding, pelvic muscle weakening, and uterine prolapse.

Family history

Because some reproductive problems tend to be familial, ask about family reproductive history. Ask the patient if she or anyone in her family ever had reproductive problems, hypertension, diabetes mellitus (including gestational diabetes mellitus), obesity, heart disease, or gynecologic surgery. Next, ask her if she's having problems that she believes are related to her reproductive system or other problems not yet covered during the interview. Finally, answer any questions she may have about her reproductive organs or sexual activity.

Psychosocial history

Ask the patient if she's sexually active. If so, ask her when she last had intercourse and if she's sexually active with more than one partner. Finally, ask if her sexual partner has any signs or symptoms of infection, such as genital sores, warts, or penile discharge.

Physical assessment

To perform a physical assessment of the female GU system, use the techniques of inspection, auscultation, percussion, and palpation to evaluate the urinary and reproductive systems.

Urinary system assessment

Begin the physical examination by documenting baseline vital signs and weighing the patient. Comparing subsequent weight measurements to this baseline may reveal a developing problem, such as dehydration or fluid retention.

The urinary system affects many body functions, so a thorough assessment includes examination of multiple, related body systems using inspection, auscultation, percussion, and palpation techniques.

Observing the patient's behavior can give you clues about her mental status. For example, study the patient for concentration problems, memory loss, or disorientation.

CRITICAL POINT *If the patient has kidney dysfunction, she may experience poor concentration, memory loss, or disorientation. If she has progressive, chronic kidney failure, her signs and symptoms may include lethargy, confusion, disorientation, stupor, convulsions, and coma.*

Ask the patient to urinate into a specimen cup. Assess the sample for color, odor, and clarity. Then have the patient undress, providing her with a gown and drapes, and proceed with a systematic physical examination.

Inspection

Urinary system inspection includes examination of the abdomen and urethral meatus.

Abdomen. Help the patient assume a supine position with her arms relaxed at her sides. Make sure she's comfortable and draped appropriately. Expose the patient's abdomen from the xiphoid process to the symphysis pubis and inspect the abdomen for gross enlargements or fullness by comparing the left and right sides, noting asymmetrical areas. In a normal adult, the abdomen is smooth, flat or scaphoid (concave), and symmetrical. Abdominal skin should be free from scars, lesions, bruises, and discolorations.

If your patient has extremely prominent veins, she may also have other vascular signs associated with renal dysfunction, such as hypertension or renal artery bruits. Distention, skin tightness and glistening, and striae (streaks or linear scars caused by rapidly developing skin tension) may signal fluid retention. If you suspect ascites, which may suggest nephrotic syndrome, perform the fluid wave test. (See chapter 11, Gastrointestinal system.)

Urethral meatus. Help the patient feel more at ease during your inspection by examining

EXPERT TECHNIQUE

PERFORMING FIST PERCUSSION

To assess the kidneys by indirect fist percussion, ask the patient to sit up with her back to you. Tell the patient that she'll feel a "blow to the kidneys." Place one hand at the costovertebral angle and strike it with the ulnar surface of your other hand, as shown.

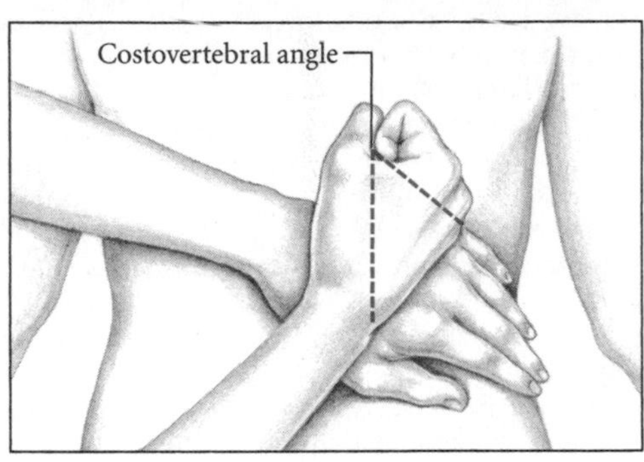

the urethral meatus last and by explaining beforehand how this assessment is accomplished. Make sure you wear gloves. Inspect the urethral meatus for inflammation, discharge, and ulceration.

CRITICAL POINT *Inflammation and discharge displayed during inspection of the urethral meatus may signal urethral infection. Ulceration usually indicates an STD.*

Auscultation

Auscultate the renal arteries in the left and right upper abdominal quadrants by pressing the stethoscope bell lightly against the abdomen and instructing the patient to exhale deeply. Begin auscultating at the midline and work to the left. Then return to the midline and work to the right.

Whooshing sounds, also known as *systolic bruits,* or other unusual sounds heard during auscultation may signal potentially significant abnormalities. For example, in a patient with hypertension, the presence of systolic bruits suggests renal artery stenosis.

Percussion

Kidney percussion checks for costovertebral angle tenderness that occurs with inflammation. To percuss over the kidneys, have the patient sit up. Place the ball of your nondominant hand on her back at the costovertebral angle of the 12th rib. Strike the ball of that hand with the ulnar surface of your other hand. Use just enough force to cause a painless but perceptible thud. (See *Performing fist percussion.*)

To percuss the bladder, first ask the patient to empty it. Then have her lie in the supine position. Start at the symphysis pubis and percuss upward toward the bladder and over it. Tympany is heard with an empty bladder.

Tenderness and pain elicited during kidney percussion may suggest glomerulonephritis or glomerulonephrosis. A dull sound heard on bladder percussion in a patient who has just urinated may indicate urine retention, reflecting bladder dysfunction or infection.

Palpation

Because the kidneys lie behind other organs and are protected by muscle, they normally aren't palpable unless they're enlarged. However, in very thin patients, you may be able to feel the lower end of the right kidney as a smooth round mass that drops on inspiration. (See *Palpating the kidneys.*)

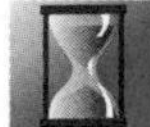

AGE ISSUE *In elderly patients, you may be able to palpate both kidneys because of decreased muscle tone and elasticity. If the kidneys feel enlarged, the patient may have hydronephrosis, cysts, or tumors.*

A lump, mass, or tenderness found during kidney palpation may indicate a tumor or cyst. A soft kidney may reflect chronic renal disease; a tender kidney, acute infection. Unequal kidney size may reflect hydro-

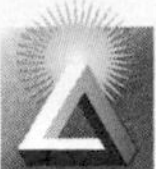

EXPERT TECHNIQUE

PALPATING THE KIDNEYS

To palpate the kidneys, first have the patient lie in a supine position. To palpate the right kidney, stand on her right side. Place your left hand under her back and your right hand on her abdomen.

Instruct her to inhale deeply, so her kidney moves downward. As she inhales, press up with your left hand and down with your right, as shown.

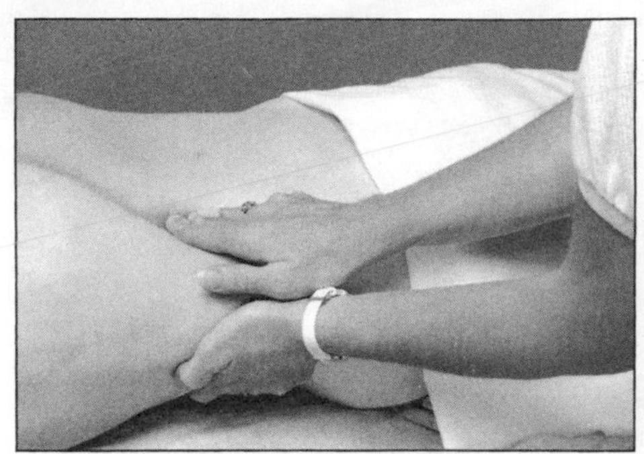

nephrosis, a cyst, a tumor, or another disorder. Bilateral enlargement suggests polycystic kidney disease.

Normally, the bladder isn't palpable unless it's distended. With the patient in a supine position, use the fingers of one hand to palpate the lower abdomen in a light dipping motion. A distended bladder will feel firm and relatively smooth.

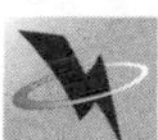

CRITICAL POINT *In pregnant patients at 12 weeks' gestation or more, you may actually be feeling the fundus of the uterus, palpable just above the symphysis pubis.*

A lump or mass found during bladder palpation may signal a tumor or cyst; tenderness may stem from infection.

Reproductive system assessment

Before beginning the reproductive system assessment, gather the necessary equipment and supplies. These include gloves, several different sizes and types of specula, a lubricant, a spatula, swabs, an endocervical brush, glass slides and cover slips, a cytologic fixative, culture bottles or plates, a sponge, forceps, a mirror, and a light source.

The examination room should be comfortable, and no one other than the health care provider, assistants, and the patient should be present.

Keep in mind that many women become anxious when undergoing a gynecologic assessment. Some feel uncomfortable or embarrassed exposing their genitalia. Others are afraid because of their lack of knowledge about the examination, past painful examinations, or accounts of painful experiences.

It's almost impossible to accurately assess a tense patient. Merely telling her to relax is ineffective. To help her calm down, ask if this is her first gynecologic assessment. If it is, explain the procedure so that she knows what to expect. If it isn't, ask her about previous assessment experiences, which may help her express her feelings. Consider using pictures and the equipment to explain the examination procedure, even if the patient has had previous gynecologic assessments. Provide supportive assurances. Stand next to the examination table, talk to her during the assessment, explain what's occurring and what will occur next, and avoid using such words as "hurt" and "pain".

Preparation and positioning

Ask the patient to empty her bladder before the examination begins.

The patient must assume the lithotomy position for the physical assessment. Her heels should be secure in the stirrups and her knees comfortably placed in the knee supports if they're used. Adjust the foot and knee supports so that her legs are equally and comfortably separated and symmetrically balanced.

The patient's buttocks must extend about 2½" (6.5 cm) over the end of the table. Because this position is precarious, offer help and direction. The hips and knees will be flexed and the thighs abducted. A pillow placed beneath her head may help her to relax her abdominal muscles. Her arms should be at her sides or over her chest; this also reduces abdominal muscle tension. Sit on a movable swivel stool an arm's length away from and between the patient's abducted legs. In this way, equipment can be reached and the genitalia seen and palpated easily.

If the patient can't assume the lithotomy position because of age, arthritis, back pain, or other reasons, place her in Sims' (left lateral) position instead. To assume this position, the patient should lie on her left side almost prone, with her buttocks close to the edge of the examination table, her left leg straight, and her right leg slightly bent in front of her left leg.

Privacy and adequate draping give the patient a sense of security. Positioning the drape low on the patient's abdomen allows her to see you and exchange visual cues. If the patient prefers no draping, respect her choice. Raising the head of the examination table helps maintain eye contact and doesn't hinder the examination.

To help the patient relax, describe what she'll feel before each new step. For example, she'll feel her inner thigh being touched, then her labia, then a finger inserted slightly into the vaginal opening and pressing on the bulbocavernous muscle in the lower vaginal wall. Explain that it's normal to tighten this muscle when tense, and show the patient how to relax by inhaling slowly and deeply through the nose, exhaling through the mouth, and concentrating on breathing regularly to relax the muscle. If the patient begins to tense up and hold her breath, remind her to breathe and relax. A celing poster or mobile in the examination room may help to distract her.

Assure the patient that the assessment takes little time. Also, keep in mind that gentle words and actions soothe; jerky movements alarm. Idle conversation may also make the patient feel more tense.

If the patient is extremely nervous, more than one appointment may be needed to complete the physical assessment. The decision of whether to perform the assessment over two or three visits will be based on the urgency of the patient's chief complaint and her anxiety. A nervous patient can be coached during a difficult assessment; however, a tranquilizer or even a general anesthetic may be necessary. The latter is especially true with young children or women who have been sexually abused.

If the health care provider is male, a female assistant should always be present during the examination for the patient's emotional comfort and the health care provider's legal protection.

External genitalia inspection

Occasionally only the patient's external genitalia need to be inspected to determine the origin of lesions or itching. Wash your hands, and then follow these steps.

Place the patient in a supine position with the pubic area uncovered, and begin the assessment by determining sexual maturity. Inspect pubic hair for amount and pattern. It's usually thick and appears on the mons pubis as well as the inner aspects of the upper thighs.

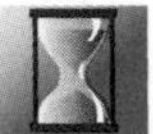

AGE ISSUE *Throughout a woman's life, pubic hair changes in density, color, and texture. Before adolescence, the pubic area is covered only with body hair. In adolescence, this hair grows thicker, darker, coarser, and curlier. In full maturity, it spreads over the symphysis pubis and inner thighs. In later years, the hair grows thin, gray, and brittle.*

Using a gloved index finger and thumb, gently spread the labia majora and look for the labia minora. The labia should be pink and moist with no lesions. Normal cervical discharge varies in color and consistency. It's clear and stretchy before ovulation, white and opaque after ovulation, and usually odorless and nonirritating to the mucosa. No other discharge should be present.

Examine the vestibule, especially the area around the Bartholin's and Skene's glands. Check for swelling, redness, lesions, discharge, and unusual odor. If you detect any of these conditions, obtain a specimen for culture. Finally, inspect the vaginal opening, noting whether the hymen is intact or perforated.

If your patient displays a male pubic hair distribution pattern (extending upward in a "line" toward the navel), note the clitoral size as well as other masculinization signs such as a deepened voice. You may need to refer your patient to an endocrinologist.

SPECULUM TYPES

Specula are available in various shapes and sizes. A Graves' speculum is typically used; however, if the patient has an intact hymen, has never given birth through the vaginal canal, or has a contracted introitus from menopause, use a Pederson speculum. These illustrations show the parts of a typical speculum and three types of specula available.

PARTS OF A SPECULUM

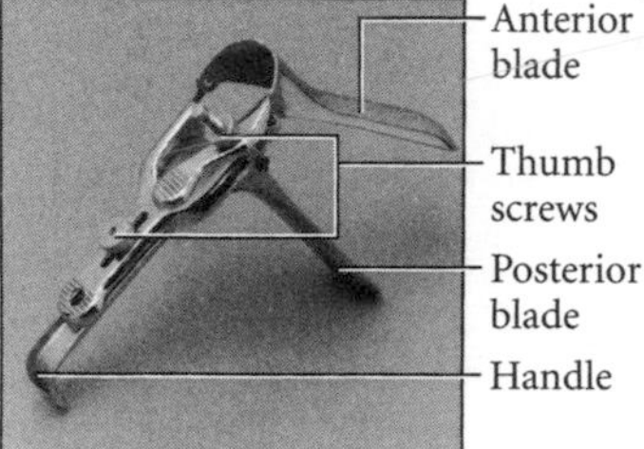

TYPES OF SPECULA

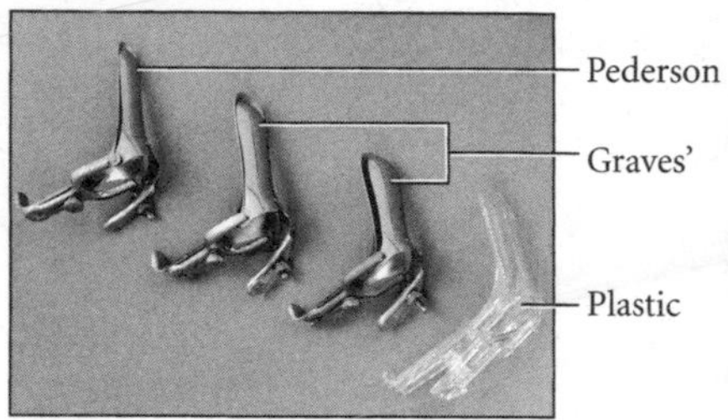

Other abnormalities include:

- varicosities, which are distended superficial vessels on the labia, that can indicate increased pressure in the pelvic region, as seen in pregnant patients and in those with uterine tumors.
- lesions, such as ulcerations or wartlike growths, which can indicate human papillomavirus.
- edema of the mons pubis, labia majora, labia minora, urethral orifice, vaginal introitus, or the surrounding skin.
- organisms, such as Candida, a yeastlike infection that may cause an inflamed vulva with a cheeselike discharge; *Chlamydia trachomatis,* which may cause a heavy gray-white discharge; *Haemophilus* or *Trichomonas,* which may cause a frothy, malodorous, green or gray watery discharge; *Neisseria gonorrhoeae,* which may cause a purulent, green-yellow urethral or vaginal discharge; and *Pediculus pubis* (lice) or nits (minute white louse eggs attached to pubic hairs), which may be present without symptoms, or with symptoms of another infection.

Specimens of all discharges should be cultured or examined microscopically in the laboratory.

External genitalia palpation

Spread the labia with one hand and palpate with the other. The labia should feel soft. Note swelling, hardness, or tenderness. If you detect a mass or lesion, palpate it to determine its size, shape, and consistency.

If you find swelling or tenderness, attempt to palpate Bartholin's glands, which normally aren't palpable. To do this, insert your finger carefully into the patient's posterior introitus, and place your thumb along the lateral edge of the swollen or tender labium. Gently squeeze the labium. Swollen or tender Bartholin's glands could indicate infection. Culture any glandular discharge.

If the urethra is inflamed, milk it and the area of Skene's glands. First, moisten your gloved index finger with water. Then separate the labia with your other hand, and insert your index finger about 1¼″ (3 cm) into the anterior vagina. With the pad of your finger, gently press and pull outward. Continue palpating down to the introitus. This procedure shouldn't cause the patient discomfort. Culture the discharge.

Internal genitalia inspection

Inspection of the internal genitalia requires advanced skill. Begin by selecting the appropriate speculum for your patient. (See *Speculum types.*)

EXPERT TECHNIQUE

INSERTING A SPECULUM

Proper positioning and insertion of the speculum are important for the comfort of the patient and for proper visualization of the internal structures. These illustrations show the proper angle and hand position for speculum insertion.

Initial insertion

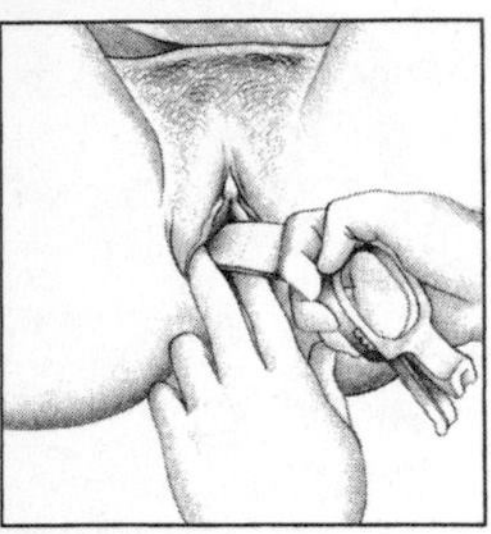

Place the index and middle fingers of your nondominant hand about 1″ (2.5 cm) into the vagina and spread the fingers to exert pressure on the posterior vagina. Hold the speculum in your dominant hand, and insert the blades between your fingers as shown above.

Deeper insertion

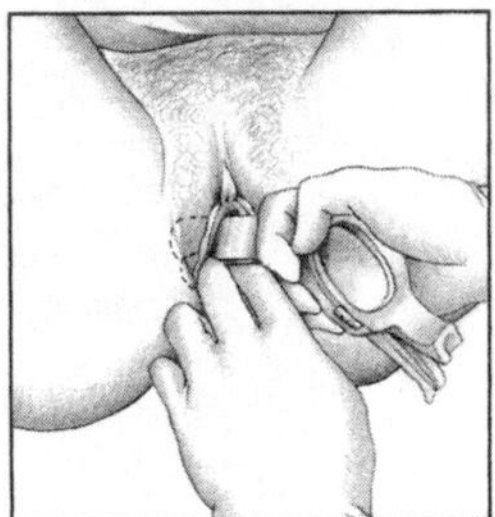

Ask the patient to bear down to open the introitus and relax the perineal muscles. Point the speculum slightly downward, and insert the blades until the base of the speculum touches your fingers, inside the vagina.

Final insertion

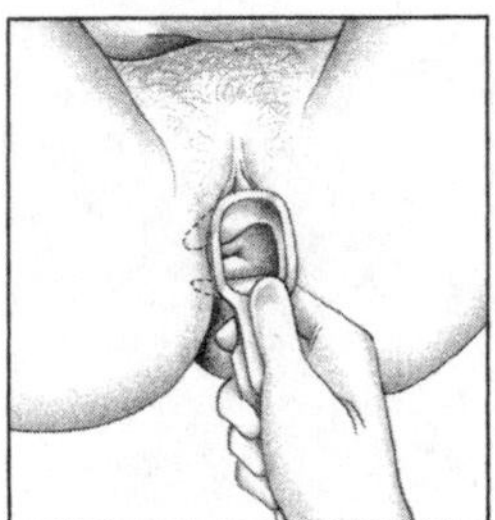

Rotate the speculum in the same plane as the vagina, and withdraw your fingers. Open the blades as far as possible and lock them. You should now be able to view the cervix clearly.

Hold the speculum under warm, running water to lubricate and warm the blades. Don't use lubricants; many are bacteriostatic and can alter Pap test results.

Sit or stand at the foot of the examination table. Tell the patient she'll feel internal pressure and possibly some slight, transient discomfort as you insert and open the speculum.

Using your dominant hand, hold the speculum by the base with the blades anchored between your index and middle fingers. This keeps the blades from accidentally opening during insertion. Encourage the patient to take slow, deep breaths during insertion to relax her abdominal muscles. (See *Inserting a speculum.*) Insert your fingers first and allow the pelvic floor muscles to relax, and then insert the speculum. Ease insertion by asking the patient to bear down.

After inserting the speculum, observe the color, texture, and integrity of the vaginal lining.

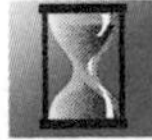

AGE ISSUE *In a postmenopausal patient, the vaginal mucosa may be pale with rugae loss due to estrogen deficiency.*

A thin, white, odorless discharge on the vaginal walls is normal. However, if a vaginal discharge is observed, note the color, consistency and character. For example:

- vaginitis, which usually results from an overgrowth of infectious organisms and causes redness, itching, dyspareunia or painful intercourse, dysuria, and a malodorous discharge

- bacterial vaginosis, which causes a fishy odor and a thin, grayish white discharge
- Candida albicans, which causes pruritus and a thick, white, curdlike discharge that appears in patches on the cervix and vaginal walls and has a yeastlike odor
- trichomoniasis, which may cause an abundant malodorous discharge (either yellow or green and frothy or watery) as well as redness and red papules on the cervix and vaginal walls, commonly known as a "strawberry" cervix
- *Chlamydia trachomatis,* which is a common but, in many cases, subtle STD that causes a mucopurulent cervical discharge and cystitis.

CRITICAL POINT *In cases of gonorrhea, note that 3 out of 4 women have no symptoms; however, it may cause a purulent green-yellow discharge and cystitis. It's now recommended to screen all sexually active women regardless of symptoms.*

Using the thumb of the hand holding the speculum, press the lower lever to open the blades. Lock them in the open position by tightening the thumbscrew above the lever.

Examine the cervix for color, position, size, shape, mucosal integrity, and discharge. It should be smooth and round. The central cervical opening, or cervical os, is circular in a woman who hasn't given birth vaginally and a horizontal slit in a woman who has. Expect to see a clear, watery cervical discharge during ovulation and a slightly bloody discharge just before menstruation. (See *The normal os.*)

THE NORMAL OS

These illustrations show the difference between the os of a woman who has never given birth vaginally (nulliparous) and the os of a woman who has (parous).

NULLIPAROUS

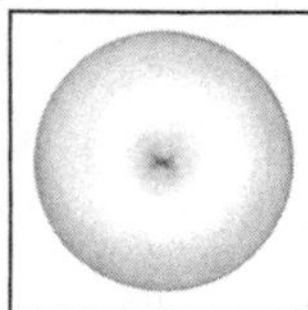

PAROUS

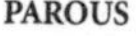

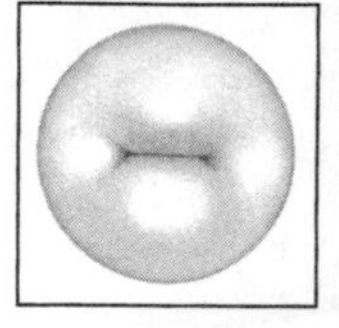

During pregnancy the cervix is enlarged. A cyanotic cervix can indicate pelvic congestion from a tumor or pregnancy. Infection may give the cervix a bright red or spotted red appearance or erythema. A cervix projecting low into the vagina or visible at the introitus can indicate uterine prolapse, which is displacement of the uterus from its normal position, caused by weak pelvic muscles or ligaments. A less severe prolapse may occur when the patient bears down; urine leakage indicates stress incontinence. A laterally placed cervix can indicate a uterine tumor or uterine adhesion to the peritoneum.

Obtain a specimen for a Pap test and perform other tests at this time, including cultures for sexually transmitted infections. Finally, unlock and close the blades and withdraw the speculum.

Internal genitalia palpation

To palpate the internal genitalia, lubricate the index and middle fingers of your gloved dominant hand. Stand at the foot of the examination table and position the hand for insertion into the vagina by extending your thumb, index, and middle fingers and curling your ring and little finger toward your palm.

Use the thumb and index finger of your other hand to spread the labia majora. Insert your two lubricated fingers into the vagina, exerting pressure posteriorly to avoid irritating the anterior wall and urethra.

When your fingers are fully inserted, note tenderness or nodularity in the vaginal wall. Ask the patient to bear down so you can assess the support of the vaginal outlet. Bulging of the patient's vaginal wall may indicate a cystocele or a rectocele.

To palpate the cervix, sweep your fingers from side to side across the cervix and around the os. The cervix should be smooth and firm and protrude ¼″ to 1¼″ (0.5 to 3 cm) into the vagina. If you palpate nodules or irregularities, the patient may have cysts, tumors, or other lesions.

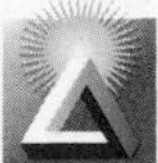

EXPERT TECHNIQUE

PERFORMING A BIMANUAL EXAMINATION

During a bimanual examination, palpate the uterus and ovaries from the inside and the outside simultaneously. These illustrations show how to perform such an examination.

Proper position

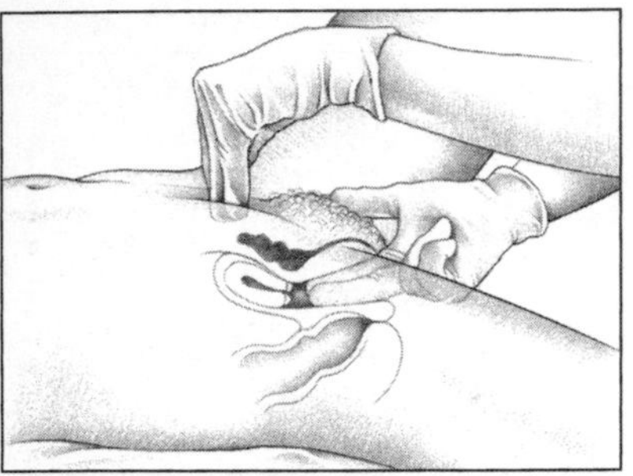

After putting on gloves, place the index and third finger of your dominant hand in the patient's vagina and move them up to the cervix. Place the fingers of your other hand on the patient's abdomen between the umbilicus and the symphysis pubis, as shown.

Elevate the cervix and uterus by pressing upward with the two fingers inside the vagina. At the same time, press down and in with the hand on the abdomen. Try to grasp the uterus between your hands.

Note the position

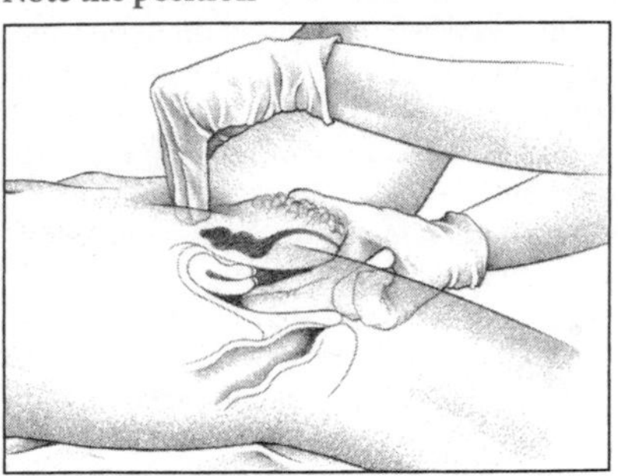

Now move your fingers into the posterior fornix, pressing upward and forward to bring the anterior uterine wall up to your nondominant hand. Use your dominant hand to palpate the lower portion of the uterine wall. Note the position of the uterus.

Next, place your fingers into the recessed area around the cervix. The cervix should move in all directions.

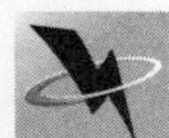

CRITICAL POINT *If the patient reports pain during this part of the examination, she may have inflammation of the uterus or adnexa—ovaries, fallopian tubes, and ligaments of the uterus. A patient with pelvic inflammatory disease may experience severe pain when you manipulate her cervix.*

Bimanual palpation

A bimanual examination allows palpation of the uterus and ovaries. Usually, bimanual palpation requires advanced skill. (See *Performing a bimanual examination.*)

CRITICAL POINT *In a pregnant patient with hyperplasia and increasing blood supply, the uterus softens and normally feels somewhat tender; however, when a tumor is suspected, the uterus may feel hard, especially if cancerous. Excessive tenderness usually indicates disease, particularly infection. In postmenopausal or prepubescent females, a palpable ovary is abnormal. Abnormal ovarian enlargement in a patient of any age warrants medical evaluation. Although common and usually benign in young fertile women, ovarian cysts should also be evaluated.*

Rectovaginal palpation

Rectovaginal palpation, the last step in a reproductive system assessment, examines the

Palpate the walls

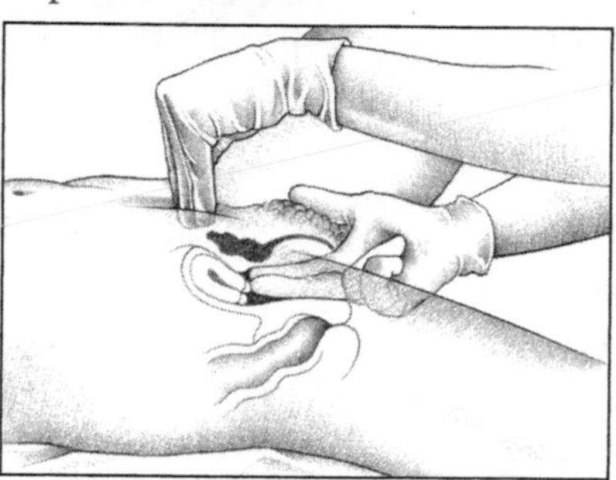

Slide your fingers farther into the anterior section of the fornix, the space between the uterus and cervix. You should feel part of the posterior uterine wall with this hand. You should also feel part of the anterior uterine wall with the fingertips of your nondominant hand. Note the size, shape, surface characteristics, consistency, and mobility of the uterus as well as tenderness.

Palpate the ovaries

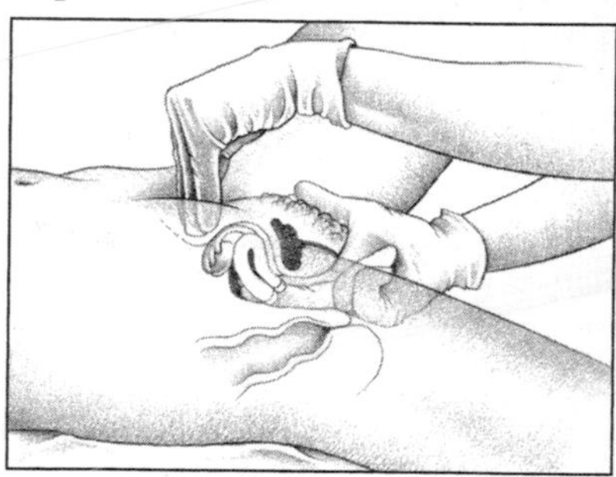

After palpating the anterior and posterior walls of the uterus, move your nondominant hand toward the right lower quadrant of the abdomen. Slip the fingers of your dominant hand into the right fornix and palpate the right ovary. Then palpate the left ovary. Note the size, shape, and contour of each ovary. They should be unpalpable in postmenopausal women. Remove your hand from the patient's abdomen and your fingers from her vagina, and discard your gloves.

posterior part of the uterus and the pelvic cavity. Warn the patient that this procedure may be uncomfortable.

Put on a new pair of gloves and apply water-soluble lubricant to the index and middle fingers of your gloved dominant hand. Instruct the patient to bear down with her vaginal and rectal muscles; then insert your index finger a short way into her vagina and your middle finger into her rectum.

Use your middle finger to assess rectal muscle and sphincter tone. Insert your finger deeper into the rectum, and palpate the rectal wall with your middle finger. Sweep the rectum with your fingers, assessing for masses or nodules.

Palpate the posterior wall of the uterus through the anterior wall of the rectum, evaluating the uterus for size, shape, tenderness, and masses. The rectovaginal septum, the wall between the rectum and the vagina, should feel smooth and springy, without any masses.

Place your nondominant hand on the patient's abdomen at the symphysis pubis. With your index finger in the vagina, palpate deeply to feel the posterior edge of the cervix and the lower posterior wall of the uterus.

When you're finished, discard the gloves and wash your hands. Help the patient to a sitting position, and provide privacy for dressing and personal hygiene.

Abnormal findings

A patient may seek care for a number of signs and symptoms related to the female GU system. The most significant findings include amenorrhea, anuria, dysmenorrhea, dyspareunia, dysuria, menorrhagia, metrorrhagia, nocturia, oliguria, urinary frequency, urinary incontinence, and vaginal discharge. Polyuria may also be a common finding and is discussed in chapter 12, Endocrine system. The following history, physical assessment, and analysis summaries will help you assess each finding quickly and accurately. After obtaining further information, begin to interpret the findings. (See *Female GU system: Interpreting your findings.*)

Amenorrhea

The absence of menstrual flow, amenorrhea can be classified as primary or secondary. With primary amenorrhea, menstruation fails to begin before age 16. With secondary amenorrhea, it begins at an appropriate age but later ceases for 3 or more months in the absence of normal physiologic changes, such as pregnancy, lactation, or menopause.

History

Begin by determining whether the amenorrhea is primary or secondary. If it's primary, ask the patient at what age her mother first menstruated because age of menarche is fairly consistent in families. Form an overall impression of the patient's physical, mental, and emotional development because these factors, as well as heredity and climate, may delay menarche until after age 16.

If menstruation began at an appropriate age but has since ceased, determine the frequency and duration of the patient's previous menses. Ask her about the onset and nature of any changes in her normal menstrual pattern and determine the date of her last menses. Find out if she has noticed any related signs, such as breast swelling or weight fluctuations.

Determine when the patient last had a physical examination. Review her health history, noting especially any long-term illnesses, such as anemia, or the use of hormonal contraceptives. Ask about exercise habits, especially running, and whether she experiences stress at her job or at home. Probe the patient's eating habits, including number and size of daily meals and snacks, and ask if she has gained weight recently.

Physical assessment

Perform a complete physical examination. Observe the patient for the appearance of secondary sex characteristics or signs of virilization. If you're responsible for performing a pelvic examination, check for anatomic aberrations of the outflow tract, such as cervical adhesions, fibroids, or an imperforate hymen.

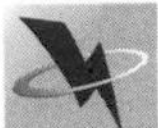

CRITICAL POINT *In patients with secondary amenorrhea, physical and pelvic examinations must rule out pregnancy before diagnostic testing begins.*

Analysis

Pathologic amenorrhea results from anovulation or physical obstruction to menstrual outflow, such as from an imperforate hymen, cervical stenosis, or intrauterine adhesions. Anovulation itself may result from hormonal imbalance, debilitating disease, stress or emotional disturbances, strenuous exercise, malnutrition, obesity, or anatomic abnormalities, such as congenital absence of the ovaries or uterus. Amenorrhea may also result from drug or hormonal treatments. Hormonal contraceptives may cause anovulation and amenorrhea after discontinuation. Irradiation of the abdomen may destroy the endometrium or ovaries, causing amenorrhea. Surgical removal of both ovaries or the uterus produces amenorrhea.

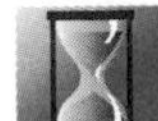

AGE ISSUE *Adolescent girls are especially prone to amenorrhea caused by emotional upsets, typically stemming from school, social, or family problems. In women older than age 50, amenorrhea usually represents the onset of menopause.*

Anuria

Anuria is clinically defined as urine output of less than 100 ml in 24 hours. It's rare because, even in renal failure, the kidneys usually produce at least 75 ml of urine daily.

History

Obtain a complete health history. First, ask about any changes in her voiding pattern. Determine the amount of fluid she normally ingests each day, the amount of fluid she

(Text continues on page 405.)

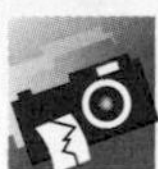

CLINICAL PICTURE

FEMALE GU SYSTEM: INTERPRETING YOUR FINDINGS

After you assess the female patient, a group of findings may lead you to suspect a particular genitourinary (GU) system disorder. The chart below shows you some common groups of findings for major signs and symptoms related to the female GU system, along with their probable causes.

Sign or symptom and findings	Probable cause
Amenorrhea	
■ Primary or secondary amenorrhea ■ Significant weight loss ■ Thin or emaciated appearance ■ Compulsive behavior patterns ■ Blotchy or sallow complexion ■ Constipation ■ Reduced libido ■ Decreased pleasure in once-enjoyable activities ■ Dry skin ■ Loss of scalp hair ■ Lanugo on face and arms ■ Skeletal muscle atrophy ■ Sleep disturbances	Anorexia nervosa
■ Primary or secondary amenorrhea due to deficient thyroid hormone levels ■ Fatigue ■ Forgetfulness ■ Cold intolerance ■ Unexplained weight gain ■ Constipation ■ Bradycardia ■ Decreased mental acuity ■ Dry, flaking, inelastic skin ■ Puffy face, hands, and feet ■ Hoarseness ■ Periorbital edema ■ Ptosis ■ Dry, sparse hair ■ Thick brittle nails	Hypothyroidism
Amenorrhea *(continued)*	
■ Menarche at normal age followed by irregular menstrual cycles, oligomenorrhea, and secondary amenorrhea ■ Periods of profuse bleeding alternating with periods of amenorrhea ■ Obesity ■ Hirsutism ■ Slight deepening of voice ■ Enlarged "oyster-like" ovaries	Polycystic ovary disease
Anuria	
■ Oliguria and possibly anuria preceding the onset of diuresis evidenced as polyuria ■ Hyperkalemia causing muscle weakness and cardiac arrhythmias ■ Uremia causing anorexia, nausea, vomiting, confusion lethargy, twitching, convulsions, pruritus, uremic frost and Kussmaul's respirations ■ Heart failure causing edema, jugular vein distention, crackles, and dyspnea	Acute tubular necrosis

(continued)

FEMALE GU SYSTEM: INTERPRETING YOUR FINDINGS *(continued)*

Sign or symptom and findings	Probable cause
Anuria *(continued)*	
■ Acute and sometimes total anuria (complete obstruction) alternating with or preceded by burning and pain on urination and overflow incontinence or dribbling ■ Increased urinary frequency and nocturia ■ Voiding small amounts or altered urine stream ■ Bladder distention ■ Pain and sensation of fullness in lower abdomen and groin ■ Upper abdominal and flank pain ■ Nausea and vomiting	Urinary tract obstruction
■ Occasionally anuria ■ Malaise ■ Myalgia ■ Polyarthralgia ■ Fever ■ Elevated blood pressure ■ Hematuria ■ Proteinuria ■ Arrhythmia ■ Pallor ■ Possible skin lesions ■ Urticaria ■ Purpura	Vasculitis
Dysmenorrhea	
■ Steady, aching pain that begins before menses and peaks at the height of menstrual flow; may occur between menstrual periods ■ Pain may radiate to the perineum or rectum ■ Premenstrual spotting ■ Dyspareunia ■ Infertility ■ Nausea and vomiting ■ Tender, fixed adrenal mass palpable on bimanual examination	Endometriosis
■ Severe abdominal pain ■ Fever ■ Malaise ■ Foul-smelling, purulent vaginal discharge ■ Menorrhagia ■ Cervical motion tenderness and bilateral adnexal tenderness on pelvic examination	Pelvic inflammatory disease
■ Cramping pain that begins with menstrual flow and diminishes with decreasing flow ■ Abdominal bloating ■ Breast tenderness ■ Depression ■ Irritability ■ Headache ■ Diarrhea	Premenstrual syndrome

FEMALE GU SYSTEM: INTERPRETING YOUR FINDINGS *(continued)*

Sign or symptom and findings	Probable cause
Dyspareunia	
■ Inadequate vaginal lubrication and dyspareunia (in postmenopausal and breast-feeding women due to decreased estrogen secretion) ■ Dyspareunia intensifying during intercourse (and as it continues) ■ Pruritus ■ Burning ■ Bleeding ■ Vaginal tenderness	Atrophic vaginitis
■ Severe pain on deep penetration unrelieved by changing coital positions ■ Uterine tenderness with gentle thrusting or during pelvic examination ■ Fever ■ Malaise ■ Foul-smelling, purulent vaginal discharge ■ Menorrhagia ■ Dysmenorrhea ■ Severe abdominal pain ■ Cervical motion tenderness	Pelvic inflammatory disease
■ Dyspareunia with vulvar pain, burning, and itching during and for several hours after coitus ■ Possible aggravation with sexual arousal aside from intercourse ■ Vaginal discharge	Vaginitis
Dysuria	
■ Urinary frequency ■ Nocturia ■ Straining to void ■ Hematuria ■ Perineal or low back pain ■ Fatigue ■ Low-grade fever	Cystitis
■ Dysuria throughout voiding ■ Bladder distention ■ Diminished urinary stream ■ Urinary frequency and urgency ■ Sensation of bloating or fullness in the lower abdomen or groin	Urinary system obstruction
■ Urinary urgency ■ Hematuria ■ Cloudy urine ■ Bladder spasms ■ Feeling of warmth or burning during urination	Urinary tract infection
Menorrhagia	
■ Menorrhagia with dysmenorrhea ■ Suprapubic pain ■ Dysuria ■ Nausea and vomiting ■ Abdominal cramps ■ Cyclic pelvic pain ■ Infertility ■ Tender, fixed, adnexal mass on bimanual palpation	Endometriosis

(continued)

FEMALE GU SYSTEM: INTERPRETING YOUR FINDINGS *(continued)*

Sign or symptom and findings	Probable cause
Menorrhagia *(continued)*	
▪ Menorrhagia with dysmenorrhea or leukorrhea ▪ Abdominal pain ▪ Feeling of abdominal heaviness ▪ Backache ▪ Constipation ▪ Urinary urgency or frequency ▪ Enlarged uterus, usually nontender	Uterine fibroids
Metrorrhagia	
▪ Spontaneous bleeding, spotting or posttraumatic bleeding ▪ Red granular irregular lesions on external cervix ▪ Purulent vaginal discharge with or without odor ▪ Lower abdominal pain ▪ Fever	Cervicitis
▪ Abnormal bleeding not caused by pregnancy or major gynecologic disorder ▪ Profuse or scant, intermittent or constant bleeding	Dysfunctional uterine bleeding
▪ Metrorrhagia occurring as a early sign of cervical or uterine cancer ▪ Weight loss ▪ Pelvic pain ▪ Fatigue ▪ Possible abdominal mass	Gynecologic cancer
Nocturia	
▪ Nocturia with frequent small voidings accompanied by dysuria and tenesmus ▪ Urgency ▪ Hematuria ▪ Fatigue ▪ Suprapubic, perineal, flank, and low back pain ▪ Occasional low-grade fever	Cystitis, bacterial
▪ Nocturia characterized by infrequent voiding of moderate amounts of urine that may appear cloudy ▪ High sustained fever with chills ▪ Fatigue ▪ Unilateral or bilateral flank pain ▪ Costovertebral tenderness ▪ Weakness ▪ Dysuria ▪ Hematuria ▪ Urinary frequency and urgency ▪ Tenesmus	Pyelonephritis

FEMALE GU SYSTEM: INTERPRETING YOUR FINDINGS *(continued)*

Sign or symptom and findings	Probable cause
Nocturia *(continued)*	
■ Early onset of nocturia, characterized by infrequent voiding of moderate amounts of urine ■ Progression possible to oliguria and anuria ■ Fatigue ■ Ammonia breath odor ■ Kussmaul's respirations ■ Peripheral edema ■ Elevated blood pressure ■ Decreased level of consciousness ■ Confusion ■ Emotional lability ■ Muscle twitching ■ Anorexia ■ Metallic taste in the mouth ■ Constipation or diarrhea	Renal failure, chronic
Oliguria	
■ Oliguria or anuria from stones that lodge in urinary tract or kidneys ■ Urinary frequency and urgency ■ Dysuria ■ Hematuria or pyuria ■ Renal colic radiating from costovertebral angle to flank, suprapubic region, and external genitalia	Calculi
Oliguria *(continued)*	
■ Oliguria or anuria ■ Mild fever ■ Fatigue ■ Gross hematuria ■ Proteinuria ■ Generalized edema ■ Elevated blood pressure ■ Headache ■ Nausea and vomiting ■ Flank and abdominal pain ■ Pulmonary congestion	Glomerulonephritis, acute
■ Oliguria secondary to decreased circulating blood volume ■ Orthostatic hypotension ■ Apathy ■ Lethargy ■ Fatigue ■ Gross muscle weakness ■ Anorexia ■ Nausea ■ Profound thirst ■ Dizziness ■ Sunken eyeballs ■ Poor skin turgor ■ Dry mucous membranes	Hypovolemia
Urinary frequency	
■ Urinary frequency, urgency, dribbling, and nocturia ■ Gross painless intermittent hematuria ■ Suprapubic or pelvic pain from bladder spasms due to invasive lesions	Bladder cancer

(continued)

FEMALE GU SYSTEM: INTERPRETING YOUR FINDINGS *(continued)*

Sign or symptom and findings	Probable cause
Urinary frequency *(continued)*	
■ Urinary frequency, urgency, and incontinence, wax and wane ■ Visual problems ■ Sensory impairment ■ Constipation ■ Muscle weakness ■ Paralysis, spasticity, and hyperreflexia ■ Intention tremor ■ Ataxic gait ■ Dysarthria ■ Emotional lability	Multiple sclerosis
■ Urinary frequency with possible urgency, dysuria, hematuria, and cloudy urine ■ Bladder spasms or feeling of warmth during urination ■ Fever ■ Suprapubic or pelvic pain	Urinary tract infection
Urinary incontinence	
■ Urge or overflow incontinence ■ Hematuria ■ Dysuria ■ Nocturia ■ Urinary frequency ■ Suprapelvic pain from bladder spasms ■ Palpable mass on bimanual examination	Bladder cancer
■ Overflow incontinence ■ Painless bladder distention ■ Episodic diarrhea or constipation ■ Orthostatic hypotension ■ Syncope ■ Dysphagia	Diabetic neuropathy
Urinary incontinence *(continued)*	
■ Vision problems ■ Sensory impairment ■ Constipation ■ Muscle weakness ■ Emotional lability	Multiple sclerosis
Vaginal discharge	
■ Profuse, white, curdlike discharge with a yeasty, sweet odor ■ Exudate may be lightly attached to the labia and vaginal walls ■ Vulvar redness and edema ■ Intense labial itching and burning ■ External dysuria	Candidiasis
■ Yellow, mucopurulent, odorless, or acrid discharge ■ Dysuria ■ Dyspareunia ■ Vaginal bleeding after douching or coitus	Chlamydia infection
■ Yellow or green, foul-smelling discharge that's expressed from the Bartholin's or Skene's ducts ■ Dysuria ■ Urinary frequency and incontinence ■ Vaginal redness and swelling	Gonorrhea

ingested in the last 24 to 48 hours, and the time and amount of her last urination. Review her medical history, especially noting previous kidney disease, urinary tract obstruction or infection, renal calculi, neurogenic bladder, or congenital abnormalities. Ask about drug use and about any abdominal, renal, or urinary tract surgery.

Physical assessment

Inspect and palpate the abdomen for asymmetry, distention, or bulging. Inspect the flank area for edema or erythema, and percuss and palpate the bladder. Palpate the kidneys anteriorly and posteriorly, and percuss them at the costovertebral angle. Auscultate over the renal arteries, listening for bruits.

Analysis

Anuria indicates either urinary tract obstruction or acute renal failure due to various mechanisms. Because urine output is easily measured, anuria rarely goes undetected. However, without immediate treatment, it can rapidly cause uremia and other complications of urine retention. Many classes of drugs can cause anuria or, more commonly, oliguria through their nephrotoxic effects. Antibiotics, especially the aminoglycosides, are the most commonly seen nephrotoxins. Anesthetics, heavy metals, ethyl alcohol, and organic solvents can also be nephrotoxic. Adrenergics and anticholinergics can also cause anuria by affecting the nerves and muscles of micturition to produce urine retention.

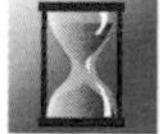

AGE ISSUE *In neonates, anuria is defined as the absence of urine output for 24 hours and can be classified as primary or secondary. Primary anuria results from bilateral renal agenesis, aplasia, or multicystic dysplasia. Secondary anuria, associated with edema or dehydration, results from renal ischemia, renal vein thrombosis, or congenital anomalies of the GU tract. Anuria in children commonly results from loss of renal function. In elderly patients, anuria is a gradually occurring sign of underlying disorders. Hospitalized or bedridden elderly patients may be unable to generate the necessary pressure to void if they remain in a supine position.*

Dysmenorrhea

Dysmenorrhea — painful menstruation — affects over 50% of menstruating women; in fact, it's the leading cause of lost time from school and work among women of childbearing age. Dysmenorrhea may involve sharp, intermittent pain or dull, aching pain. It's usually characterized by mild to severe cramping or colicky pain in the pelvis or lower abdomen that may radiate to the thighs and lower sacrum. This pain may precede menses by several days or may accompany it. The pain gradually subsides as bleeding tapers off.

History

If the patient complains of dysmenorrhea, have her describe it fully. Find out if the pain is intermittent or continuous and if it's sharp, cramping, or aching. Ask where the pain is located and whether it's bilateral. Find out how long she has been experiencing it. Ask her when the pain begins and ends and when it's severe. Also ask her if it radiates to her back. Explore associated signs and symptoms, such as nausea and vomiting, altered bowel or urinary habits, bloating, pelvic or rectal pressure, and unusual fatigue, irritability, or depression.

Then obtain a menstrual and sexual history. Ask the patient if her menstrual flow is heavy or scant. Have her describe any vaginal discharge between menses. Find out if she experiences pain during sexual intercourse and if it occurs with menses. Find out what relieves her cramps such as taking pain medication and, if so, if it's effective. Note her method of contraception, and ask about a history of pelvic infection. Determine if she has signs or symptoms of urinary system obstruction, such as pyuria, urine retention, or incontinence. Determine how she copes with stress.

Physical assessment

Perform a focused physical examination. Inspect the abdomen for distention, and palpate for tenderness and masses. Note costovertebral angle tenderness.

Analysis

Dysmenorrhea may be idiopathic, as in premenstrual syndrome and primary dysmenorrhea. It commonly results from endometriosis and other pelvic disorders. It may also result from structural abnormalities, such as an imperforate hymen. Stress and poor health may aggravate dysmenorrhea. Rest and mild exercise may relieve it.

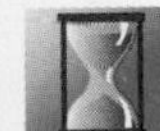

AGE ISSUE *Dysmenorrhea is rare during the first year of menses, before the cycle becomes ovulatory. However, generally, more adolescents experience dysmenorrhea than older women.*

Dyspareunia

A major obstacle to sexual enjoyment, dyspareunia is painful or difficult coitus. Although most sexually active women occasionally experience mild dyspareunia, persistent or severe dyspareunia is cause for concern. Dyspareunia may occur with attempted penetration or during or after coitus. It may stem from friction of the penis against perineal tissue or from jarring of deeper adnexal structures. The location of pain helps determine its cause.

History

Begin by asking the patient to describe the pain. Ask her if it occurs with attempted penetration or deep thrusting. Find out how long the pain lasts and if it's intermittent or if it always accompanies intercourse. Ask whether changing coital position or using vaginal lubrication relieves the pain.

Next, ask about a history of pelvic, vaginal, or UTI. Determine if the patient has signs and symptoms of a current infection. Have her describe any discharge. Also ask about malaise, headache, fatigue, abdominal or back pain, nausea and vomiting, and diarrhea or constipation.

Obtain a sexual and menstrual history. Determine whether dyspareunia is related to the patient's menstrual cycle. Find out if her cycles are regular. Ask about dysmenorrhea and metrorrhagia.

Find out if the patient has given birth and, if so, if she had an episiotomy. Note whether she's breast-feeding. Ask about previous abortion, sexual abuse, or pelvic surgery. Find out what contraceptive method the patient uses. Find out if the patient or her partner uses condoms. Ask if she has a possible or known latex allergy. Then try to determine her attitude toward sexual intimacy. Ask her if she feels tense during coitus, if she's satisfied with the length of foreplay, and if she usually achieves orgasm. Ask about a history of rape, incest, or sexual abuse as a child.

Physical assessment

Perform a physical examination. Take the patient's vital signs. Palpate her abdomen for tenderness, pain, or masses and for inguinal lymphadenopathy. Finally, inspect the genitalia for lesions and vaginal discharge.

Analysis

Dyspareunia commonly accompanies pelvic disorders. However, it may also result from diminished vaginal lubrication associated with aging, the effects of drugs, and psychological factors — most notably, fear of pain or injury. A cycle of fear, pain, and tension may become established, in which repeated episodes of painful coitus condition the patient to anticipate pain, causing fear, which prevents sexual arousal and adequate vaginal lubrication. Contraction of the pubococcygeus muscle also occurs, making penetration still more difficult and traumatic.

Other psychological factors include guilty feelings about sex, fear of pregnancy or of injury to the fetus during pregnancy, and anxiety caused by a disrupted sexual relationship or by a new sexual partner. Inadequate vaginal lubrication associated with insufficient foreplay and mental or physical fatigue may also cause dyspareunia. Some spermicidal jellies, douches, and vaginal creams and deodorants cause irritation and edema, resulting in dyspareunia. An ill-fitting diaphragm may produce cramps during intercourse. An incorrectly placed intrauterine device may cause dyspareunia during orgasm. Antihistamines, decongestants, and nonsteroidal anti-inflammatories may cause insufficient lubrication. If an episiotomy scar constricts the vaginal introitus or narrows the vaginal barrel, the patient may experience perineal pain with coitus.

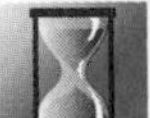

AGE ISSUE *Dyspareunia can also be an adolescent problem. Although about 40% of adolescents are sexually active by age 19, most are reluctant to initiate a frank sexual discussion. Obtain a thorough sexual history by asking the patient direct but nonjudgmental questions. In postmenopausal women, the absence of estrogen reduces vaginal diameter and elasticity, which causes tearing of the vaginal mucosa during*

intercourse. These tears, as well as inflammatory reactions to bacterial invasion, cause fibrous adhesions that occlude the vagina. Dyspareunia can result from any or all of these conditions.

Dysuria

Dysuria — painful or difficult urination — is commonly accompanied by urinary frequency, urgency, or hesitancy. This symptom usually reflects a lower UTI — a common disorder, especially in women.

History

If the patient complains of dysuria, have her describe its severity and location. Find out when she first noticed it. Ask what precipitated it and if any measures aggravate or alleviate it.

Next, ask about previous UTIs or genital infections. Find out if the patient has recently undergone an invasive procedure, such as a cystoscopy or urethral dilatation. Also ask if she has a history of intestinal disease. Ask about menstrual disorders and use of products that irritate the urinary tract, such as bubble bath salts, feminine deodorants, contraceptive gels, or perineal lotions. Also ask about vaginal discharge or pruritus.

Physical assessment

During the physical examination, inspect the urethral meatus for discharge, irritation, or other abnormalities. A pelvic or rectal examination may be necessary.

Analysis

Dysuria results from lower urinary tract irritation or inflammation, which stimulates nerve endings in the bladder and urethra. The pain's onset provides clues to its cause; for example, pain just before voiding usually indicates bladder irritation or distention, whereas pain at the start of urination typically results from bladder outlet irritation. Pain at the end of voiding may indicate bladder spasms or vaginal candidiasis.

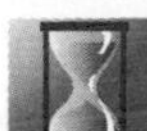

AGE ISSUE *Be aware that elderly patients tend to under-report their symptoms, even though postmenopausal women are more likely to experience noninfectious dysuria.*

Menorrhagia

Abnormally heavy or long menstrual bleeding, menorrhagia may occur as a single episode or a chronic sign. In menorrhagia, bleeding is heavier than the patient's normal menstrual flow; menstrual blood loss is 80 ml or more per menses.

History

When the patient's condition permits, obtain a health history. Determine her age at menarche, the duration of menstrual periods, and the interval between them. Establish the date of the patient's last menses, and ask about any recent changes in her normal menstrual pattern. Have the patient describe the character and amount of bleeding. For example, ask how many pads or tampons the patient uses. Find out if she has noted clots or tissue in the blood. Also ask about the development of other signs and symptoms before and during the menstrual period.

Next, ask if the patient is sexually active. Find out if she uses a method of birth control and, if so, what type. Ask the patient if she could possibly be pregnant. Be sure to note the number of pregnancies, the outcome of each, and any pregnancy-related complications. Find out the dates of her most recent pelvic examination and Pap test and the details of any previous gynecologic infections or neoplasms. Also, be sure to ask about any previous episodes of abnormal bleeding and the outcome of any treatment. If possible, obtain a pregnancy history of the patient's mother, and determine if the patient was exposed in utero to diethylstilbestrol, which has been linked to vaginal adenosis.

Be sure to ask the patient about her general health and medical history. Particularly note if the patient or her family has a history of thyroid, adrenal, or hepatic disease; blood dyscrasias; or tuberculosis because these may predispose the patient to menorrhagia.

Ask about the patient's past surgical procedures and any recent emotional stress. Find out if the patient has undergone X-ray or other radiation therapy because this may indicate prior treatment for menorrhagia. Obtain a thorough drug and alcohol history, noting the use of anticoagulants or aspirin.

Physical assessment
Perform a pelvic examination, and obtain blood and urine samples for pregnancy testing.

Analysis
A form of dysfunctional uterine bleeding, menorrhagia can result from endocrine and hematologic disorders, stress, and certain drugs and procedures. Use of a hormonal contraceptive may cause sudden onset of profuse, prolonged menorrhagia. Anticoagulants have also been associated with excessive menstrual flow. Injectable or implanted contraceptives may cause menorrhagia in some women. Herbal remedies such as ginseng can cause postmenopausal bleeding.

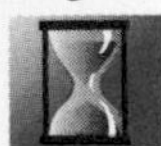

AGE ISSUE *In young females, irregular menstrual function may be accompanied by hemorrhage and resulting anemia. In postmenopausal women, menorrhagia can't occur. In such patients, vaginal bleeding is usually caused by endometrial atrophy. Malignancy must be ruled out in these cases.*

Metrorrhagia
Metrorrhagia — uterine bleeding that occurs irregularly between menstrual periods — is usually light. However, it can range from staining to hemorrhage.

History
Begin your evaluation by obtaining a thorough menstrual history. Ask the patient when she began menstruating and about the duration of menstrual periods, the interval between them, and the average number of tampons or pads she uses. Find out if metrorrhagia usually occurs in relation to her period. Ask if she experiences other signs or symptoms. Find out the date of her last menses, and ask about any other recent changes in her normal menstrual pattern. Get details of any previous gynecologic problems. If applicable, obtain a contraceptive and obstetric history. Record the dates of her last Pap test and pelvic examination. Ask the patient when she last had sexual intercourse and whether she was protected. Next, ask about her general health and any recent changes. Find out if she's under emotional stress. If possible, obtain a pregnancy history of the patient's mother. Find out if the patient was exposed in utero to diethylstilbestrol, which has been linked to vaginal adenosis.

Physical assessment
Perform a pelvic examination if indicated, and obtain blood and urine samples for pregnancy testing.

Analysis
Usually, metrorrhagia is a common sign that reflects slight physiologic bleeding from the endometrium during ovulation. However, metrorrhagia may be the only indication of an underlying gynecologic disorder and can result from stress, drugs, treatments, and intrauterine devices. Anticoagulants and oral, injectable, or implanted contraceptives may cause metrorrhagia. Cervical conization and cauterization also may cause metrorrhagia.

Nocturia
Nocturia — excessive urination at night — may result from disruption of the normal diurnal pattern of urine concentration or from overstimulation of the nerves and muscles that control urination. Normally, more urine is concentrated during the night than during the day. As a result, most people excrete three to four times more urine during the day, and can sleep for 6 to 8 hours during the night without being awakened. The patient with nocturia may awaken one or more times during the night to empty her bladder and excrete 700 ml or more of urine.

History
Begin by exploring the history of the patient's nocturia. Ask when it began, how it occurs, and if she can identify a specific pattern. Find out if there are any precipitating factors. Also note the volume of urine voided. Ask the patient about changes in the color, odor, or consistency of her urine. Find out if the patient has changed her usual pattern or volume of fluid intake. Next, explore associated symptoms. Ask about pain or burning on urination, difficulty initiating a urine stream, costovertebral angle tenderness, and flank, upper abdominal, or suprapubic pain.

Determine if the patient or her family has a history of renal or urinary tract disorders or endocrine and metabolic diseases, particularly diabetes. Find out if she's taking a drug that increases urine output, such as a diuretic, cardiac glycoside, or an antihypertensive.

Physical assessment
Focus your physical examination on palpating and percussing the kidneys, the costovertebral angle, and the bladder. Carefully inspect the urinary meatus. Obtain a urine specimen and inspect it for color, odor, and the presence of sediment.

Analysis
Although nocturia usually results from renal and lower urinary tract disorders, it may result from certain cardiovascular, endocrine, and metabolic disorders. This common sign may also result from drugs that induce diuresis, particularly when they're taken at night, and from the ingestion of large quantities of fluids, especially caffeinated beverages or alcohol, at bedtime. Any drug that mobilizes edematous fluid or produces diuresis (for example, a diuretic or a cardiac glycoside) may cause nocturia; obviously, this effect depends on when the drug is administered.

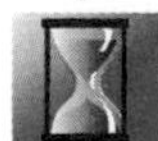

AGE ISSUE *In children, nocturia may be voluntary or involuntary. The latter is commonly known as enuresis, or bedwetting. Children with nocturia due to pyelonephritis are more susceptible to sepsis, which may display as fever, irritability, and poor skin perfusion. In addition, young females may experience vaginal discharge and vulvar soreness or pruritus. Postmenopausal women have decreased bladder elasticity, but urine output remains constant, resulting in nocturia.*

Oliguria
A cardinal sign of renal and urinary tract disorders, oliguria is clinically defined as urine output of less than 400 ml in 24 hours. Typically, this sign occurs abruptly and may herald serious — possibly life-threatening — hemodynamic instability.

History
Begin by asking the patient about her usual daily voiding pattern, including frequency and amount. Find out when she first noticed changes in this pattern and in the color, odor, or consistency of her urine. Ask about pain or burning on urination. Find out if the patient has had a fever. Note her normal daily fluid intake. Ask if she has recently been drinking more or less than usual. Find out if her caffeine or alcohol intake has changed drastically. Ask about recent episodes of diarrhea or vomiting that might cause fluid loss. Next, explore associated complaints, especially fatigue, loss of appetite, thirst, dyspnea, chest pain, or recent weight gain or loss due to dehydration.

Check for a history of renal, urinary tract, or cardiovascular disorders. Note recent traumatic injury or surgery associated with significant blood loss, as well as recent blood transfusions. Find out if the patient was exposed to nephrotoxic agents, such as heavy metals, organic solvents, anesthetics, or radiographic contrast media. Next, obtain a drug history.

Physical assessment
Begin the physical examination by taking the patient's vital signs and weighing her. Assess her overall appearance for edema. Palpate both kidneys for tenderness and enlargement, and percuss for costovertebral angle tenderness. Also inspect the flank area for edema or erythema. Auscultate the heart and lungs for abnormal sounds, and the flank area for renal artery bruits. Assess the patient for edema or signs of dehydration such as dry mucous membranes.

Obtain a urine sample and inspect it for abnormal color, odor, or sediment. Use reagent strips to test for glucose, protein, and blood. Measure specific gravity.

Analysis
The causes of oliguria can be classified as prerenal, resulting in decreased renal blood flow; intrarenal, resulting in intrinsic renal damage; or postrenal, resulting in urinary tract obstruction. Oliguria associated with a prerenal or postrenal cause is usually promptly reversible with treatment, although it may lead to intrarenal damage if untreated. However, oliguria associated with an intrarenal cause is usually more persistent and may be irreversible.

Radiographic studies that use contrast media may cause nephrotoxicity and oliguria. Oliguria may also result from drugs that cause decreased renal perfusion such as diuretics; nephrotoxicity, most notably due to aminoglycosides and chemotherapeutic drugs; urine retention due to adrenergics and anticholinergics; or urinary obstruction associated with precipitation of urinary crystals due to sulfonamides and acyclovir.

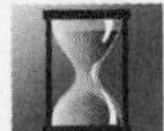

AGE ISSUE *In the neonate, oliguria may result from edema or dehydration. Major causes include congenital heart disease, respiratory distress syndrome, sepsis, congenital hydronephrosis, acute tubular necrosis, and renal vein thrombosis. Common causes of oliguria in children between ages 1 and 5 are acute poststreptococcal glomerulonephritis and hemolytic-uremic syndrome. After age 5, causes of oliguria are similar to those in adults. In elderly patients, oliguria may result from the gradual progression of an underlying disorder. It may also result from overall poor muscle tone secondary to inactivity, poor fluid intake, and infrequent voiding attempts.*

Urinary frequency

Urinary frequency refers to an increased incidence of the urge to void without an increase in the total volume of urine produced.

History

Ask the patient how many times a day she voids. Find out how this compares to her previous pattern of voiding. Ask about the onset and duration of the abnormal frequency and about any associated urinary signs or symptoms, such as dysuria, urgency, incontinence, hematuria, discharge, or lower abdominal pain with urination. Ask also about neurologic symptoms, such as muscle weakness, numbness, or tingling. Explore her medical history for UTI, other urologic problems or recent urologic procedures, and neurologic disorders. Ask whether she is or could be pregnant.

Physical assessment

Obtain a clean-catch midstream sample for urinalysis and culture and sensitivity tests. Then palpate the patient's suprapubic area, abdomen, and flanks, noting any tenderness. Examine her urethral meatus for redness, discharge, or swelling.

If the patient's medical history reveals symptoms or a history of neurologic disorders, perform a neurologic examination.

Analysis

Usually resulting from decreased bladder capacity, urinary frequency is a cardinal sign of UTI. However, it can also stem from another urologic disorder, neurologic dysfunction, or pressure on the bladder from a nearby tumor or from organ enlargement, as with pregnancy. Excessive intake of coffee, tea, and other caffeinated beverages leads to urinary frequency. These substances, which include caffeine, reduce the body's total volume of water and salt by increasing urine excretion. Radiation therapy may cause bladder inflammation, leading to urinary frequency.

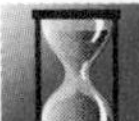

AGE ISSUE *In children, especially females, UTIs are a common cause of urinary frequency. Congenital anomalies that can cause UTIs include a duplicated ureter, congenital bladder diverticulum, and an ectopicureteral orifice.*

Urinary incontinence

Incontinence, the uncontrollable passage of urine, results from either a bladder abnormality or a neurologic disorder. A common urologic sign, incontinence may be transient or permanent and may involve large volumes of urine or scant dribbling.

History

Ask the patient when she first noticed the incontinence and whether it began suddenly or gradually. Have her describe her typical urinary pattern. Find out if the incontinence usually occurs during the day or at night. Ask her if she has any urinary control or if she's totally incontinent. If she sometimes urinates with control, ask her the usual times and amounts voided. Determine her normal fluid intake. Ask about other urinary problems, such as hesitancy, frequency, urgency, nocturia, and decreased force or interruption of the urinary stream.

Also ask if she has ever sought treatment for incontinence or found a way to deal with it herself. Obtain a medical history, especially noting UTI, childbirth, spinal injury or tumor, stroke, or surgery involving the bladder or pelvic floor.

Physical assessment

After completing the health history, have the patient empty her bladder. Inspect the urethral meatus for obvious inflammation or anatomic defect. Have her bear down; note any urine leakage. Gently palpate the abdomen for bladder distention, which signals urine retention. Perform a complete neurologic assessment, noting motor and sensory function and obvious muscle atrophy.

Analysis
Urinary incontinence can be classified as stress, overflow, urge, or total incontinence. Stress incontinence refers to intermittent leakage resulting from a sudden physical strain, such as a cough, sneeze, or quick movement. Overflow incontinence is a dribble resulting from urine retention, which fills the bladder and prevents it from contracting with sufficient force to expel a urinary stream. Urge incontinence refers to the inability to suppress a sudden urge to urinate. Total incontinence is continuous leakage resulting from the bladder's inability to retain any urine.

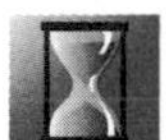

AGE ISSUE *In children, causes of incontinence include infrequent or incomplete voiding. These may also lead to UTI. In elderly patients, diagnosing a UTI can be problematic because many present only with urinary incontinence or changes in mental status, anorexia, or malaise. In addition, many elderly patients without UTIs present with dysuria, frequency, urgency, or incontinence.*

Vaginal discharge
Common in women of childbearing age, physiologic vaginal discharge is mucoid, clear or white, nonbloody, and odorless. Produced by the cervical mucosa and, to a lesser degree, by the vulvar glands, this discharge may occasionally be scant or profuse due to estrogenic stimulation and changes during menses. However, a marked increase in discharge or a change in discharge color, odor, or consistency can signal disease.

History
Ask the patient to describe the onset, color, consistency, odor, and texture of her vaginal discharge. Find out how the discharge differs from her usual vaginal secretions. Ask her if the onset is related to her menstrual cycle. Also ask about associated symptoms, such as dysuria and perineal pruritus and burning. Find out if she has spotting after coitus or douching. Ask about recent changes in sexual habits and hygiene practices. Find out if she is or could possibly be pregnant. Next, ask if she has had vaginal discharge before or has ever been treated for a vaginal infection. Find out what treatment was given and if she completed the course of medication. Ask about current use of medications, especially antibiotics, oral estrogens, and contraceptives.

Physical assessment
Examine the external genitalia and note the character of the discharge. Observe vulvar and vaginal tissues for redness, edema, and excoriation. Palpate the inguinal lymph nodes to detect tenderness or enlargement, and palpate the abdomen for tenderness. A pelvic examination may be required. Obtain vaginal discharge specimens for testing.

Analysis
The discharge may result from an infection, a sexually transmitted or reproductive tract disease, a fistula, or use of certain drugs. In addition, the prolonged presence of a foreign body, such as a tampon or diaphragm, in the patient's vagina can cause irritation and an inflammatory exudate, as can frequent douching, feminine hygiene products, contraceptive products, bubble baths, and colored or perfumed toilet papers.

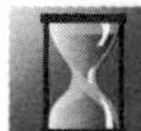

AGE ISSUE *Female neonates who have been exposed to maternal estrogens in utero may have a white mucous vaginal discharge for the first month after birth; a yellow mucous discharge indicates a pathologic condition. In the older child, a purulent, foul-smelling, and bloody vaginal discharge may result if a foreign object is placed in the vagina. The possibility of sexual abuse should be considered in this instance. In postmenopausal women, the vaginal mucosa becomes thin due to decreased estrogen levels. Together with a rise in vaginal pH, this reduces resistance to infectious agents, increasing the incidence of vaginitis.*

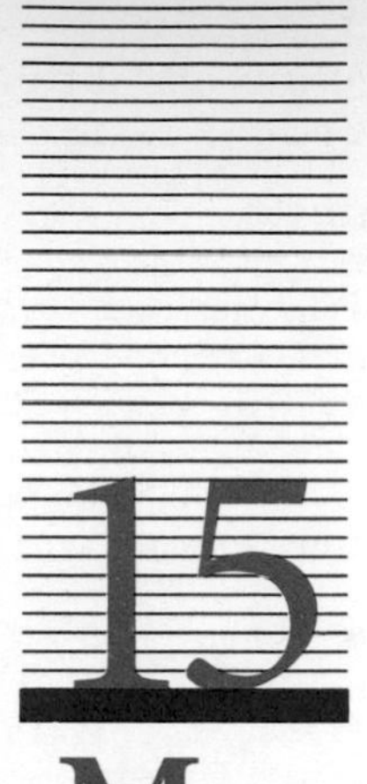

15 Male genitourinary system

Any disorder of the male urinary tract or reproductive system can have far-reaching consequences and can influence other body systems. These disorders have a great potential to challenge the quality of a man's life, including his self-esteem and sense of well-being.

Despite the potential compromises and general changes in social behavior, men remain reluctant to discuss their genitourinary (GU) system problems with health care providers. Therefore, it's essential that you gain insight into the cultural background of your patient and conduct yourself in a professional manner at all times. Providing a setting where both you and the patient are comfortable in the examination will allow openness in the evaluation of your patient's needs.

To thoroughly and accurately assess your patient's GU system, you'll need to review and have an understanding of the anatomy and physiology of the urinary and reproductive systems.

Urinary system

The urinary system helps maintain homeostasis by regulating fluid and electrolyte balance. It consists of the kidneys, ureters, bladder, and urethra. (For more information on these organs and their functions, see chapter 14, Female genitourinary system.) The essential functions of the urinary system, such as forming urine and maintaining homeostasis, occur in the highly vascular kidneys. This process involves filtration, reabsorption, and secretion.

Although the male and female urinary systems function in the same way, a man's urethra is 6″ (15.2 cm) longer than a

STRUCTURES OF THE MALE REPRODUCTIVE SYSTEM

This illustration shows the structures of the male reproductive system.

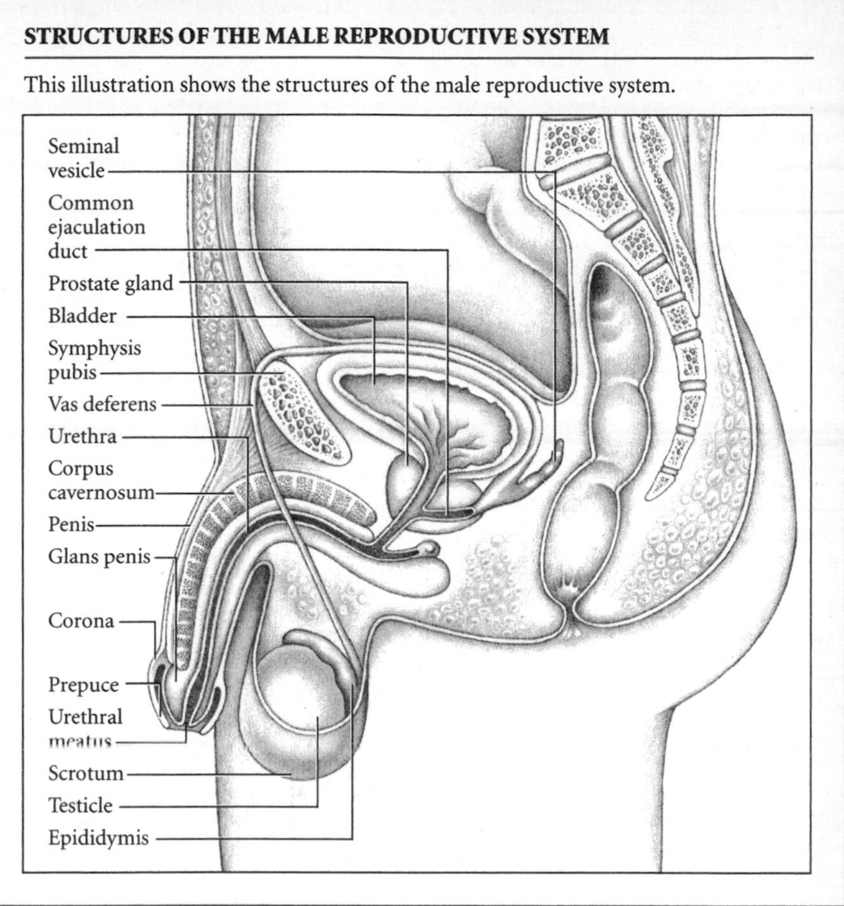

woman's. That's because it must pass through the erectile tissue of the penis. In the male, the urethra is about 8″ (20 cm) long, with the urethral meatus located at the end of the glans penis.

Reproductive system

The male reproductive system consists of the organs that produce, transfer, and introduce mature sperm into the female reproductive tract, where fertilization occurs. In addition to supplying male sex cells, called *spermatogenesis*, the male reproductive system plays a part in the secretion of male sex hormones.

In men, the urethra is also part of the reproductive system, carrying semen as well as urine. Contraction of the muscle fibers that surround the urethra inhibits the retrograde flow of semen into the bladder during ejaculation. The male reproductive system also includes the penis, scrotum, testicles, epididymis, vas deferens, seminal vesicles, and prostate gland. (See *Structures of the male reproductive system.*)

Penis

The penis consists of the shaft, glans, urethral meatus, corona, and prepuce. The skin of the penis is hairless and usually darker than the skin on other parts of the body.

The shaft contains three columns of vascular erectile tissue. The glans is located at the end of the penis. The urethral meatus, which is the slitlike opening, is located ventrally at the tip of the glans. The corona is formed by the junction of the glans and the shaft. The prepuce, the loose skin covering the glans, is commonly removed shortly after birth in a surgical procedure called circumcision.

When the penile tissues are engorged with blood, the erect penis can discharge sperm. During sexual activity, sperm and semen are forcefully ejaculated from the urethral meatus.

Scrotum

The scrotum is located at the base of the penis. It's a loose, wrinkled, deeply pigmented pouch that consists of a muscle layer covered by skin. Each of its two compartments contains a testicle, epididymis, and portions of the spermatic cord. The left side of the scrotum is usually lower than the right because the left spermatic cord is longer.

Testicles

The testicles are oval, rubbery structures suspended vertically and slightly forward in the scrotum. They produce testosterone and sperm.

Testosterone stimulates the changes that occur during puberty, which begins between ages 9½ and 13½. The testicles enlarge, pubic hair grows, and penis size increases. Secondary sex characteristics appear, such as facial and body hair, muscle development, and voice changes.

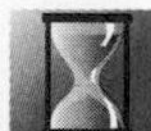

AGE ISSUE *In young males, the first sign of pubescent changes is the enlargement of the testicles, along with pubic hair and increased size of the penis. These stages of development are documented in Tanner's sexuality ratings.*

Epididymis

The epididymis is a reservoir for maturing sperm. It curves over the posterolateral surface of each testicle, creating a visible bulge on the surface. In a small number of males, the epididymis is located anteriorly.

Vas deferens

The vas deferens — a storage site and the pathway for sperm — begins at the lower end of the epididymis, climbs the spermatic cord, travels through the inguinal canal, and ends in the abdominal cavity where it rests on the fundus of the bladder.

Seminal vesicles

A pair of saclike glands, the seminal vesicles are found on the lower posterior surface of the bladder in front of the rectum. Secretions from the seminal vesicles help form seminal fluid.

Prostate gland

A walnut-shaped gland about 2½″ (6.5 cm) long, the prostate surrounds the urethra like a doughnut, just below the bladder. It produces a thin, milky, alkaline fluid that mixes with seminal fluid during ejaculation. During sexual activity, prostatic fluid adds volume to the semen and enhances sperm motility and, possibly, fertility by neutralizing the acidity of the urethra and of the woman's vagina.

Inguinal structures

The spermatic cord travels from the testis through the inguinal canal, exiting the scrotum through the external inguinal ring and entering the abdominal cavity through the internal inguinal ring. The external inguinal ring is located just above and lateral to the pubic tubercle; the internal ring, about ½″ (1 cm) above the midpoint of the inguinal ligament, between the pubic tubercle of the symphysis pubis and the anterior superior iliac spine. Between the two rings lies the inguinal canal. Lymph nodes from the penis, scrotal surface, and anus drain into the inguinal lymph nodes. Lymph nodes from the testes drain into the lateral aortic and preaortic lymph nodes in the abdomen.

Spermatogenesis

Sperm formation, or spermatogenesis, begins when a male reaches puberty and normally continues throughout life. Spermatogenesis occurs in four stages:

- In the first stage, the primary germinal epithelial cells, called *spermatogonia,* grow and develop into primary spermatocytes. Both spermatogonia and primary spermatocytes contain 46 chromosomes, consisting of 44 autosomes and the two sex chromosomes, X and Y.
- In the second stage, primary spermatocytes divide to form secondary spermatocytes. No new chromosomes are formed in

this stage; the pairs only divide. Each secondary spermatocyte contains half the number of autosomes, 22; one secondary spermatocyte contains an X chromosome, the other, a Y chromosome.

- In the third stage, each secondary spermatocyte divides again to form spermatids also called *spermatoblasts.*
- In the fourth and final stage, the spermatids undergo a series of structural changes that transform them into mature spermatozoa, or sperm. Each spermatozoa has a head, neck, body, and tail. The head contains the nucleus, the tail, a large amount of actenosine triphosphate, which provides energy for sperm motility.

Newly mature sperm pass from the seminiferous tubules through the vasa recta into the epididymis. Only a small number of sperm can be stored in the epididymis. Most of them move into the vas deferens, where they're stored until sexual stimulation triggers emission.

Sperm cells retain their potency in storage for many weeks. After ejaculation, sperm survive for 24 to 72 hours at body temperature.

Hormones

Androgens, or male sex hormones, are produced in the testes and the adrenal glands. Androgens are responsible for the development of male sex organs and secondary sex characteristics. Major androgens include testosterone, luteinizing hormone (LH), and follicle-stimulating hormone (FSH).

Leydig's cells, located in the testes between the seminiferous tubules, secrete testosterone, the most significant male sex hormone.

Testosterone is responsible for the development and maintenance of male sex organs and secondary sex characteristics, such as facial hair and vocal cord thickness. Testosterone is also required for spermatogenesis.

Testosterone secretion begins approximately 2 months after conception, when the release of chorionic gonadotropins from the placenta stimulates Leydig's cells in the male fetus. The presence of testosterone directly affects sexual differentiation in the fetus. With testosterone, fetal genitalia develop into a penis, scrotum, and testes; without testosterone, genitalia develop into a clitoris, vagina, and other female organs.

During the last 2 months of gestation, testosterone normally causes the testes to descend into the scrotum. If the testes don't descend after birth, exogenous testosterone may correct the problem.

Other hormones also affect male sexuality. Two of these, LH—also called *interstitial cell-stimulating hormone*—and FSH, directly affect secretion of testosterone.

During early childhood, a young male doesn't secrete gonadotropins and thus has minimal circulating testosterone. Secretion of gonadotropins from the pituitary gland, which usually occurs between ages 11 and 14, marks the onset of puberty. These pituitary gonadotropins stimulate testis functioning as well as testosterone secretion.

During puberty, the penis and testes enlarge and the male reaches full adult sexual and reproductive capability. Puberty also marks the development of male secondary sex characteristics that includes distinct body hair distribution; skin changes, such as increased secretion by sweat and sebaceous glands; deepening of the voice, from laryngeal enlargement; increased musculoskeletal development; and other intracellular and extracellular changes.

After a male achieves full physical maturity, usually by age 20, sexual and reproductive function remain fairly consistent throughout life.

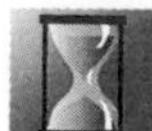

AGE ISSUE *With aging, males may experience subtle changes in sexual function, but they don't lose the ability to reproduce. For example, elderly males may require more time to achieve an erection, experience less firm erections, and have reduced ejaculatory volume. After ejaculation, they may also take longer to regain an erection.*

Health history

Obtaining a health history about the male GU system requires a sensitive, considerate, nonjudgmental approach. Men can be sensitive when questioned about sexual performance; they tend to equate sexual and reproductive functioning with manhood and may view sexual problems as signs of diminished masculinity.

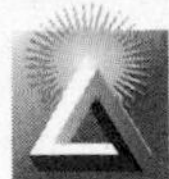

EXPERT TECHNIQUE

EASING PATIENT DISCOMFORT

Here are some steps to take for helping your male patients feel more comfortable during the health history interview:

- Make sure that the room is private and that there are no interruptions.
- Phrase your questions in a clear and tactful manner.
- Tell the patient that his answers are and will remain confidential.
- Begin with less sensitive questions about his urinary function, and then lead up to more sensitive areas such as sexual function.
- Don't rush or omit important facts because the patient displays embarrassment.
- Be sensitive to the older patient's responses during the interview because he may view decreases in sexual prowess as a sign of declining health.
- When asking questions, keep in mind that many male patients view sexual problems as a sign of diminished masculinity. Phrase your questions carefully and offer reassurance as needed.
- Consider the patient's educational and cultural background. If he uses slang or euphemisms to talk about his sexual organs or their function, make sure you're both discussing the same subject.

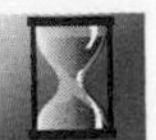

AGE ISSUE *Older men may view diminishing sexual ability as a sign of lost youth and declining health.*

A patient with sexual dysfunction may feel uncomfortable discussing it. Assure him that his replies to your questions will be kept strictly confidential. To put him at ease, begin the interview with general questions about his health as it relates to the male reproductive system. Reserve questions about sexual function until the end of the health history.

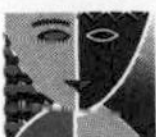

CULTURAL INSIGHT *Remember that the patient has his own view of sexuality and reproduction, largely influenced by his cultural and religious background. Consider these views and remain nonjudgmental and supportive.*

During the assessment, use terminology that the patient can understand. Medical terminology may be confusing, especially to a younger patient. On the other hand, using too much slang may render the interview process too informal to be effective. (See *Easing patient discomfort.*)

Chief complaint

Ask the patient about his chief complaint. Document his answer using his own words. If he can't identify a single reason, ask more specific questions about his current and past health status.

Common complaints about the male GU system include changes in voiding patterns, pain during urination, scrotal or inguinal mass, sexual impotence, and infertility.

Current health history

Explore the patient's chief complaint in detail. Find out how the patient's symptoms developed and progressed. Ask if they began suddenly or gradually and if they occur continuously or intermittently. If intermittent, ask about the frequency and length of each episode. Ask the patient how long he has had the problem and how it affects his daily routine. Also ask about related signs and symptoms.

If he has had pain, ask about its location, radiation, intensity, and duration. Find out what precipitates, exacerbates, or relieves it. Ask him which, if any, self-help remedies and over-the-counter (OTC) medications he has used.

Ask the patient if he has diabetes or hypertension. Review the patient's chief complaint and obtain detailed information about it.

Changes in voiding patterns

If the patient voices a change in voiding patterns, ask him if he has to wait longer than a few seconds before urine flow begins. Find out if he strains to urinate and if he has a feeling of urgency to urinate. Ask him if his urinary stream seems smaller in caliber or less forceful than usual. Also ask him if he has been urinating more frequently or if he wakes up in the middle of the night to urinate.

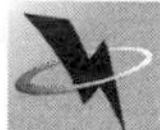

CRITICAL POINT *An obstructed or decreased urinary flow or an increase in urinary frequency, including nocturia, is commonly caused by an enlarged prostate gland. Also consider that the patient may have a urinary system disorder.*

Finally, ask the patient what color his urine is and if he has noticed any blood in it.

CRITICAL POINT *A patient with hematuria may have brown or bright red urine. Bleeding at the end of urination signals a disorder of the bladder neck, urethra, or prostate gland.*

Urethral discharge

If the patient complains of a discharge from his urethra, ask about the amount and if it's present only during urination or if it occurs continuously. Find out what color it is and its consistency.

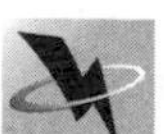

CRITICAL POINT *Large quantities of thick, creamy, yellow-green discharge usually indicate gonorrhea. A thin, watery discharge may suggest a nonspecific urethritis or a prostate infection. A bloody discharge may indicate an infection or cancer in the urinary or reproductive tract.*

Next, ask the patient about sores, lumps, or ulcers that may appear on his penis. Ask him if he has noticed bleeding from the opening where urine comes out. Find out he has noticed any swelling in his scrotum.

Also question the patient about the appearance of his reproductive organs. Find out if he has noticed changes in the color of the skin on his penis or scrotum. If he's uncircumcised, ask him if he can retract and replace the foreskin easily.

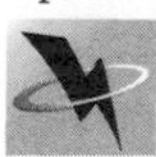

CRITICAL POINT *An inability to retract the prepuce, or foreskin, is called* phimosis; *an inability to replace it is called* paraphimosis. *Untreated, these conditions can impair local circulation and lead to edema and even gangrene.*

Pain or tenderness

Ask the patient if urination is painful. This may suggest a nonspecific urinary tract infection (UTI) or a sexually transmitted disease (STD). Ask if the painful passage of urine is accompanied by spasms, or strangury. This may result from bladder or prostate infection. Find out if dull, aching scrotal pain worsens when he strains to urinate. This could indicate an inguinal hernia. Ask the patient if he has urinary frequency, hesitancy, or dribbling; or pain in the area between his rectum and penis or his hips or lower back.

CRITICAL POINT *Extreme scrotal pain that begins suddenly suggests testicular torsion. Gradual onset of acute pain accompanied by warmth, heat, and swelling, usually indicates an infection. Flank pain suggests renal calculi.*

Scrotal or inguinal mass

If the patient reports a mass in the scrotal or inguinal area, ask him if the mass disappears when he lies flat on his back. Commonly, this indicates an inguinal hernia. Also ask the patient if has recently received an injury to his genitals. This may cause a hematocele.

Ask about the duration of the mass. Ask him how long the mass has been present and if there are associated symptoms such as pain or tenderness. Although benign conditions may be painless, testicular cancer must be considered.

Sexual impotence

Begin your questions about sexual impotence by stating to the patient that it has different meanings for each individual. Then ask him to describe what sexual impotence means to him. Clarifying the patient's understanding of impotence is important, because sexual terms are frequently misunderstood and misused. First, ask him if he has difficulty achieving and maintaining an erection during sexual activity and, if so, find out if he has erections at other times such as on awakening. Ask him if he has nocturnal or morning erections. Find out if he has difficulty with ejaculation and if he ever experiences pain from erection or ejaculation. Ask the patient what his lifestyle was like at the time the problem began. Ask if the problem began suddenly or gradually. Sudden impotence that occurs during a stressful time in the patient's life most likely originates psychogenically. Finally, ask the patient if he can achieve an erection through fantasizing or masturbation. Patients with psychogenic impotence usually retain these capabilities.

Ask the patient about the medications that he takes, including prescription, OTC, and illicit drugs. Many drugs affect the male reproductive system. For example, anticonvulsants, antidepressants, antihypertensives, beta-adrenergic blockers, antipsychotics, anticholinergics, and androgenic steroids can cause impotence. Antidepressants, antihypertensives, antipsychotics, beta-adrenergic blockers, benzodiazepines, and androgenic steroids can cause changes in libido. Antidepressants and beta-adrenergic blockers can also cause ejaculatory failure.

Infertility

If your patient and his partner are experiencing infertility, find out how long he and his partner have been trying to achieve pregnancy. Suspect infertility only if the couple has engaged regularly in intercourse, without using birth control, for at least 1 year. Gather additional information by finding out if the patient has a low sex drive, premature ejaculation, or impotence. Ask if his sexual development was normal. Also ask if he has had any infections or injuries to his testes.

Past health history

Information about the patient's past illnesses is important; past reproductive system problems or dysfunctions in other body systems may affect present reproductive function. Start by asking your patient if he has fathered any children and, if so, how many and their current ages. Find out if the patient has ever had a problem with infertility and if it's currently a concern. Ask him if he has ever been diagnosed with a low sperm count. If so, hot baths, frequent bicycle riding, and tight underwear or athletic supporters can elevate scrotal temperature and temporarily decrease sperm count.

Next, ask the patient if he has ever had surgery on the GU tract and, if so, where, when, and why. Find out if he experienced any postoperative complications. Ask about any trauma to the GU tract and, if so, what happened, when did it occur, and what symptoms have developed as a result. Ask the patient if he has ever experienced blood in the urine, difficulty urinating, an excessive urge to urinate, dribbling, or difficulty maintaining the urine stream.

Ask the patient if he has ever been diagnosed as having an STD or other infection in the GU tract. If so, find out what the specific problem was and how long it lasted. Ask him about treatment and if any associated complications developed. Also find out if he has ever been tested for human immunodeficiency virus, the virus that causes acquired immunodeficiency syndrome (AIDS).

Ask the patient if he has diabetes mellitus, cardiovascular disease, neurologic disease, or cancer of the GU tract. Find out if there's a history of undescended testes or an endocrine disorder. Ask him if he has ever had the mumps and, if so, did the disease affect his testes.

Finally, ask the patient if he examines his testes periodically. Make sure that he has been taught the proper procedure for doing so.

Family history

Questions about family health history can provide clues to disorders with known familial tendencies. Ask the patient if anyone in his family has had infertility problems or a hernia. Also ask him if anyone in his family has ever had cancer of the reproductive tract.

Psychosocial history

Obtain information about the patient's lifestyle and relationships with others. First, find out if the patient is sexually active and, if so, does he have more than one partner. Ask how many partners he has had during the last month. Multiple partners can lead to increased incidence of STDs, hepatitis, and AIDS.

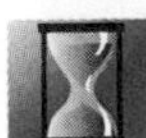

AGE ISSUE *Elderly adults who are sexually active with multiple partners have as high a risk of developing an STD, as do younger adults. However, because of decreased immunity, poor hygiene, poor symptom reporting and, possibly, several concurrent conditions, they may seek treatment for different symptoms.*

Next, find out if the patient's sexual practices are homosexual, bisexual, or heterosexual. Ask him if he takes precautions to prevent contracting an STD or AIDS. If so, find out what he does. Ask about his employment and if he has ever been exposed to radiation or toxic chemicals.

Ask the patient if he engages in sports or in activities that require heavy lifting or straining. If so, ask him if he wears any protective or supportive devices, such as a jock strap, protective cup, or truss.

Ask the patient if he's under a lot of stress. Find out how he perceives himself and if he considers himself to be attractive to others.

Find out about his cultural and religious backgrounds and if cultural or religious factors affect his beliefs or practices regarding sexuality and reproduction.

Finally, ask the patient if he has a supportive relationship with another person. Also find out if he's experiencing sexual difficulty and if it's affecting his emotional and social relationships.

Physical assessment

To perform a physical assessment of the male GU system, use the techniques of inspection, percussion, palpation, and auscultation. Assessment of the urinary system may be done at this time or as part of the GI assessment.

Urinary system assessment

In many ways, assessing the male urinary system is similar to assessing the female urinary system. Before examining specific structures, check the patient's blood pressure and weight and observe the patient's skin.

Inspect the patient's overall appearance of the skin. A patient with decreased renal function may be pale because of a low hemoglobin level or may even have uremic frost — snowlike crystals on the skin from metabolic wastes. Also look for signs of fluid imbalance, such as dry mucous membranes, sunken eyeballs, edema, or ascites.

Before performing an assessment, ask the patient to urinate. If appropriate, obtain a urinalysis. Help him into the supine position with his arms at his sides. As you proceed, expose only the areas being examined.

Inspection

First, inspect the patient's abdomen. When he's supine, his abdomen should be smooth, flat or concave, and symmetrical. The skin should be free from lesions, bruises, discolorations, and prominent veins.

Watch for abdominal distention with tight, glistening skin and striae — silvery streaks caused by rapidly developing skin tension.

CRITICAL POINT *Abdominal distention with tight, glistening skin and striae indicates ascites, which may accompany nephrotic syndrome. This syndrome is characterized by edema, increased urine protein levels, and decreased serum albumin levels.*

Percussion and palpation

First, tell the patient what you're going to do; otherwise, he may be startled, and you could mistake his reaction for a feeling of acute tenderness. Next, percuss the kidneys to check for pain or tenderness and the bladder to elicit tympany or dullness.

If a patient experiences pain or tenderness upon kidney percussion and palpation, this may suggest a kidney infection. (See chapter 14, Female genitourinary system, page 390, which discusses performing fist percussion.)

Remember to percuss both sides of the body to assess both kidneys. If you hear a dull sound instead of the normal tympany, this may indicate urine retention in the bladder caused by bladder dysfunction or infection.

Also palpate the bladder to check for distention. Because the kidneys aren't usually palpable, detecting an enlarged kidney may prove to be important. Kidney enlargement may accompany hydronephrosis, a cyst, or a tumor.

Auscultation

Auscultate the renal arteries to rule out bruits, which signal renal artery stenosis. You can perform this now or as part of an abdominal assessment.

Reproductive system assessment

Before examining the reproductive system, or any part of the body, first wash your hands and ask the patient if he has a latex allergy; if he doesn't, put on examination gloves. Make sure the patient is as comfortable as possible and ensure that the privacy curtain is drawn and the door is closed.

MALE GENITAL LESIONS

Several types of lesions may affect the male genitalia. Some of the more common lesions are described here.

Penile cancer

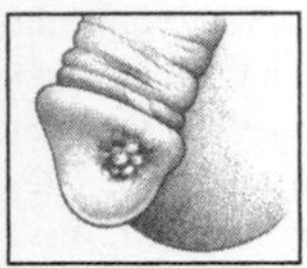

Penile cancer causes a painless, ulcerative lesion on the glans or foreskin, possibly accompanied by discharge. It's generally associated with genital herpes viral infections. The cancer presents as a local mass or bleeding ulcer and metastasizes early.

Genital herpes

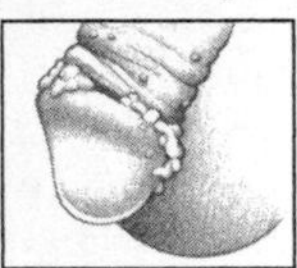

Genital herpes causes a painful, reddened group of small vesicles or blisters on the foreskin, shaft, or glans. Although lesions eventually disappear, the virus can remain latent in the nervous tissues and stress may reactivate their reoccurrence. The vesicles are associated with itching or pain.

Genital warts

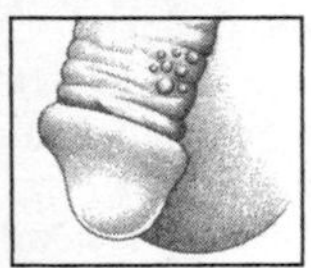

Genital warts appear as small, soft, moist, pink or red, swollen papillary growths that may be painless and appear as cauliflower-like groups. They are caused by the human papillomavirus and are sexually transmitted. Atypical warts may possibly be related to carcinoma.

Syphilis

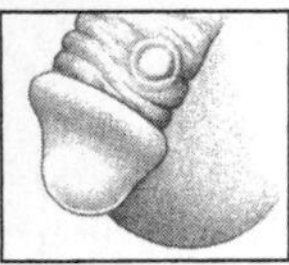

Syphilis causes a hard, round papule—usually on the glans penis. When palpated, this syphilitic chancre may feel like a button. Eventually, the papule erodes into an ulcer. You may also note swollen lymph nodes in the inguinal area. Syphilis occurs in three stages: the primary stage produces a bloodless ulcer known as a *chancre,* which contains spirochetes. This lesion spontaneously heals in 10 to 40 days and may not be of concern to the patient; the secondary and tertiary stages involve the other body systems and become more debilitating with the disease's progress.

Inspection

Inspect the penis, scrotum, and testicles, as well as the inguinal and femoral areas.

Penis. Start by examining the penis. Penis size depends on the patient's age and overall development.

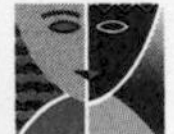

CULTURAL INSIGHT *The penile skin should be slightly wrinkled and the color should be pink to light brown in Whites and light brown to dark brown in Blacks.*

Ask an uncircumcised patient to retract his prepuce, or foreskin, to expose the glans penis. Normally, he can do this easily to reveal a glans with no ulcers or lesions and then easily replace it over the glans after inspection.

Check the penile shaft and glans for lesions, nodules, inflammation, and swelling. Inflammation of the glans is called *balanitis;* inflammation of the glans and prepuce is called *balanoposthitis*. Lesions on the penis can vary in appearance. A hard, nontender nodule, especially on the glans or inner lip of the prepuce, may indicate penile cancer. (See *Male genital lesions.*) Also check the

EXPERT TECHNIQUE

EXAMINING THE URETHRAL MEATUS

To inspect the urethral meatus, compress the tip of the glans, as shown.

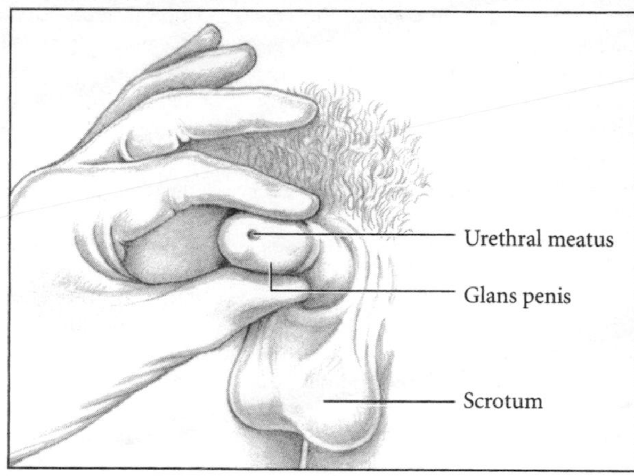

glans for smegma, a cheesy secretion commonly found beneath the prepuce.

Next, gently compress the tip of the glans to open the urethral meatus. It should be located in the center of the glans and be pink and smooth. When the urethral meatus is located on the underside of the penis, the condition is called *hypospadias.* When the urethral meatus is placed on the top of the penis, it's called *epispadias.* Both conditions are congenital.

Inspect the penis for swelling, discharge, lesions, inflammation and, especially, genital warts. If you note discharge, obtain a culture specimen. (See *Examining the urethral meatus.*) A profuse, yellow discharge from the penis suggests gonococcal urethritis. Other symptoms include urinary frequency, burning, and urgency. Without treatment, the prostate gland, epididymis, and periurethral glands will become inflamed. A copious, watery, purulent urethral discharge may indicate chlamydial infection; a bloody discharge may indicate infection or cancer in the urinary or reproductive tract.

Scrotum and testicles. To inspect the scrotum, first evaluate the amount, distribution, color, and texture of pubic hair. Hair should cover the symphysis pubis and scrotum.

The absence of pubic hair or presence of bald spots is abnormal. So are lesions, ulcers, induration, or reddened areas, which may indicate infection or inflammation. Lack of pubic hair may indicate a vascular or hormonal problem.

Have the patient hold his penis away from his scrotum so you can observe the scrotum's general size and appearance. The skin here is darker than on the rest of the body. Spread the surface of the scrotum, and examine the skin for swelling, nodules, redness, ulceration, and distended veins.

Sebaceous cysts — firm, white to yellow, nontender cutaneous lesions — are a normal finding. Also check for pitting edema, a sign of cardiovascular disease. Spread the pubic hair and check the skin for lesions and parasites.

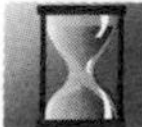

AGE ISSUE *Before palpating a boy's scrotum for a testicular examination, explain what you'll be doing and why. Make sure he's comfortable and warm and as relaxed as possible. Cold and anxiety may cause his testicles to retract so that you can't palpate them. Having a parent in the room may offer support. If you see an enlarged scrotum in a boy younger than age 2, suspect a scrotal extension of an inguinal hernia, a hydrocele, or both. Hydroceles, typically*

associated with inguinal hernias, are common in children of this age-group. To differentiate between the two, remember that hydroceles transilluminate and aren't tender or reducible. An obese adolescent boy may appear to have an abnormally small penis. You may have to retract the fat over the symphysis pubis to properly assess penis size. Have the child hold up any excessive adipose tissue, or have him lay down on the examination table.

Inguinal and femoral areas. Have the patient stand. Check the inguinal area for obvious bulges—a sign of hernias. Then ask the patient to bear down as you inspect again. This maneuver increases intra-abdominal pressure, which pushes any herniation downward and makes it more easily visible. Also check for enlarged lymph nodes which, if present, could suggest an infection.

Palpation

Palpate the penis, testicles, epididymis, spermatic cords, inguinal and femoral areas, and prostate gland.

Penis. Use your thumb and forefinger to palpate the entire penile shaft. It should be somewhat firm, and the skin should be smooth and movable. Note swelling, nodules, or indurations.

Testicles. Gently palpate both testicles between your thumb and first two fingers. Assess their size, shape, and response to pressure. A normal response is a deep visceral pain. The testicles should be equal in size, move freely in the scrotal sac, and feel firm, smooth, and rubbery.

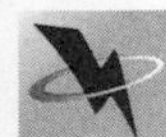

CRITICAL POINT *If you note hard, irregular areas or lumps, transilluminate them by darkening the examination room and pressing the head of a flashlight against the scrotum, behind the lump. The testicle and any lumps, masses, warts, or blood-filled areas will appear as opaque shadows. Transilluminate the other testicle to compare your findings.*

A painless scrotal nodule that can't be transilluminated may be a testicular tumor. This disorder is most common in men ages 20 to 35. The tumor can grow, enlarging the testicle.

Use this opportunity to reinforce the methods and importance of doing a monthly testicular self-examination.

Scrotal swelling occurs when a condition affecting the testicles, epididymis, or scrotal skin produces edema or a mass; the penis may not be involved. Scrotal swelling can affect males at any age. It can be unilateral or bilateral and painful or painless and can result from an inguinal hernia, hydrocele, or trauma to the scrotum.

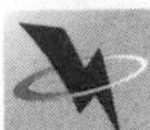

CRITICAL POINT *The sudden onset of painful scrotal swelling suggests torsion of a testicle or testicular appendages, especially in a prepubescent male. This emergency requires immediate surgery to untwist and stabilize the spermatic cord or to remove the appendage.*

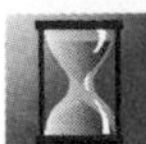

AGE ISSUE *In children up to age 1, a hernia or hydrocele of the spermatic cord may stem from abnormal fetal development. In infants, scrotal swelling may stem from ammonia-related dermatitis, if diapers aren't changed often enough. Other disorders that can produce scrotal swelling in children include epididymitis, which is rare in those younger than age 10; orchitis from contact sports; and mumps, which usually occurs after puberty.*

An enlarged scrotum may suggest hydrocele, or a collection of fluid in the testicle. Hydrocele is associated with conditions that cause poor fluid reabsorption, such as cirrhosis, heart failure, and testicular tumor. A hydrocele can be transilluminated.

The absence of a testis may result from temporary migration. The cremaster muscle surrounding the testes contracts in response to such stimuli as cold air, cold water, or touching the inner thigh. This contraction raises the contents of the scrotum toward the inguinal canal. When the muscle relaxes, the scrotal contents resume their normal position. This temporary migration is normal and may occur at any time during the assessment.

Epididymis. Next, palpate the epididymis, which is usually located in the posterolateral area of the testicle. It should be smooth, discrete, nontender, and free from swelling and induration.

Spermatic cords. Palpate both spermatic cords, which are located above each testicle.

EXPERT TECHNIQUE

PALPATING FOR AN INDIRECT INGUINAL HERNIA

To palpate for an indirect inguinal hernia, place your gloved finger on the neck of the scrotum and insert it into the inguinal canal, as shown. Then ask the patient to bear down.

If the patient has a hernia, you'll feel a soft mass at your fingertip.

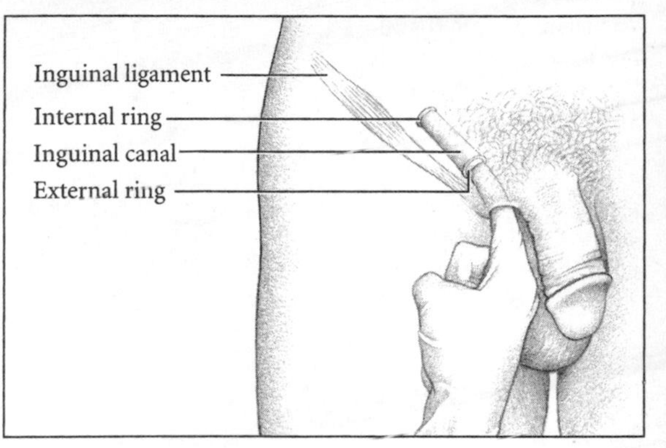

Palpate from the base of the epididymis to the inguinal canal. The vas deferens is a smooth, movable cord inside the spermatic cord. If you feel swelling, irregularity, or nodules, transilluminate the problem area as described earlier. If serous fluid is present, you won't see this glow.

Palpation of multiple tortuous veins in the spermatic cord area, usually on the left, suggests a varicocele.

Inguinal area. To assess the patient for a direct inguinal hernia, place two fingers over each external inguinal ring and ask the patient to bear down. If the patient has a hernia, you'll feel a bulge. It also feels like a mass of tissue that withdraws when it meets the finger.

To assess the patient for an indirect inguinal hernia, examine him while he's standing and then while he's in a supine position with his knee flexed on the side you're examining. (See *Palpating for an indirect inguinal hernia.*)

Place your index finger on the neck of the scrotum and gently push upward into the inguinal canal. The inguinal ring should feel like a triangular, slitlike opening. You may be able to place your finger into the canal. If you can insert your finger, do so as far as possible and then ask the patient to bear down or cough.

A direct inguinal hernia emerges from behind the external inguinal ring and protrudes through it. This type of hernia seldom descends into the scrotum and usually affects men older than age 40.

An indirect inguinal hernia is the most common type of hernia, and it occurs in men of all ages. It can be palpated in the internal inguinal canal with its tip in or beyond the canal, or the hernia may descend into the scrotum.

Femoral area. Although you can't palpate the femoral canal, you can estimate its location to help detect a femoral hernia. Place your right index finger on the right femoral artery with your finger pointing toward the patient's head. Keep your other fingers close together. Your middle finger will rest on the femoral vein; your ring finger, on the femoral canal. Note tenderness or masses. Use your left hand to check the patient's left side.

A femoral hernia feels like a soft tumor below the inguinal ligament in the femoral area. It may be difficult to distinguish from a lymph node and is uncommon in men.

Prostate gland. Tell the patient that he'll feel some pressure or urgency during this examination. Have him stand and lean over the examination table. If he can't do this, have him lie on his left side, with his right

EXPERT TECHNIQUE

PALPATING THE PROSTATE GLAND

To palpate the prostate gland, insert your gloved, lubricated index finger into the patient's rectum. Then palpate the prostate through the anterior rectal wall, just past the anorectal ring, as shown.

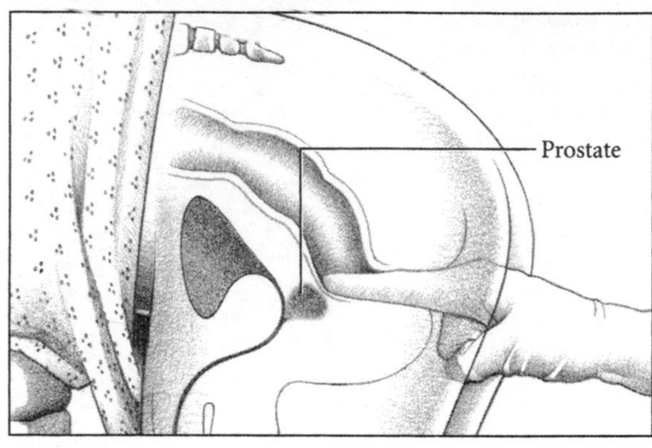

knee and hip flexed or with both knees drawn toward his chest. Inspect the skin of the perineal, anal, and posterior scrotal areas. It should be smooth and unbroken, with no protruding masses.

Tell the patient that you're going to place your finger into his rectum. Have him relax as much as possible. If he maintains anal sphincter tension, have him bear down as if having a bowel movement and gently insert your finger into his rectum. With your finger, rotate and palpate the entire muscular ring. The canal should be smooth. There should be no pain, only mild discomfort with this examination. The prostate gland is on the anterior wall just past the anorectal ring. The gland should feel smooth, rubbery, and about the size of a walnut. A test for occult blood would be appropriate at this time. (See *Palpating the prostate gland.*)

If the patient's prostate gland protrudes into the rectal lumen, it's probably enlarged. The enlargement is classified from grades 1 (protruding less than ⅜″ [1 cm] into the rectal lumen) to 4 (protruding more than 1¼″ [3 cm] into the rectal lumen). Also note tenderness or nodules.

A smooth, firm, symmetrical enlargement of the prostate gland indicates benign prostatic hyperplasia, which typically starts after age 50. This finding may be associated with nocturia, urinary hesitancy and frequency, and recurring UTIs.

Abnormal findings

A patient may seek care for a number of signs and symptoms related to the male GU system. The most significant findings are bladder distention, genital lesions, hematuria, impotence, scrotal swelling, urethral discharge, and urinary hesitancy. Polyuria may also be a common finding and is discussed in chapter 12, Endocrine system. The following history, physical assessment, and analysis summaries will help you assess each one quickly and accurately. After obtaining further information, begin to interpret the findings. (See *Male GU system: Interpreting your findings.*)

Bladder distention

Bladder distention — abnormal enlargement of the bladder — results from an inability to excrete urine, which results in its accumulation.

Distention usually develops gradually, but it occasionally has a sudden onset. Gradual distention usually doesn't produce symptoms until stretching of the bladder produces discomfort. Acute distention produces suprapubic fullness, pressure, and pain. If severe distention isn't corrected promptly by catheterization or massage, the bladder rises within the abdomen, its walls become thin, and renal function can be impaired.

(Text continues on page 428.)

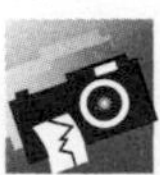

CLINICAL PICTURE

MALE GU SYSTEM: INTERPRETING YOUR FINDINGS

After you assess the male patient, a group of findings may lead you to suspect a particular genitourinary (GU) system disorder. The chart below shows you some common groups of findings for major signs and symptoms related to the male GU system, along with their probable causes.

Sign or symptom and findings	Probable cause
Bladder distention	
■ Gradual onset of bladder distention (but can occur acutely) ■ Urinary hesitancy ■ Straining and frequency ■ Reduced force of and the inability to stop urine stream ■ Nocturia ■ Postvoiding dribbling ■ Sensations of suprapubic fullness and incomplete bladder emptying, perineal pain, constipation, and hematuria as prostate enlarges	Benign prostatic hyperplasia
■ Eventual development of bladder distention ■ Dysuria ■ Urinary frequency and urgency ■ Nocturia ■ Weight loss ■ Fatigue ■ Perineal pain ■ Constipation ■ Induration of prostate or a rigid irregular prostate on digital rectal examination	Prostate cancer
Hematuria	
■ Gross hematuria ■ Possible pain in bladder rectum, pelvis, flank, back, or legs ■ Nocturia ■ Dysuria ■ Urinary frequency and urgency ■ Vomiting ■ Diarrhea ■ Insomnia	Bladder cancer
■ Macroscopic hematuria, usually at the end of urination ■ Urinary frequency and urgency ■ Dysuria followed by visible bladder distention ■ Malaise ■ Myalgia ■ Polyarthralgia ■ Fever with chills ■ Nausea and vomiting ■ Perineal and low back pain ■ Decreased libido ■ Tender, swollen, boggy, and firm prostate on rectal palpation	Prostatitis, acute

(continued)

MALE GU SYSTEM: INTERPRETING YOUR FINDINGS *(continued)*

Sign or symptom and findings	Probable cause
Hematuria *(continued)*	
▪ Grossly bloody hematuria, possibly accompanied by intense flank pain, costovertebral angle tenderness, abdominal rigidity, and colicky pain ▪ Oliguria or anuria ▪ Pyuria ▪ Fever and chills ▪ Vomiting ▪ Hypoactive bowel sounds ▪ Arthralgia ▪ Hypertension	Renal cancer
Impotence	
▪ Bending of penis making erection painful and penetration difficult, eventually impossible (Peyronie's disease) ▪ Prevention of erection due to constriction of foreskin (phimosis)	Penile disorders
▪ Progressive impotence ▪ Bladder distention with overflow incontinence ▪ Orthostatic hypotension ▪ Syncope ▪ Paresthesia ▪ Muscle weakness ▪ Leg atrophy	Peripheral neuropathy, diabetic
Impotence	
▪ Impotence ▪ Depression ▪ Traumatic recall of memories associated with sexual experiences ▪ Conflicts related to morality or religion ▪ Difficulties involving sexual or emotional relationships	Psychological distress
Male genital lesions	
▪ Fluid-filled vesicles on the glans penis, foreskin, or penile shaft ▪ Painful ulcers ▪ Tender inguinal lymph nodes ▪ Fever ▪ Malaise ▪ Dysuria	Genital herpes
▪ Painless warts (tiny pink swellings that grow and become pedunculated) near the urethral meatus ▪ Lesions spread to the perineum and the perianal area ▪ Cauliflower appearance of multiple swellings	Genital warts
▪ Sharply defined, slightly raised, scaling patches on the inner thigh or groin (bilaterally), or the scrotum or penis ▪ Severe pruritus	Tinea cruris (jock itch)

MALE GU SYSTEM: INTERPRETING YOUR FINDINGS *(continued)*

Sign or symptom and findings	Probable cause
Scrotal swelling	
▪ Swollen scrotum that's soft or unusually firm ▪ Bowel sounds may be auscultated in the scrotum	Hernia
▪ Gradual scrotal swelling ▪ Scrotum may be soft and cystic or firm and tense ▪ Painless ▪ Round, nontender scrotal mass on palpation ▪ Glowing when transilluminated	Hydrocele
▪ Scrotal swelling with sudden and severe pain ▪ Unilateral elevation of the affected testicle ▪ Nausea, vomiting	Testicular torsion
Urethral discharge	
▪ Purulent or milky urethral discharge ▪ Fever and chills ▪ Lower back pain ▪ Myalgia ▪ Perineal fullness ▪ Arthralgia ▪ Urinary frequency and urgency ▪ Cloudy urine ▪ Dysuria ▪ Tense, boggy, very tender, and warm prostate palpated on digital rectal examination	Prostatitis
▪ Painless, opaque, gray, yellowish, or blood-tinged discharge ▪ Dysuria ▪ Eventual anuria	Urethral neoplasm
Urethral discharge *(continued)*	
▪ Scant or profuse urethral discharge that's either thin and clear, mucoid, or thick and purulent ▪ Urinary hesitancy, frequency, and urgency ▪ Dysuria ▪ Itching and burning around the meatus	Urethritis
Urinary hesitancy	
▪ Reduced caliber and force of urinary stream ▪ Perineal pain ▪ A feeling of incomplete voiding ▪ Inability to stop the urine stream ▪ Urinary frequency ▪ Urinary incontinence ▪ Bladder distention	Benign prostatic hyperplasia
▪ Urinary frequency and dribbling ▪ Nocturia ▪ Dysuria ▪ Bladder distention ▪ Perineal pain ▪ Constipation ▪ Hard, nodular prostate palpated on digital rectal examination	Prostate cancer
▪ Dysuria ▪ Urinary frequency and urgency ▪ Hematuria ▪ Cloudy urine ▪ Bladder spasms ▪ Costovertebral angle tenderness ▪ Suprapubic, lower back, pelvic, or flank pain ▪ Urethral discharge	Urinary tract infection

History

If distention isn't severe, begin by reviewing the patient's voiding patterns. Find out the time and amount of the patient's last voiding and the amount of fluid consumed since then. Ask if he has difficulty urinating. Find out if he uses Valsalva's or Credé's maneuver to initiate urination. Ask if he urinates with urgency or without warning. Find out if urination is painful or irritating. Ask about the force and continuity of his urine stream and whether he feels that his bladder is empty after voiding.

Explore the patient's history of urinary tract obstruction or infections; venereal disease; neurologic, intestinal, or pelvic surgery; lower abdominal or urinary tract trauma; and systemic or neurologic disorders. Note his drug history, including his use of OTC drugs.

Physical assessment

Take the patient's vital signs, and percuss and palpate his bladder. Remember that if the bladder is empty, it can't be palpated through the abdominal wall. Inspect the urethral meatus, and measure its diameter. Describe the appearance and amount of any discharge. Finally, test for perineal sensation and anal sphincter tone; in male patients, digitally examine the prostate gland.

Analysis

Distention can be caused by a mechanical or anatomic obstruction, neuromuscular disorder, or the use of certain drugs. Relatively common in all ages and both sexes, it's most common in older men with prostate disorders that cause urine retention. Bladder distention is aggravated by the intake of caffeine, alcohol, large quantities of fluid, and diuretics. Bladder or prostate cancer also may be a cause.

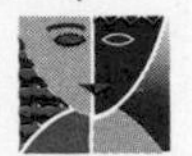

CULTURAL INSIGHT *Bladder cancer is twice as common in Whites as in Blacks. It's relatively uncommon among Asians, Hispanics, and Native Americans. Prostate cancer is more common in Blacks than in other ethnic groups.*

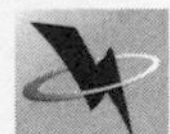

CRITICAL POINT *Using an indwelling urinary catheter can result in urine retention and bladder distention. While the catheter is in place, inadequate drainage due to kinked tubing or an occluded lumen may lead to urine retention. In addition, a misplaced urinary catheter or irritation with catheter removal may cause edema, thereby blocking urine outflow. Parasympatholytics, anticholinergics, ganglionic blockers, sedatives, anesthetics, and opiates can produce urine retention and bladder distention.*

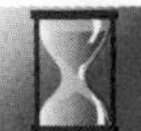

AGE ISSUE *In infants who fail to void normal amounts, look for urine retention and bladder distention. In the first 48 hours of life, an infant excretes about 60 ml of urine; during the next week, he excretes about 300 ml of urine daily. In males, posterior urethral valves, meatal stenosis, phimosis, spinal cord anomalies, bladder diverticula, and other congenital defects may cause urinary obstruction and resultant bladder distention.*

Hematuria

Hematuria is the abnormal presence of blood in the urine. Strictly defined, it means three or more red blood cells (RBCs) per high-power microscopic field in the urine. Microscopic hematuria is confirmed by an occult blood test, whereas macroscopic hematuria is immediately visible. However, macroscopic hematuria must be distinguished from pseudohematuria. Macroscopic hematuria may be continuous or intermittent, is often accompanied by pain, and may be aggravated by prolonged standing or walking.

History

Obtain a pertinent health history. If hematuria is macroscopic, ask the patient when he first noticed blood in his urine. Find out it varies in severity between voidings and if it worsens at the beginning, middle, or end of urination. Ask the patient if it has occurred before. Find out if he's passing clots. To rule out artifactitious hematuria, ask about bleeding hemorrhoids. Ask if there's pain or burning with the episodes of hematuria.

Ask about recent abdominal or flank trauma. Find out if the patient has been exercising strenuously. Note a history of renal, urinary, prostatic, or coagulation disorders. Then obtain a drug history, noting anticoagulants or aspirin.

Physical assessment

Begin the physical examination by palpating and percussing the abdomen and flanks. Next, percuss the costovertebral angle to elicit tenderness. Check the urinary meatus for bleeding or other abnormalities. Using a chemical reagent strip, test a urine specimen for protein. A digital rectal examination may be necessary.

Analysis

Hematuria is a cardinal sign of renal and urinary tract problems. It may be classified by the stage of urination it predominantly affects. Bleeding at the start of urination — initial hematuria — usually indicates urethral disease; bleeding at the end of urination — terminal hematuria — usually indicates disease of the bladder neck, posterior urethra, or prostate; bleeding throughout urination — total hematuria — usually indicates disease above the bladder neck.

Hematuria may result from one of two mechanisms: rupture or perforation of vessels in the renal system or urinary tract or impaired glomerular filtration, which allows RBCs to seep into the urine. The color of the bloody urine provides a clue to the source of the bleeding. Generally, dark or brownish blood indicates renal or upper urinary tract bleeding, whereas bright red blood indicates lower urinary tract bleeding.

Although hematuria usually results from renal and urinary tract disorders, it may also result from certain GI, prostate, or coagulation disorders, or from the effects of certain drugs. Invasive therapy and diagnostic tests that involve manipulation or instrumentation of the renal and urologic systems may also cause hematuria. Nonpathologic hematuria may result from hypercatabolic states. Transient hematuria may follow strenuous exercise.

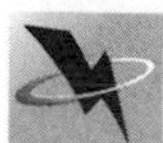

CRITICAL POINT *The patient receiving anticoagulants, who's also using herbal medications, such as garlic and ginkgo biloba, may also develop adverse reactions, including excessive bleeding and hematuria.*

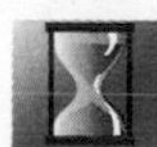

AGE ISSUE *In children, many of the causes seen in adults also produce hematuria. However, cyclophosphamide is more likely to cause hematuria in children than in adults. In children, common causes of hematuria include congenital anomalies, such as obstructive uropathy and renal dysplasia; birth trauma; hematologic disorders, such as vitamin K deficiency, hemophilia, and hemolytic-uremic syndrome; certain neoplasms, such as Wilms' tumor, bladder cancer, and rhabdomyosarcoma; allergies; and foreign bodies in the urinary tract. Artifactual hematuria may result from recent circumcision.*

Impotence

Impotence is the inability to achieve and maintain penile erection sufficient to complete satisfactory sexual intercourse; ejaculation may or may not be affected. Impotence varies from occasional and minimal to permanent and complete. Occasional impotence occurs in about one-half of adult American men, whereas chronic impotence affects about 10 million American men.

History

If the patient complains of impotence or of a condition that may be causing it, let him describe his problem without interruption. Then begin your examination in a systematic way, moving from less sensitive to more sensitive matters. Begin with a psychosocial history. Find out if the patient is married, single, or widowed. Ask the patient how long he has been married or had a sexual relationship. Find out the age and health status of his sexual partner. Find out about past marriages, if any, and ask him why he believes they ended. If you can do so discreetly, ask about sexual activity outside his marriage or primary sexual relationship. Also ask about his employment history, his typical daily activities, and his living situation. Find out how well he gets along with others in his household.

Focus your medical history on the causes of erectile dysfunction. Find out if the patient has type 2 diabetes mellitus, hypertension, or heart disease. If so, ask about its onset and treatment. Also ask about neurologic diseases such as multiple sclerosis. Obtain a surgical history, emphasizing neurologic, vascular, and urologic surgery. If trauma may be causing the patient's impotence, find out the date of the injury as well as its severity, associated effects, and treatment. Ask about intake of alcohol, drug use or abuse, smoking, diet, and exercise. Obtain a urologic history, including voiding problems and past injury.

Next, ask the patient when his impotence began. Find out how it progressed and its current status. Make your questions specific, but remember that many patients have difficulty discussing sexual problems, and many don't understand the physiology involved.

To yield helpful data, ask the patient when was the first time he remembers not being able to initiate or maintain an erection. Find out how often he wakes in the morning or at night with an erection and if he has wet dreams. Ask the patient if his sexual drive has changed. Find out how often he attempts to have intercourse with his partner and how often he would like to. Ask him if he can ejaculate with or without an erection. Also ask him if he experiences orgasm with ejaculation.

Ask the patient to rate the quality of a typical erection on a scale of 0 to 10, with 0 being completely flaccid and 10 being completely erect. Using the same scale, also ask him to rate his ability to ejaculate during sexual activity, with 0 being never and 10 being always.

Physical assessment

Next, perform a brief physical examination. Inspect and palpate the genitalia and prostate for structural abnormalities. Assess the patient's sensory function, concentrating on the perineal area. Next, test motor strength and deep tendon reflexes in all extremities, and note other neurologic deficits. Take the patient's vital signs and palpate his pulses for quality. Note any signs of peripheral vascular disease, such as cyanosis and cool extremities. Auscultate for abdominal aortic, femoral, carotid, or iliac bruits, and palpate for thyroid gland enlargement.

Analysis

Impotence can be classified as primary or secondary. A man with primary impotence has never been potent with a sexual partner but may achieve normal erections in other situations. This uncommon condition is difficult to treat. Secondary impotence carries a more favorable prognosis because, despite his present erectile dysfunction, the patient has completed satisfactory intercourse in the past. Penile erection involves increased arterial blood flow secondary to psychological, tactile, and other sensory stimulation. Trapping of blood within the penis produces increased length, circumference, and rigidity. Impotence results when any component of this process — psychological, vascular, neurologic, or hormonal — malfunctions.

Organic causes of impotence include vascular disease, diabetes mellitus, hypogonadism, a spinal cord lesion, alcohol and drug abuse, and surgical complications. The incidence of organic impotence associated with other medical problems increases after age 50.

Psychogenic causes range from performance anxiety and marital discord to moral or religious conflicts. Fatigue, poor health, age, and drugs can also disrupt normal sexual function.

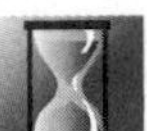

AGE ISSUE *Most people erroneously believe that sexual performance normally declines with age. Many also believe that elderly people are incapable of or aren't interested in sex or that they can't find elderly partners who are interested in sex. Organic disease must be ruled out in elderly people who suffer from sexual dysfunction before counseling to improve sexual performance can begin.*

Male genital lesions

Among the diverse lesions that may affect the male genitalia are warts, papules, ulcers, scales, and pustules. These common lesions may be painful or painless, singular or multiple. They may be limited to the genitalia or may also occur elsewhere on the body.

History

Begin by asking the patient when he first noticed the lesion. Find out if it erupted after he began taking a new drug or after a trip out of the country. Ask the patient if he has had similar lesions before. If so, ask if he received medical treatment for them. Find out if he has been treating the lesion himself and, if so, how he has been treating them. Ask if the lesions itch and, if so, ask if the itching is constant or does it bother him only at night. Note whether the lesion is painful. Next, take a complete sexual history, noting the frequency of relations and the number of sexual partners.

Physical assessment

Before you examine the patient, observe his clothing. For example, observe if his pants fit properly. Tight pants or underwear, especially those made of nonabsorbent fabrics, can promote the growth of bacteria and fungi. Examine the entire skin surface, noting the location, size, color, and pattern of the lesions. Observe the genital lesions to see if they resemble those on other parts of the body. Palpate for nodules, masses, and tenderness. Also look for bleeding, edema, or signs of infection such as erythema.

Analysis

Genital lesions may result from infection, neoplasms, parasites, allergy, or the use of certain drugs. These lesions can profoundly affect the patient's self-image. In fact, the patient may hesitate to seek medical attention because he fears cancer or an STD.

Genital lesions that arise from an STD could mean that the patient is at risk for HIV. Genital ulcers make HIV transmission between sexual partners more likely. Unfortunately, if the patient is treating himself, he may alter the lesions, making differential diagnosis especially difficult.

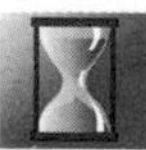

AGE ISSUE *In infants, contact dermatitis, also called "diaper rash" may produce minor irritation or bright red, weepy, excoriated lesions. The use of disposable diapers and careful cleaning of the penis and scrotum can help reduce diaper rash. In children, impetigo may cause pustules with thick, yellow, weepy crusts. Like adults, children may develop genital warts, but they'll need more reassurance that the treatment (excision) won't hurt or castrate them. Children with an STD must be evaluated for signs of sexual abuse. Adolescents ages 15 to 19 have a high incidence of STDs and related genital lesions. Syphilis, however, may also be congenital.*

Scrotal swelling

Scrotal swelling occurs when a condition affecting the testicles, epididymis, or scrotal skin produces edema or a mass. The penis may also be involved. It can affect males of any age. It can be unilateral or bilateral, painful or painless.

History

If the patient isn't in distress, proceed with the health history. Ask about injury to the scrotum, urethral discharge, cloudy urine, increased urinary frequency, and dysuria. Ask the patient if he's sexually active and when he had his last sexual contact. Find out about recent illnesses, particularly mumps. Ask the patient if he has a history of prostate surgery or prolonged catheterization. Find out if changing his body position or level of activity affects the swelling.

Physical assessment

Palpate the patient's abdomen for tenderness. Then examine the entire genital area. Assess the scrotum with the patient in supine and standing positions. Note its size and color. Determine if the swelling is unilateral or bilateral. Note if there are visible signs of trauma or bruising. Gently palpate the scrotum for a cyst or a lump. Especially note tenderness or increased firmness. Check the position of the testicles in the scrotum. Finally, transilluminate the scrotum to distinguish a fluid-filled cyst from a solid mass; a solid mass can't be transilluminated.

Analysis

Scrotal swelling can result from an inguinal hernia, hydrocele, or trauma to the scrotum. The sudden onset of painful scrotal swelling suggests torsion of a testicle or testicular appendages, especially in a prepubescent male. This emergency requires immediate surgery to untwist and stabilize the spermatic cord or to remove the appendage.

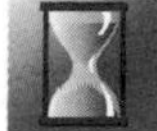

AGE ISSUE *For children with scrotal swelling, a thorough physical assessment is especially important, because they may be unable to offer clues about their medical history. In children up to age 1, a hernia or hydrocele of the spermatic cord may stem from abnormal fetal development. In infants, scrotal swelling may stem from ammonia-related dermatitis, if diapers aren't changed often enough. In prepubescent males, it usually results from torsion of the spermatic cord.*

Urethral discharge

Discharge from the urinary meatus may be purulent, mucoid, or thin; sanguineous or clear; and scant or profuse. It usually develops suddenly.

History
Ask the patient when he first noticed the discharge, and have him describe its color, consistency, and quantity. Find out if the patient has pain on urination. Ask him if he has difficulty initiating a urinary stream. Also ask the patient about other associated signs and symptoms, such as fever, chills, and perineal fullness. Explore his history for prostate problems, STDs, or UTIs. Find out if the patient has had recent sexual contacts or a new sexual partner.

Physical assessment
Inspect the patient's urethral meatus for inflammation and swelling. Using proper technique, obtain a culture specimen. Then obtain a urine sample. The prostate gland may also have to be palpated for inflammation and swelling.

Analysis
Urethral discharge is most common in men with a prostate infection. Other causes may include urethral neoplasm (a rare cancer) and urethritis (an inflammatory disorder that can be sexually transmitted).

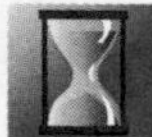

AGE ISSUE *Carefully evaluate a child with urethral discharge for evidence of sexual and physical abuse. In elderly males, urethral discharge usually isn't related to an STD.*

Urinary hesitancy
Hesitancy — difficulty starting a urinary stream — usually arises gradually, commonly going unnoticed until urine retention causes bladder distention and discomfort.

History
Ask the patient when he first noticed hesitancy and whether he has ever had the problem before. Ask about other urinary problems, especially reduced force or interruption of the urinary stream. Ask if he has ever been treated for a prostate problem, UTI, or obstruction. Obtain a drug history.

Physical assessment
Inspect the patient's urethral meatus for inflammation, discharge, and other abnormalities. Examine the anal sphincter, and test sensation in the perineum. Obtain a clean-catch sample for urinalysis. Palpate the prostate gland.

Analysis
Hesitancy can result from a UTI, a partial lower urinary tract obstruction, a neuromuscular disorder, or the use of certain drugs. Occurring at all ages and in both sexes, it's most common in older men with prostatic enlargement.

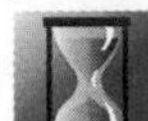

AGE ISSUE *In male infants, the most common cause of urinary obstruction is posterior strictures in the prostatic urethra. Infants with this problem may have a less forceful urinary stream and may also present with fever caused by a UTI, failure to thrive, or a palpable bladder.*

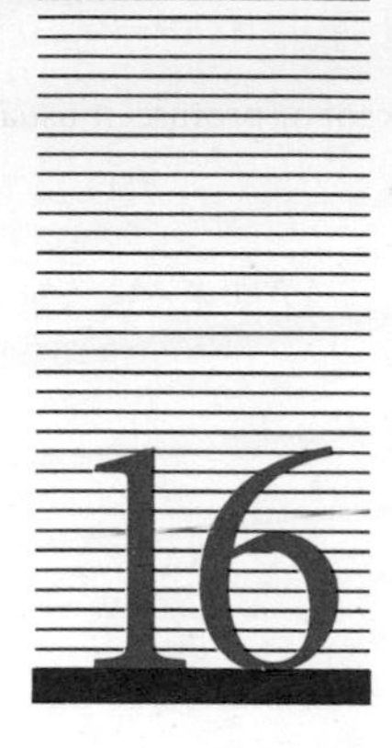

Musculoskeletal system

The musculoskeletal system consists of bones, muscles, tendons, ligaments, cartilage, joints, and bursae. These structures work together to produce skeletal movement.

During a musculoskeletal assessment, use sight, hearing, and touch to determine the health of the patient's bones, muscles, joints, and connective tissue, including tendons, and ligaments. These structures give the human body its shape and ability to move. Sharp assessment skills will help uncover musculoskeletal abnormalities and evaluate the patient's ability to perform activities of daily living.

Bones

Classified by shape and location, bones may be long, such as the humerus, radius, femur, and tibia; short, such as the carpals and tarsals; flat, such as the scapula, ribs, and skull; irregular, such as the vertebrae and mandible; or sesamoid such as the patella. Bones of the axial skeleton, the head and trunk, include the facial and cranial bones, hyoid bone, vertebrae, ribs, and sternum; bones of the appendicular skeleton, which involve the extremities, include the clavicle, scapula, humerus, radius, ulna, metacarpals, pelvic bone, femur, patella, fibula, tibia, and metatarsals. (See *Structures of the skeletal system,* pages 434 and 435.)

Bone function

Bones perform various anatomic, or mechanical, and physiologic functions. They protect internal tissues and organs, for example, the 33 vertebrae surround and protect the spinal cord. Bones stabilize and support the body and provide a surface for

(Text continues on page 436.)

STRUCTURES OF THE SKELETAL SYSTEM

Of the 206 bones in the human skeletal system, 80 form the axial skeleton and 126 form the appendicular skeleton. Shown below are the body's major bones.

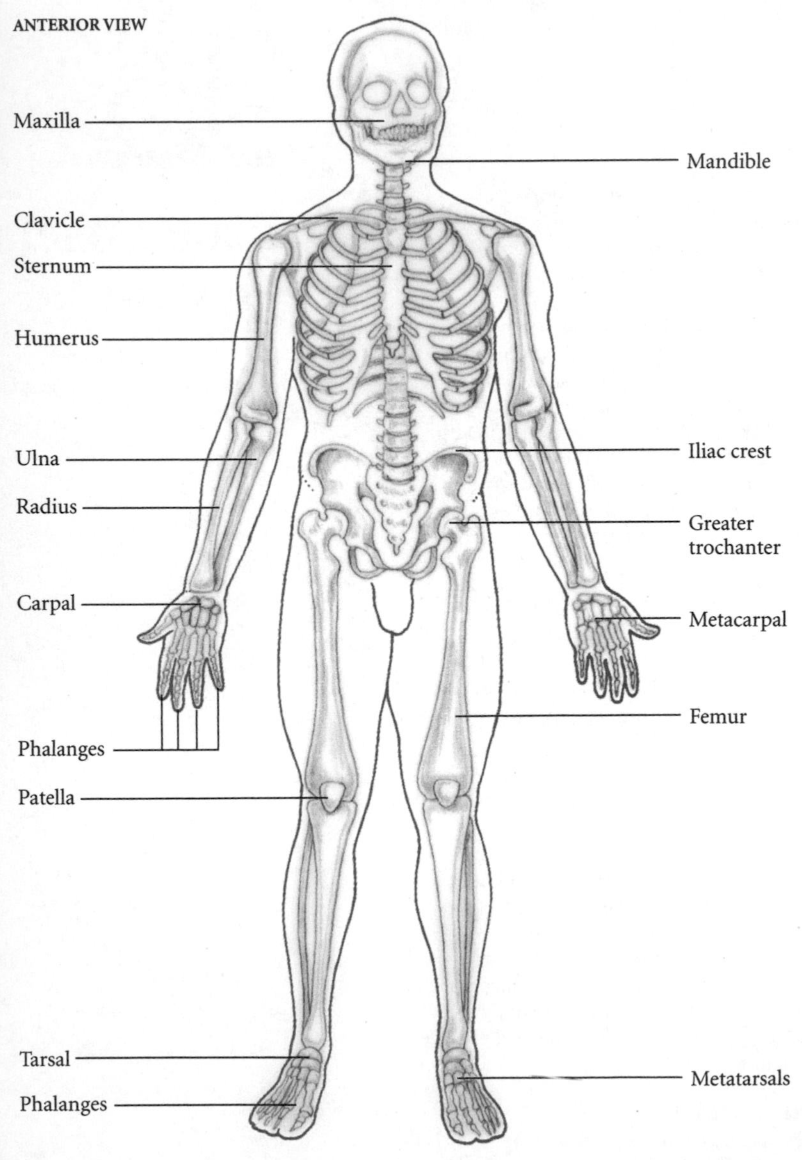

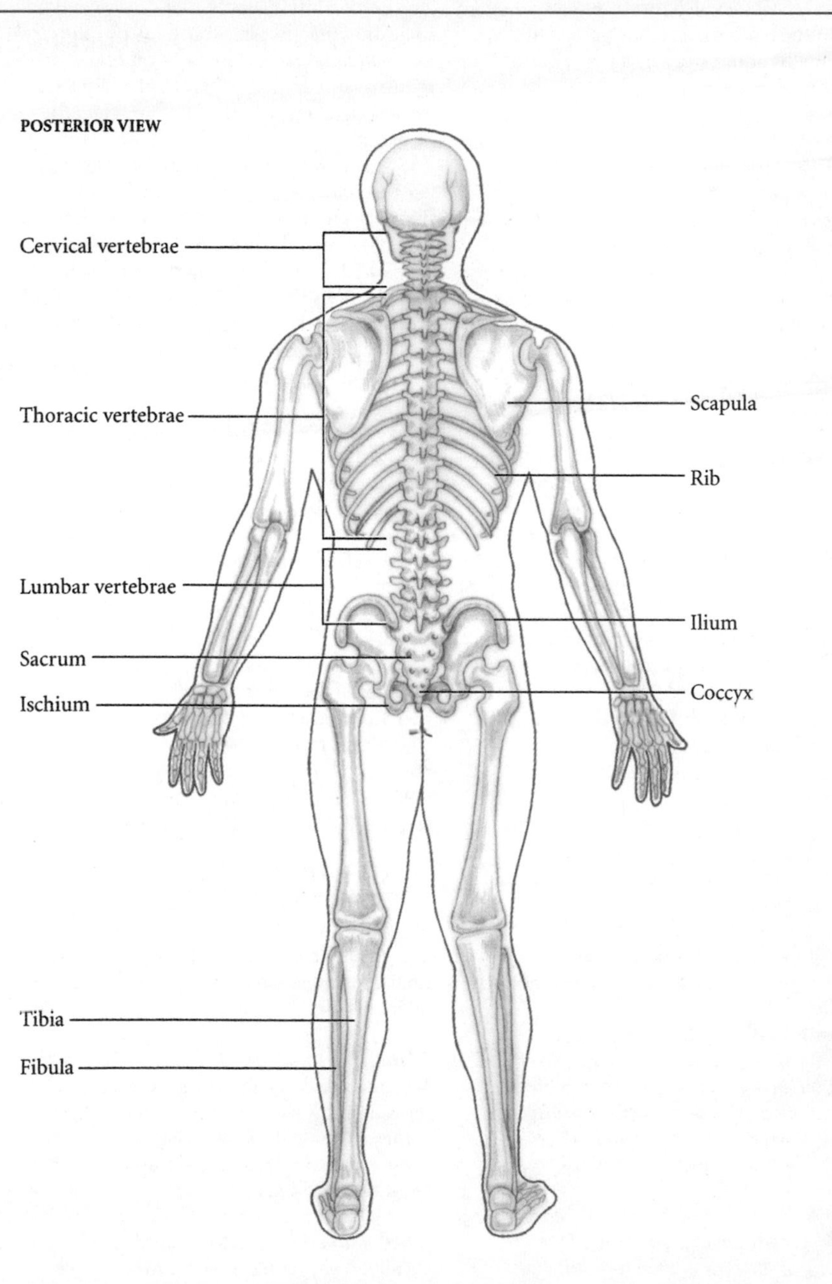
POSTERIOR VIEW
Cervical vertebrae
Thoracic vertebrae
Lumbar vertebrae
Sacrum
Ischium
Tibia
Fibula
Scapula
Rib
Ilium
Coccyx

muscle, ligament, and tendon attachment. They move through "lever" action when contracted. Bones also produce red blood cells in the bone marrow, called *hematopoiesis.* Finally, bones store mineral salts, for example, about 99% of the body's calcium.

Bone formation

Cartilage composes the fetal skeleton at 3 months in utero. By about 6 months, the fetal cartilage has been transformed into bony skeleton. However, some bones ossify after birth, most notably the carpals and tarsals. The change results from endochondral ossification, a process by which bone-forming cells, called *osteoblasts,* produce a collagenous material, called *osteoid,* that ossifies.

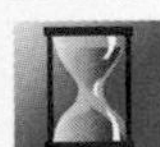

AGE ISSUE *A child's bones grow at a much faster rate and their bones are more porous and flexible than those of an adult. Thus, a child's bones heal more rapidly.*

Two types of osteocytes, osteoblasts and osteoclasts, are responsible for remodeling—the continuous process whereby bone is created and destroyed. Osteoblasts deposit new bone and osteoclasts increase long-bone diameter through reabsorption of previously deposited bone. These activities promote longitudinal bone growth, which continues until the epiphyseal growth plates, located at the bone ends, close in adolescence.

Researchers are currently studying the role of the endocrine system in bone formation. Estrogen secretion plays a significant role not only in calcium uptake and release but also in osteoblastic activity regulation. Researchers think that decreased estrogen levels lead to diminished osteoblastic activity.

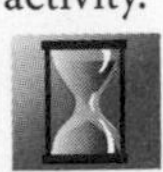

AGE ISSUE *A patient's age, race, and sex affect bone mass, structural integrity, and bone loss. Bone density and structural integrity decrease after age 30 in women and age 45 in men. Thereafter, a relatively steady quantitative loss of bone matrix occurs.*

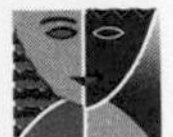

CULTURAL INSIGHT *Blacks typically have denser bones than Whites, and men typically have denser bones than women.*

Muscles

The body contains three major muscle types including the visceral, known as *involuntary* or *smooth;* skeletal, known as *voluntary* or *striated;* and cardiac. This chapter discusses only skeletal muscle, which is attached to bone.

Skeletal muscles are groups of contractile cells or fibers. These fibers contract and produce skeletal movement when they receive a stimulus from the central nervous system.

Viewed through the microscope, skeletal muscle looks like long bands or strips called *striations.* Skeletal muscle is voluntary; its contraction can be controlled at will.

The human body has about 600 skeletal muscles. (See *Viewing the major skeletal muscles.*)

The muscles of the axial skeleton are essential for respiration. These include the muscles of the face, tongue, and neck; the muscles of mastication; and the muscles of the vertebral column situated along the spine.

The appendicular skeleton includes the muscles of the shoulder, abdominopelvic cavity, and upper and lower extremities. Muscles of the upper extremities are classified according to the bones they move. Those that move the arm are further categorized into those with an origin on the axial skeleton and those with an origin on the scapula.

Muscle growth

Muscle develops when existing muscle fibers hypertrophy. Exercise, nutrition, gender, and genetic constitution account for variations in muscle strength and size among individuals.

Muscle movements

Skeletal muscle can permit several types of movement. A muscle's functional name comes from the type of movement it permits. For example, a flexor muscle permits bending, called *flexion;* an adductor muscle permits movement away from the body axis, called *adduction;* and a circumductor muscle allows a circular movement, called *circumduction.*

VIEWING THE MAJOR SKELETAL MUSCLES

This illustration shows anterior and posterior views of some of the major skeletal muscles in the body.

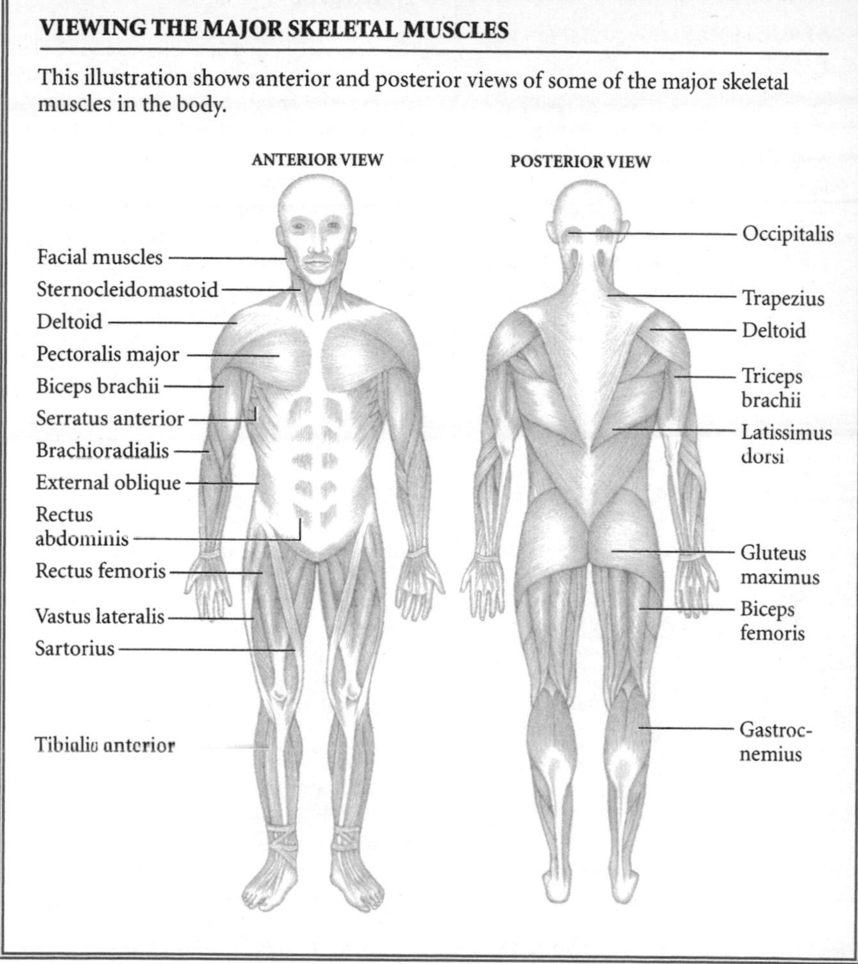

Connective tissue

In the musculoskeletal system, the connective tissue is the supporting or framework tissue of the human body. Connective tissue includes the tendons, ligaments, and cartilage.

Tendons

Tendons are bands of fibrous connective tissue that attach muscles to the periosteum, the fibrous membrane covering the bone. They enable bones to move when skeletal muscles contract.

Ligaments

Ligaments are dense, strong, flexible bands of fibrous connective tissue that tie bones to other bones. The ligaments of concern in a musculoskeletal system assessment connect the joint, or articular, ends of bones, serving to limit or facilitate movement as well as provide stability.

Cartilage

Cartilage is a dense connective tissue that consists of fibers embedded in a strong, gel-like substance. It's found primarily in the joints, the walls of the thorax, and tubular structures such as the larynx, air passages,

STRUCTURES OF A SYNOVIAL JOINT

In synovial joints, a layer of resilient cartilage covers the surface of opposing bones. This cartilage cushions the bones and allows full joint movement by making the surfaces of the bones smooth. The synovial joint cushions the end of each bone and synovial fluid fills the joint space, lubricating the joint and easing movement.

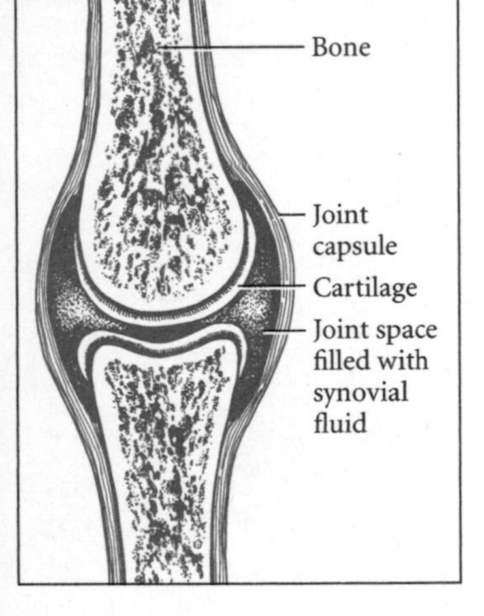

and ears. Cartilage is avascular and lacks innervation.

Cartilage may be fibrous, hyaline, or elastic. Fibrous cartilage forms the symphysis pubis and the intervertebral disks. Hyaline cartilage covers the articular bone surfaces, where one or more bones meet at a joint; connects the ribs to the sternum; and appears in the trachea, bronchi, and nasal septum. Elastic cartilage is located in the auditory canal, external ear, and epiglottis.

Cartilage supports and shapes various structures, such as the auditory canal and intervertebral disks. It also cushions and absorbs shock, preventing direct transmission to the bone.

Joints

The junction of two or more bones is called a *joint*. Joints stabilize the bones and allow a specific type of movement. A joint can be functionally classified as synarthrosis (immovable), amphiarthrosis (slightly movable), and diarthrosis (freely movable).

Joints also may be classified by their structure as nonsynovial (fibrous and cartilaginous) and synovial. In *nonsynovial* joints, the bones are connected by fibrous tissue or cartilage. The bones may be immovable, like the sutures in the skull, or slightly movable, like the vertebrae. *Synovial* joints move freely and thus are functionally classified as diarthrodial joints. The bones are separate from each other and meet in a cavity filled with synovial fluid, a lubricant. (See *Structures of a synovial joint.*)

Synovial joints are surrounded by a fibrous capsule that stabilizes the joint structures. The capsule also surrounds the joint's ligaments—the tough, fibrous bands that join one bone to another. Types of synovial joints include ball-and-socket joints, hinge joints, gliding joints, pivot joints, condylar joints, and saddle joints.

Ball-and-socket joints

Ball-and-socket joints get their name from the way their bones connect. The spherical head of one bone fits into a concave "socket" of another bone. Ball-and-socket joints—the shoulders and hips being the only examples of this type—allow for flexion, extension, adduction, and abduction. These joints also rotate in their sockets and are assessed by their degree of internal and external rotation.

Hinge joints

In hinge joints, a convex portion of one bone fits into a concave portion of another. The movement of a hinge joint resembles that of a metal hinge.

Hinge joints, such as the knee and elbow, normally move in flexion and extension only.

Gliding joints

Gliding joints have flat or slightly curved articular surfaces and allow gliding movements. However, because they're bound by ligaments, they may not allow movement in all directions. Examples of gliding joints are the intertarsal and intercarpal joints of the hands and feet.

Pivot joints

A rounded portion of one bone in a pivot joint fits into the groove of another bone. Pivot joints allow only uniaxial rotation of the first bone around the second. An example of a pivot joint is the head of the radius, which rotates within the groove of the ulna.

Condylar joints

In condylar joints, an oval surface of one bone fits into a concavity in another bone. Condylar joints allow flexion, extension, abduction, adduction, and circumduction. Examples include the radiocarpal and metacarpophalangeal joints of the hand.

Saddle joints

Saddle joints resemble condylar joints but allow greater freedom of movement. The only saddle joints in the body are the carpometacarpal joints of the thumb.

Bursae

Located at friction points around joints between tendons, ligaments, and bones, bursae are small synovial fluid sacs that act as cushions, thereby decreasing stress to adjacent structures. Examples of bursae include the subacromial bursa, located in the shoulder, and the prepatellar bursa, located in the knee.

Skeletal movement

Although skeletal movement results primarily from muscle contractions, other musculoskeletal structures are also involved. To contract, skeletal muscle, which is richly supplied with blood vessels and nerves, needs an impulse from the nervous system along with oxygen and nutrients from the circulatory system.

When a skeletal muscle contracts, force is applied to the tendon. Then one bone is pulled toward, moved away from, or rotated around a second bone, depending on the type of muscle contracted. Typically, one bone moves less than the other. The muscle tendon attached to the more stationary bone is called the origin. The muscle tendon attached to the more movable bone is called the insertion site. The *origin* usually lies on the proximal end of the bone and the *insertion site* on the distal end.

In skeletal movement, the bones act as levers and the joints act as fulcrums, or fixed points. Each bone's function is partially determined by the location of the fulcrum, which establishes the relation between resistance, a force to be overcome, and effort, a force to be resisted. Most body movement uses groups of muscles rather than one muscle. (See *Basics of body movement,* pages 440 and 441.)

Health history

Musculoskeletal assessment typically represents a small part of an overall physical assessment, especially when the patient's chief complaint involves a different body system. However, when the patient's health history or physical findings suggest musculoskeletal involvement, perform a complete assessment of this system, beginning with a thorough health history.

During the patient interview, use open-ended questions to assess broad areas quickly and identify specific problems that require further attention. Ask questions systematically to avoid missing important data. Keep in mind that the entire history doesn't need to be completed all at once; as long as the necessary information is obtained and incorporated into the patient's care plan, dividing up the interview and completing it as time permits is appropriate. Also take into account the patient's emotional and physical condition when conducting the interview.

During the interview, cover the chief complaint, current health, past health history, family history, and psychosocial history.

Chief complaint

Ask your patient what made him seek medical care. Encourage him to describe his problem in detail. Patients with musculoskeletal problems commonly complain of joint pain, joint stiffness, deformity or immobility, redness and swelling, and general

BASICS OF BODY MOVEMENT

Body movement is generated by muscles. The diarthrodial joints allow 13 angular and circular movements that form the basis of the musculoskeletal assessment. The jaw demonstrates retraction and protraction; the shoulder, abduction and adduction; the hip, external and internal rotation; the ankle, dorsiflexion and plantar flexion; the foot, eversion and inversion; the arm, circumduction; the wrist, extension and flexion; and the hand, supination and pronation.

RETRACTION AND PROTRACTION
Moving backward and forward

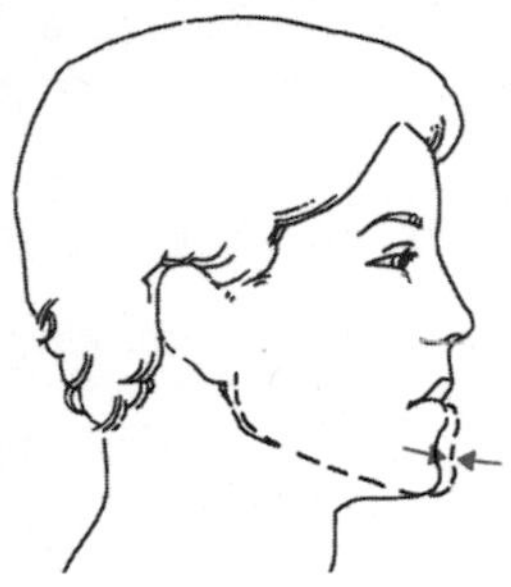

ABDUCTION AND ADDUCTION
Moving away from midline, and moving toward midline

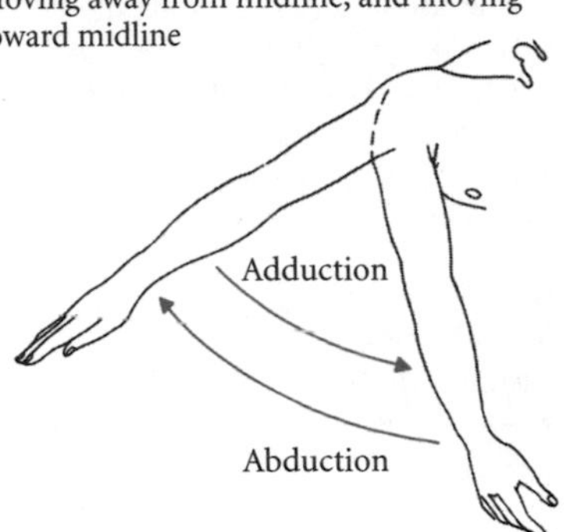

EXTERNAL ROTATION
Turning away from midline

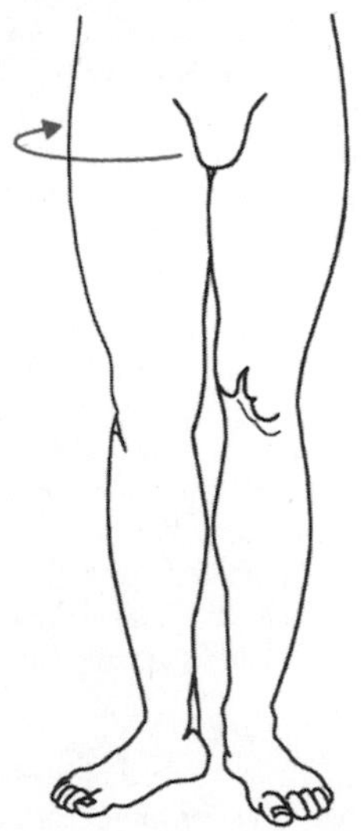

INTERNAL ROTATION
Turning toward midline

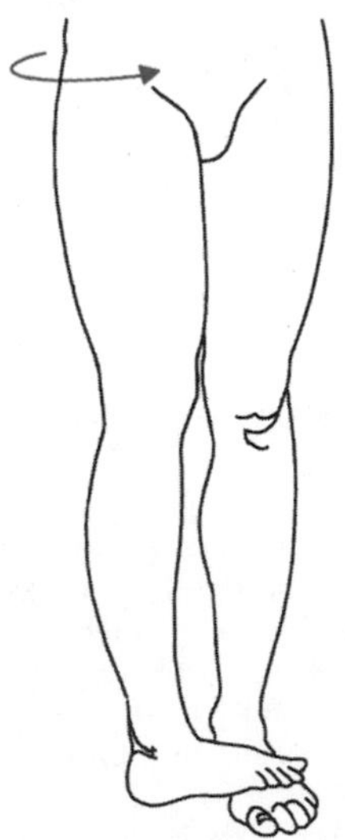

BASICS OF BODY MOVEMENT *(continued)*

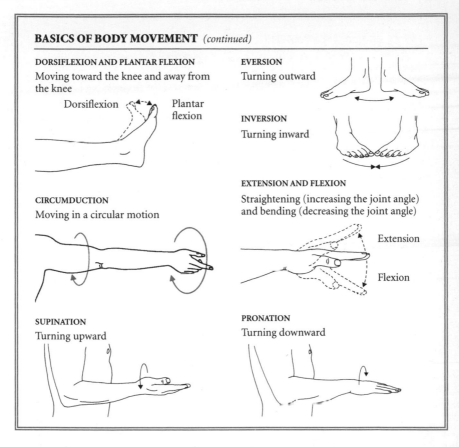

DORSIFLEXION AND PLANTAR FLEXION

Moving toward the knee and away from the knee

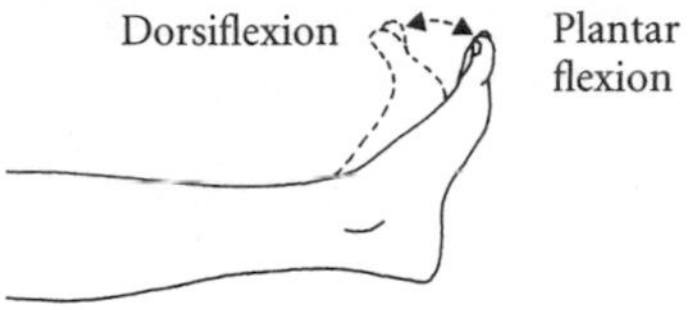

Dorsiflexion

Plantar flexion

EVERSION

Turning outward

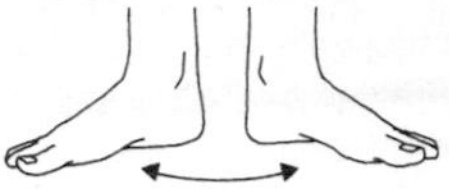

INVERSION

Turning inward

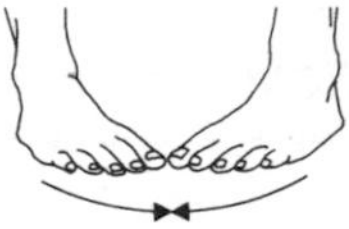

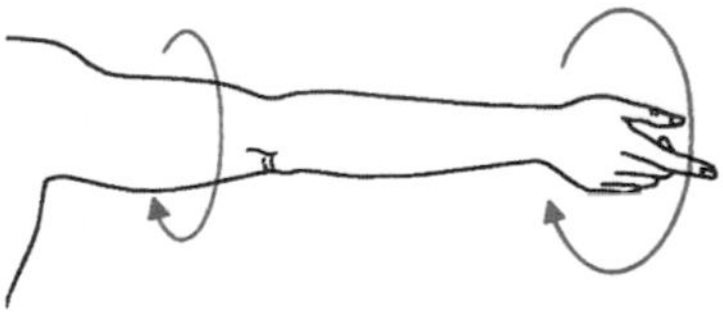

EXTENSION AND FLEXION

Straightening (increasing the joint angle) and bending (decreasing the joint angle)

Extension

Flexion

CIRCUMDUCTION

Moving in a circular motion

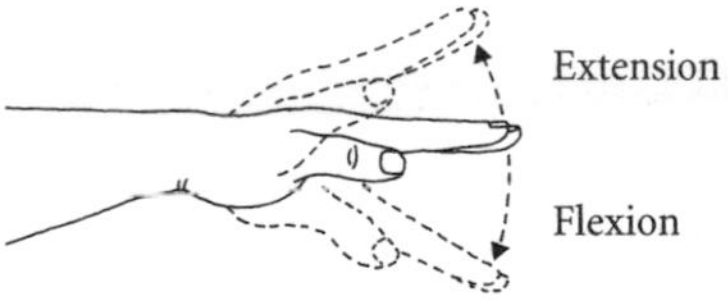

SUPINATION

Turning upward

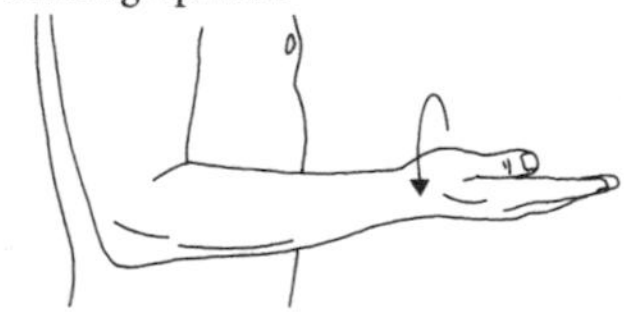

PRONATION

Turning downward

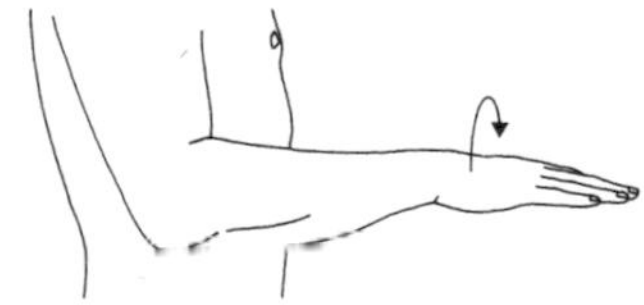

systemic problems, such as fever and malaise.

CRITICAL POINT *If the patient has experienced musculoskeletal trauma, quickly assess the 5 P's.* *(See* Assessing the 5 P's of musculoskeletal injury, *page 442.)*

Analyze the patient's chief complaint. Ask him to describe its onset, location, duration, timing, and quality. Also ask about exacerbating and alleviating factors and any associated symptoms.

Ask the patient to pinpoint when the symptom first occurred and how suddenly or gradually it occurred. Find out what circumstances surrounded its occurrence. For instance, ask the patient if he hurt himself in a fall or other accident. With joint pain, ask him if the pain began suddenly or gradually.

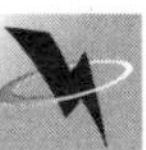

CRITICAL POINT *Joint pain that begins suddenly may indicate gout, pseudogout, infection, or trauma. Whereas joint pain that begins gradually may indicate rheumatoid arthritis, rheumatic fever, or degenerative joint disease.*

Next, determine the location of the patient's complaint. Ask him where he experiences the symptom and if he can point to the exact area. With joint pain, find out if the pain involves one joint or multiple joints. Try to determine whether joint involvement is symmetrical, asymmetrical, or migratory.

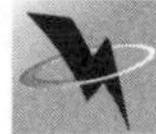

CRITICAL POINT *Pain that's located in one joint may indicate trauma, gout, pseudogout, or infectious arthritis. If pain is located in multiple joints this may indicate rheumatoid disease, juvenile-onset arthritis, or psoriatic arthritis. Symmetrical joint pain may indicate rheumatoid arthritis, whereas asymmetrical*

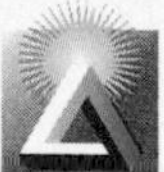

EXPERT TECHNIQUE

ASSESSING THE 5 P'S OF MUSCULOSKELETAL INJURY

If you uncover a musculoskeletal injury during your assessment, remember to check for the 5 P's—pain, paresthesia, paralysis, pallor, and pulse.

Pain
Ask the patient whether he feels pain. If he does, assess the pain's location, severity, and quality.

Paresthesia
Assess the patient for loss of sensation by touching the injured area with the tip of an open safety pin. Abnormal sensation or loss of sensation indicates neurovascular involvement.

Paralysis
Assess whether the patient can move the affected area. If he can't, he might have nerve or tendon damage.

Pallor
Assess the injured site for paleness, discoloration, and coolness, which may indicate neurovascular compromise.

Pulse
Check all pulses distal to the injury site. If a pulse is decreased or absent, blood supply to the area is reduced.

joint pain may indicate psoriatic arthritis, spondyloarthropathies, or polyarticular osteoarthritis. Lastly, pain that migrates through the joint may indicate rheumatic fever, gonococcal arthritis or, sometimes, Reiter's syndrome.

Evaluate the duration of the patient's symptom. Find out how long he has had this symptom. With joint pain, ask him if the pain has lasted for 1 to 2 days or for several weeks. Joint pain lasting 1 to 2 days may indicate gout, pseudogout, or infection. Joint pain that lasts for several weeks may indicate rheumatoid arthritis or degenerative joint disease.

Assess the timing of the symptom. Find out when the symptom is worst. With joint pain or stiffness, ask the patient if it hurts more in the morning on arising or after activity. Joint pain or stiffness that's worse in the morning suggests rheumatoid arthritis; whereas joint pain or stiffness that's worse after activity suggests simple joint dysfunction.

Determine the quality of the patient's symptom and any factors that alleviate or exacerbate it, for example, pain. Find out if the patient has a deep, throbbing, aching pain or if it's sharp and intermittent. Deep, throbbing, aching pain suggests serious bone or joint disease; sharp and intermittent pain suggests a relatively mild joint problem. Ask the patient what makes the symptom worse, what relieves it, and if medication, rest, and activity have any effect on his pain.

Question the patient further about any other symptoms that may be occurring. Find out if other symptoms occur along with the primary symptom. Remember, associated symptoms may be wide ranging, depending on the primary disease involved.

Current health history

Ask the patient to elaborate on his primary complaint, using open-ended questions to focus the interview. Ascertain if the patient is experiencing any problems with his activities of daily living (ADLs) due to the complaint. Also question the patient about any measures used to treat the problem.

Joint pain

Assess the patient's complaint of joint pain, asking him to point to its exact location. Deep, poorly localized pain usually indicates damage to blood vessels, fascia, joints, or periosteum. Inquire about how the patient describes the pain, for example, as an ache or as sharp, constant, or throbbing. Pain arising in the bones is commonly described as throbbing. A patient will usually characterize muscle and joint pain as an ache.

Ask the patient if the pain worsens with movement, with temperature changes, or if he's carrying something heavy. Pain that increases with motion indicates a joint disorder. The pain of degenerative joint disease of the hip occurs with weight bearing. Leg pain that worsens with standing, walking, or exercise and that persists for longer than 10 minutes after the patient stops the activity is probably caused by a degenerative hip or knee joint problem. Bending or lifting can elicit leg or back pain in a patient with a herniated lumbar disk. Pain associated with carpal tunnel syndrome worsens after extensive use of the hands. Cold and damp weather increases osteoarthritis pain.

Ask the patient if his pain is worse at any particular time of day. The pain caused by inflammation of the tendons and bursae may become intolerable at night. Joint discomfort from degenerative disease is usually most intense at the end of the day. Find out if his pain is relieved by rest. Pain from most forms of degenerative joint disease is relieved by rest. Ask the patient if aspirin relieves the pain. Aspirin relieves joint pain caused by inflammation. Find out if the patient has recently fallen or been injured. Trauma causes such injuries as fractures, torn ligaments, and back problems.

Joint stiffness

Ask the patient to identify which joints feel stiff and clarify with him how many joints are involved. The patient's answers will help identify the cause of his problem. Ask him if stiffness and pain in the joints stops for extended periods, such as for several weeks, and then recurs. Certain joint diseases, such as ankylosing spondylitis, have characteristic patterns of exacerbation and remission.

Ask the patient if he experiences stiffness when he wakes up in the morning and, if so, find out how long it lasts. In a patient with degenerative joint disease, inactivity during sleep causes stiffness that diminishes with joint use during the day. Find out if the stiffness is relieved or aggravated by temperature changes. Heat relieves joint stiffness by alleviating muscle spasms. However, in a traumatic joint injury, heat applied immediately after the injury may aggravate stiffness by increasing bleeding into the joint. Generally, failure to use the joint and exposure to cold and dampness exacerbate joint stiffness.

Find out from the patient if the stiffness is accompanied by locking of the joint. Ask him if he can feel or hear the bones rubbing together. Locking indicates poor bone alignment with the joint. Crepitus can occur in a fracture or from destruction of the joint cushioning structures.

Redness and swelling

First, determine how long the patient has noted the swelling. Then ask if pain occurred at the same time. Edema and pain commonly occur simultaneously with traumatic injuries to muscles and bone. They're also present simultaneously in certain forms of bursitis, called *housemaid's knee.* Swelling associated with degenerative joint disease can occur weeks or months after the pain because of proliferative changes in cartilage and bone. Ask the patient if the swelling limits his motion. Swelling of soft tissue over a joint may act as a splint and immobilize it. Swelling within a joint also inhibits motion.

Ask the patient if rest or elevation relieves the swelling. Elevation relieves swelling from a fresh injury because it facilitates blood return and prevents fluid from pooling in the extremity. Find out if a cast or splint has been removed from the affected part recently. This may have caused the swelling because the loss of muscle tone that normally occurs in a casted extremity impairs venous blood return. Find out if the affected area has ever appeared red or warm. Redness and warmth are signs of acute inflammation, infection, or recent trauma. These signs don't usually occur in degenerative joint disease.

Also ask the patient about any sensory changes. Find out if he has noticed any loss of feeling and if it's associated with pain. Swelling can put pressure on a nerve, causing a loss of sensation in the area distal to the affected site. Compression of nerves or of blood vessels by a tumor or fracture also can cause a loss of feeling. Sensory changes sometimes accompany arm or hand pain.

Deformity and immobility

Ask the patient if he noticed the deformity recently, or if it has been gradually increasing in size. A slow-growing mass may be a tumor. Gradual bony enlargement of a joint causes deformity.

Find out if the deformity limits his movement. Ask the patient if it's always present, or if it's more evident at certain times, such as after he has been active or when his body is in a particular position. In a patient with degenerative joint disease, movement limitation depends on the joints involved and the disease's progression. A patient with contracture of the hand, for example, can't extend his fingers. Ask the patient if his deformity or limitation of movement interferes with his daily activities. Find out what specific ways he has had to alter his routine because of these restrictions. Knowledge of how the patient carries out his ADLs helps determine how the deformity affects his ability to function.

Find out from the patient if he needs, or prefers to use, any support equipment, such as crutches or elastic bandages. This information will give a general idea of the severity of the patient's limitation of movement.

Past health history

The patient's past health history will give you clues to his present condition. Inquire whether he has ever had gout, arthritis, tuberculosis, or cancer, which may have bony metastasis. Ask the patient if he has been diagnosed with osteoporosis. Find out if he has ever had a sexually transmitted infection. If so, find out what type and when it occurred.

Ask whether he has had a recent blunt or penetrating trauma. If so, find out how it happened. For example, ask if he suffered any knee and hip injuries after being in an automobile accident or if he fell from a ladder and landed on his coccyx. This information will help guide your assessment and predict hidden trauma.

Also, if not already determined, ask the patient whether he uses an assistive device, such as a cane, walker, or brace. If he does, watch him use the device to assess how he moves.

Also note any history of allergies, hay fever, or asthma and ask about drug use, including herbal supplements or prescription, illicit, and over-the-counter drugs. Many drugs can affect the musculoskeletal system. For example, corticosteroids can cause muscle weakness, myopathy, osteoporosis, pathologic fractures, and avascular necrosis of the heads of the femur and humerus.

Family history

Ask the patient if any family member suffers from joint disease. Disorders with a hereditary component include gout; osteoarthritis of the distal interphalangeal joints; spondyloarthropathies, such as ankylosing spondylitis, Reiter's syndrome, psoriatic arthritis, and enteropathic arthritis; and rheumatoid arthritis.

Psychosocial history

Determine factors in the patient's lifestyle that influence his musculoskeletal status. Start with a general review of your patient's background that includes his age, sex, marital status, occupation, education, and ethnic background. Then focus on his specific problems.

Review the patient's typical diet. Poor calcium intake can lead to bone decalcification and subsequent fractures. Lack of exercise can lead to bone decalcification and muscle atrophy. A sedentary lifestyle can contribute to poor muscle tone and an increased risk of muscle strain. Additionally, sporadic exercise can be harmful, causing poorly toned muscles to be overworked, which can lead to muscle strain and spasm.

Ask the patient about his employment status, hobbies, and personal habits. Knitting, playing football or tennis, working at a computer, or doing construction work can all cause repetitive stress injuries or injure the musculoskeletal system in other ways. Even carrying a heavy knapsack or purse can cause injury or increase muscle size.

Physical assessment

Because the central nervous system and the musculoskeletal system are interrelated, assess them together.

To assess the musculoskeletal system, use the techniques of inspection and palpation to test all the major bones, joints, and muscles. Perform a complete examination if the patient has generalized symptoms such as aching in several joints. Perform an abbreviated examination if he has pain in only one body area such as his ankle.

Before starting the assessment, have the patient undress down to his underwear and put on a hospital gown. Be sure to explain each procedure as you perform it. The only special equipment you'll need is a tape measure. Begin the examination with a general observation of the patient and then measure his height.

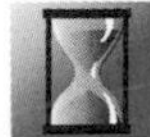

AGE ISSUE *With aging, elderly people commonly experience a decrease in height. It usually results from exaggerated spinal curvatures and narrowing intervertebral spaces, which shorten the person's trunk and make the arms appear longer.*

Next, systematically assess the patient's entire body, beginning at the head and ending at the toe, from proximal to distal structures. Because muscles and joints are interdependent, interpret these findings together. As you work your way down the body, note the size and shape of joints, limbs, and body regions. Inspect and palpate the skin and tissues around the joint, limbs, and body regions. Have the patient perform active range-of-motion (ROM) exercises of a joint if possible. If he can't, use passive ROM. During passive ROM exercises, support the joint firmly on either side, and move it gently to avoid causing pain or spasm.

Posture, gait, and coordination assessment

Your assessment begins the moment you have contact with the patient. Good observation skills provide a wealth of information, such as approximate muscle strength, facial muscle movement, body symmetry, and obvious physical or functional deformities or abnormalities. They also help in assessing children who are unable or unwilling to follow directions.

Assess the patient's overall body symmetry as he assumes different postures and makes diverse movements. Note marked dissimilarities in side-to-side size, shape, and motion. Observing his posture, gait, and coordination will provide important information in your assessment.

Posture

Evaluating posture — the attitude, or position, that body parts assume in relation to other body parts and to the external environment — includes inspecting spinal curvature and knee positioning.

Spinal curvature. To assess spinal curvature, instruct the patient to stand as straight as possible. While standing to the patient's side, back, and front, respectively, inspect the spine for alignment and the shoulders, iliac crests, and scapulae for symmetry of position and height. Then have the patient bend forward from the waist with arms relaxed and dangling. Standing behind him, inspect the spine's straightness, noting flank and thorax position and symmetry. Normally, convex curvature characterizes the thoracic spine and concave curvature characterizes the lumbar spine in a standing patient.

Other normal findings include a midline spine without lateral curvatures; a concave lumbar curvature that changes to a convex curvature in the flexed position; and iliac crests, shoulders, and scapulae at the same horizontal level.

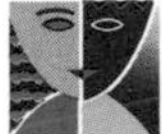

CULTURAL INSIGHT *Race can lead to differences in spinal curvature; for example, some blacks have pronounced lumbar lordosis.*

Knee positioning. To assess knee positioning, have the patient stand with his feet together. Note the relation of one knee to the other. They should be bilaterally symmetrical and located at the same height in a forward-facing position. Normally, the knees are less than 1″ (2.5 cm) apart and the medial malleoli, or the ankle bones, are less than 1⅛″ (2.9 cm) apart.

Gait

To assess gait, direct the patient to walk away, turn around, and walk back toward you. Observe and evaluate his posture; movement, such as pace and length of stride; foot position; coordination; and balance. During the stance phase, the foot on the floor should flatten completely and be able to bear the body's weight. As the patient pushes off, the toes should be flexed. In the swing phase, the foot in midswing should clear the floor and pass the opposite leg in its stance phase. When the swing phase ends, the patient should be able to control the swing as it stops, as the foot again contacts the floor.

Other normal findings include smooth, coordinated movements, the head leading the body when turning, and erect posture with approximately 2″ to 4″ (5 to 10 cm) of space between the feet.

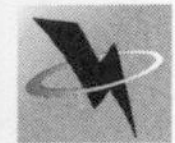

CRITICAL POINT *During the gait assessment, remain close to an elderly or infirm patient, and be ready to help if he should stumble or start to fall.*

Abnormal gait results from joint stiffness and pain, muscle weakness, deformities, and orthopedic devices such as leg braces. Other abnormal gait findings may also include an abnormally wide support base, which, in adults, may indicate central nervous system dysfunction; toeing in or out; arms held out to the side or in front; jerky or shuffling motions; and the ball of the foot, rather than the heel, striking the floor first.

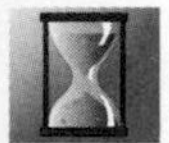

AGE ISSUE *Aging affects the elderly patient's nervous system, which, in turn, may cause difficulty in tandem walking. Typically, the elderly person walks with shorter steps and a wider leg stance to achieve better balance and stable weight distribution.*

Coordination

Evaluate how well a patient's muscles produce movement by observing his coordination. Coordination results from neuromuscular integrity. When the patient lacks muscular or nervous system integrity, or both, the ability to make voluntary and productive movements is impaired.

Assess gross motor skills by having the patient perform any body action involving the muscles and joints in natural directional movements, such as lifting the arm to the side and other ROM exercises. Assess fine motor coordination by asking the patient to pick up a small object from a desk or table. Examples of coordination problems associated with voluntary movement include ataxia, causing impaired movement coordination that's characterized by unusual or erratic muscular activity; spasticity, causing awkward, jerky, and stiff movements; and tremor, causing muscular quivering.

Bone and joint assessment

Perform a head-to-toe evaluation of the patient's bones and joints using inspection and palpation. Then perform ROM exercises to help determine whether the joints are healthy.

Head, jaw, and neck

First, inspect the patient's face for swelling, symmetry, and evidence of trauma. The mandible should be in the midline, not shifted to the right or left.

Next, evaluate ROM in the temporomandibular joint (TMJ). Place the tips of your first two or three fingers in front of the middle of the ear. Ask the patient to open and close his mouth. Then place your fingers into the depressed area over the joint, and note the motion of the mandible. The patient should be able to open and close his jaw and protract and retract his mandible easily, without pain or tenderness.

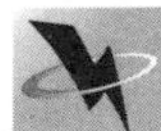

CRITICAL POINT *If you hear or palpate a click as the patient's mouth opens, suspect an improperly aligned jaw. TMJ dysfunction may also lead to swelling of the area, crepitus, or pain.*

Inspect the front, back, and sides of the patient's neck, noting muscle asymmetry or masses. Palpate the spinous processes of the cervical vertebrae and supraclavicular fossae for tenderness, swelling, or nodules.

To palpate the neck area, stand facing the patient with your hands placed lightly on the sides of the neck. Ask him to turn his head from side to side, flex his neck forward, and then extend it backward. Feel for any lumps or tender areas.

As the patient moves his neck, listen and palpate for crepitus. This is an abnormal crunching or grating sound, not the occasional "crack" that's heard from the joints. Crepitus is heard and felt when a joint with roughened articular surfaces moves. It occurs in patients with rheumatoid arthritis or osteoarthritis or when broken pieces of bone rub together.

Now, check ROM in the neck. Ask the patient to try touching his right ear to his right shoulder and his left ear to his left shoulder. The usual ROM is 40 degrees on each side. Next, ask him to touch his chin to his chest and then to point his chin toward the ceiling. The neck should flex forward 45 degrees and extend backward 55 degrees.

To assess rotation, ask the patient to turn his head to each side without moving his trunk. His chin should be parallel to his shoulders. Finally, ask him to move his head in a circle—normal rotation is 70 degrees.

Spine

Ask the patient to remove his examination gown so you can observe his spine. First check his spinal curvature as he stands in profile. In this position, the spine has a reverse S shape. (See *Recognizing kyphosis and lordosis.*)

Next, observe the spine posteriorly. It should be in midline position, without deviation to either side. Lateral deviation suggests scoliosis. You also may notice that one shoulder is lower than the other.

To assess for scoliosis, have the patient bend at the waist. This position makes deformities more apparent. Normally, the spine remains at midline. (See *Testing for scoliosis,* page 448.)

Next, assess the range of spinal movement. Ask the patient to straighten up, and use the measuring tape to measure the distance from the nape of his neck to his waist. Then ask him to bend forward at the waist. Continue to hold the tape at his neck, letting it slip through your fingers slightly to accommodate the increased distance as the spine flexes.

The length of the spine from neck to waist usually increases by at least 2″ (5 cm) when the patient bends forward. If it doesn't, the patient's mobility may be impaired, and you'll need to assess him further.

Finally, palpate the spinal processes and the areas lateral to the spine. Have the patient bend at the waist and let his arms hang loosely at his sides. Palpate the spine with your fingertips. Then repeat the palpation using the side of your hand, lightly striking the areas lateral to the spine. Note tenderness, swelling, or spasm.

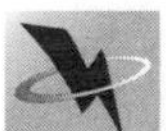

CRITICAL POINT *A lateral forward bending posture accompanied by low back pain radiating to the buttock, leg, and foot and sciatic pain or muscle spasms suggests a herniated disk. To help confirm this suspicion, perform the straight leg test. First, have the patient lie in a supine position and ask him to raise one leg while keeping his knee extended. Then, ask him to dorsiflex his foot. If this movement triggers posterior leg pain (sciatica), he probably has a herniated disk.*

RECOGNIZING KYPHOSIS AND LORDOSIS

These illustrations show the difference between kyphosis and lordosis.

Kyphosis

If the patient has a pronounced kyphosis, the thoracic curve is abnormally rounded, as shown.

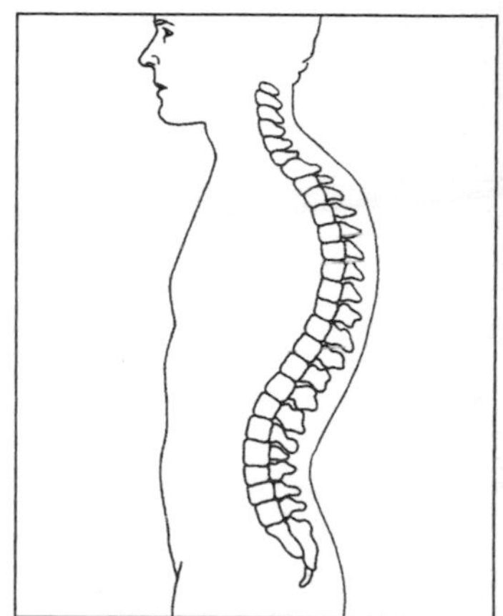

Lordosis

If the patient has a pronounced lordosis, the lumbar spine is abnormally concave, as shown. Lordosis, as well as a waddling gait, is normal in pregnant women and young children.

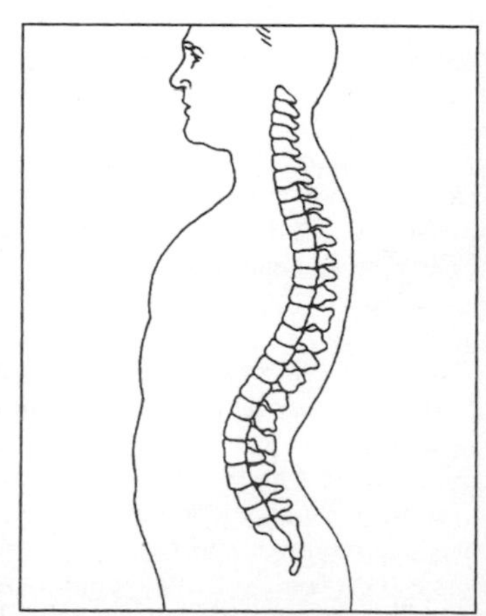

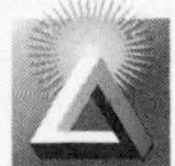

EXPERT TECHNIQUE

TESTING FOR SCOLIOSIS

When testing for scoliosis, have the patient remove the examination gown and stand as straight as possible with her back to you. Observe for:

- uneven shoulder height and shoulder blade prominence
- unequal distance between the arms and the body
- asymmetrical waistline
- uneven hip height
- sideways lean.

Next, have her bend forward, keeping her head down and palms together. Observe for:

- asymmetrical thoracic spine or prominent rib cage, or rib hump, on either side
- asymmetrical waistline.

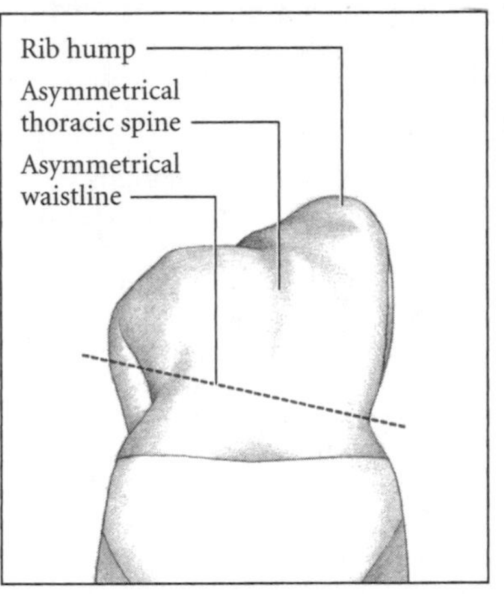

Shoulders and elbows

Start by observing the patient's shoulders, noting asymmetry, muscle atrophy, or deformity. Swelling or loss of the normal rounded shape could mean that one or more bones are dislocated or out of alignment.

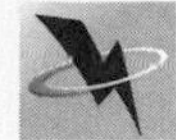

CRITICAL POINT *If the patient's chief complaint is shoulder pain, keep in mind that the problem may not have originated there. Shoulder pain may be referred from other sources and may be due to a heart attack or ruptured ectopic pregnancy. Either of these conditions requires emergency intervention.*

Palpate the patient's shoulders with the palmar surfaces of the fingers to locate bony landmarks; note crepitus or tenderness. Using the entire hand, palpate the shoulder muscles for firmness and symmetry of size. Also palpate the elbow and the ulna for subcutaneous nodules that occur with rheumatoid arthritis. Palpate the acromion process and biceps tendon and assess for tenderness.

If shoulder joint palpation produces pain in the greater humeral tuberosity area, calcium deposits or trauma-related inflammation may be the cause. If you have difficulty abducting the patient's arm and pain occurs in the deltoid muscle or over the supraspinatus tendon insertion site during palpation, this may indicate a rotator cuff tear.

If the patient's shoulders don't appear dislocated, assess rotation. Start with the patient's arm straight at his side—the neutral position. Ask him to lift his arm straight up from his side to shoulder level and then to bend his elbow horizontally until his forearm is at a 90-degree angle to his upper arm. His arm should be parallel to the floor, and his fingers should be extended with palms down.

To assess external rotation, have him bring his forearm up until his fingers point toward the ceiling. To assess internal rotation, have him lower his forearm until his fingers point toward the floor. Normal ROM is 90 degrees in each direction.

To assess flexion and extension, start with the patient's arm in the neutral position, at his side. To assess flexion, ask him to move his arm anteriorly over his head, as if reaching for the sky. Full flexion is 180 degrees. To assess extension, have him move his arm from the neutral position posteriorly as far as possible. Normal extension ranges from 30 to 50 degrees.

To assess abduction, ask the patient to move his arm from the neutral position laterally as far as possible. Normal ROM is 180 degrees. To assess adduction, have the patient move his arm from the neutral position across the front of his body as far as possible. Normal ROM is 50 degrees.

Next, assess the elbows for flexion and extension. Have the patient rest his arm at his side. Ask him to flex his elbow from this position and then extend it. Normal ROM is 90 degrees for both flexion and extension.

To assess supination and pronation of the elbow, have the patient place the side of his hand on a flat surface with the thumb on top. Ask him to rotate his palm down toward the table for pronation and upward for supination. The normal angle of elbow rotation is 90 degrees in each direction.

Wrists and hands

Inspect the patient's wrists and hands for contour, and compare them for symmetry. Also check for nodules, redness, swelling, deformities, and webbing between fingers.

Use the thumb and index finger to palpate both wrists and each finger joint. Note any tenderness, nodules, or bogginess.

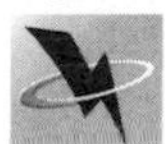

CRITICAL POINT *To avoid causing pain, be especially gentle with elderly patients and those with arthritis.*

Assess ROM in the wrist. Ask the patient to rotate his wrist by moving his entire hand — first laterally, then medially — as if he's waxing a car. Normal ROM is 55 degrees laterally and 20 degrees medially.

Observe the wrist while the patient extends his fingers up toward the ceiling and down toward the floor, as if he's flapping his hand. He should be able to extend his wrist 70 degrees and flex it 90 degrees. If these movements cause pain or numbness, the patient may have carpal tunnel syndrome. (See *Testing for carpal tunnel syndrome.*)

To assess extension and flexion of the metacarpophalangeal joints, ask the patient to keep his wrist still and move only his fingers — first up toward the ceiling, then down toward the floor. Normal extension is 30 degrees; normal flexion, 90 degrees.

Next, ask the patient to touch his thumb to the little finger of the same hand. He should be able to fold or flex his thumb across the palm of his hand so that it touch-

EXPERT TECHNIQUE

TESTING FOR CARPAL TUNNEL SYNDROME

To diagnose carpal tunnel syndrome, perform these two tests — for Tinel's sign and Phalen's sign — as described here.

Tinel's sign

Lightly percuss the transverse carpal ligament over the median nerve where the patient's palm and wrist meet. If this action produces discomfort, such as numbness and tingling shooting into the palm and finger, the patient has Tinel's sign, which suggests carpal tunnel syndrome.

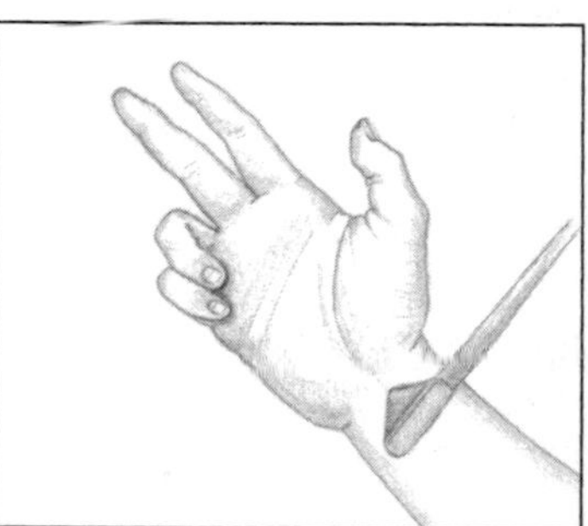

Phalen's sign

If flexing the patient's wrist for about 30 seconds causes pain or numbness in his hand or fingers, he has Phalen's sign. The more severe the carpal tunnel syndrome, the more rapidly symptoms develop.

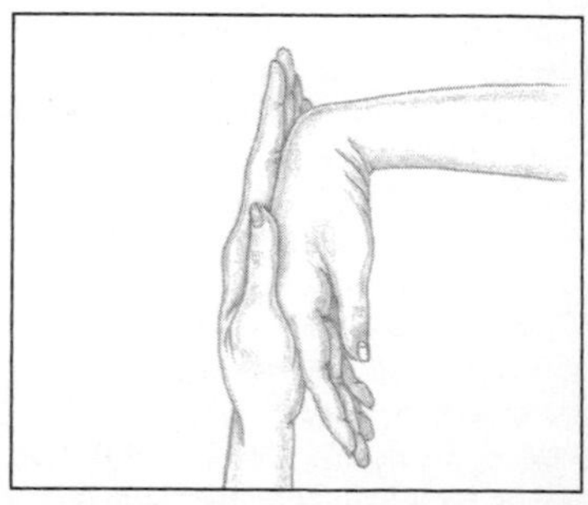

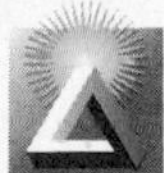

EXPERT TECHNIQUE

ASSESSING FOR BULGE SIGN

The bulge sign indicates excess fluid in the joint. To assess the patient for this sign, ask him to lie down so that you can palpate his knee. Then give the medial side of his knee two to four firm strokes, as shown, to displace excess fluid.

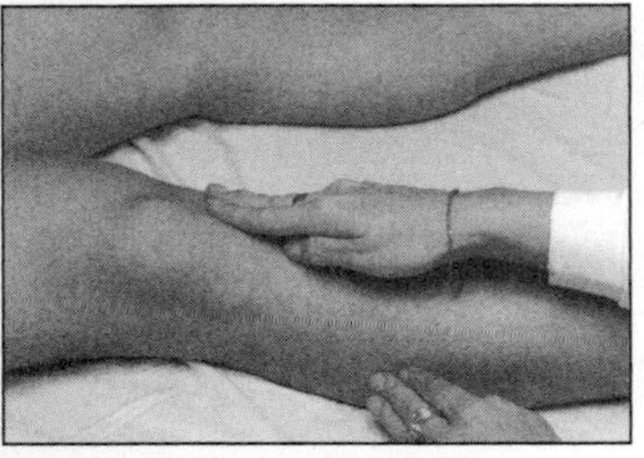

Lateral check
Next, tap the lateral aspect of the knee while checking for a fluid wave on the medial aspect, as shown.

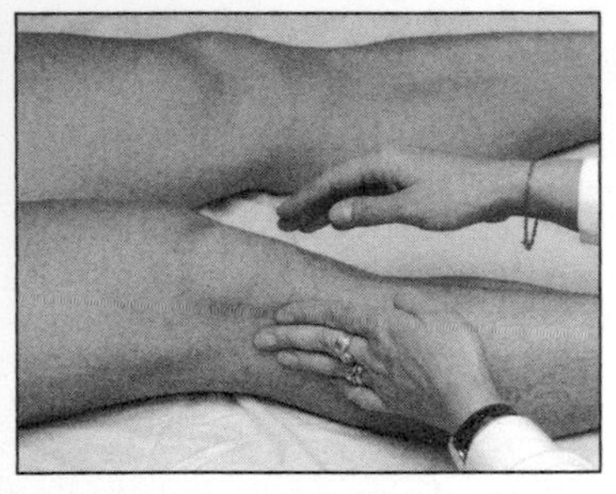

es or points toward the base of his little finger.

To assess flexion of all of the fingers, ask the patient to form a fist. Then have him spread his fingers apart to demonstrate abduction and draw them back together to demonstrate adduction.

If you suspect that one arm is longer than the other, take measurements. Put one end of the measuring tape at the acromial process of the shoulder and the other on the tip of the middle finger. Drape the tape over the outer elbow. The difference between the left and right extremities should be no more than 3/8" (1 cm).

Hips and knees

Inspect the hip area for contour and symmetry. Inspect the position of the knees, noting whether the patient is "bowlegged", with knees that point out, or "knock-kneed", with knees that turn in. Then watch the patient walk.

Palpate both knees. They should feel smooth, and the tissues should feel solid. Swelling over the patella suggests prepatellar bursitis. (See *Assessing for bulge sign.*)

Assess ROM in the hip. These exercises are usually done with the patient in the supine position.

To assess hip flexion, have the patient bend each knee up to the chest and pull it firmly against the abdomen. Place your hand under the patient's lumbar spine. Note when the back touches your hand. To assess hip extension, extend the thigh toward you in a posterior direction while the patient is lying face down.

To assess abduction, stabilize the pelvis by pressing down on the opposite anterior superior iliac spine with one hand. With the other hand, grasp the ankle and abduct the extended leg. To assess adduction, stabilize the pelvis and move the leg medially across the body while holding the ankle. Normal ROM is about 45 degrees for abduction and 30 degrees for adduction.

To assess internal and external rotation of the hip, flex the leg to 90 degrees at the hip and knee, stabilize the thigh with one hand, and swing the lower leg medially and laterally. Normal ROM for internal rotation is 40 degrees; for external rotation, 45 degrees.

CRITICAL POINT *Restriction of internal rotation is a sensitive indicator of arthritis in the hip.*

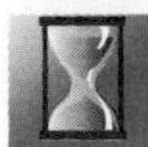

AGE ISSUE *For a child, inspect the gluteal folds for asymmetry, which might suggest a hip dislocation. If this condition is suspected, perform Ortolani's maneuver (see chapter 19, Assessing the neonate). Also observe the child's legs for shape, length, symmetry, and alignment. Bowlegs are common in children between ages 1½ and 2½; knock-knees is common in preschoolers. Test for bowlegs by having the child stand straight with his ankles touching. In this position, the knees shouldn't be more 1" (2.5 cm)*

apart; test for knock-knees by having the child stand straight with his knees touching. The ankles shouldn't be more than 1" (2.5 cm) apart. Also, look for the pattern of wear on the child's shoes. Wear on the outside of the heel suggests bowlegs; on the inside of the heel, knock-knees.

Assess ROM in the knee. If the patient is standing, ask him to bend his knee as if trying to touch his heel to his buttocks. Normal ROM for flexion is 120 to 130 degrees. If the patient is lying down, have him draw his knee up to his chest. His calf should touch his thigh.

Knee extension returns the knee to a neutral position of 0 degrees; however, some knees may normally be hyperextended 15 degrees.

If the patient can't extend his leg fully or if his knee "pops" audibly and painfully, consider the response abnormal. Other abnormalities include pronounced crepitus, which may signal a degenerative disease of the knee, and sudden buckling, which may indicate a ligament injury.

Ankles and feet

Inspect the patient's ankles and feet for swelling, redness, nodules, and other deformities. Check the arch of the foot and look for toe deformities. Also note edema, calluses, bunions, corns, ingrown toenails, plantar warts, trophic ulcers, hair loss, or unusual pigmentation.

Use the fingertips to palpate the bony and muscular structures of the ankles and feet. Palpate each toe joint by compressing it with the thumb and fingers.

To examine the ankle, have the patient sit in a chair or on the side of a bed. To test plantar flexion, ask him to point his toes toward the floor. Test dorsiflexion by asking him to point his toes toward the ceiling. Normal ROM for plantar flexion is about 45 degrees; for dorsiflexion, 20 degrees.

Next, assess ROM in the ankle. Ask the patient to demonstrate inversion by turning his feet inward, and eversion by turning his feet outward. Normal ROM for inversion is 45 degrees; for eversion, 30 degrees.

To assess the metatarsophalangeal joints, ask the patient to flex his toes and then straighten them. If you suspect that one leg is longer than the other, take measurements. Put one end of the tape at the medial malleolus at the ankle and the other end at the anterior iliac spine. Cross the tape over the medial side of the knee.

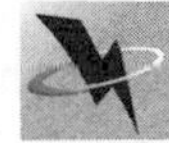

CRITICAL POINT *A difference of more than ⅜" (1 cm) in one leg is abnormal.*

Muscle assessment

Start by inspecting all major muscle groups for tone, strength, asymmetry, and other abnormalities. If a muscle appears atrophied or hypertrophied, measure it by wrapping a tape measure around the largest circumference of the muscle on each side of the body and comparing the two numbers.

Abnormalities of muscle appearance include contracture and abnormal movements, such as spasms, tics, tremors, or fasciculation.

Muscle tone

Muscle tone describes muscular resistance to passive stretching. To test the patient's arm muscle tone, move his shoulder through passive ROM exercises. You should feel a slight resistance. Then let his arm drop. It should fall easily to his side.

Test leg muscle tone by putting the patient's hip through passive ROM exercises and then letting the leg fall to the examination table or bed. Like the arm, the leg should fall easily.

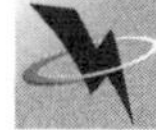

CRITICAL POINT *Muscle rigidity indicates increased muscle tone, possibly caused by an upper motor neuron lesion such as from a stroke. Muscle flaccidity may result from a lower motor neuron lesion.*

Muscle strength

Observe the patient's gait and movements to form an idea of his general muscle strength. To test specific muscle groups, ask him to move the muscles while you apply resistance; then compare the contralateral muscle groups. (See *Testing muscle strength,* pages 452 and 453.)

Grade muscle strength on a scale of 0 to 5, with 0 representing no strength and 5 representing maximum strength. Document the results as a fraction, with the score as the numerator and maximum strength as the denominator.

(Text continues on page 454.)

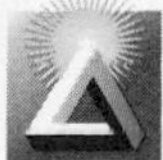

EXPERT TECHNIQUE

TESTING MUSCLE STRENGTH

Obtain an overall picture of your patient's motor function by testing strength in 10 selected muscle groups in the arms and legs. Ask the patient to attempt normal range-of-motion movements against your resistance. If the muscle group is weak, vary the amount of resistance as required to permit accurate assessment. If necessary, position the patient so his limbs don't have to resist gravity, and repeat the test.

ARM MUSCLES

Biceps. With your hand on the patient's hand, have him flex his forearm against your resistance. Watch for biceps contraction.

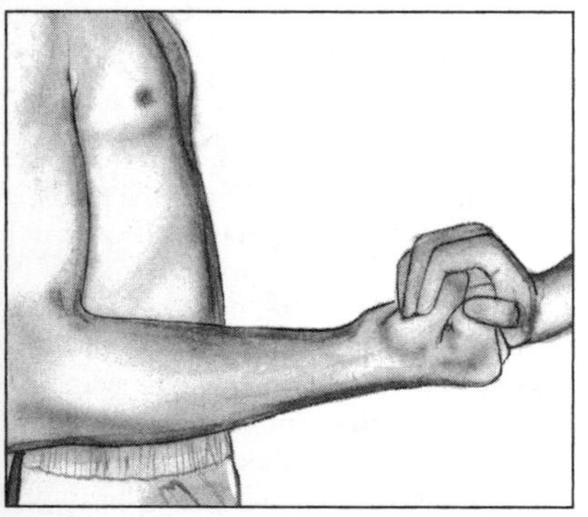

Deltoid. With the patient's arm fully extended, place one hand over his deltoid muscle and the other on his wrist. Ask him to abduct his arm to a horizontal position against your resistance; as he does so, palpate for deltoid contraction.

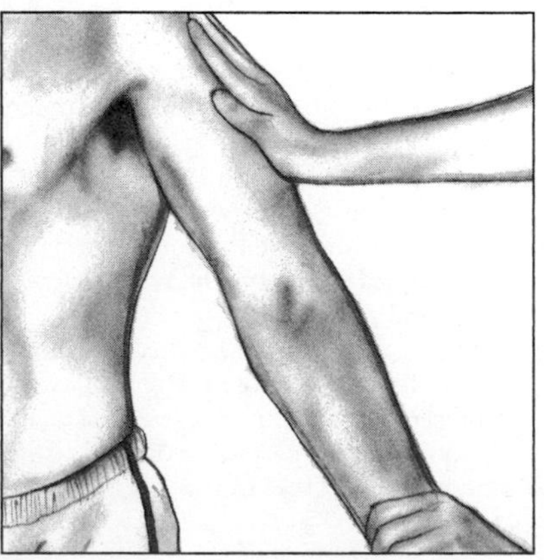

Triceps. Have the patient abduct and hold his arm midway between flexion and extension. Hold and support his arm at the wrist, and ask him to extend it against your resistance. Watch for triceps contraction.

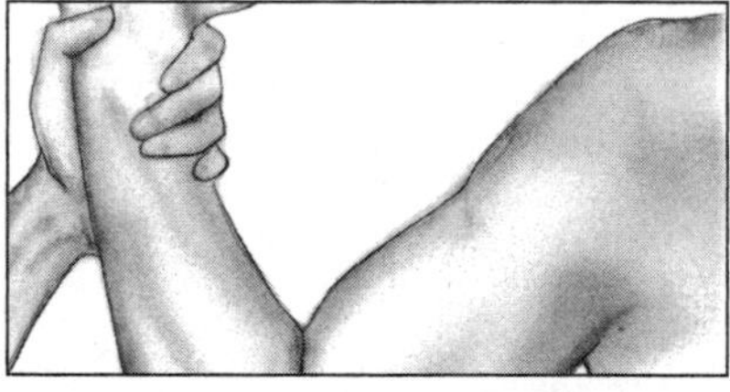

Dorsal interossei. Have the patient extend and spread his fingers, and tell him to try to resist your attempt to squeeze them together.

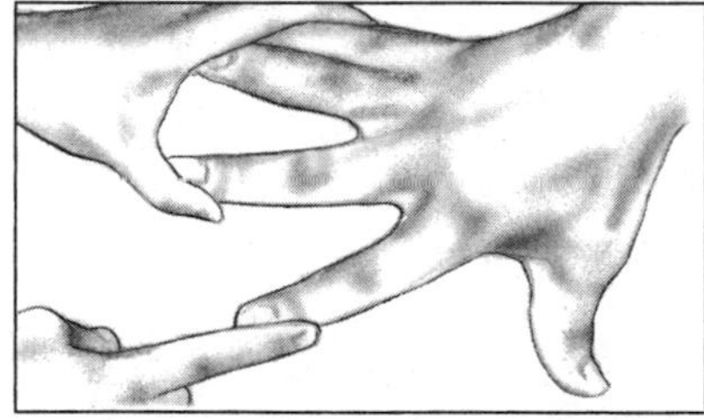

Forearm and hand (grip). Have the patient grasp your middle and index fingers and squeeze as hard as he can. To prevent pain or injury to the examiner, the examiner should cross his fingers.

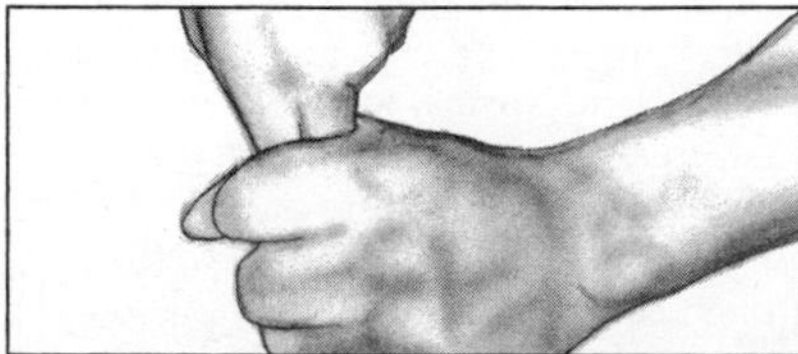

Rate muscle strength on a scale from 0 to 5:
0 = Total paralysis
1 = Visible or palpable contraction, but no movement
2 = Full muscle movement with force of gravity eliminated
3 = Full muscle movement against gravity, but no movement against resistance
4 = Full muscle movement against gravity; partial movement against resistance
5 = Full muscle movement against both gravity and resistance — normal strength

LEG MUSCLES

Anterior tibial. With the patient's leg extended, place your hand on his foot and ask him to dorsiflex his ankle against your resistance. Palpate for anterior tibial contraction.

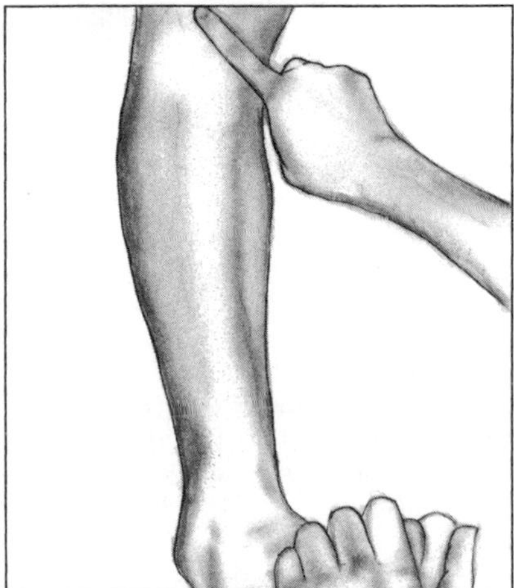

Psoas. While you support his leg, have the patient raise his knee and then flex his hip against your resistance. Watch for psoas contraction.

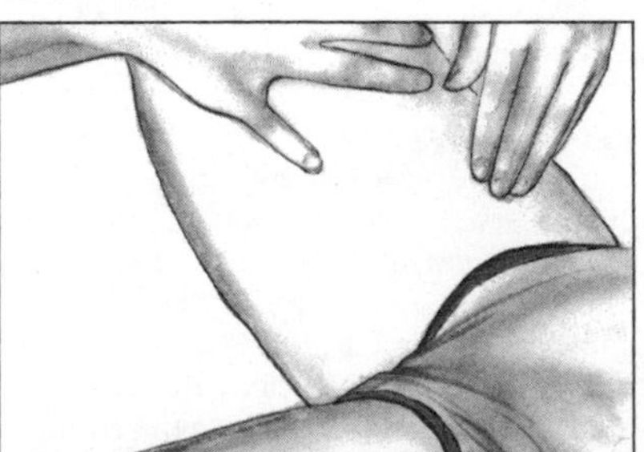

Extensor hallucis longus. With your finger on the patient's great toe, have him dorsiflex the toe against your resistance. Palpate for extensor hallucis contraction.

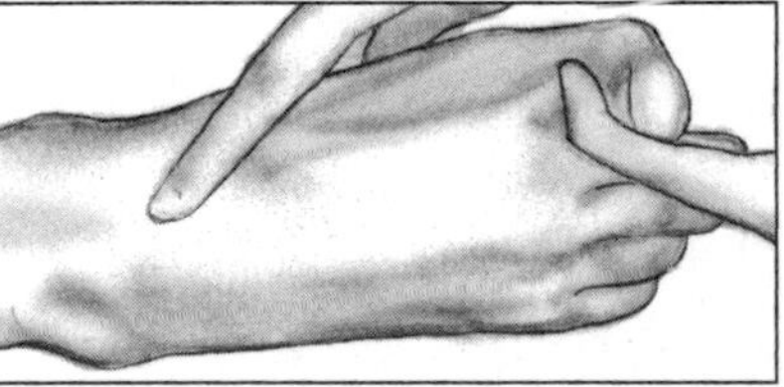

Quadriceps. Have the patient bend his knee slightly while you support his lower leg. Then ask him to extend the knee against your resistance; as he's doing so, palpate for quadriceps contraction.

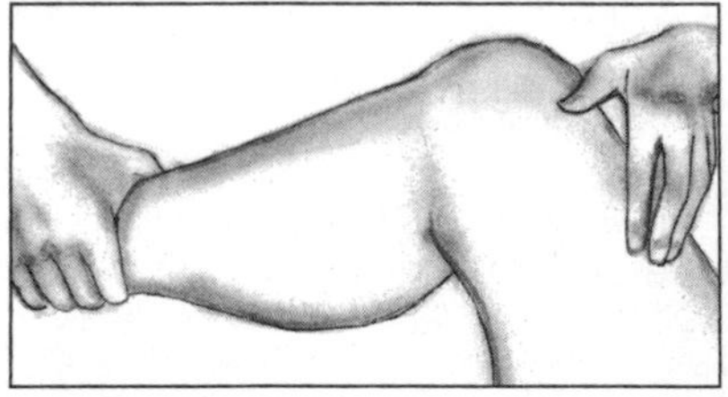

Gastrocnemius. With the patient on his side, support his foot and ask him to plantarflex his ankle against your resistance. Palpate for gastrocnemius contraction.

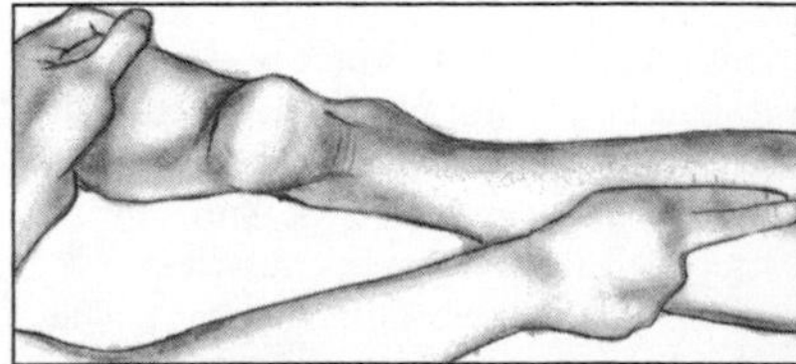

Shoulder, arm, wrist, and hand strength. Test the strength of the patient's shoulder girdle by asking him to extend his arms with the palms up and hold this position for 30 seconds. If the patient can't lift both of his arms equally and keep his palms up, or if one arm drifts down, he probably has shoulder girdle weakness on that side.

If he passes the first part of the test, gauge his strength by lacing your hands on his arms and applying downward pressure as he resists you.

Next, have the patient hold his arm in front of him with the elbow bent. To test biceps strength, pull down on the flexor surface of his forearm as he resists. To test triceps strength, have him try to straighten his arm as you push upward against the extensor surface of his forearm.

Assess the strength of the patient's flexed wrist by pushing against it. Test the strength of the extended wrist by pushing down on it. Test the strength of finger abduction, thumb opposition, and handgrip the same way.

Leg strength. Ask the patient to lie in a supine position on the examination table or bed and lift both legs at the same time. Note whether he lifts both legs at the same time and to the same distance. To test quadriceps strength, have him lower his legs and raise them again while you press down on his anterior thighs.

Then ask the patient to flex his knees and put his feet flat on the bed. Assess lower-leg strength by pulling his lower leg forward as he resists and then by pushing it backward as he extends his knee.

Finally, assess ankle strength by having the patient push his foot down against your resistance and then pull his foot up as you try to hold it down.

Abnormal findings

A patient's chief complaint may be due to several signs and symptoms related to the musculoskeletal system. The most significant findings are arm pain, back pain, jaw pain, leg pain, muscle atrophy, muscle spasm, muscle weakness, and neck pain. The following history, physical assessment, and analysis summaries will help you assess each one quickly and accurately. After obtaining further information, begin to interpret the findings. (See *Musculoskeletal system: Interpreting your findings.*)

Arm pain

Arm pain usually results from musculoskeletal disorders, but it can also stem from neurovascular or cardiovascular disorders. In some cases, it may be referred pain from another area, such as the chest, neck, or abdomen.

History

If the patient reports arm pain after an injury, take a brief history of the injury. Then quickly assess him for severe injuries requiring immediate treatment. If you've ruled out severe injuries, check pulses, capillary refill time, sensation, and movement distal to the affected area because circulatory impairment or nerve injury may require immediate surgery. Inspect the arm for deformities, assess the level of pain, and immobilize the arm to prevent further injury.

If the patient reports continuous or intermittent arm pain, ask him to describe it and relate when it began. Ask him if the pain is associated with repetitive or specific movements or positions. Ask him to point out other painful areas because arm pain may be referred. For example, arm pain commonly accompanies the characteristic chest pain of myocardial infarction, and right shoulder pain may be referred from the right-upper-quadrant abdominal pain of cholecystitis. Ask the patient if the pain worsens in the morning or in the evening, if it prevents him from performing his job, and if it restricts movement. Also ask if heat, rest, or medications relieve it. Finally, ask about any preexisting illnesses, a family history of gout or arthritis, and current medication therapy.

Physical assessment

Next, perform a focused physical examination. Observe the way the patient walks, sits, and holds his arm. Inspect the entire arm, comparing it with the opposite arm for symmetry, movement, and muscle atrophy. It's important to know whether the patient is right- or left-handed. Palpate the entire arm for swelling, nodules, and tender areas.

(Text continues on page 459.)

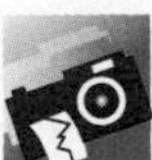

CLINICAL PICTURE

MUSCULOSKELETAL SYSTEM: INTERPRETING YOUR FINDINGS

After you assess the patient, a group of findings may lead you to suspect a particular musculoskeletal disorder. The chart below shows you some common groups of findings for major signs and symptoms related to the musculoskeletal system, along with their probable causes.

Sign or symptom and findings	Probable cause
Arm pain	
▪ Pain radiating through the arm ▪ Pain worsens with movement ▪ Crepitus, felt and heard ▪ Deformity, if bones are misaligned ▪ Local ecchymosis and edema ▪ Impaired distal circulation ▪ Paresthesia	Fracture
▪ Left arm pain ▪ Deep and crushing chest pain ▪ Weakness ▪ Pallor ▪ Dyspnea ▪ Diaphoresis ▪ Apprehension	Myocardial infarction
▪ Severe arm pain with passive muscle stretching ▪ Impaired distal circulation ▪ Muscle weakness ▪ Decreased reflex response ▪ Paresthesia ▪ Edema ▪ Ominous signs, such as paralysis and absent pulse	Compartment syndrome

Sign or symptom and findings	Probable cause
Back pain	
▪ Sacroiliac pain radiating up the spine and aggravated by lateral pressure on the pelvis; most severe in the morning or after a period of inactivity and not relieved by rest ▪ Abnormal lumbar spine rigidity with forward flexion ▪ Local tenderness ▪ Fatigue ▪ Fever ▪ Anorexia ▪ Weight loss ▪ Occasional iritis	Ankylosing spondylitis
▪ Colicky pain from costovertebral angle to the flank, suprapubic region, and external genitalia of varying intensity; may be dull and constant flank pain ▪ Nausea and vomiting ▪ Urinary urgency ▪ Hematuria ▪ Agitation due to pain	Renal calculi

(continued)

MUSCULOSKELETAL SYSTEM: INTERPRETING YOUR FINDINGS *(continued)*

Sign or symptom and findings	Probable cause
Back pain *(continued)*	
■ Initially painless becoming painful, which is aggravated by weight bearing and local tenderness ■ Possible referred pain in the lumbar area, if thoracic vertebra involved	Vertebral compression fracture
Jaw pain	
■ Jaw pain usually radiating from the substernal area and left arm pain; commonly triggered by exertion, emotional stress, or ingestion of a heavy meal; subsiding with rest and nitroglycerin ■ Shortness of breath ■ Nausea and vomiting ■ Tachycardia ■ Dizziness ■ Diaphoresis ■ Belching ■ Palpitations	Angina pectoris
■ Painful muscle contractions of the jaw and mouth ■ Paresthesia and carpopedal spasm ■ Weakness and fatigue ■ Palpitations ■ Hyperreflexia and positive Chvostek's and Trousseau's signs ■ Muscle twitching ■ Choreiform movements ■ Muscle cramps ■ Laryngeal spasms, if severe, with stridor	Hypocalcemic tetany
Jaw pain *(continued)*	
■ Jaw pain at the temporomandibular (TMJ) joint; unilateral, localized pain possibly radiating to other head and neck areas ■ Spasm and pain of the masticating muscle ■ Clicking, popping, or crepitus of the TMJ ■ Restricted jaw movement ■ Teeth clenching ■ Bruxism ■ Emotional stress	TMJ syndrome
Leg pain	
■ Severe, acute leg pain, particularly with movement ■ Ecchymosis and edema ■ Leg can't bear weight ■ Impaired neurovascular status distal to injury ■ Deformity, crepitus, and muscle spasms	Fracture
■ Shooting, aching, or tingling pain that radiates down the leg ■ Pain exacerbated by activity and relieved by rest ■ Limping ■ Difficulty moving from a sitting to standing position	Sciatica

MUSCULOSKELETAL SYSTEM: INTERPRETING YOUR FINDINGS
(continued)

Sign or symptom and findings	Probable cause
Leg pain *(continued)*	
▪ Discomfort ranging from calf tenderness to severe pain ▪ Edema and a feeling of heaviness in the affected leg ▪ Warmth ▪ Fever, chills, malaise, muscle cramps ▪ Positive Homans' sign	Thrombophlebitis
Muscle atrophy	
▪ Initially muscle weakness and atrophy beginning in one hand and spreading to the arm, then developing in other hand and arm ▪ Weakness and atrophy progressing to trunk, neck, tongue, larynx, pharynx, and legs ▪ Progressive respiratory muscle weakness ▪ Muscle flaccidity ▪ Fasciculations ▪ Hyperactive deep tendon reflexes ▪ Slight leg muscle spasticity ▪ Dysphagia ▪ Impaired speech ▪ Excessive drooling ▪ Depression	Amyotrophic lateral sclerosis
Muscle atrophy *(continued)*	
▪ Muscle weakness, disuse of, and ultimate atrophy due to pressure on nerve roots ▪ Severe lower back pain possibly radiating to buttocks, legs, and feet, and commonly accompanied by muscle spasms ▪ Diminished reflexes ▪ Sensory changes	Herniated disk
▪ Contralateral or bilateral weakness with eventual atrophy of arms, legs, face, and tongue ▪ Associated signs and symptoms depend on site and extent of vascular damage, including apraxia, agnosia, and ipsilateral paresthesia or sensory loss ▪ Vision disturbances ▪ Altered level of consciousness (LOC) ▪ Personality changes ▪ Emotional lability ▪ Bowel and bladder dysfunction	Stroke

(continued)

MUSCULOSKELETAL SYSTEM: INTERPRETING YOUR FINDINGS *(continued)*

Sign or symptom and findings	Probable cause
Muscle spasms	
▪ Spasms and intermittent claudication ▪ Loss of peripheral pulses ▪ Pallor or cyanosis ▪ Decreased sensation ▪ Hair loss ▪ Dry or scaling skin ▪ Edema ▪ Ulcerations	Arterial occulsive disease
▪ Localized spasms and pain ▪ Swelling ▪ Limited mobility ▪ Bony crepitation	Fracture
▪ Tetany (muscle cramps and twitching, carpopedal and facial muscle spasms, and seizures) ▪ Positive Chvostek's and Trousseau's signs ▪ Paresthesia of the lips, fingers, and toes ▪ Choreiform movements ▪ Hyperactive deep tendon reflexes ▪ Fatigue ▪ Palpitations ▪ Cardiac arrhythmias	Hypocalcemia
Muscle weakness	
▪ Unilateral or bilateral weakness of the arms, legs, face, or tongue ▪ Dysarthria ▪ Aphasia ▪ Paresthesia or sensory loss ▪ Vision disturbances ▪ Bowel and bladder dysfunction	Stroke
▪ Muscle weakness, disuse, and possible atrophy ▪ Altered LOC ▪ Personality changes ▪ Severe low back pain, possibly radiating to buttocks, legs, and feet, usually unilateral ▪ Diminished reflexes ▪ Sensory changes	Herniated disk
▪ Muscle weakness in one or more limbs which may lead to atrophy, spasticity, and contractures ▪ Diplopia, blurred vision, or vision loss ▪ Hyperactive deep tendon reflexes ▪ Paresthesia or sensory loss ▪ Incoordination ▪ Intention tremors	Multiple sclerosis

MUSCULOSKELETAL SYSTEM: INTERPRETING YOUR FINDINGS
(continued)

Sign or symptom and findings	Probable cause
Neck pain	
▪ Posterior neck pain restricting movement and aggravated by movement; radiating to either arm ▪ Paresthesia ▪ Weakness ▪ Stiffness	Cervical spondylosis
▪ Variable neck pain restricting movement and aggravated by movement ▪ Referred pain along a specific dermatome ▪ Paresthesia ▪ Sensory disturbances ▪ Arm weakness	Herniated cervical disk
***Neck pain** (continued)*	
▪ Neck pain accompanied by nuchal rigidity ▪ Fever ▪ Headache ▪ Photophobia ▪ Positive Brudzinski's and Kernig's signs ▪ Decreased LOC	Meningitis
▪ Pain ▪ Slight swelling ▪ Stiffness ▪ Restricted range of motion ▪ Pain, marked swelling, ecchymosis, muscle spasms, and nuchal rigidity with head tilt, ligament rupture	Neck sprain

In both arms, compare active range of motion (ROM), muscle strength, and reflexes.

If the patient reports numbness or tingling, check his sensation to vibration, temperature, and pinprick. Compare bilateral hand grasps and shoulder strength to detect weakness.

If a patient has a cast, splint, or restrictive dressing, check for circulation, sensation, and mobility distal to the dressing. Ask him if he has experienced edema and if the pain has worsened within the last 24 hours. Also ask which activities he has been performing.

Examine the patient's neck for pain on motion, point tenderness, muscle spasms, or arm pain when the neck is extended with the head toward the involved side.

Analysis

The location, onset, and character of the patient's arm pain provide clues to its cause. The pain may affect the entire arm or only the upper arm or forearm. It may occur suddenly or gradually and be constant or intermittent. Arm pain can be described as sharp or dull, burning or numbing, and shooting or penetrating. Diffuse arm pain, though, may be difficult to describe, especially if it isn't associated with injury.

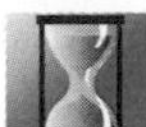

AGE ISSUE *In children, arm pain commonly results from fractures, muscle sprain, muscular dystrophy, or rheumatoid arthritis. In young children especially, the pain's exact location may be difficult to establish. Watch for nonverbal clues, such as wincing or guarding. If the child has a fracture or sprain, obtain a complete account of the injury. Closely observe interactions between the child and his family, and don't rule out the possibility of child abuse. Elderly patients with osteoporosis may experience fractures from simple trauma or even from heavy lifting or unexpected movements. They're also prone to degenerative joint disease that can involve several joints in the arm or neck.*

Back pain

Back pain affects an estimated 80% of the U.S. population; in fact, it's the second leading reason — after the common cold — for lost time from work. The onset, location, and distribution of pain and its response to activity and rest provide important clues about the cause. Pain may be acute or chronic, constant or intermittent. It may remain localized in the back or radiate along the spine or down one or both legs. Pain may be exacerbated by activity — usually, bending, stooping, lifting — and alleviated by rest, or it may unaffected by either.

History

If life-threatening causes of back pain are ruled out, continue with a complete health history and physical examination. Be aware of the patient's expressions of pain during the assessment. Obtain a medical history, including past injuries and illnesses, and a family history. Ask about diet and alcohol intake. Also, take a drug history, including past and present prescriptions and over-the-counter drugs.

CRITICAL POINT *If the patient reports acute, severe back pain, quickly take his vital signs; then perform a rapid evaluation to rule out life-threatening causes. Ask him when the pain began and if he can relate it to any causes. For example, find out if the pain occurred after eating or after slipping on an icy surface. Have the patient describe the pain, such as if it's burning, stabbing, throbbing, or aching. Find out if it's constant or intermittent and if it radiates to the buttocks or legs. Ask him if he has leg weakness. Find out if the pain originates in the abdomen and radiates to the back. Ask him if he has had this pain before. Find out what makes it better or worse and if it's affected by activity or rest. Ask the patient if the pain is worse in the morning or evening and if it wakes him up. Typically, visceral-referred back pain is unaffected by activity and rest. In contrast, spondylogenic referred back pain worsens with activity and improves with rest. Pain of neoplastic origin is usually relieved by walking and worsens at night.*

Physical assessment

Next, perform a thorough physical examination. Observe skin color, especially in the patient's legs, and palpate skin temperature. Palpate femoral, popliteal, posterior tibial, and pedal pulses. Ask about unusual sensations in the legs, such as numbness and tingling. Observe the patient's posture if pain doesn't prohibit standing. Note if he stands erect or tends to lean toward one side. Observe the level of the shoulders and pelvis and the curvature of the back. Ask the patient to bend forward, backward, and from side to side while you palpate for paravertebral muscle spasms. Note rotation of the spine on the trunk. Palpate the dorsolumbar spine for point tenderness. Then ask the patient to walk — first on his heels, then on his toes; protect him from falling as he does so. Weakness may reflect a muscular disorder or spinal nerve root irritation. Place the patient in a sitting position to evaluate and compare patellar tendon (knee), Achilles tendon, and Babinski's reflexes. Evaluate the strength of the extensor hallucis longus by asking the patient to hold up his big toe against resistance. Measure leg length and hamstring and quadriceps muscles bilaterally. Note a difference of more than ⅜″ (1 cm) in muscle size, especially in the calf.

To reproduce leg and back pain, position the patient in a supine position on the examination table. Grasp his heel and slowly lift his leg. If he feels pain, note its exact location and the angle between the table and his leg when it occurs. Repeat this maneuver with the opposite leg. Pain along the sciatic nerve may indicate disk herniation or sciatica. Also, note the ROM of the hip and knee.

CRITICAL POINT *If the patient describes deep lumbar pain unaffected by activity, palpate for a pulsating epigastric mass. If this sign is present, suspect dissecting abdominal aortic aneurysm. If the patient describes severe epigastric pain that radiates through the abdomen to the back, assess him for absent bowel sounds and for abdominal rigidity and tenderness. If these occur, suspect perforated ulcer or acute pancreatitis.*

Palpate the flanks and percuss with the fingertips or perform fist percussion to elicit costovertebral angle tenderness.

Analysis

Although back pain may herald a spondylogenic disorder, it may also result from a genitourinary, GI, cardiovascular, or neoplastic disorder. Postural imbalance associated with pregnancy may also cause back pain.

Intrinsic back pain results from muscle spasm, nerve root irritation, fracture, or a combination of these mechanisms. It usually occurs in the lower back, or lumbosacral area. Back pain may also be referred from the abdomen or flank, possibly signaling a life-threatening perforated ulcer, acute pancreatitis, or dissecting abdominal aortic aneurysm.

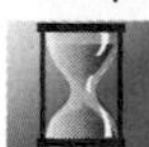

AGE ISSUE *Because a child may have difficulty describing back pain, be alert for nonverbal clues, such as wincing or refusal to walk. Closely observe family dynamics during history taking for clues suggesting child abuse. Back pain in the child may stem from intervertebral disk inflammation (diskitis), neoplasms, idiopathic juvenile osteoporosis, and spondylolisthesis. Disk herniation typically doesn't cause back pain. Scoliosis, a common disorder in adolescents, rarely causes back pain. Suspect metastatic cancer — especially of the prostate, colon, or breast — in older patients with a recent onset of back pain that usually isn't relieved by rest and worsens at night.*

Jaw pain

Jaw pain may arise from either of the two bones that hold the teeth in the jaw — the maxilla, known as the upper jaw, and the mandible, known as the lower jaw. Jaw pain also includes pain in the temporomandibular joint (TMJ), where the mandible meets the temporal bone.

Jaw pain may develop gradually or abruptly and may range from barely noticeable to excruciating, depending on its cause. Jaw pain is seldom a primary indicator of any one disorder; however, some causes are medical emergencies.

History

Begin the patient's health history by asking him to describe the pain's character, intensity, and frequency. Ask him when he first noticed the jaw pain and where on the jaw he feels the pain. Find out if the pain radiates to other areas. Sharp or burning pain arises from the skin or subcutaneous tissues. Causalgia, an intense burning sensation, usually results from damage to the fifth cranial, or trigeminal, nerve. This type of superficial pain is easily localized, unlike dull, aching, boring, or throbbing pain, which originates in muscle, bone, or joints. Also ask about aggravating or alleviating factors.

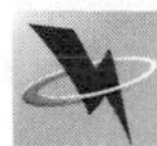

CRITICAL POINT *Sudden severe jaw pain, especially when associated with chest pain, shortness of breath, or arm pain, requires prompt evaluation because it may herald a life-threatening disorder. Jaw pain may accompany more characteristic signs and symptoms of life-threatening disorders, such as chest pain in a patient with a myocardial infarction (MI).*

Ask about recent trauma, surgery, or procedures, especially dental work. Ask about associated signs and symptoms, such as joint or chest pain, dyspnea, palpitations, fatigue, headache, malaise, anorexia, weight loss, intermittent claudication, diplopia, and hearing loss.

Physical assessment

Focus the physical examination on the patient's jaw. Inspect the painful area for redness, and palpate for edema or warmth. Facing the patient directly, look for facial asymmetry indicating swelling. Check the TMJs by placing your fingertips just anterior to the external auditory meatus and asking the patient to open and close, and to thrust out and retract his jaw. Note the presence of crepitus, an abnormal scraping or grinding sensation in the joint. Clicks heard when the jaw is widely spread apart are normal. Observe how wide the patient can open his mouth. Less than 1⅛″ (3 cm) or more than 2″ (5.1 cm) between upper and lower teeth is abnormal. Next, palpate the parotid area for pain and swelling, and inspect and palpate the oral cavity for lesions, elevation of the tongue, or masses.

Analysis

Jaw pain usually results from disorders of the teeth, soft tissue, or glands of the mouth or throat or from local trauma or infection. Systemic causes include musculoskeletal, neurologic, cardiovascular, endocrine, immunologic, metabolic, and infectious disorders. Life-threatening disorders, such as MI and tetany, also produce jaw pain, as do certain medications, especially phenothiazines that affect the extrapyramidal tract, causing dyskinesias; others cause tetany of the jaw secondary to hypocalcemia and dental or surgical procedures.

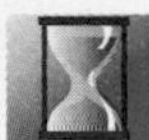

AGE ISSUE *Be alert for nonverbal signs of jaw pain in patients, such as rubbing the affected area or wincing while talking or swallowing. In infants, initial signs of tetany from hypocalcemia include episodes of apnea and generalized jitteriness progressing to facial grimaces and generalized rigidity. Finally, seizures may occur. In children, jaw pain sometimes stems from disorders uncommon in adults. Mumps, for example, causes unilateral or bilateral swelling from the lower mandible to the zygomatic arch. Parotiditis due to cystic fibrosis also causes jaw pain. When trauma causes jaw pain in children, always consider the possibility of abuse.*

Leg pain

Although leg pain commonly signifies a musculoskeletal disorder, it can also result from more serious vascular or neurologic disorders. The pain may occur suddenly or gradually and may be localized or affect the entire leg. Constant or intermittent, it may feel dull, burning, sharp, shooting, or tingling.

History

If the patient's condition permits, ask him when the pain began and have him describe its intensity, character, and pattern. Find out if the pain is worse in the morning, at night, or with movement. If it doesn't prevent him from walking, find out if he relies on a crutch or other assistive device. Also, ask him about the presence of other signs and symptoms.

Find out if the patient has a history of leg injury or surgery, and if he or a family member has a history of joint, vascular, or back problems. Also, ask what medications he's taking and whether they've helped to relieve leg pain.

Physical assessment

Begin the physical examination by watching the patient walk, if his condition permits. Observe how he holds his leg while standing and sitting. Palpate the legs, buttocks, and lower back to determine the extent of pain and tenderness. If fracture has been ruled out, test ROM in the hip and knee. Also, check reflexes with the patient's leg straightened and raised, noting any action that causes pain. Then compare both legs for symmetry, movement, and active ROM. Also, assess sensation and strength. If the patient wears a leg cast, splint, or restrictive dressing, carefully check distal circulation, sensation, and mobility, and stretch his toes to elicit any associated pain.

Analysis

Leg pain typically affects movement, limiting weight bearing. Severe leg pain that follows cast application for a fracture may signal limb-threatening compartment syndrome. Sudden onset of severe leg pain in a patient with underlying vascular insufficiency may signal acute deterioration, possibly requiring an arterial graft or amputation.

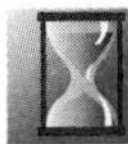

AGE ISSUE *Common pediatric causes of leg pain include fracture, osteomyelitis, and bone cancer. If parents fail to give an adequate explanation for a leg fracture, consider the possibility of child abuse.*

Muscle atrophy

Muscle atrophy, or wasting, results from denervation or prolonged muscle disuse. When deprived of regular exercise, muscle fibers lose both bulk and length, producing a visible loss of muscle size and contour and apparent emaciation or deformity in the affected area. Even slight atrophy usually causes some loss of motion or power.

History

Ask the patient when and where he first noticed the muscle wasting and how it has progressed. Also ask about associated signs and symptoms, such as weakness, pain, loss of sensation, and recent weight loss. Review the patient's medical history for chronic illnesses; musculoskeletal or neurologic disorders, including trauma; and endocrine and metabolic disorders. Ask about his use of alcohol and drugs, particularly steroids.

Physical assessment

Begin the physical examination by determining the location and extent of atrophy. Visually evaluate small and large muscles. Check major muscle groups for size, tonicity, and strength. Measure the circumference of all limbs, comparing sides. Check for muscle contractures in all limbs by fully extending joints and noting any pain or resistance. Complete the examination by palpating peripheral pulses for quality and rate, assessing sensory function in and around the atrophied area, and testing deep tendon reflexes.

Analysis

Atrophy usually results from neuromuscular disease or injury. However, it may also stem from certain metabolic and endocrine disorders and prolonged immobility. Some muscle atrophy also occurs with aging. Prolonged steroid therapy interferes with muscle metabolism and leads to atrophy, most prominently in the limbs. Prolonged immobilization from bed rest, casts, splints, or traction may cause muscle weakness and atrophy.

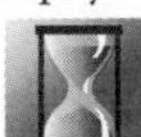

AGE ISSUE *In young children, profound muscle weakness and atrophy can result from muscular dystrophy. Muscle atrophy may also result from cerebral palsy and poliomyelitis, and from paralysis associated with meningocele and myelomeningocele.*

Muscle spasms

Muscle spasms, or cramps, are strong, painful contractions. They can occur in virtually any muscle but are most common in the calf and foot.

History

If the patient isn't in distress, ask when the spasms began. Find out how long they lasted and how painful they were. Ask the patient what measures, if any, worsened or lessened the pain. Ask about other symptoms, such as weakness, sensory loss, or paresthesia.

Physical assessment

Evaluate muscle strength and tone. Then check all major muscle groups, and note whether any movements precipitate spasms. Test the presence and quality of all peripheral pulses, and examine the limbs for color and temperature changes. Test capillary refill time, and inspect for edema, especially in the involved area. Finally, test reflexes and sensory function in all extremities.

Analysis

Muscle spasms typically occur with simple muscle fatigue, after exercise, and during pregnancy. However, they may also result from an electrolyte imbalance such as hypocalcemia, a neuromuscular disorder, or use of certain drugs. They're typically precipitated by movement, and they can usually be relieved by slow stretching.

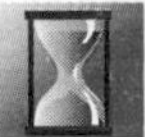

AGE ISSUE *In children, muscle spasms rarely occur. However, their presence may indicate hypoparathyroidism, osteomalacia, rickets or, rarely, congenital torticollis.*

Muscle weakness

Muscle weakness may be reported to you by the patient, or it may be detected by observing and measuring the strength of an individual muscle or muscle group.

History

Begin by determining the location of the patient's muscle weakness. Ask if he has difficulty with specific movements such as rising from a chair. Find out when he first noticed the weakness; ask him whether it worsens with exercise or as the day progresses. Ask about related symptoms, especially muscle or joint pain, altered sensory function, and fatigue. Obtain a medical history, noting especially chronic disease, such as hyperthyroidism; musculoskeletal or neurologic problems, including recent trauma; family history of chronic muscle weakness, especially in men; and use of alcohol or certain drugs.

Physical assessment

Focus your physical examination on evaluating muscle strength. Test all major muscles bilaterally. When testing, make sure the patient's effort is constant; if it isn't, suspect pain or other reluctance to make the effort. If the patient complains of pain, ease or discontinue testing, and have him try the movements again. Remember that the patient's dominant arm, hand, and leg are somewhat stronger than their nondominant counterparts.

Besides testing individual muscle strength, test for ROM at all major joints, including the shoulder, elbow, wrist, hip, knee, and ankle. Also test sensory function in the involved areas, and test deep tendon reflexes bilaterally.

Analysis

Muscle weakness can result from a malfunction in the cerebral hemispheres, brain stem, spinal cord, nerve roots, peripheral nerves, or myoneural junctions and within the muscle itself. Muscle weakness occurs in certain neurologic, musculoskeletal, metabolic, endocrine, and cardiovascular disorders; as a response to certain drugs; and after prolonged immobilization.

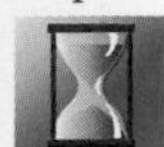

AGE ISSUE *In children, muscular dystrophy, typically the Duchenne type, is a major cause of muscle weakness.*

Neck pain

Neck pain may originate from any neck structure, ranging from the meninges and cervical vertebrae to its blood vessels, muscles, and lymphatic tissue. This symptom can also be referred from other areas of the body. Its location, onset, and pattern help determine its origin and underlying causes.

History

If the patient hasn't sustained trauma, find out the severity and onset of his neck pain. Ask him where specifically in the neck he feels the pain. Find out what relieves or worsens it. Ask him if any particular event precipitates the pain. Also, ask about the development of other symptoms such as headaches. Next, focus on the patient's current and past illnesses and injuries, diet, drug history, and family health history.

CRITICAL POINT *If the patient's neck pain is due to trauma, first ensure proper cervical spine immobilization, preferably with a long backboard and a Philadelphia collar.*

Physical assessment

Thoroughly inspect the patient's neck, shoulders, and cervical spine for swelling, masses, erythema, and ecchymoses. Assess active ROM in his neck by having him perform flexion, extension, rotation, and lateral side bending. Note the degree of pain produced by these movements. Examine his posture, and test and compare bilateral muscle strength. Check the sensation in his arms, and assess his hand grasp and arm reflexes. Attempt to elicit Brudzinski's and Kernig's signs if there isn't a history of neck trauma, and palpate the cervical lymph nodes for enlargement.

Analysis

Neck pain usually results from trauma and degenerative, congenital, inflammatory, metabolic, and neoplastic disorders.

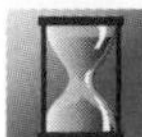

AGE ISSUE *In children, the most common causes of neck pain are meningitis and trauma. A rare cause of neck pain is congenital torticollis.*

17 Neurologic system

The neurologic system serves as the body's communication network. It processes information from the outside world, through the sensory portion, and coordinates and organizes the functions of all other body systems. Its far-reaching effects can be seen when patients, who suffer from diseases of other body systems, develop neurologic impairments related to the disease. For example, the patient who has heart surgery could suffer a stroke.

Because the neurologic system is so complex, evaluating it can seem overwhelming. Although tests for neurologic status are extensive, they're also basic and straightforward. In fact, you may routinely include some of these tests in your practice.

Just talking with a patient helps assess his orientation, level of consciousness, and ability to formulate and produce speech. Having him perform a simple task, such as walking, allows you to evaluate motor ability. Knowledge of neurologic anatomy, physiology, and assessment will enhance patient care and may save a patient from irreversible neurologic damage.

The neurologic system is divided into the central nervous system, the peripheral nervous system, and the autonomic nervous system. Through complex and coordinated interactions, these three parts integrate all physical, intellectual, and emotional activities. Understanding how each part works is essential to conducting an accurate neurologic assessment.

Nervous system cells

Two major cell types, neurons and neuroglia, compose the nervous system. The conducting cells of the central nervous system (CNS), neurons, also called *nerve cells,* detect and transmit stimuli by electromechanical messages. These specialized cells don't reproduce themselves.

Neuroglial cells, or glial cells (derived from the Greek word for glue because they hold the neurons together), serve as the supportive cells of the CNS and form roughly 40% of the brain's bulk. The four types of neuroglial cells include:

- Astroglia, or astrocytes, exist throughout the nervous system and form part of the blood-brain barrier. They supply nutrients to the neurons and help maintain their electrical potential.
- Ependymal cells line the brain's four ventricles and the choroid plexus and help produce cerebrospinal fluid.
- Microglia phagocytize waste products from injured neurons and are deployed throughout the nervous system.
- Oligodendroglia support and electrically insulate CNS axons by forming protective myelin sheaths.

Central nervous system

The central nervous system (CNS) includes the brain and the spinal cord. These two major structures of the CNS collect and interpret voluntary and involuntary motor and sensory stimuli. (See *Major structures of the central nervous system.*)

Brain

The brain consists of the cerebrum or cerebral cortex, the brain stem, the cerebellum, the limbic system, and the reticular activating system (RAS). It collects, integrates, and interprets all stimuli and initiates and monitors voluntary and involuntary motor activity.

Cerebrum

The cerebrum, the largest portion of the brain, houses the nerve center that controls motor and sensory functions and intelligence. It's encased by the skull and enclosed by three membrane layers called *meninges.* If blood or fluid accumulates between these layers, pressure builds inside the skull and compromises brain function.

The cerebrum is divided into hemispheres, consisting of a left and a right hemisphere joined by the corpus callosum, a mass of nerve fibers that allows communication between corresponding centers in the right and left hemispheres. Each hemisphere is divided into four lobes, based on anatomic landmarks and functional differences. The lobes are named for the cranial bones that lie over them, the frontal, temporal, parietal, and occipital. The cerebral cortex, the surface layer of the cerebrum, is composed of gray matter, which are unmyelinated cell bodies. The cerebrum has a rolling surface made up of convolutions, called gyri, and creases or fissures, called sulci.

The frontal lobe influences personality, judgment, abstract reasoning, social behavior, language expression, and movement. The temporal lobe controls hearing, language comprehension, and the storage and recall of memories, although some memories are stored throughout the brain. The parietal lobe interprets and integrates sensations, including pain, temperature, and touch. It also interprets size, shape, distance, and texture. The parietal lobe of the nondominant hemisphere, usually the right, is especially important for awareness of body schema or shape. The occipital lobe functions primarily in interpreting visual stimuli.

In addition, cranial nerves I and II originate in the cerebrum. The cerebrum is considered the area involving upper motor neuron function. (See *The cerebrum and its functions,* page 468.)

The diencephalon, a division of the cerebrum, contains the thalamus and hypothalamus. The thalamus is a relay station for sensory impulses as they ascend to the cerebral cortex. Its functions include primitive awareness of pain, screening of incoming stimuli, and focusing of attention. The hypothalamus has many regulatory functions, including temperature control, pituitary hormone production, and water balance.

Brain stem

The brain stem lies below the diencephalon and is divided into the midbrain, pons, and medulla. It's continuous with the cerebrum above and with the spinal cord below. The brain stem relays messages between the parts of the nervous system. It has three main functions that include producing the rigid autonomic behaviors necessary for

MAJOR STRUCTURES OF THE CENTRAL NERVOUS SYSTEM

This illustration shows a cross section of the major structures of the central nervous system—the brain and spinal cord. The brain joins the spinal cord at the base of the skull and ends between the first and second lumbar vertebrae. Note the H-shaped mass of gray matter in the spinal cord.

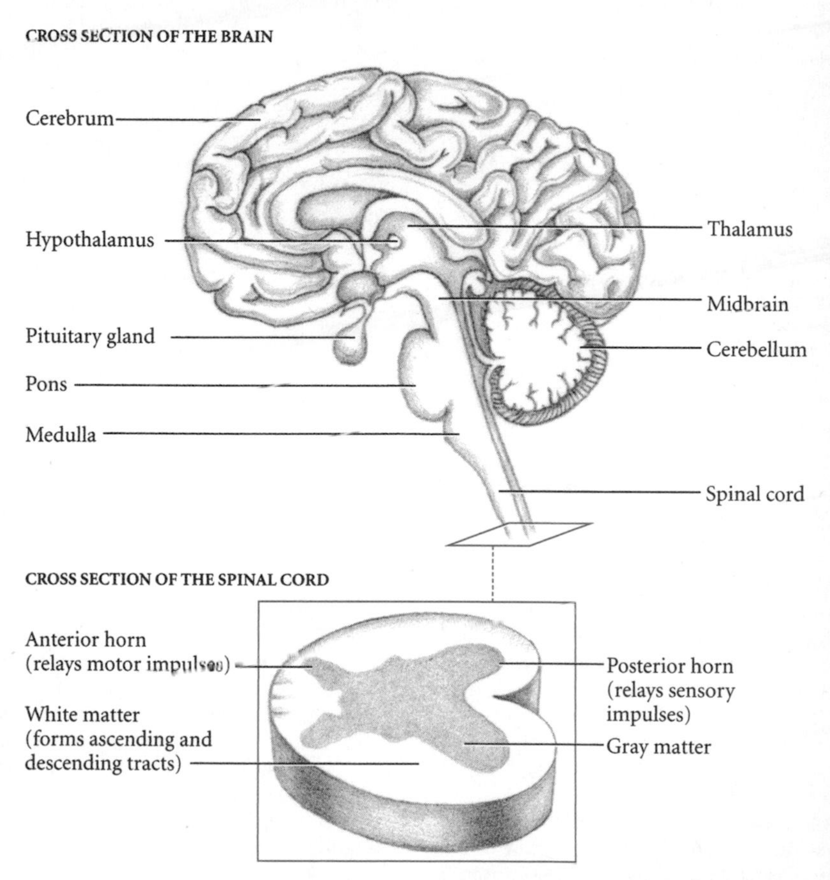

survival, such as increasing the heart rate and stimulating the adrenal medulla to produce epinephrine; providing the pathways for nerve fibers between higher and lower neural centers; and serving as the origin for 10 of the 12 pairs of cranial nerves.

The three parts of the brain stem provide two-way conduction between the spinal cord and brain. The midbrain is the origination site for cranial nerves III and IV and the corticospinal tract, which is the main motor pathway from the cerebrum. The midbrain mediates the auditory and visual reflexes. The pons is the origination area for cranial nerves V, VI, and VII and it contains one of the respiratory centers. The pons connects the cerebellum to the cerebrum and the midbrain to the medulla. The pons mediates actions such as chewing, taste, saliva secretion, hearing and equilibrium.

The medulla is the origination area for cranial nerves VIII to XII. It joins the spinal cord at the level of the foramen magnum, an opening in the occipital portion of the

THE CEREBRUM AND ITS FUNCTIONS

The cerebrum is divided into four lobes, based on anatomic landmarks and functional differences. The lobes—parietal, occipital, temporal, and frontal—are named for the cranial bones that lie over them.

This illustration shows the locations of the cerebral lobes and explains their functions. It also shows the location of the cerebellum.

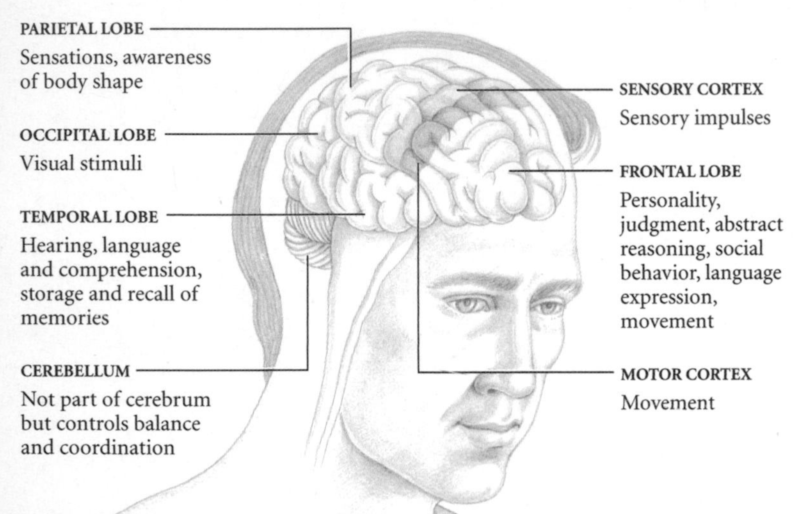

skull. The medulla regulates respiratory, vasomotor, and cardiac function. It's the center for vomiting, coughing, and hiccupping reflexes. Areas below the cerebrum are considered the areas involving lower motor neuron function.

Cerebellum

The cerebellum, the most posterior part of the brain lying behind and below the cerebrum, is the brain's second largest region. It contains the major motor and sensory pathways. It facilitates smooth, coordinated muscle movement and helps to maintain equilibrium.

Limbic system

The limbic system is a primitive brain area deep within the temporal lobe. In addition to initiating basic drives, such as hunger, aggression, and emotional and sexual arousal, the limbic system screens all sensory messages traveling to the cerebral cortex.

Reticular activating system

The RAS is a diffuse network of hyperexcitable neurons. It fans out from the brain stem through the cerebral cortex. After screening all incoming sensory information, the RAS channels it to appropriate areas of the brain for interpretation. It functions as the arousal, or alerting, system for the cerebral cortex, and its functioning is crucial for maintaining consciousness.

Vascular supply

Four major arteries—two vertebral and two carotid—supply the brain with oxygenated blood. The two vertebral arteries, which are branches of the subclavians, converge to become the basilar artery. The basilar artery supplies oxygen to the posterior brain.

The common carotids branch into the two internal carotids, which divide further to supply oxygen to the anterior brain and the middle brain. These arteries interconnect through the circle of Willis, an anastomosis at the base of the brain. The circle of

Willis ensures that oxygen is continuously circulated to the brain despite interruption of any of the brain's major vessels.

Spinal cord

The spinal cord is the primary pathway for messages traveling between the body's peripheral areas and the brain. It extends from the upper border of the first cervical vertebrae to the lower border of the first lumbar vertebrae. The spinal cord is encased in the spinal column by the uninterrupted meningeal linings and spinal fluid that protect the brain. Further protection of the spinal cord is provided by the bony vertebrae and the intervertebral disks. The spinal nerves arise from the spinal cord. At the spinal cord's inferior end, nerve roots cluster in the cauda equina.

A cross section of the spinal cord reveals a central H-shaped mass of gray matter divided into dorsal (posterior) and ventral (anterior) horns. These horns consist mainly of neuron cell bodies. Cell bodies in the two dorsal horns primarily relay sensory, or afferent, impulses; those in the two ventral horns relay motor, or efferent, impulses, thus playing a part in voluntary and reflex motor activity. White matter surrounds the horns and consists of myelinated axons of sensory and motor nerve fibers grouped in vertical columns, or tracts, which form the ascending and descending tracts.

Sensory pathways

Sensory impulses travel via the afferent, also called *sensory* or *ascending,* neural pathways to the sensory cortex in the brain's parietal lobe. Here, the impulses are interpreted using two major pathways: the dorsal horn and the ganglia.

Pain and temperature sensations enter the spinal cord through the dorsal horn. After immediately crossing over to the opposite side of the spinal cord, these impulses then travel to the thalamus via the spinothalamic tract.

Touch, pressure, and vibration sensations enter the spinal cord via relay stations called *ganglia.* Ganglia are knotlike masses of nerve cell bodies on the dorsal roots of spinal nerves. Impulses travel up the spinal cord in the dorsal column to the medulla, where they cross to the opposite side and enter the thalamus. The thalamus relays all incoming sensory impulses, except olfactory impulses, to the sensory cortex for interpretation.

Motor pathways

Motor impulses travel from the brain to the muscles via the efferent, also known as the *motor* or *descending,* neural pathways. Motor impulses originate in the motor cortex of the frontal lobe and reach the lower motor neurons of the peripheral nervous system via upper motor neurons.

Upper motor neurons originate in the brain and form two major systems that include the pyramidal system and extrapyramidal system.

The *pyramidal system,* or corticospinal tract, is responsible for fine, skilled movements of skeletal muscle. Impulses in this system travel from the motor cortex through the internal capsule to the medulla. At the medulla they cross to the opposite side and continue down the spinal cord.

The *extrapyramidal system,* or extracorticospinal tract, controls gross motor movements. Impulses originate in the premotor area of the frontal lobes and travel to the pons. At the pons the impulses cross to the opposite side. Then the impulses travel down the spinal cord to the anterior horns, where they're relayed to the lower motor neurons. These neurons, in turn, carry the impulses to the muscles. (See *How neurotransmission occurs,* page 470.)

Reflexes

The spinal cord mediates the sensory-to-motor transmission path known as the *reflex arc.* Because the reflex arc enters and exits the spinal cord at the same level, reflex pathways don't need to travel up and down as other stimuli. Reflex responses occur automatically, without brain involvement, to protect the body. For example, if the brain can't send a message to a patient's leg after a severe spinal cord injury, a stimulus can still cause a knee jerk, or patellar, reflex as long as the spinal cord remains intact at the level of the reflex. (See *Functioning of the reflex arc,* page 471.)

Spinal nerves, which have both sensory and motor portions, mediate deep tendon reflexes (involuntary contractions of a muscle after brief stretching caused by tendon percussion), superficial reflexes (withdrawal

HOW NEUROTRANSMISSION OCCURS

Neurotransmission occurs when sensory and motor impulses travel through different pathways to the brain for interpretation. Typically, these impulses trigger sensations, such as touch, pressure, and vibration as well as muscle movement.

Sensory pathways
Sensory impulses travel through two major sensory (afferent, or ascending) pathways to the sensory cortex in the cerebrum.

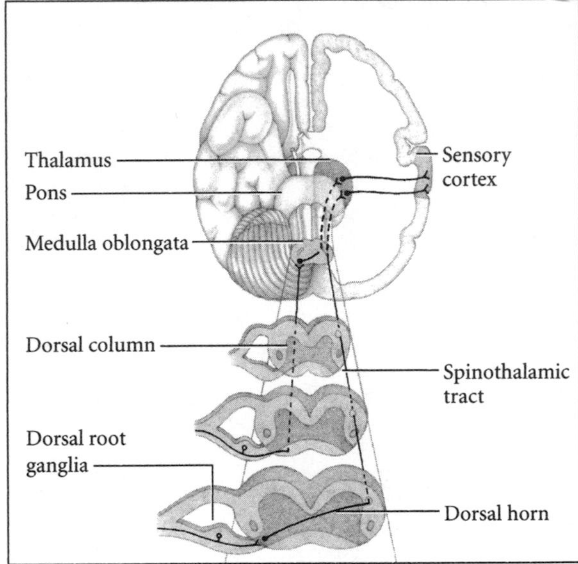

Motor pathways
Motor impulses travel from the motor cortex in the cerebrum to the muscles via motor (efferent, or descending) pathways.

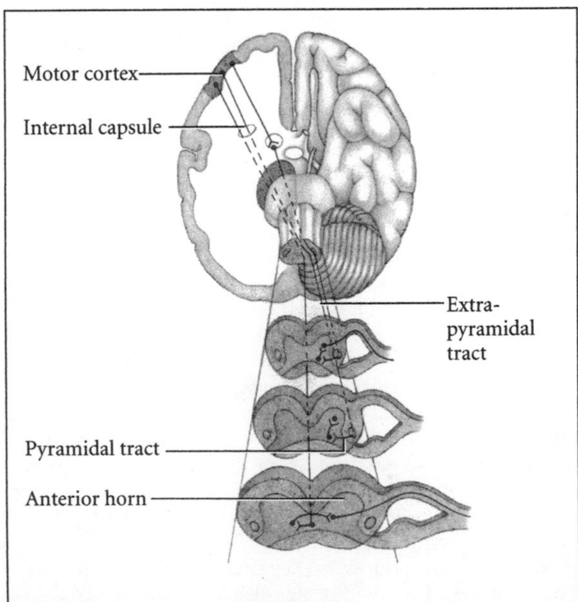

FUNCTIONING OF THE REFLEX ARC

Spinal nerves, which have sensory and motor portions, control deep tendon and superficial reflexes. A simple reflex arc requires a sensory, or afferent, neuron and a motor, or efferent, neuron. The knee jerk, or patellar, reflex illustrates the sequence of events in a normal reflex arc.

First, a sensory receptor detects the mechanical stimulus produced by the reflex hammer striking the patellar tendon. Then the sensory neuron carries the impulse along its axon by way of the spinal nerve to the dorsal root, where it enters the posterior horn of the spinal cord.

Next, in the anterior horn of the spinal cord, illustrated here, the sensory neuron joins with a motor neuron, which carries the impulse along its axon by way of spinal nerve to the muscle. The motor neuron transmits the impulse to the muscle fibers through stimulation of the motor end plate. This triggers the muscle to contract and the leg to extend.

PATELLAR REFLEX ARC

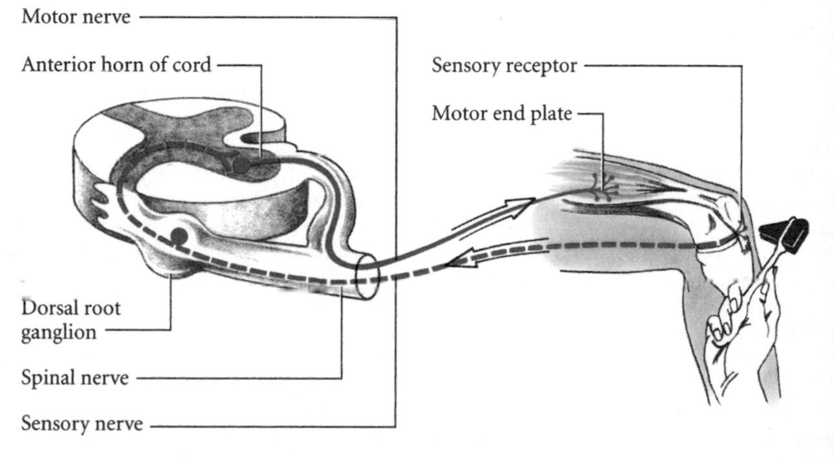

reflexes elicited by noxious or tactile stimulation of the skin, cornea, or mucous membranes), and, in infants, primitive reflexes.

Deep tendon reflexes include reflex responses of the biceps, triceps, brachioradialis, patellar, and Achilles tendons. The biceps reflex contracts the biceps muscle and forces flexion of the forearm, whereas the triceps reflex contracts the triceps muscle and forces extension of the forearm. The brachioradialis reflex causes supination of the hand and flexion of the forearm at the elbow. The patellar reflex forces contraction of the quadriceps muscle in the thigh with extension of the leg. Lastly, the Achilles reflex forces plantar flexion of the foot at the ankle.

Superficial reflexes are reflexes of the skin and mucous membranes. Successive attempts to stimulate these reflexes provoke increasingly limited responses. Superficial reflexes include the plantarflexion of the toes, cremasteric reflex, and the abdominal reflex. Plantarflexion of the toes occurs when the lateral sole of an adult's foot is stroked from heel to great toe with a tongue blade. Babinski's reflex causes upward movement of the great toe and fanning of the little toes in children under age 2 in response to stimulation of the outer margin of the sole of the foot. In men, the cremasteric reflex is stimulated by stroking the inner thigh. This forces the contraction of the cremaster muscle and elevation of the testicle on the side of the stimulus. Abdominal reflex is induced by stroking the sides of the abdomen above and below the umbilicus, moving from the periphery toward the midline. Movement of the umbilicus toward the stimulus is normal.

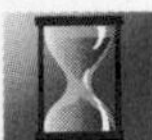

AGE ISSUE *Primitive reflexes are abnormal in adults but normal in infants, whose central nervous systems are immature. As the neurologic system matures, these reflexes disappear. Primitive reflexes include grasping, sucking, and glabella. Grasping involves the application of gentle pressure to an infant's palm, which results in grasping. The infantile sucking reflex to ingest milk is a primitive response to oral stimuli. The glabella reflex is elicited by repeatedly tapping the bridge of the infant's nose, with a normal response being persistent blinking.*

Dermatomes

For the purpose of documenting sensory function, the body is divided into dermatomes. Each dermatome represents an area supplied with afferent, or sensory, nerve fibers from an individual spinal root—cervical, thoracic, lumbar, or sacral. This body "map" is used when testing sensation and trying to identify the source of a lesion. (See *Identifying dermatomes.*)

Protective structures

Bone, meninges, and cerebrospinal fluid (CSF) protect the brain and the spinal cord from shock and infection.

Bone

Formed of cranial bones, the skull completely surrounds the brain and opens at the base, called the *foramen magnum,* where the spinal cord exits.

The vertebral column protects the spinal cord. It consists of 30 vertebrae, each separated by an intervertebral disk that allows flexibility.

Meninges

The meninges cover and protect the cerebral cortex and spinal column. They consist of three layers of connective tissue that include the dura mater, the arachnoid membrane, and the pia mater. (See *Protecting the central nervous system,* page 474.)

Dura mater. The dura mater, a fibrous membrane, lines the skull and forms folds, called reflections, that descend into the brain's fissures and provide stability. The dural folds include the falx cerebri, which lies in the longitudinal fissure and separates the cerebrum's hemispheres; the tentorium cerebelli, which separates the cerebrum from the cerebellum; and the falx cerebelli, which separates the two cerebellar lobes. The arachnoid villi, projections of the dura mater into the superior sagittal and transverse sinuses, serve as the exit points for CSF drainage into venous circulation.

Arachnoid membrane. A fragile, fibrous layer with moderate vascularity, the arachnoid membrane lies between the dura and pia mater. Injury to its blood vessels during head trauma, lumbar puncture, or cisternal puncture may cause hemorrhage.

Pia mater. An extremely thin and highly vascular membrane, the pia mater closely covers the brain's surface and extends into its fissures. Its intimate invaginations help form the choroid plexuses of the brain's ventricular system.

Additional layers. Three layers of space further cushion the brain and spinal cord against injury. The epidural space (a potential space) lies over the dura mater. The subdural space lies between the dura mater and the arachnoid membrane and is commonly the site of hemorrhage after head trauma. The subarachnoid space, which is filled with CSF, lies between the arachnoid membrane and the pia mater.

Cerebrospinal fluid

CSF nourishes cells, transports metabolic waste, and cushions the brain. This colorless fluid circulates through the ventricular system, into the subarachnoid space of the brain and spinal cord, and back to the venous sinuses on top of the brain where it's reabsorbed. The ependymal cells that cover the surface of the choroid plexus, which is a tangled mass of tiny blood vessels lining the ventricles, constantly produce CSF at a rate of about 150 ml/day.

IDENTIFYING DERMATOMES

Knowledge of dermatomes is useful to localize neurologic lesions. These illustrations demonstrate the patterns of dermatomes on the body.

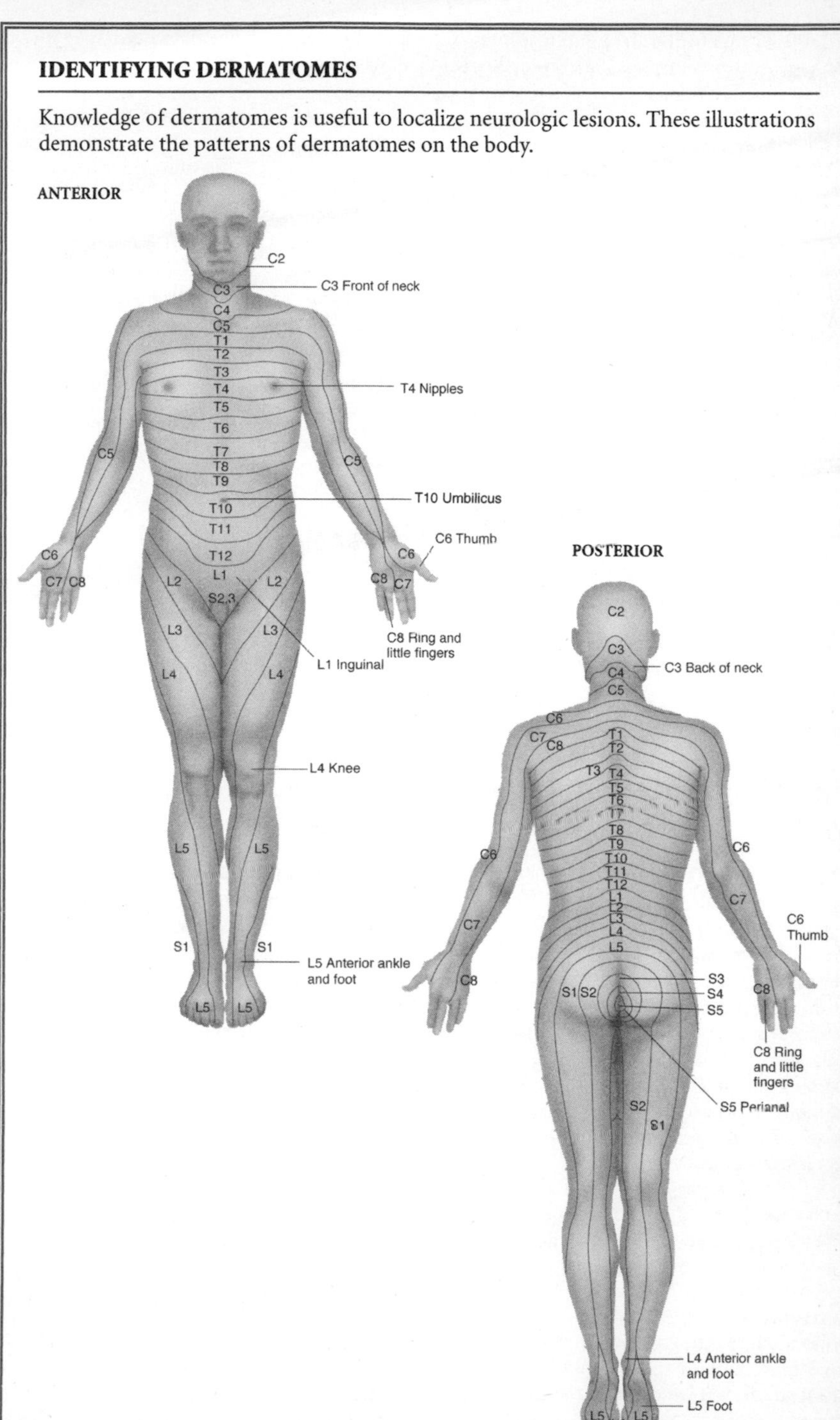

PROTECTING THE CENTRAL NERVOUS SYSTEM

Three primary membranes, or meninges, help protect the central nervous system: the dura mater, the arachnoid membrane, and the pia mater.

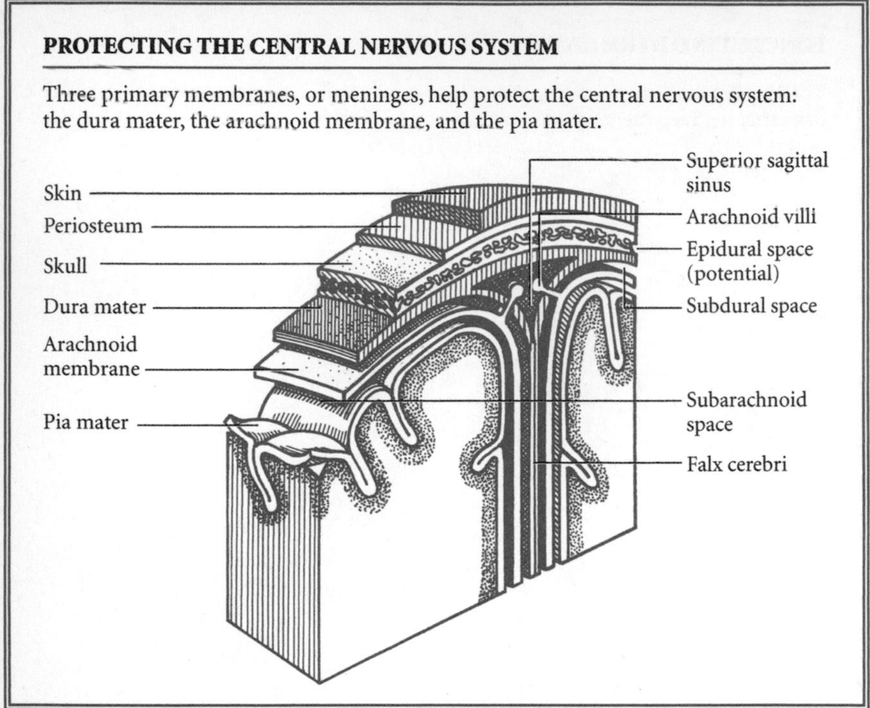

Peripheral nervous system

The peripheral nervous system consists of the peripheral and cranial nerves.

Peripheral nerves

Peripheral sensory nerves transmit stimuli to the spinal cord's dorsal horn from sensory receptors located in the skin, muscles, sensory organs, and viscera. The upper motor neurons of the brain and the lower motor neurons of the cell bodies in the spinal cord's ventral horn carry impulses that affect movement.

Cranial nerves

The 12 pairs of cranial nerves transmit motor or sensory messages, or both, primarily between the brain or brain stem and the head and neck. All cranial nerves, except the olfactory and optic nerves, exit from the midbrain, pons, or medulla oblongata of the brain stem. (See *Functions of the cranial nerves.*)

Autonomic nervous system

The vast autonomic nervous system (ANS) enervates all internal organs. Also known as the *visceral efferent nerves,* the nerves of the ANS carry messages to the viscera from the brain stem and neuroendocrine system. The ANS has two major divisions that include the sympathetic nervous system and the parasympathetic nervous system.

Sympathetic nervous system

Sympathetic nerves, called *preganglionic neurons,* exit the spinal cord between the first thoracic and second lumbar vertebrae. After these nerves leave the spinal cord, they enter small relay stations, the ganglia, near the spinal cord. The ganglia form a chain that disseminates the impulse to postganglionic neurons. These neurons reach many organs and glands and can produce widespread, generalized responses.

The physiologic effects of sympathetic activity include vasoconstriction; elevated blood pressure; enhanced blood flow to

FUNCTIONS OF THE CRANIAL NERVES

The 12 pairs of cranial nerves (CNs) transmit motor or sensory messages, or both, primarily between the brain or brain stem and the head and neck. All cranial nerves, except for the olfactory and optic nerves, exit from the midbrain, pons, or medulla of the brain stem.

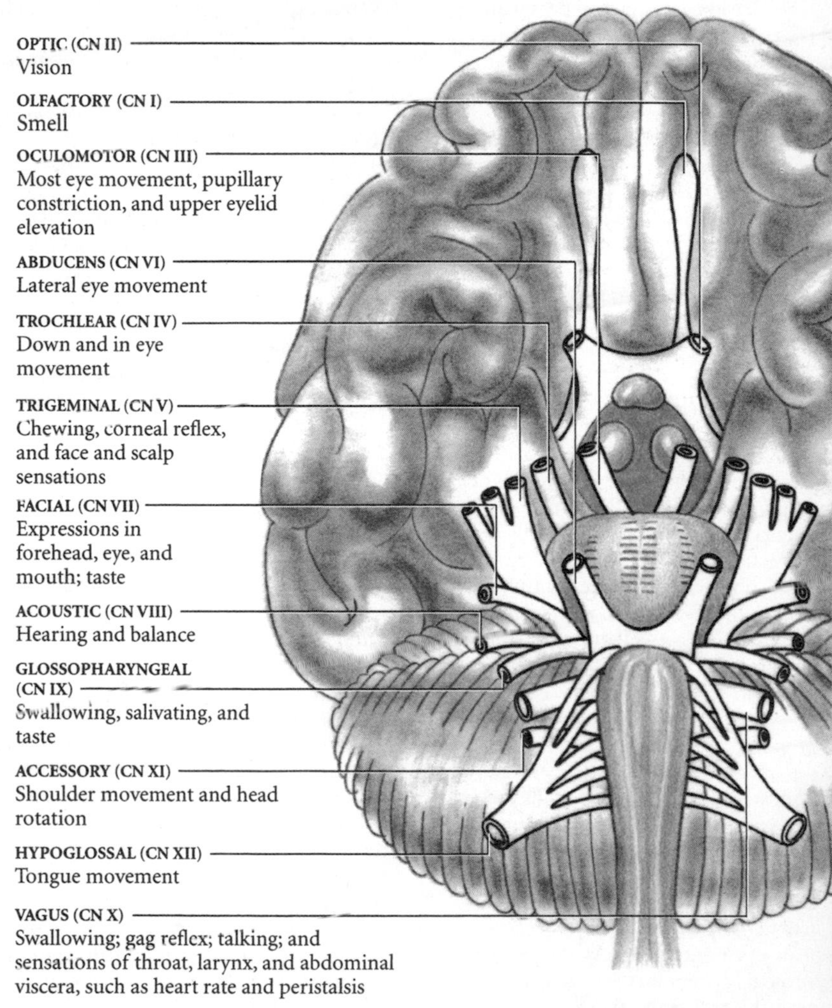

skeletal muscles; increased heart rate and contractility; heightened respiratory rate; smooth-muscle relaxation of the bronchioles, GI tract, and urinary tract; sphincter contraction; pupillary dilation and ciliary muscle relaxation; increased sweat gland secretion; and reduced pancreatic secretion.

Parasympathetic nervous system

The fibers of the parasympathetic nervous system leave the central nervous system (CNS) via the cranial nerves from the midbrain and medulla and from the spinal nerves between the second and fourth sacral vertebrae (S2 to S4).

After leaving the CNS, the long preganglionic fiber of each parasympathetic nerve travels to a ganglion near a particular organ or gland; the short postganglionic fiber enters the organ or gland. This creates a more specific response involving only one organ or gland.

The physiologic effects of parasympathetic system activity include reduced heart rate, contractility, and conduction velocity; bronchial smooth-muscle constriction; increased GI tract tone and peristalsis with sphincter relaxation; urinary system sphincter relaxation and increased bladder tone; vasodilation of external genitalia, causing erection; pupillary constriction; and increased pancreatic, salivary, and lacrimal secretions. The parasympathetic system has a minimal effect on mental or metabolic activity.

Health history

Begin the health history by asking about the patient's chief complaint. Then gather details about his current illness, past illnesses, family history, and psychosocial history. Also perform a body systems review.

If possible, include the patient's family members or close friends when taking the history. Don't assume that the patient remembers accurately; corroborate the details with others to get a clearer picture.

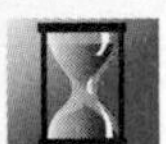

AGE ISSUE *When obtaining a child's health history, ask questions about the child's development, including a prenatal history up to the present. Also evaluate the child's achievement of developmental milestones, such as sitting up, walking, and talking at the appropriate age.*

Chief complaint

The most common complaints about the neurologic system include headache, dizziness, disturbances in balance and gait, and changes in mental status or level of consciousness (LOC). When documenting the patient's chief complaint, record the information in the patient's own words.

When learning of the patient's chief complaint, ask him about the problem's onset and frequency, what precipitates or exacerbates it, and what alleviates it. Ask whether other symptoms accompany the problem and whether he has had adverse effects from treatments.

Current health history

Ask the patient to elaborate on his primary complaint, using questions to focus the interview. Determine if the patient is experiencing problems with his activities of daily living (ADLs) due to the complaint. Also question the patient about measures used to treat the problem.

Make sure you ask about other aspects of his current health. Help the patient describe problems by asking pertinent focused questions.

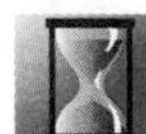

AGE ISSUE *Keep in mind that some neurologic changes, such as decreased reflexes, hearing, and vision, are a normal part of aging. Additionally, because neurons undergo various degenerative changes, aging can lead to diminished reflexes, decreased hearing, vision, taste, and smell, slowed reaction time, decreased agility, decreased vibratory sense in the ankles, and the development of muscle tremors, such as in the head and hands. Remember that not all neurologic changes in elderly patients are caused by aging and that certain drugs can cause changes as well. Find out if the changes are symmetric, indicating a pathologic condition, or if other abnormalities need further investigation.*

Headache

Ask the patient whether he has headaches. If so, ask him how often they occur and what seems to bring them on. Find out if light bothers his eyes during a headache. Also find out what other symptoms occur with the headache.

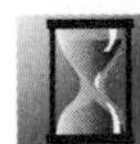

AGE ISSUE *In children older than age 3, headache is the most common symptom of a brain tumor. In a school-age child, ask the parents about recent scholastic performance and about any problems at home that may produce a tension headache. Twice as many young boys have migraine headaches as girls.*

Attempt to gather additional information about the headache to aid in ascertaining the possible cause. First, ask the patient where the pain is located, such as across his forehead, on one side of his head, or at the back of his head and neck. Pain that emanates from specific areas of the head characterizes certain types of headaches. For example, tension headaches are usually located in the occipital area, and migraine pain tends to be unilateral.

Ask the patient if the pain is tight, bandlike, boring, throbbing, steady, or dull. Headaches can be identified by the quality of pain they produce. A dull, steady pain may indicate a tension, or muscle, headache; severe or throbbing pain may indicate a vascular problem such as a migraine headache.

Find out from the patient if the pain's onset is sudden or gradual. Migraine headaches may develop suddenly, with no warning, but are usually preceded by a prodromal disturbance. Headaches associated with hemorrhage characteristically occur suddenly and with increasing severity.

Ask the patient how long the pain usually lasts and if it's continuous or recurrent. Tension headaches may last from several hours to several days. Migraine headaches may also last this long. Cluster headaches last about an hour. Also, find out if the headaches are occurring more frequently. A change in headache pattern may signal a developing condition.

Next, find out when the headaches occur, such as in the evening or if they wake him up during the night. Ask the patient if the headaches worsen when he wakes up in the morning. Although tension headaches usually occur in the evening, a person may awaken in the morning with the headache. A patient who suffers from headaches caused by hypertension, inflammation, or tumors may awaken anytime with the pain. Cluster headaches typically awaken the patient a few hours after he has fallen asleep.

Ask the patient if he sees flashing lights or shining spots or feels tingling, weakness, or numbness immediately before the headache occurs. These are common characteristics of the prodromal (premonitory) neurologic disturbance that commonly precedes a migraine headache.

Ask the patient if the pain worsens when he coughs, sneezes, or bends over. Valsalva's maneuver may exacerbate a headache caused by an intracranial lesion, such as a subarachnoid hemorrhage. Find out if he becomes nauseated or vomits during the headache. Such GI distress may accompany a migraine headache or a brain tumor or hemorrhage.

Ask the patient about any recent stress. Find out if he's experiencing any feelings of anxiety or depression. Headaches that occur daily for a prolonged period may be related to stress or depression.

Find out about any measures, such as medication, he takes for the headache and whether it's effective. Ask about other approaches — lying down, applying heat, sleeping — and if they relieve the headache.

Finally, have your patient describe the last headache he experienced by rating it on a scale of 1 to 10 with 1 being no pain and 10 being the worst headache he has ever had. How a particular headache differs from headaches a patient typically experiences can provide valuable clues to the possible cause.

Dizziness

Ask the patient about complaints of feeling dizzy. Find out if he has dizziness, numbness, tingling, seizures, tremors, weakness, or paralysis. Ask how often it occurs and how long each episode lasts. Find out if the dizziness abates spontaneously or if it leads to loss of consciousness. Ask him if the dizziness is triggered by sitting or standing up suddenly or stooping over. Find out if being in a crowd makes the patient feel dizzy. Ask about emotional stress. Find out if the patient has been irritable or anxious lately. Ask him if he has insomnia or difficulty concentrating. Look for fidgeting and eyelid twitching. Observe the patient to see if he startles easily. Also, ask about palpitations, chest pain, diaphoresis, shortness of breath, and chronic cough.

Balance and gait disturbances

Find out if the patient has problems with his senses or with walking and keeping his balance. Then ask him when his balance or gait impairment first developed and whether it has recently worsened. Find out if the problem occurred gradually over time or developed suddenly. Because he may have difficulty remembering, attempt to gain information from family members or friends, if possible. Find out if the problem has remained constant or if it's getting progressively worse. Ask about environmental changes such as hot weather, or other conditions, such as fatigue or warm baths or showers that could make his problem worse.

Such exacerbation typically is associated with multiple sclerosis. Also, find out if anyone in his family has experienced a similar type of problem.

Obtain a thorough drug history, including both medication type and dosage. Ask the patient if he has been taking antianxiety agents, especially phenothiazines. If he knows he has Parkinson's disease and has been taking levodopa, pay particular attention to the dosage because an overdose can cause acute exacerbation of signs and symptoms. If Parkinson's disease isn't a known or suspected diagnosis, ask the patient if he has been acutely or routinely exposed to carbon monoxide or manganese.

Mental status or LOC changes

First ask the patient how he would rate his memory and ability to concentrate. Ask him if he ever has trouble speaking or understanding people. Find out if he has difficulty reading or writing. If so, find out how much the problems interfere with his ADLs.

If the patient complains of problems with mental status, such as confusion, ask him how long he has felt confused and how quickly it occurred. Depending on the patient's degree of change, family members may need to be questioned to determine the true nature of the problem. Find out if the change occurred gradually or developed suddenly. An acute onset of confusion can indicate metabolic encephalopathy or delirium; gradual onset usually indicates a degenerative disorder. Ask if the confusion fluctuates. This question can help distinguish between an extracerebral disorder, such as metabolic encephalopathy, and a subdural hematoma caused by intracerebral impairment, such as arteriosclerosis or senile dementia.

If the patient was found unconscious, note where he was found. This answer will provide clues to the cause of the unconsciousness, such as a possible reaction to drugs or alcohol. Ask him if unconsciousness occurred abruptly or gradually. Find out if his LOC has fluctuated. Abrupt loss of consciousness may indicate a stroke. Gradual onset could result from metabolic, extracerebral, toxic, or systemic causes.

A fluctuating LOC can signal that systemic hypotension is affecting the brain. Find out what could have happened to the patient recently that could have exacerbated an existing condition, resulting in unconsciousness. An infection or a break in treatment of an existing condition can result in unconsciousness.

Past health history

Explore all of the patient's previous major illnesses, recurrent minor illnesses, accidents or injuries, surgical procedures, and allergies. Also explore his health and dietary habits. Find out if he exercises daily, smokes, drinks alcohol, or uses illicit drugs.

Ask the patient if he's taking prescription or over-the-counter drugs or herbal preparations. If so, document the name and dosage of each drug or preparation, the duration of therapy, and the reason for it. If the patient can't remember which medications or herbal preparations he's taking, find out if he has brought any with him. If he has, examine the label and contents yourself.

Family history

Information about the patient's family may help uncover hereditary disorders. Ask him if anyone in his family has had diabetes, cardiac or renal disease, high blood pressure, cancer, bleeding disorders, mental disorders, or a stroke.

Some genetic diseases are degenerative; others cause muscle weakness. For example, seizures are more common in patients whose family history shows idiopathic epilepsy, and more than 50% of patients with migraine headaches have a family history of the disorder.

Psychosocial history

Always consider the patient's cultural and social background when planning his care. Find out what religion he practices and if he actively practices his beliefs. Also note the patient's education level and occupation. Find out if he has a stable or erratic employment history. Find out if his employment involves possible exposure to toxic substances such as heavy metals or carbon monoxide. Ask him if he lives alone or with someone. Find out what his hobbies are. Ask him how he views his illness. Assess the patient's self-image while gathering this information.

Physical assessment

A complete neurologic examination can be extremely time consuming and detailed making it difficult to perform one in its entirety. However, if initial screening examination suggests a neurologic problem, you may want to perform a more detailed neurologic assessment.

Always examine the patient's neurologic system in an orderly fashion.

Vital signs

The central nervous system (CNS), primarily by way of the brain stem and the autonomic nervous system (ANS), controls the body's vital functions including body temperature; heart rate and rhythm; blood pressure; and respiratory rate, depth, and pattern. However, because these vital control centers lie deep within the cerebral hemispheres and in the brain stem, changes in vital signs — temperature, heart rate, blood pressure, and respiration — aren't usually early indicators of CNS deterioration. When evaluating the significance of vital sign changes, consider each sign individually as well as in relation to the others.

Temperature

Normal body temperature ranges from 96.7° F to 100.5° F (35.9° C to 38.1° C), depending upon the route used for measurement. Damage to the hypothalamus or upper brain stem can impair the body's ability to maintain a constant temperature, resulting in profound hypothermia (temperature below 94° F [34.4° C]) or hyperthermia (temperature above 106° F [41.1° C]). Such damage can result from petechial hemorrhages in the hypothalamus or brain stem; trauma, causing pressure, twisting, or traction; or destructive lesions.

Heart rate

Because the ANS controls heart rate and rhythm, pressure on the brain stem and cranial nerves slows the heart rate by stimulating the vagus nerve. Bradycardia occurs in patients in the later stages of increasing intracranial pressure (ICP) and with cervical spinal cord injuries; it's usually accompanied by rising systolic blood pressure, widening pulse pressure, and bounding pulse. Tachycardia occurs in patients with acutely increased ICP or a brain injury; it signals decompensation, a condition in which the body has exhausted its compensatory measures for managing ICP, which rapidly leads to death.

Blood pressure

Pressor receptors in the medulla continuously monitor blood pressure.

CRITICAL POINT *In a patient with no history of hypertension, rising systolic blood pressure may signal rising ICP. If ICP continues to rise, the patient's pulse pressure widens as his systolic pressure climbs and diastolic pressure remains stable or falls. In the late stages of acutely elevated ICP, blood pressure plummets as cerebral perfusion fails, resulting in the patient's death.*

Hypotension accompanying a brain injury is also an ominous sign. In addition, cervical spinal cord injuries may interrupt sympathetic nervous system pathways, causing peripheral vasodilation and hypotension.

Respiration

Respiratory centers in the medulla and pons control the rate, depth, and pattern of respiration. Neurologic dysfunction, particularly when it involves the brain stem or both cerebral hemispheres, commonly alters respirations. Assessment of respiration provides valuable information about a CNS lesion's site and severity. (See *Respiratory patterns associated with neurologic impairment,* page 480.)

Mental status assessment

The mental status assessment begins when interviewing the patient during the health history. How he responds to your questions gives clues to his orientation and memory and guides the physical assessment.

Ask the patient questions that require more than yes-or-no answers. Otherwise, confusion or disorientation might not be immediately apparent. If you have doubts about a patient's mental status, perform a screening examination. (See *Screening mental status,* page 481.)

Another guide during the physical assessment is the patient's health history and chief complaint. For example, if he complains about confusion or memory problems,

RESPIRATORY PATTERNS ASSOCIATED WITH NEUROLOGIC IMPAIRMENT

Several patterns displaying impaired respiration due to neurologic dysfunction include:

- Cheyne-Stokes respiration — a waxing and waning period of hyperpnea that alternates with a shorter period of apnea, which usually indicates increased intracranial pressure from a deep cerebral or brain stem lesion, or a metabolic disturbance in the brain.
- Central neurogenic hyperventilation — a type of hyperpnea that indicates damage to the lower midbrain or upper pons, which may occur as a result of severe head injury.
- Apneustic respiration — an irregular breathing pattern characterized by prolonged, gasping inspiration, with a pause at full inspiration followed by expiration; there can also be a pause after expiration; an important localizing sign of severe brain stem damage.
- Biot's respiration — late signs of neurologic deterioration, which are rare and may appear abruptly; characterized by irregular and unpredictable rate, rhythm, and depth of respiration, they may reflect increased pressure on the medulla coinciding with brain stem compression.
- Respiration impairment — varying degrees can occur due to spinal cord damage above C7, which could weaken or paralyze the respiratory muscles.

you'll want to concentrate on the mental status part of the examination.

The mental status examination consists of checking level of consciousness (LOC), orientation, appearance, behavior, communication, cognitive function, and constructional ability.

Level of consciousness

In performing an initial assessment, first evaluate the patient's LOC.

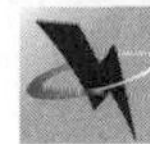

CRITICAL POINT *A change in the patient's LOC is the earliest and most sensitive indicator that his neurologic status has altered.*

If the patient's behavior is threatening while performing this initial assessment, he may not be in immediate danger, but as the health care provider, you may be at risk. Therefore, you may need to change the order of the assessment. Always consider the environment and physical condition. For example, an elderly patient admitted to the health care facility for several days may not be oriented to time, especially if he's bedridden. Also, consider the patient's vital signs and need for immediate lifesaving care.

Speak the patient's name in a normal tone of voice and note the response to an auditory stimulus. If he doesn't respond, use a tactile stimulus, such as touching him gently, squeezing his hand, or shaking his shoulder.

A fully awake patient is alert, open-eyed, and attentive to environmental stimuli. A less-awake patient appears drowsy, has reduced motor activity, and seems less attentive to environmental stimuli. Decreased arousal commonly precedes disorientation.

Use painful stimuli only to assess a patient who's unconscious or who has a markedly decreased LOC and doesn't respond to other stimuli. To test response to pain, apply firm pressure over the patient's nail bed with a blunt, hard object such as a pen. Other acceptable methods include squeezing the trapezius muscle, applying supraorbital pressure, applying mandibular pressure, performing a sternal rub, and applying nail-bed pressure.

Next, note the type and intensity of stimulus required to elicit a response. Observe if the response is verbally appropriate, if it consists of unintelligible mumbling, body movement or eye opening, or if he exhibits no response at all. After you remove the stimulus, observe the patient's level of alertness, for example, if he's wide awake, drowsy, or drifting to sleep.

After assessing the patient's level of alertness, compare the findings with results of previous assessments. Note trends, for example, if he's lethargic more often than usu-

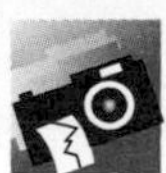

CLINICAL PICTURE

SCREENING MENTAL STATUS

To screen patients for disordered thought processes, ask the questions presented here. An incorrect answer to any question may indicate the need for a complete mental status examination.

Question	Function screened
What's your name?	Orientation to person
What's your mother's name?	Orientation to other people
What year is it?	Orientation to time
Where are you now?	Orientation to place
How old are you?	Memory
Where were you born?	Remote memory
What did you have for breakfast?	Recent memory
Who's the U.S. president?	General knowledge
Can you count backward from 20 to 1?	Attention span and calculation skills

al. Consider factors that could affect patient responsiveness. For example, a normally alert patient may become drowsy after administration of such CNS depressant medications as sedatives and opioids.

Describe a patient's responsiveness objectively. For example, describe a lethargic patient's responses this way: "awakened when called loudly, then immediately fell asleep."

Many terms are used to describe LOC, but their definitions may differ slightly among health care providers. To avoid confusion, clearly describe the patient's response to various stimuli using these guidelines:

- alert — follows commands and responds completely and appropriately to stimuli
- lethargic — is drowsy; has delayed responses to verbal stimuli; may drift off to sleep during examination
- stuporous — requires vigorous stimulation for a response
- comatose — doesn't respond appropriately to verbal or painful stimuli; can't follow commands or communicate verbally.

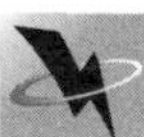

CRITICAL POINT *If the patient has sustained a skull fracture, but appears lucid, and later has a decreased LOC, this could indicate an arterial epidural bleed that requires immediate surgery.*

To minimize the subjectivity of LOC assessment and to establish a greater degree of reliability, use the Glasgow Coma Scale. This scale evaluates the patient's LOC according to three objective behaviors: eye opening, verbal responsiveness (which includes orientation), and motor response. (See *Using the Glasgow Coma Scale,* page 482.)

Consciousness is the most sensitive indicator of neurologic dysfunction and may be a valuable adjunct to other findings. Several disorders can affect the cerebral hemisphere of the brain stem — and consciousness can be impaired by any one of them. When assessing LOC, be sure to provide a stimulus that's strong enough to get a true picture of the patient's baseline.

A change in the patient's LOC commonly serves as the earliest indication of a brain

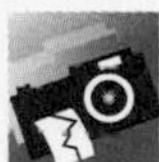

CLINICAL PICTURE

USING THE GLASGOW COMA SCALE

The Glasgow Coma Scale describes a patient's baseline mental status and helps to detect and interpret changes from baseline findings. When using the Glasgow Coma Scale, test the patient's ability to respond to verbal, motor, and sensory stimulation, and grade your findings according to the scale. A score of 15 indicates that the patient is alert, can follow simple commands, and is oriented to time, place, and person. A decreased score in one or more categories may signal an impending neurologic crisis. A score of 7 or less indicates severe neurologic damage.

Test	Score	Response
Eye opening response		
Spontaneously	4	Opens eyes spontaneously
To speech	3	Opens eyes when told to
To pain	2	Opens eyes only to painful stimulus
None	1	Doesn't open eyes in response to stimuli
Motor response		
Obeys	6	Shows two fingers when asked
Localizes	5	Reaches toward painful stimulus and tries to remove it
Withdraws	4	Moves away from painful stimulus
Abnormal flexion	3	Assumes a decorticate posture (shown below)
Abnormal extension	2	Assumes a decerebrate posture (shown below)
None	1	No response; just lies flaccid (an ominous sign)
Verbal response (to question, "What year is this?")		
Oriented	5	Tells correct year
Confused	4	Tells incorrect year
Inappropriate words	3	Replies randomly with incorrect words
Incomprehensible	2	Moans or screams
No response	1	No response
Total score		

disorder. Disorders that affect LOC include toxic encephalopathy; hemorrhage; extensive, generalized cortical atrophy; and tumor or intracranial hemorrhage. Rapid deterioration of LOC, from minutes to hours, usually indicates an acute neurologic disorder requiring immediate intervention. A gradually decreasing LOC, from weeks to months, may reflect a progressive or degenerative neurologic disorder.

Orientation

The orientation portion of the mental status assessment measures the ability of the cerebral cortex to receive and accurately interpret sensory stimuli. It includes three aspects: orientation to person, place, and time. Always ask questions that require the patient to provide information, rather than a yes-or-no answer. First, find out if the patient is aware of his identity by asking the patient's name, and note the response. A patient disoriented to person may not be able to tell his name. When asked, he may look baffled or may stammer and finally produce an unintelligible or inaccurate answer. Self-identity usually remains intact until late in decreasing LOC, making disorientation to person an ominous sign.

Next, ask the patient about place. Find out if he can correctly state his location. For example, when looking around the room, note if he concludes that he's in a health care facility, or if he thinks he's at home.

A patient in the health care facility disoriented to place most commonly confuses the health care facility's room with home or some other familiar surrounding; a patient who isn't in a health care facility, yet is still disoriented to place, such as a patient with Alzheimer's disease, may fail to recognize familiar home surroundings and may wander off in search of something familiar.

The patient oriented to place may not be able to name the health care facility, especially if he has been admitted through the emergency department. However, if a patient states the full name of the health care facility and later can't recall its name, he may be becoming disoriented to place.

Finally, to ask about orientation to time, ask the patient to state the year, month, and date. Most people usually answer correctly and can also differentiate day from night if their environment provides enough information; for example, if the room has a window.

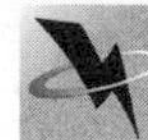

CRITICAL POINT *A patient's orientation to time is usually disrupted first and his orientation to person is disrupted last.*

If disorientation to time arises from a physiologic problem, the patient is likely to mistake unfamiliar surroundings or people for familiar ones. For example, he may confuse the health care facility's room with his bedroom or mistake a health care provider for a relative. If the disorientation originates from psychiatric disturbances, such as schizophrenia, he may have an unusually bizarre confusion pattern. For example, he may think the current year is 1972. Bizarre answers, such as 1756 or 2054, may indicate a psychiatric disturbance—or a lack of cooperation.

Appearance

Note how the patient behaves, dresses, and grooms himself. Observe him for his appearance and if he acts appropriately. Note his personal hygiene. If you observe negative findings, discuss them with family members to determine whether this is a change. Even subtle changes in a patient's behavior can signal a new onset of a chronic disease or a more acute change that involves the frontal lobe.

Look at the patient's color, facial expressions, mobility, deformities, and nutritional state. Observe the patient's gait, posture, and ability to rise from a chair. Note if he needs assistance to walk, rise from a chair, or get undressed. Observe if he can hear and see you when you're talking. Observe him for raccoon eyes. Note if he has otorrhea, cerebrospinal fluid leaking from his ears.

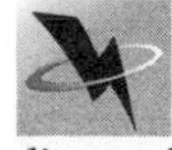

CRITICAL POINT *Raccoon eyes could indicate bleeding into the periorbital tissue. Otorrhea could indicate a basilar skull fracture. If the brain stem is lacerated or contused, immediate death can occur. Smaller leakages can resolve in 2 to 10 days.*

Behavior

Assess the patient's thought content by evaluating the clarity and cohesiveness of his ideas. Observe his conversation for smoothness, with logical transitions between ideas. Note if he has hallucinations, which are sensory perceptions that lack appropriate stimuli; or delusions, which are beliefs not supported by reality. Disordered thought patterns may indicate delirium or psychosis.

Test the patient's ability to think abstractly by asking him to interpret a common proverb such as "A stitch in time saves nine." A patient with dementia may interpret a common proverb literally.

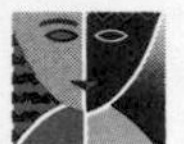

CULTURAL INSIGHT *If the patient's primary language isn't English, he'll probably have difficulty interpreting a common proverb. Engage the assistance of family members when English isn't the patient's primary language. Have them ask the patient to explain a saying in his native language.*

Test the patient's judgment by asking him how he would respond to a hypothetical situation. For example, ask him what he would do if he was in a public building and the fire alarm sounded. Evaluate the appropriateness of his answer.

Throughout the interview, assess the patient's emotional status. Note his mood, his emotional stability or lability, and the appropriateness of his emotional responses. Also assess his mood by asking how he feels about himself and his future.

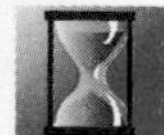

AGE ISSUE *In elderly patients, symptoms of depression may be atypical—for example, decreased function or increased agitation may occur rather than the usual sad affect.*

Communication

Assess the patient's ability to comprehend speech, writing, numbers, and gestures. Language skills include learning and recalling the parts of the language (such as words), organizing word relationships according to grammatical rules, and structuring message content logically. Speech involves neuromuscular actions of the mouth, tongue, and oropharynx.

Verbal responsiveness. During the interview and physical assessment, observe the patient when you ask a question. If you suspect a decreased LOC, call the patient's name or gently shake his shoulder to try to elicit a verbal response. Note how much the patient says. For example, if he speaks in complete sentences, in phrases, or in single words; note if he communicates spontaneously or if he rarely speaks.

Note the quality of the patient's speech, such as if it's unusually loud or soft. Observe the patient for clear articulation, or if his words are difficult to understand. Note the rate and rhythm of his speech and what language he speaks. If you can't speak his language, seek help from an interpreter or family member.

Note if the patient's verbal responses are appropriate. Observe him for the words he chooses to express thoughts, or for any problems finding or articulating his words. Also, note if he uses made-up words, or neologisms.

Test the patient to see if he can understand and follow commands. Give him a multistep command and note if he remembers to follow the steps in sequence.

If communication problems arise, note if the patient is aware of them. If he appears frustrated or angry when communication fails, note if he continues to attempt to talk, unaware that you don't comprehend.

If you suspect a language difficulty, show the patient a common object, such as a cup or a book, and ask him to name it. Ask the patient to repeat a word that you say, such as dog or breakfast. If the patient appears to have difficulty understanding spoken language, ask him to follow a simple instruction such as "Touch your nose." If the patient succeeds, then try a two-step command such as "Touch your right knee, then touch your nose." Keep in mind that language performance tends to fluctuate with the time of day and changes in physical condition. A healthy individual may experience language difficulty when ill or fatigued. Increasing language difficulties may indicate deteriorating neurologic status, warranting further evaluation.

Speech impairment or impaired language function can occur from dysphasia, which is the impaired ability to use or understand language, and aphasia, which is the inability to use or understand language, or both, that's caused by injury to the cerebral cortex. Several types of aphasia exist, including:

- expressive or Broca's aphasia—impaired fluency; difficulty finding words; impairment located in the frontal lobe, the anterior speech area

- receptive or Wernicke's aphasia—inability to understand written words or speech; use of made-up words; impairment located in the posterior speech cortex, which involves the temporal and parietal lobes
- global aphasia—lack of both expressive and receptive language; impairment of both speech areas
- facial muscle paralysis—difficulty in articulation and slurred speech
- dysarthria—impairment of neuromuscular speech
- dysphonia—impairment of voice.

Formal language skills evaluation. The formal language skills evaluation identifies the extent and characteristics of the patient's language deficits. Usually performed by a speech pathologist, it may help pinpoint the site of a CNS lesion. For example, identifying expressive aphasia, when the patient knows what he wants to say but can't speak the words, may help diagnose a frontal lobe lesion.

When evaluating the patient, include assessment of these language skills:

- spontaneous speech—After showing the patient a picture, ask him to describe what's going on.
- comprehension—Ask the patient a series of simple yes-or-no questions and evaluate his answers. Use questions with obvious answers. For example: "Does it snow in July?"
- naming—Show the patient various common objects, one at a time, and then ask him to name each one. Typical objects include a comb, ball, cup, and pencil.
- repetition—Ask him to repeat words or phrases such as "no ifs, ands, or buts."
- vocabulary—Have the patient explain the meaning of each of a series of words.
- reading—Ask him to read printed words on cards and perform the action described. For example: "Raise your hand."
- writing—Ask the patient to write something, perhaps a story describing a scene or a picture.
- copying figures—Show the patient several figures, one at a time, and then ask him to copy them. The figures usually become increasingly complex, starting with a circle, an X, and a square and proceeding to a triangle and a star.

Cognitive function

Assessing cognitive function involves testing the patient's memory, orientation, attention span, calculation ability, thought content, abstract thinking, judgment, insight, and emotional status.

To test your patient's orientation, memory, and attention span, use the mental status screening questions discussed previously. Always consider the patient's environment and physical condition when assessing orientation. Also, when the person is intubated and can't speak, ask questions that require only a nod, such as "Do you know you're in the hospital?" and "Are we in Pennsylvania?" The patient with an intact short-term memory can generally repeat five to seven nonconsecutive numbers right away and again 10 minutes later.

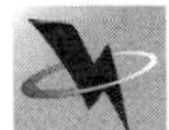

CRITICAL POINT *Short-term memory is commonly affected first in patients with neurologic disease.*

When testing attention span and calculation skills, keep in mind that lack of mathematical ability and anxiety can affect the patient's performance. If he has difficulty with numerical computation, ask him to spell the word "world" backward. While he's performing these functions, note his ability to pay attention.

Constructional ability

The patient's ability to perform simple tasks and use various objects reflects constructional ability. Assess constructional ability by asking the patient to draw a clock or a square. Apraxia and agnosia are two types of constructional disorders.

Commonly associated with parietal lobe dysfunction, *apraxia* is the inability to perform purposeful movements and make proper use of objects. Apraxia can appear in any of four types. Ideomotor agnosia is loss of the ability to understand the effect of motor activity; ability to perform simple activities but without awareness of performing them; inability to perform actions on command. Ideational apraxia is the awareness of actions that need to be done accompanied by an inability to perform them. Constructional apraxia is the inability to copy a design such as the face of a clock. Finally, dressing apraxia is the inability to understand the meaning of various articles of clothing or the sequence of actions required to get dressed.

The inability to identify common objects — called *agnosia* — may indicate a lesion in the sensory cortex. Agnosia types include visual, which is the inability to identify common objects unless they're touched; auditory, the inability to identify common sounds; and body image, the inability to identify body parts by sight or touch, inability to localize a stimulus, or denial of existence of half of the body.

Cranial nerve assessment

There are 12 pairs of cranial nerves (CNs). These nerves transmit motor or sensory messages, or both, primarily between the brain and brain stem and the head and neck. CN assessment provides valuable information about the condition of the CNS, particularly the brain stem.

Olfactory (CN I)

To assess the olfactory nerve, first check the patency of both nostrils, then instruct the patient to close his eyes. Occlude one nostril and hold a familiar, pungent-smelling substance — such as coffee, tobacco, soap, or peppermint — under his nose and ask its identity. Repeat this technique with the other nostril.

If the patient reports detecting the smell but can't name it, offer a choice such as "Do you smell lemon, coffee, or peppermint?" The patient should be able to detect and identify the smell correctly. The location of the olfactory nerve makes it especially vulnerable to damage from facial fractures and head injuries.

Damage to CN I may be due to disorders of the base of the frontal lobe, such as tumors or arteriosclerotic changes.

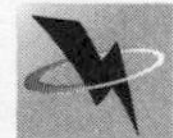

CRITICAL POINT *The sense of smell remains intact as long as one of the two olfactory nerves exists; it's permanently lost (anosmia) if both nerves are affected. Anosmia can also result from nonneurologic causes, such as nasal congestion, sinus infection, smoking, and cocaine use, and impair the sense of taste. A complaint about food taste may signal CN I damage.*

Optic (CN II) and oculomotor (CN III)

To assess the optic nerve, check visual acuity, visual fields, and the retinal structures. To assess the oculomotor nerve, check pupil size, pupil shape, and pupillary response to light.

To test visual acuity quickly and informally, have the patient read a newspaper, starting with large headlines and moving to small print.

Test visual fields with a technique called *confrontation*. To do this, stand 2′ (0.6 m) in front of the patient, and have him cover one eye. Then close one of your eyes and bring your moving fingers into the patient's visual field from the periphery. Ask him to tell you when he sees the object. Test each quadrant of the patient's visual field, and compare his results with your own. Chart any defects you find. (See *Detecting visual field defects.*)

A visual field defect may signal stroke, head injury, or brain tumor. The area and extent of the loss depend on the lesion's location.

When assessing pupil size, look for trends. For example, watch for a gradual increase in the size of one pupil or the appearance of unequal pupils in a patient whose pupils were previously equal. The pupils should be equal, round, and reactive to light.

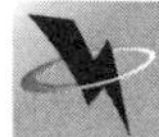

CRITICAL POINT *In a blind patient with a nonfunctional optic nerve, light stimulation will fail to produce either a direct or a consensual pupillary response. However, a legally blind patient may have some optic nerve function, which causes the blind eye to respond to direct light. In a patient who's totally blind in only one eye, the pupil of the eye with the intact optic nerve will react to direct light stimulation, whereas the blind eye, because it receives sensory messages from the functional optic nerve, will respond consensually.*

Pupil size can be affected by increased ICP that puts pressure on the oculomotor nerve causing a change in responsiveness or pupil size on the affected side that results in dilation of the pupil ipsilateral to the mass lesion; as the ICP rises, the other oculomotor nerve becomes affected, causing both pupils to become oval or react sluggishly to light shortly before dilating; but, without treatment, both pupils become fixed and di-

DETECTING VISUAL FIELD DEFECTS

Here are some examples of visual field defects. The black areas represent vision loss.

	Left	Right
1. Blindness of right eye		
2. Bitemporal hemianopsia, or loss of half the visual field		
3. Left homonymous hemianopsia		
4. Left homonymous hemianopsia, superior quadrant		

lated. The hippus phenomenon causes brisk pupil constriction in response to light followed by a pulsating dilation and constriction, which may be normal in some patients but may also reflect early oculomotor nerve compression. Optic and oculomotor nerve damage can also affect pupil size by impairing the pupillary response to light, which indicates neurologic demise. Lastly, anisocoria, or unequal pupils, which are normal in about 20% of people, occurs when pupil size doesn't change with the amount of illumination. (See *Understanding pupillary changes*, page 488.)

Oculomotor (CN III), trochlear (CN IV), and abducens (CN VI)

To test the coordinated function of the oculomotor, trochlear, and abducens nerves, assess them simultaneously by evaluating the patient's extraocular eye movement. (See chapter 7, Ears, nose, and throat, for additional information.)

The patient's eyes should move smoothly and in a coordinated manner through all six directions of eye movement including left superior, left lateral, left inferior, right superior, right lateral, and right inferior.

Observe each eye for rapid oscillation, known as *nystagmus,* movement not in unison with that of the other eye, called *disconjugate movement,* or inability to move in certain directions, known as *ophthalmoplegia.* Also, note any complaint of double vision, or *diplopia.* Nystagmus may indicate a disorder of the brain stem, the cerebellum, or the vestibular portion of CN VIII. It can also imply drug toxicity such as from the anticonvulsant phenytoin.

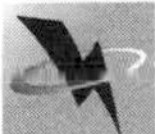

CRITICAL POINT *Increased ICP can put pressure on CN IV, causing impaired extraocular eye movement inferiorly and medially, and CN VI, causing impaired extraocular eye movement laterally.*

The oculomotor nerve is also responsible for eyelid elevation and pupillary constriction. Drooping of the patient's eyelid, or ptosis, can result from a defect in the oculomotor nerve. To assess ptosis more accurately, have the patient sit upright.

Trigeminal (CN V)

To assess the sensory portion of the trigeminal nerve, gently touch the right side and the left side of the patient's forehead with a cotton ball while his eyes are closed. Instruct him to state the moment the cotton touches the area. Compare his response on both sides. Repeat the technique on the right and left cheek and on the right and left jaw. Next, repeat the entire procedure using a sharp object. The cap of a disposable ballpoint pen can be used to test light touch with the dull end and sharp stimuli with the sharp end. If an abnormality appears, also test for temperature sensation by touching

UNDERSTANDING PUPILLARY CHANGES

Use this chart as a guide when observing your patient for pupillary changes.

Pupillary change	Possible causes
Unilateral, dilated (4 mm), fixed, and nonreactive 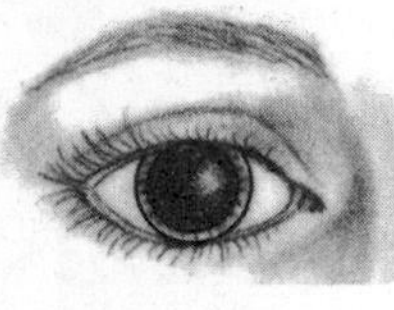 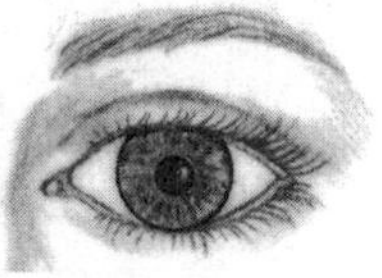	▪ Uncal herniation with oculomotor nerve damage ▪ Brain stem compression ▪ Increased intracranial pressure ▪ Tentorial herniation ▪ Head trauma with subdural or epidural hematoma ▪ May be normal in some people
Bilateral, dilated (4 mm), fixed, and nonreactive 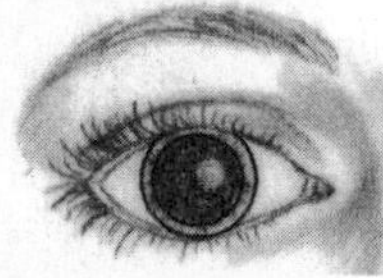 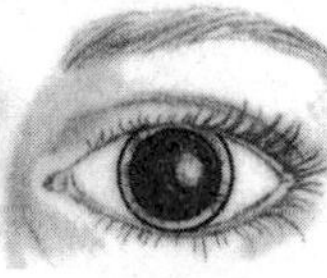	▪ Severe midbrain damage ▪ Cardiopulmonary arrest (hypoxia) ▪ Anticholinergic poisoning
Bilateral, midsize (2 mm), fixed, and nonreactive 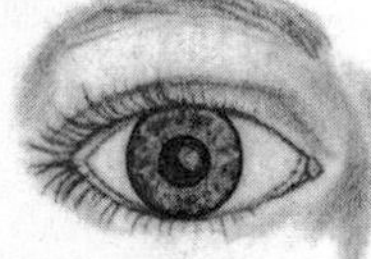 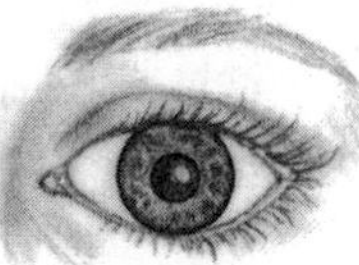	▪ Midbrain involvement caused by edema, hemorrhage, infarctions, lacerations, contusions
Bilateral, pinpoint (< 1 mm), and usually nonreactive 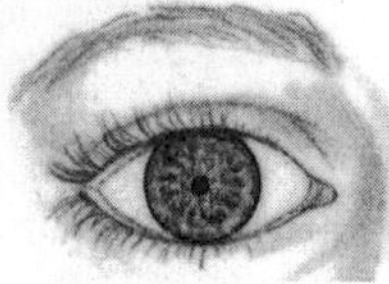 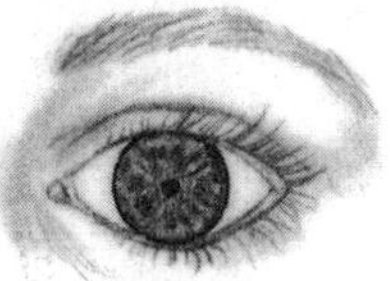	▪ Lesions of pons, usually after hemorrhage
Unilateral, small (1.5 mm), and nonreactive 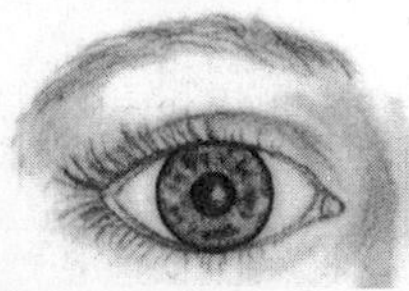 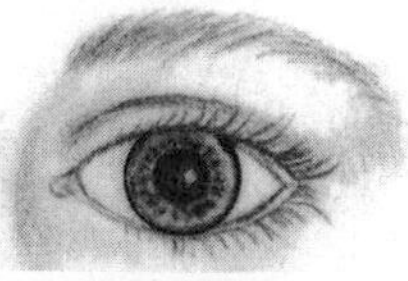	▪ Disruption of sympathetic nerve supply to the head caused by spinal cord lesion above the first thoracic vertebra

the patient's skin with test tubes filled with hot and cold water and asking the patient to differentiate between them. The patient should report feeling both light touch and sharp stimuli in all three areas, the forehead, cheek, and jaw, on both sides of the face.

Peripheral nerve damage can create a loss of sensation in any or all three regions supplied by the trigeminal nerve that includes the forehead, cheek, and jaw. Trigeminal neuralgia causes severe, piercing, or stabbing pain over one or more of the facial dermatomes. A lesion in the cervical spinal cord or brain stem can produce impaired sensory function in each of the three areas.

To assess the motor portion of the trigeminal nerve, ask the patient to clench his jaws. Palpate the temporal and masseter muscles bilaterally, checking for symmetry. Try to open his clenched jaws. Next, watch the patient while he's opening and closing his mouth for asymmetry. The jaws should clench symmetrically and remain closed against resistance.

A lesion in the cervical spinal cord or brain stem can produce impaired motor function in regions supplied by the trigeminal nerve, weakening the patient's jaw muscles, causing the jaw to deviate toward the affected side when chewing, and allowing residual food to collect in the affected cheek.

To assess the patient's corneal reflex, stroke a wisp of cotton lightly across a cornea. The lids of both eyes should close. (See *Eliciting the corneal reflex.*) An absent corneal reflex may result from peripheral nerve or brain stem damage. However, a diminished corneal reflex commonly occurs in patients who wear contact lenses.

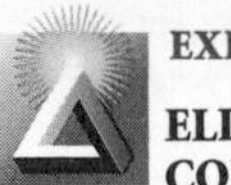

EXPERT TECHNIQUE

ELICITING THE CORNEAL REFLEX

To elicit the corneal reflex, have the patient turn her eyes away from you to avoid involuntary blinking during the procedure. Then approach the patient from the opposite side, out of her line of vision, and brush the cornea lightly with a fine wisp of sterile cotton. Repeat the procedure on the other eye. The lids of both eyes should close.

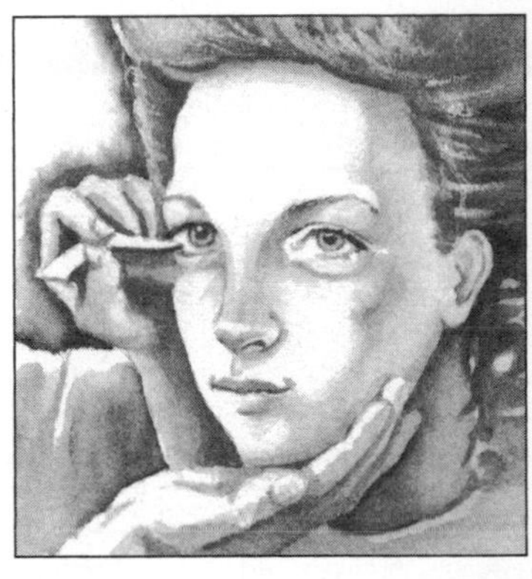

Facial (CN VII)

To test the motor portion of the facial nerve, ask the patient to wrinkle his forehead, raise and lower his eyebrows, smile to show teeth, and puff out his cheeks. Also, with the patient's eyes tightly closed, attempt to open the eyelids. With each of these movements, observe closely for symmetry. Facial movements should be symmetrical.

Unilateral facial weakness can reflect an upper motor neuron problem, such as a stroke or a tumor that has damaged neurons in the facial control area of the motor strip in the cerebral cortex. If the weakness originates in the cerebral cortex, the patient will retain the ability to wrinkle his forehead because the forehead receives motor messages from both hemispheres of the brain—which explains why when one side is damaged, such as in a stroke, the other side takes over. However, if CN VII is damaged, the weakness will extend to the forehead, and the eye on the affected side won't close.

To test the sensory portion of the facial nerve, which supplies taste sensation to the anterior two-thirds of the tongue, first prepare four marked, closed containers, with one containing salt; another sugar; a third, vinegar (or lemon); and a fourth, quinine (or bitters). Then, with the patient's eyes closed, place salt on the anterior two-thirds of his tongue using a cotton swab or dropper. Ask him to identify the taste as sweet, salty, sour, or bitter. Rinse his mouth with water. Repeat this procedure, alternating flavors and sides of the tongue, until all four flavors have been tested on both sides. Taste sensations to the posterior third of the tongue are supplied by the glossopharyngeal nerve (CN IX) and are usually tested at the same time. The patient should have symmetrical taste sensations.

An impaired sense of taste can signify damage to the patient's facial or glossopharyngeal nerve, or it may simply reflect a part of the normal aging process. Chemotherapy or head and neck radiation can also alter taste by damaging taste bud receptors.

Acoustic (CN VIII)

To assess the acoustic portion of the acoustic nerve, test the patient's hearing acuity. To test hearing, ask the patient to cover one ear, and then stand on his opposite side and whisper a few words. See whether he can repeat what you said. Test the other ear the same way.

To assess the vestibular portion of this nerve, observe for nystagmus and disturbed balance and note reports of dizziness or the room spinning.

The patient should be able to hear a whispered voice, rubbing of fingers, or a watch ticking. He should have normal eye movement and balance and no dizziness or vertigo. With sensorial hearing loss, the patient may have trouble hearing high-pitched sounds, or he may have a total loss of hearing in the affected ear due to lesions of the cochlear branch of CN VIII. With nystagmus and vertigo, the patient may have a disturbance of the vestibular centers. If it's caused by a peripheral lesion, vertigo and nystagmus will occur 10 to 20 seconds after the patient changes position, and symptoms will gradually lessen with the repetition of the position change. If the vertigo is of central origin, there's no latent period, and the symptoms don't diminish with repetition.

Glossopharyngeal (CN IX) and vagus (CN X)

To assess the glossopharyngeal and vagus nerves, which have overlapping functions, first listen to the patient's voice for indications of a hoarse or nasal quality. Then watch his soft palate when he says "ah." Next, test the gag reflex after warning him. To evoke this reflex, touch the posterior wall of the pharynx with a cotton swab or tongue blade.

The patient's voice should sound strong and clear. The soft palate and the uvula should rise when he says "ah," and the uvula should remain midline. The palatine arches should remain symmetrical during movement and at rest. The gag reflex should be intact. If it diminishes or the pharynx moves asymmetrically, evaluate each side of the posterior pharyngeal wall to confirm integrity of both cranial nerves.

Glossopharyngeal neuralgia produces paroxysmal pain, which radiates from the patient's throat to his ear. Damage to the CN IX or CN X impairs swallowing. Furthermore, during swallowing, the palate fails to rise and close off the nasal passageways, allowing nasal regurgitation of fluids.

A damaged CN X can also cause loss of the gag reflex and a hoarse or nasal-sounding voice. Finally, because the vagus nerve innervates most viscera through the parasympathetic nervous system, vagal damage can affect involuntary vital functions, producing tachycardia, other cardiac arrhythmias, and dyspnea.

Accessory (CN XI)

To assess the spinal accessory nerve, press down on the patient's shoulders while he attempts to shrug against this resistance. Note shoulder strength and symmetry while inspecting and palpating the trapezius muscle.

Then apply resistance to his turned head while he attempts to return to a midline position. Note neck strength while inspecting and palpating the sternocleidomastoid muscle. Repeat for the opposite side.

CRITICAL POINT *If the patient complains of stiffness in the neck, suspect nuchal rigidity, an early sign of meningeal irritation. Passively flex the patient's neck and touch his chin to his chest. Nuchal rigidity is present if the patient experiences pain and muscle spasms. If positive, check for Kernig's and Brudzinski's signs. (See* Eliciting Kernig's and Brudzinski's signs.*)*

Both shoulders should be able to overcome the resistance equally well. The neck should overcome resistance in both directions. Unilateral weakness, atrophy, or paralysis of the muscles innervated by the spinal accessory nerve suggests a peripheral nerve lesion. Signs include a drooping shoulder or a scapula that appears displaced toward the affected side.

Hypoglossal (CN XII)

To assess the hypoglossal nerve, observe the patient's protruded tongue for any deviation from midline, atrophy, or fasciculations, very fine muscle flickering, which indicates lower motor neuron disease.

Next, instruct the patient to move his tongue rapidly from side to side with the mouth open, to curl his tongue up toward the nose, and to curl his tongue down toward the chin. Then use a tongue blade or folded gauze pad to apply resistance to his protruded tongue and ask him to try to push the tongue blade to one side. Repeat this procedure on the other side and note the patient's tongue strength.

EXPERT TECHNIQUE

ELICITING KERNIG'S AND BRUDZINSKI'S SIGNS

If, during your spinal accessory nerve assessment (cranial nerve XI), you observe nuchal rigidity, indicating meningeal irritation, test the patient for Kernig's and Brudzinski's signs.

Kernig's sign
To elicit Kernig's sign, place the patient in a supine position. Flex the leg at the hip and knee, as shown. Then try to extend the leg while keeping the hip flexed. If the patient experiences pain and possibly spasm in the hamstring muscle and resists further extension, assume that meningeal irritation has occurred.

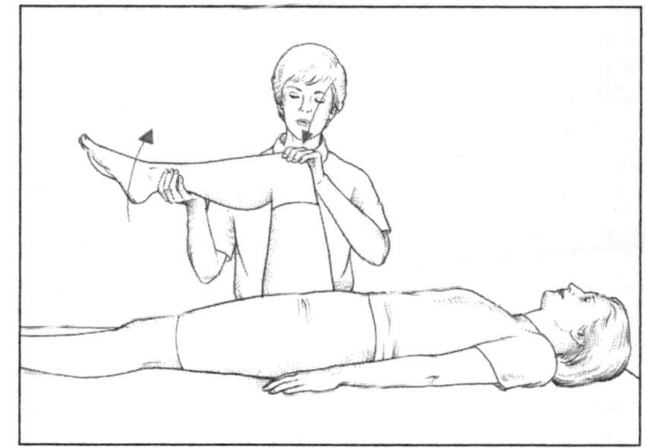

Brudzinski's sign
To test for Brudzinski's sign, place the patient in the supine position with your hands behind the neck and lift the patient's head toward the chest.

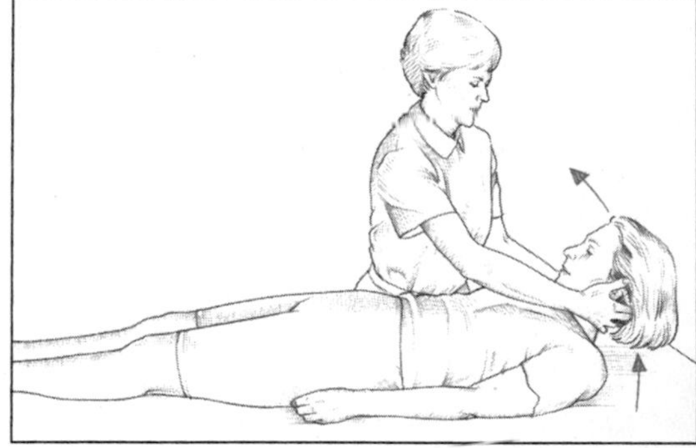

The patient with meningeal irritation will flex the hips and knees in response to passive neck flexion.

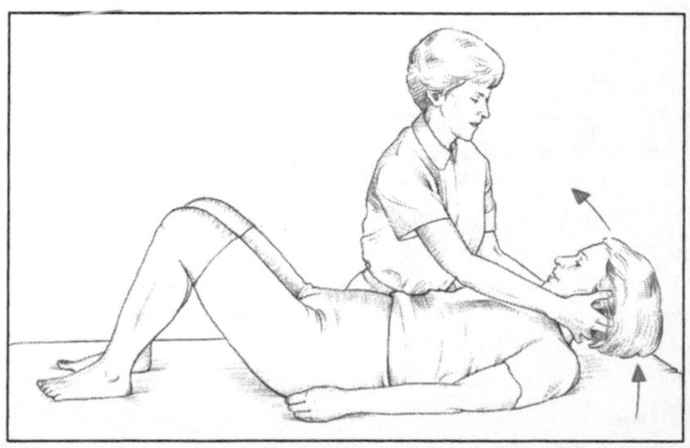

Listen to the patient's speech for the sounds "d", "n", and "t", which require use of the tongue to articulate. If his general speech suggests a problem, have him repeat a phrase or a series of words that contain these sounds such as "Round the rugged rock that ragged rascal ran." The tongue should be midline, and the patient should be able to move it right and left equally. He also should be able to move the tongue up and down. Pressure exerted by the tongue on the tongue blade should be equal on either side. Speech should be clear.

A peripheral nerve lesion creates a unilateral flaccid paralysis of the patient's tongue, atrophy of the affected side, and deviation of the tongue. A unilateral spastic paralysis of the tongue produces poorly articulated, difficult speech, or dysarthria, characterized by an explosive production of words. The tongue deviates toward the affected side.

Sensory function assessment

Evaluation of the sensory system involves assessing five areas of sensation: pain, light touch, vibration, position, and discrimination.

Pain

To test the patient for pain, have him close his eyes; then touch all the major dermatomes, first with the sharp end of a safety pin and then with the dull end. Proceed in this order: fingers, shoulders, toes, thighs, and trunk. Ask him to identify when he feels the sharp stimulus.

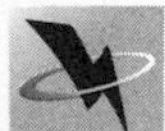

CRITICAL POINT *If the patient has major deficits, start in the area with the least sensation, and move toward the area with the most sensation. This helps you determine the level of deficit.*

Light touch

To test for the sense of light touch, follow the same routine as above, but use a wisp of cotton. Lightly touch the patient's skin — don't swab or sweep the cotton, because you might miss an area of loss. A patient with a peripheral neuropathy might retain his sensation for light touch after he has lost pain sensation.

Vibration

To test vibratory sense, apply a tuning fork over certain bony prominences while the patient keeps his eyes closed. Start at the distal interphalangeal joint of the index finger, and move proximally. Test only until the patient feels the vibration, because everything above that level will be intact. (See *Evaluating vibration.*) If vibratory sense is intact, you don't have to check position sense because the same pathway carries both.

Position

To assess position sense, have the patient close his eyes. Then grasp the sides of his big toe, move it up and down, and ask him what position it's in. To be tested for position sense, the patient needs intact vestibular and cerebellar function.

Perform the same test on the patient's upper extremities by grasping the sides of his index finger and moving it back and forth.

Discrimination

Discrimination testing assesses the ability of the cerebral cortex to interpret and integrate information. Stereognosis is the ability to discriminate an object's shape, size, weight, texture, and form by touching and manipulating it. To test stereognosis, ask the patient to close his eyes and open his hand. Then place a common object, such as a key, in his hand, and ask him to identify it. If he can't identify the key, test graphesthesia next. Have the patient keep his eyes closed and hold out his hand while you draw a large number on his palm. Ask him to identify the number. Both these tests assess the ability of the cortex to integrate sensory input.

To test point localization, have the patient close his eyes; then touch one of his limbs, and ask him where you touched him. Test two-point discrimination by touching the patient simultaneously in two contralateral areas. He should be able to identify both touches. Failure to perceive touch on one side is called extinction.

Assessment of the sensory system may reveal several abnormal findings. A reduced sensory acuity is evidenced by a need for repeated, prolonged, or excessive contact to evoke a response. Sensory deficits, indicated by repeated failure to detect tactile stimuli in one body area or a difference in sensory acuity in the same extremity on opposite sides of the body can occur. Damaged sensory nerve fibers can occur indicated by a complaint of tingling or dysesthesia in one area, even if the patient can correctly identi-

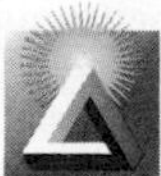

EXPERT TECHNIQUE

EVALUATING VIBRATION

To evaluate the patient's vibratory sense, apply the base of a vibrating tuning fork to the interphalangeal joint of the great toe, as shown.

Ask the patient what he feels. If he feels the sensation, he'll typically report a feeling of buzzing or vibration. If he doesn't feel the sensation at the toe, try the medial malleolus. Then continue moving proximally until he feels the sensation. Note where he feels it, and then repeat the process on the other leg.

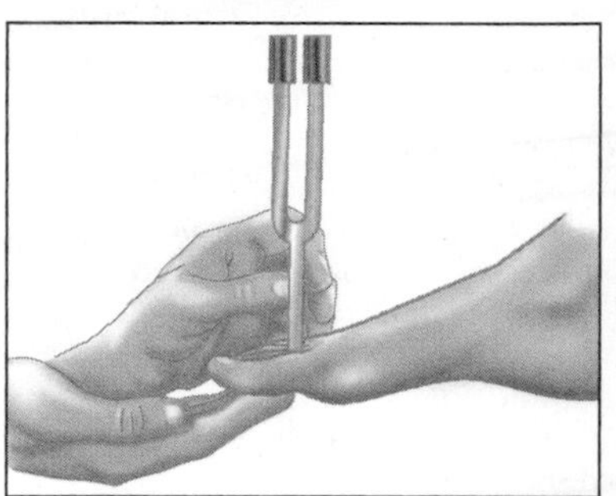

fy the tactile stimulus. A disorder in the posterior tracts, dorsal columns, of the spinal cord or a peripheral nerve or root lesion may occur as evidenced by a loss of the sense of light touch, vibration, and position. A disorder in the spinothalamic tracts can occur as indicated by impaired pain or temperature sensation. Developing peripheral neuropathy can occur that's commonly preceded by loss of the sense of vibration. A bilateral, symmetrical, distal sensory loss also suggests a peripheral neuropathy. A disorder in the dorsal columns or the sensory interpretive regions of the parietal lobe of the cerebral cortex can occur as evidenced by an impaired ability to recognize the distance between two points (discriminative sensation). In addition, lesions of the sensory cortex can occur, indicated by impaired point localization.

Motor function assessment

Assessing the patient's motor system includes inspecting the muscles and testing muscle tone and muscle strength. Cerebellar testing is also performed because the cerebellum plays a role in abnormal smooth-muscle movements, such as tics, tremors, or fasciculations.

Muscle tone

Muscle tone represents muscular resistance to passive stretching. To test arm muscle tone, move the patient's shoulder through passive range-of-motion (ROM) exercises. You should feel a slight resistance. Then let the arm drop to the patient's side. The arm should fall easily.

To test leg muscle tone, guide the hip through passive ROM exercises; then let the leg fall to the bed. If it falls into an externally rotated position, this is an abnormal finding.

Assessment may reveal abnormal muscle movements, including uncontrollable tics that involve sudden, uncontrolled movements of the face, shoulders, and extremities caused by abnormal neural stimuli. They can be normal movements that appear repetitively and inappropriately, such as blinking, shoulder shrugging, and facial twitching. Involuntary tremors may also occur, which involve repetitive, involuntary movements (such as tics) usually seen in the fingers, wrist, eyelids, tongue, and legs. These movements occur when the affected body part is at rest or with voluntary movement. For example, the patient with Parkinson's disease has a characteristic pill-rolling tremor, and the patient with cerebellar disease has an "intention tremor" when reaching for an object. In addition, small-muscle fasciculations — fine twitchings in small muscle groups — may occur, which are most commonly associated with lower motor neuron dysfunction.

Muscle strength

To perform a general examination of muscle strength, observe the patient's gait and motor activities. Assessment may reveal gait abnormalities that may result from disorders of the cerebellum, posterior columns, corticospinal tract, basal ganglia, and lower motor neurons. These abnormalities include hemiparetic, or spastic, gait with characteristics varying according to the amount of upper motor neuron damage. In severe cases, the patient walks with the affected upper extremity abducted and the elbow, wrist, and fingers flexed. The upper body is somewhat stooped, and he tilts slightly to the opposite side. As he walks, he extends his leg and inverts his foot at the ankle with the leg swinging in a circular motion.

Ataxic gait may also occur, which is caused by cerebellar damage. The patient has a wide-based and reeling walk, commonly called "drunken gait." If sensory loss occurs, the patient may not be able to feel where he's placing his foot so he partially flexes his hips and lifts up his legs and then slaps his feet down with each step.

Steppage gait is another abnormality associated with lower motor neuron disease and commonly accompanied by muscle weakness and atrophy. The patient deliberately lifts up his feet and slaps them down on the floor.

To evaluate muscle strength, ask the patient to move major muscles and muscle groups against resistance. For instance, to test shoulder girdle strength, have him extend his arms with his palms up and maintain this position for 30 seconds. If he can't maintain this position, test further by pushing down on his outstretched arms. If he lifts both arms equally, look for pronation of the hand and downward drift of the arm on the weaker side.

Cerebellar function

Cerebellar testing looks at the patient's coordination and general balance. Observe the patient to see if he can sit and stand without support. If he can, observe him as he walks across the room, turns, and walks back. Note imbalances or abnormalities.

CRITICAL POINT *With cerebellar dysfunction, the patient will have a wide-based, unsteady gait. Deviation to one side may indicate a cerebellar lesion on that side.*

Ask the patient to walk heel to toe, and observe his balance. Then perform Romberg's test.

Romberg's test. Observe the patient's balance as he stands with his eyes open, feet together, and arms at his sides. Then ask him to close his eyes. Hold your arms out on either side of him to protect him if he sways. If he falls to one side, the result of Romberg's test is positive.

Nose-to-finger test. Test extremity coordination by asking the patient to touch his nose and then touch your outstretched finger as you move it. Have him do this faster and faster. His movements should be accurate and smooth.

Rapid alternating movement tests. Other tests of cerebellar function assess rapid alternating movements. In these tests, the patient's movements should be accurate and smooth.

First, ask the patient to touch the thumb of his right hand to his right index finger and then to each of his remaining fingers. Observe the movements for accuracy and smoothness. Next, ask him to sit with his palms on his thighs. Tell him to turn his palms up and down, gradually increasing his speed.

Finally, have the patient lie in a supine position. Then stand at the foot of the table or bed and hold your palms near the soles of his feet. Ask him to alternately tap the sole of his right foot and the sole of his left foot against your palms. He should increase his speed as you observe his coordination.

Reflex assessment

Evaluating the patient's reflexes involves testing deep tendon and superficial reflexes and observing for primitive reflexes.

Deep tendon reflexes

Deep tendon reflexes (DTRs), also called *muscle-stretch reflexes,* occur when a sudden stimulus causes the muscle to stretch. Make sure the patient is relaxed and comfortable during assessment because tension or anxiety may diminish the reflex. Position the patient comfortably and encourage him to relax and become limp.

Ask the patient who seems to have depressed reflexes to perform two isometric muscle contractions. First, to improve leg reflexes, have the patient clench his hands together and tense the arm muscles during

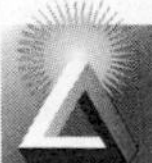

EXPERT TECHNIQUE

ASSESSING DEEP TENDON REFLEXES

During a neurologic examination, you'll assess the patient's deep tendon reflexes. Test the biceps, triceps, brachioradialis, patellar or quadriceps, and Achilles reflexes.

Biceps reflex
Position the patient's arm so his elbow is flexed at a 45-degree angle and his arm is relaxed. Place your thumb or index finger over the biceps tendon and your remaining fingers loosely over the triceps muscle. Strike your finger with the pointed end of the reflex hammer, and watch and feel for the contraction of the biceps muscle and flexion of the forearm.

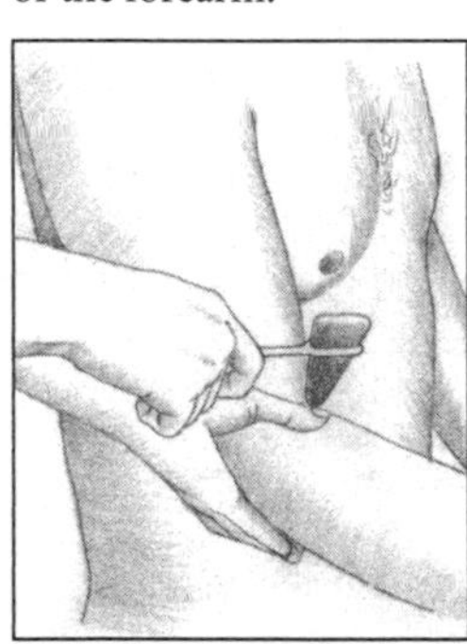

Triceps reflex
Have the patient adduct his arm and place his forearm across his chest. Strike the triceps tendon about 2″ (5 cm) above the olecranon process on the extensor surface of the upper arm. Watch for contraction of the triceps muscle and extension of the forearm.

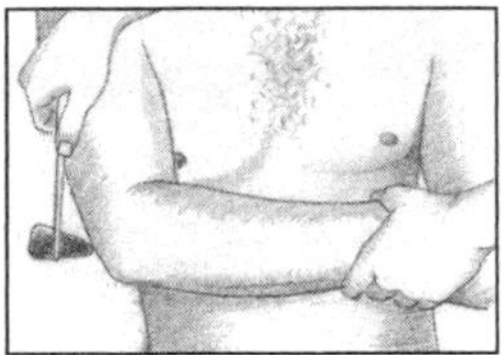

Brachioradialis reflex
Ask the patient to rest the ulnar surface of his hand on his abdomen or lap with the elbow partially flexed. Strike the radius, and watch for supination of the hand and flexion of the forearm at the elbow.

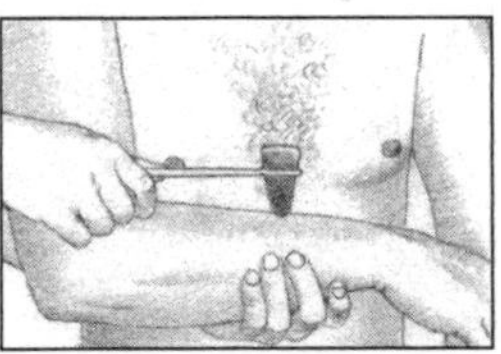

Patellar reflex
Have the patient sit with his legs dangling freely. If he can't sit up, flex his knee at a 45-degree angle, and place your nondominant hand behind it for support. Strike the patellar tendon just below the patella, and look for contraction of the quadriceps muscle in the thigh with extension of the leg.

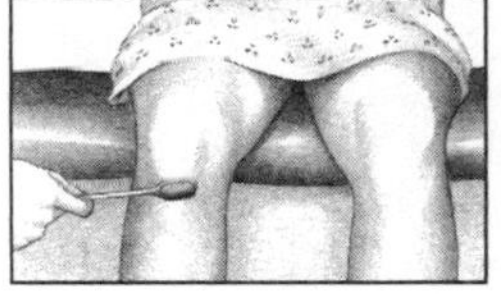

Achilles reflex
Have the patient flex his foot. Then support the plantar surface. Strike the Achilles tendon, and watch for plantar flexion of the foot at the ankle.

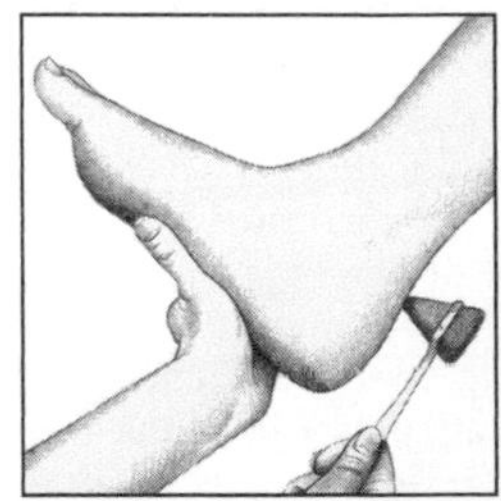

the reflex assessment. Second, to improve arm reflexes, have him clench his teeth or squeeze one thigh with the hand not being evaluated.

These maneuvers force the patient to concentrate on something other than the reflexes being tested, which can help to eliminate unintentional inhibition of the reflexes. Hold the reflex hammer loosely, yet securely, between your thumb and fingers so that it can swing freely in a controlled direction.

Place the patient's extremities in a neutral position, with the muscle you're testing in a slightly stretched position. Compare reflexes on opposite body sides for symmetry of movement and muscle strength. (See *Assessing deep tendon reflexes.*)

Grade deep tendon reflexes using a "0" for absent impulses; +1 for diminished impulses; +2 for normal impulses; +3 for increased impulses, but may be normal; and

DOCUMENTING DEEP TENDON REFLEXES

Record the patient's deep tendon reflex (DTR) scores by drawing a stick figure and entering the grades on this scale at the proper location. The figure shown here indicates hypoactive DTRs in the legs; other reflexes are normal.

Key:

0 = absent
+ = hypoactive (diminished)
++ = normal
+++ = brisk (increased)
++++ = hyperactive (clonus may be present)

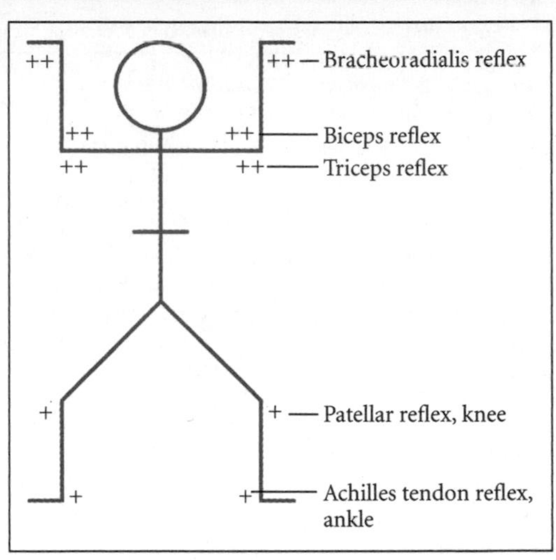

+4 for hyperactive impulses (See *Documenting deep tendon reflexes.*)

Increased or hyperactive reflexes occur with upper motor neuron disorders, where damaged CNS neurons in the cerebral cortex or corticospinal tracts prevent the brain from inhibiting peripheral reflex activity thereby allowing a small stimulus to trigger reflexes, which then tend to overrespond. Examples of hyperactive reflexes include spasticity associated with spinal cord injuries or other upper motor neuron disorders such as multiple sclerosis.

Decreased, hypoactive, or absent reflexes indicate a disorder of the lower motor neurons or the anterior horn of the spinal cord, where the peripheral nerve originates. Examples of lower motor neuron disorders characterized by hyporeflexia or areflexia include Guillain-Barré syndrome and amyotrophic lateral sclerosis.

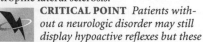

CRITICAL POINT *Patients without a neurologic disorder may still display hypoactive reflexes but these reflexes should be symmetrical. For example, a compressed spinal nerve root, which can cause a herniated intervertebral disk at L3 or L4, may diminish the patient's reflex associated with that cord such as the knee jerk reflex.*

Superficial reflexes

Stimulating the skin or mucous membranes is a method of testing superficial reflexes. Because these are cutaneous reflexes, the more you try to elicit them in succession, the less of a response you'll get. So observe carefully the first time you stimulate.

Babinski's reflex. Using an applicator stick, tongue blade, or key, slowly stroke the lateral side of the patient's sole from the heel to the great toe. The normal response in an adult is plantar flexion of the toes. Upward movement of the great toe and fanning of the little toes—called *Babinski's reflex*—is abnormal. (See *Eliciting Babinski's reflex.*)

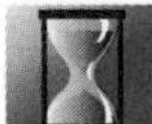

AGE ISSUE *In normal infants, Babinski's reflex can be elicited, in some cases until age 2. However, plantar flexion of the toes is seen in more than 90% of normal infants.*

Cremasteric reflex. The cremasteric reflex is tested in men by using an applicator stick to stimulate the inner thigh. Normal reaction is contraction of the cremaster muscle and elevation of the testicle on the side of the stimulus.

Abdominal reflexes. Test the abdominal reflexes with the patient in the supine position with his arms at his sides and his knees slightly flexed. Briskly stroke both sides of the abdomen above and below the umbilicus, moving from the periphery toward the midline. Movement of the umbilicus toward the stimulus is normal.

Primitive reflexes

The primitive reflexes you'll check for are the grasp, snout, sucking, and glabella reflexes.

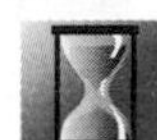

AGE ISSUE *Primitive reflexes are abnormal in adults but normal in infants, whose central nervous systems are immature. As the patient's neurologic system matures these reflexes disappear.*

Assess the grasp reflex by applying gentle pressure to the patient's palm with your fingers. If the patient grasps your fingers between his thumb and index finger, suspect cortical or premotor cortex damage.

Assess the snout reflex by lightly tapping on the patient's upper lip. If the patient's lip purses when lightly tapped, this is a positive snout reflex indicating frontal lobe damage.

Observe the patient while you're feeding him or while he has an oral airway or endotracheal tube in place. A sucking motion while the patient is being fed indicates cortical damage. This reflex is commonly seen in patients with advanced dementia.

Elicit the glabella response by repeatedly tapping the bridge of the patient's nose. If the patient responds with persistent blinking after being repeatedly tapped on the bridge of his nose, this indicates diffuse cortical dysfunction.

EXPERT TECHNIQUE
ELICITING BABINSKI'S REFLEX

To elicit Babinski's reflex, stroke the lateral aspect of the sole of the patient's foot with your thumbnail or another moderately sharp object. Normally, this elicits flexion of all toes — a negative Babinski's reflex — as shown in the top illustration. With a positive Babinski's reflex, the great toe dorsiflexes and the other toes fan out, as shown in the bottom illustration.

NORMAL TOE FLEXION

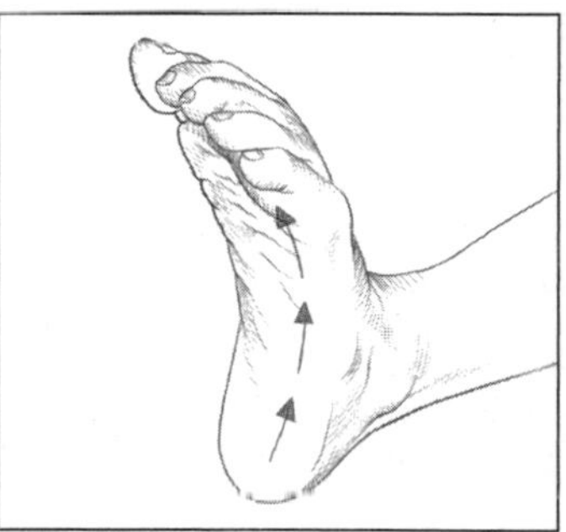

POSITIVE BABINSKI'S REFLEX

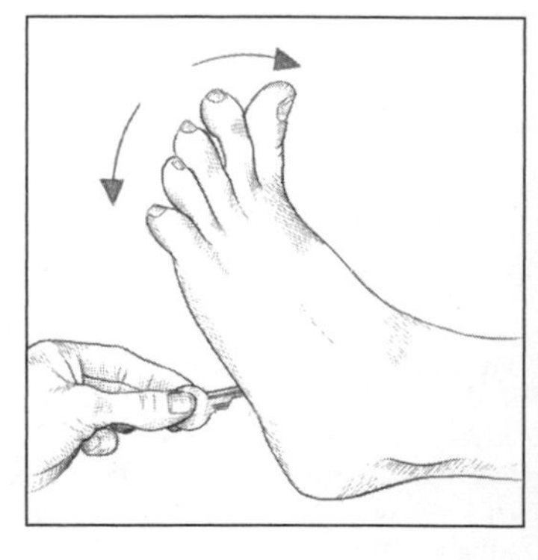

Abnormal findings

A patient may seek care for several signs and symptoms related to the neurologic system. The most significant findings are aphasia; apraxia; Babinski's reflex; Brudzinski's sign; corneal reflex, absent; deep tendon reflexes (DTRs), hyperactive or hypoactive; fasciculations; level of consciousness (LOC), deceased; headache; Kernig's sign; muscle flaccidity; muscle spasticity; paralysis; pupils, nonreactive; Romberg's sign; seizures, generalized tonic-clonic or simple partial; and tremors. The following history, physical assessment, and analysis summaries will help you assess each one quickly and accurately. After obtaining further information, begin to interpret the findings. (See *Neurologic system: Interpreting your findings,* pages 498 to 507.)

(Text continues on page 508.)

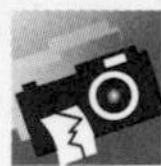

CLINICAL PICTURE

NEUROLOGIC SYSTEM: INTERPRETING YOUR FINDINGS

After you assess the patient, a group of findings may lead you to suspect a particular neurologic disorder. The chart below shows you some common groups of findings for major signs and symptoms related to the neurologic system, along with their probable causes.

Sign or symptom and findings	Probable cause
Aphasia	
▪ Wenicke's, Broca's, or global aphasia ▪ Decreased level of consciousness (LOC) ▪ Right-sided hemiparesis ▪ Homonymous hemianopsia ▪ Paresthesia and loss of sensation	Stroke
▪ Any type of aphasia occurring suddenly, may be transient or permanent ▪ Blurred or double vision ▪ Headache ▪ Cerebrospinal otorrhea and rhinorrhea ▪ Disorientation ▪ Behavioral changes ▪ Signs of increased intracranial pressure (ICP)	Head trauma
▪ Any type of aphasia occurring suddenly and resolving within 24 hours ▪ Transient hemiparesis ▪ Paresthesia ▪ Dizziness and confusion	Transient ischemic attack
Apraxia	
▪ Gradual and irreversible motor apraxia ▪ Amnesia ▪ Anomia ▪ Decreased attention span ▪ Apathy ▪ Aphasia ▪ Restlessness, agitation ▪ Paranoid delusions ▪ Incontinence ▪ Social withdrawal ▪ Ataxia ▪ Tremors	Alzheimer's disease
▪ Occasional apraxia accompanied by headache, fever, drowsiness, decreased mental acuity, aphasia ▪ Dysarthria ▪ Hemiparesis ▪ Hyperreflexia ▪ Incontinence ▪ Focal or generalized seizures ▪ Ocular disturbances such as nystagmus, visual field deficits, unequal pupils	Brain abscess

NEUROLOGIC SYSTEM: INTERPRETING YOUR FINDINGS *(continued)*

Sign or symptom and findings	Probable cause
Apraxia *(continued)*	
▪ Progressive apraxia preceded by decreased mental acuity, headache, dizziness, and seizures ▪ Increased ICP as evidenced by papillary changes ▪ Localized signs and symptoms of tumor such as aphasia, dysarthria, visual field deficits, weakness, stiffness, and hyperreflexia	Brain tumor
Babinski's reflex	
▪ Bilateral Babinski's reflex with hyperactive deep tendon reflexes (DTRs) and spasticity ▪ Fasciculations accompanied by muscle atrophy and weakness ▪ Incoordination ▪ Impaired speech ▪ Difficulty chewing, swallowing, or breathing ▪ Urinary frequency and urgency ▪ Occasional choking and drooling	Amyotrophic lateral sclerosis (ALS)

Sign or symptom and findings	Probable cause
Babinski's reflex *(continued)*	
▪ Unilateral or bilateral Babinski's reflex with hyperreflexia and spasticity ▪ Weakness and incoordination ▪ Headache ▪ Vomiting ▪ Behavioral changes ▪ Altered vital signs ▪ Decreased LOC with abnormal pupillary size and response to light	Head trauma
▪ Babinski's reflex unilateral, eventually becoming bilateral ▪ Initially paresthesia, nystagmus, and blurred or double vision ▪ Scanning speech ▪ Dysphagia ▪ Intention tremor ▪ Weakness, incoordination ▪ Spasticity ▪ Gait ataxia ▪ Seizures ▪ Paraparesis or paraplegia ▪ Bladder incontinence ▪ Occasionally, loss of pain and temperature sensation and proprioception	Multiple sclerosis

(continued)

NEUROLOGIC SYSTEM: INTERPRETING YOUR FINDINGS *(continued)*

Sign or symptom and findings	Probable cause
Babinski's reflex *(continued)*	
■ Unilateral Babinski's reflex with hemiplegia or hemiparesis, unilateral hyperactive DTRs, hemianopsia, and aphasia, if stroke involves cerebrum ■ Bilateral Babinski's reflex with bilateral weakness or paralysis, bilateral hyperreflexia, cranial nerve dysfunction, incoordination and unsteady gait if stroke involves brain stem	Stroke
Brudzinski's sign	
■ Positive sign occurring within 24 hours of onset of disorder ■ Headache ■ Positive Kernig's sign ■ Nuchal rigidity ■ Irritability ■ Deep stupor or coma ■ Vertigo ■ Fever ■ Chills, malaise ■ Hyperalgesia ■ Opisthotonos ■ Symmetrical DTRs ■ Papilledema ■ Ocular and facial palsies ■ Nausea and vomiting ■ Photophobia, diplopia, and unequal sluggish pupils	Meningitis
Brudzinski's sign *(continued)*	
■ Positive sign within minutes of onset of hemorrhage ■ Sudden onset of severe headache ■ Nuchal rigidity ■ Altered LOC ■ Dizziness ■ Photophobia ■ Cranial nerve palsies ■ Nausea and vomiting ■ Fever ■ Positive Kernig's sign	Subarachnoid hemorrhage
Corneal reflex, absent	
■ Diminished or absent corneal reflex ■ Tinnitus ■ Unilateral hearing impairment ■ Facial palsy and anesthesia ■ Palate weakness ■ Ataxia, nystagmus if tumor impinging on adjacent cranial nerves	Acoustic neuroma
■ Diminished or absent corneal reflex ■ Complete hemifacial weakness or paralysis ■ Drooling on affected side ■ Masklike appearance of affected side ■ Constant eye tearing on affected side	Bell's palsy

NEUROLOGIC SYSTEM: INTERPRETING YOUR FINDINGS *(continued)*

Sign or symptom and findings	Probable cause
Corneal reflex, absent *(continued)*	
▪ Diminished or absent corneal reflex with sudden bursts of intense pain or shooting sensation lasting from 1 to 15 minutes, possibly triggered by light touch or exposure to hot or cold temperatures ▪ Hypersensitivity around mouth and nose	Trigeminal neuralgia
Deep tendon reflexes, hyperactive	
▪ Sudden or gradual onset of hyperactive DTRs with paresthesia, muscle twitching and cramping ▪ Positive Chvostek's and Trousseau's signs ▪ Carpopedal spasm and tetany	Hypocalcemia
▪ Hyperactive DTRs preceded by weakness and paresthesia in one or both arms or legs ▪ Clonus ▪ Positive Babinski's reflex ▪ Tingling sensation down back with passive flexion of neck ▪ Ataxia ▪ Diplopia ▪ Vertigo ▪ Vomiting ▪ Urinary retention or incontinence	Multiple sclerosis
Deep tendon reflexes, hyperactive *(continued)*	
▪ Sudden onset of generalized hyperactive DTRs accompanied by tachycardia, diaphoresis, low-grade fever and painful involuntary muscle contractions ▪ Trismus ▪ Masklike grin	Tetanus
Deep tendon reflexes, hypoactive	
▪ Hypoactive DTRs ▪ Associated signs and symptoms variable depending on cause and location of the dysfunction	Cerebellar dysfunction
▪ Bilateral hypoactive DTRs progressing rapidly from hypotonia to areflexia ▪ Muscle weakness beginning in the legs and extending to the arm and possibly trunk and neck muscles ▪ Cranial nerve palsies ▪ Pain ▪ Paresthesia ▪ Signs of brief autonomic dysfunction such as sinus tachycardia or bradycardia, flushing, fluctuating blood pressure, and anhidrosis	Guillain-Barré syndrome

(continued)

NEUROLOGIC SYSTEM: INTERPRETING YOUR FINDINGS *(continued)*

Sign or symptom and findings	Probable cause
Deep tendon reflexes, hypoactive *(continued)*	
▪ Hypoactive DTRs below the level of the lesion ▪ Quadriplegia or paraplegia ▪ Flaccidity ▪ Loss of sensation below the lesion ▪ Dry pale skin ▪ Urine retention with overflow incontinence ▪ Hypoactive bowel sounds ▪ Constipation ▪ Loss of genital reflex	Spinal cord lesion
Fasciculations	
▪ Fasciculations of face and tongue early on ▪ Dysarthria ▪ Dysphagia ▪ Hoarseness ▪ Drooling ▪ Eventual spreading of weakness to respiratory muscles	Bulbar palsy
▪ Fasciculations of muscles innervated by compressed nerve roots ▪ Severe low back pain possibly radiating unilaterally to the leg and exacerbated by coughing, sneezing, bending, and straining ▪ Muscle weakness, atrophy, and spasms ▪ Paresthesia ▪ Footdrop ▪ Steppage gait ▪ Hypoactive DTRs in legs	Herniated disk
Fasciculations *(continued)*	
▪ Coarse, usually transient, fasciculations accompanied by progressive muscle weakness, spasms, and atrophy ▪ Decreased DTRs ▪ Paresthesia ▪ Coldness and cyanosis in affected limbs ▪ Bladder paralysis ▪ Dyspnea ▪ Elevated blood pressure ▪ Tachycardia	Poliomyelitis, spinal paralytic
Headache	
▪ Excruciating headache ▪ Acute eye pain ▪ Blurred vision ▪ Halo vision ▪ Nausea and vomiting ▪ Moderately dilated, fixed pupil	Acute angle-closure glaucoma
▪ Slightly throbbing occipital headache on awakening that decreases in severity during the day ▪ Atrial gallop ▪ Restlessness ▪ Blurred vision ▪ Nausea and vomiting	Hypertension
▪ Sudden onset of severe generalized or frontal headache ▪ Stabbing retro-orbital pain ▪ Weakness, diffuse myalgia ▪ Fever, chills ▪ Coughing ▪ Rhinorrhea	Influenza

NEUROLOGIC SYSTEM: INTERPRETING YOUR FINDINGS *(continued)*

Sign or symptom and findings	Probable cause
Kernig's sign	
■ Positive sign with fever, chills ■ Nuchal rigidity ■ Hyperreflexia ■ Brudzinski's sign ■ Opisthotonos ■ Headache and vomiting with increasing ICP	Meningitis
■ Positive Kernig's sign with positive Brudzinski's sign ■ Sudden onset of severe headache, initially localized but then spreads ■ Pupillary inequality ■ Nuchal rigidity ■ Decreased LOC	Subarachnoid hemorrhage
Level of consciousness, decreased	
■ Slowly decreasing LOC, from lethargy to coma ■ Apathy, behavior changes ■ Memory loss ■ Decreased attention span ■ Morning headache ■ Sensorimotor disturbances	Brain tumor
■ Slowly decreasing LOC, from lethargy to coma ■ Malaise ■ Tachycardia ■ Tachypnea ■ Orthostatic hypotension ■ Skin is hot, flushed, and diaphoretic	Heatstroke
Level of consciousness, decreased *(continued)*	
■ Lethargy, progressing to coma ■ Confusion, anxiety, and restlessness ■ Hypotension ■ Tachycardia ■ Weak pulse with narrowing pulse pressure ■ Dyspnea ■ Oliguria ■ Cool, clammy skin	Shock
Muscle flaccidity	
■ Progressive muscle weakness and paralysis accompanied by generalized flaccidity, typically beginning in one hand and spreading to arm, other hand and arm, ultimately spreading to trunk, neck, tongue, larynx, pharynx, and legs ■ Progressive respiratory muscle weakness ■ Muscle cramps and coarse fasciculations ■ Hyperactive DTRs ■ Dysphagia ■ Dysarthria ■ Excessive drooling ■ Depression	ALS

(continued)

NEUROLOGIC SYSTEM: INTERPRETING YOUR FINDINGS *(continued)*

Sign or symptom and findings	Probable cause
Muscle flaccidity *(continued)*	
▪ Generalized flaccidity or hypotonia ▪ Ataxia ▪ Dysmetria ▪ Intention tremor ▪ Slight muscle weakness ▪ Fatigue ▪ Dysarthria	Cerebellar dysfunction
▪ Symmetrical and ascending muscle flaccidity ▪ Sensory loss or paresthesia ▪ Absent DTRs ▪ Tachycardia, bradycardia ▪ Fluctuating blood pressure ▪ Diaphoresis ▪ Incontinence ▪ Dysphagia ▪ Dysarthria ▪ Hypernasality ▪ Facial diplegia	Guillain-Barré syndrome
Muscle spasticity	
▪ Bilateral limb spasticity occurring late ▪ Momentary loss of consciousness after head trauma followed by lucid interval and then rapid deterioration in LOC ▪ Unilateral hemiparesis or hemiplegia ▪ Seizures ▪ Fixed, dilated pupils ▪ High fever ▪ Decreased and bounding pulse ▪ Widened pulse pressure ▪ Elevated blood pressure ▪ Irregular respiratory pattern ▪ Decerebrate posture ▪ Positive Babinski's reflex	Epidural hemorrhage
▪ Muscle spasticity, hyperreflexia, and contractures ▪ Progressive weakness and atrophy ▪ Diplopia, blurred vision, or loss of vision ▪ Nystagmus ▪ Sensory loss or paresthesia ▪ Dysarthria ▪ Dysphagia ▪ Incoordination, ataxic gait ▪ Intention tremors ▪ Emotional lability ▪ Impotence ▪ Urinary dysfunction	Multiple sclerosis

NEUROLOGIC SYSTEM: INTERPRETING YOUR FINDINGS *(continued)*

Sign or symptom and findings	Probable cause
***Muscle spasticity** (continued)*	
■ Spastic paralysis on affected side following acute stage ■ Dysarthria ■ Aphasia ■ Ataxia ■ Apraxia ■ Agnosia ■ Ipsilateral paresthesia or sensory loss ■ Vision disturbance ■ Altered LOC ■ Amnesia ■ Personality changes ■ Emotional lability ■ Bowel and bladder dysfunction	Stroke
Paralysis	
■ Transient, unilateral, facial muscle paralysis with sagging muscles and failure of eyelid closure ■ Increased tearing ■ Diminished or absent corneal reflex	Bell's palsy
■ Transient paralysis that gradually becomes more persistent ■ May include weak eye closure, ptosis, diplopia, lack of facial mobility, and dysphagia ■ Neck muscle weakness ■ Possible respiratory distress	Myasthenia gravis
***Paralysis** (continued)*	
■ Permanent spastic paralysis below the level of back injury ■ Absent reflexes may or may not return	Spinal cord injury
Pupils, nonreactive or sluggish	
■ Initially sluggish pupils becoming dilated and nonreactive ■ Decreased accommodation and cranial nerve palsies ■ Decreased LOC ■ High fever ■ Headache ■ Vomiting ■ Nuchal rigidity	Encephalitis
■ Bilateral midposition nonreactive pupils ■ Loss of upward gaze ■ Coma ■ Central neurogenic hyperventilation ■ Bradycardia ■ Hemiparesis or hemiplegia ■ Decorticate or decerebrate posture	Midbrain lesion
■ Dilated nonreactive pupil and loss of accommodation reaction (unilateral or bilateral depending on whether palsy is unilateral or bilateral) ■ Diplopia ■ Ptosis ■ Outward deviation of eye	Oculomotor nerve palsy

(continued)

NEUROLOGIC SYSTEM: INTERPRETING YOUR FINDINGS *(continued)*

Sign or symptom and findings	Probable cause
Romberg's sign	
■ Positive Romberg's sign with nystagmus, constipation, muscle weakness, and spasticity ■ Vision changes, diplopia, and paresthesia early on ■ Hyperreflexia ■ Dysphagia ■ Dysarthria ■ Incontinence ■ Urinary frequency and urgency ■ Impotence ■ Emotional instability	Multiple sclerosis
■ Positive Romberg's sign with loss of proprioception in lower limbs ■ Gait changes ■ Muscle weakness ■ Impaired coordination ■ Paresthesia ■ Sensory loss ■ Hypoactive or hyperactive DTRs ■ Sore tongue ■ Positive Babinski's reflex ■ Fatigue ■ Blurred vision ■ Light-headedness	Anemia, pernicious
■ Positive Romberg's sign ■ Vertigo ■ Nystagmus ■ Nausea and vomiting	Vestibular disorders
Seizures, generalized tonic-clonic or simple partial	
■ Generalized seizures depending on location and type of tumor ■ Slowly decreasing LOC ■ Morning headache ■ Dizziness, confusion ■ Focal seizures ■ Vision loss ■ Motor and sensory disturbances ■ Aphasia ■ Ataxia	Brain tumor
■ Generalized seizures ■ Severe frontal headache ■ Nausea and vomiting ■ Increased blood pressure ■ Fever ■ Peripheral edema ■ Sudden weight gain ■ Oliguria ■ Irritability ■ Hyperactive DTRs ■ Decreased LOC	Eclampsia
■ Seizures early on ■ Fever ■ Headache ■ Photophobia ■ Nuchal rigidity ■ Neck pain ■ Vomiting ■ Aphasia ■ Ataxia ■ Hemiparesis ■ Nystagmus ■ Irritability ■ Cranial nerve palsies ■ Myoclonic jerks	Encephalitis

NEUROLOGIC SYSTEM: INTERPRETING YOUR FINDINGS *(continued)*

Sign or symptom and findings	Probable cause
Seizures, generalized tonic-clonic or simple partial *(continued)*	
■ Generalized seizures possible immediately after injury with partial seizures occurring months later ■ Decreased LOC ■ Soft tissue injury to the face, head, or neck ■ Clear or bloody drainage from the mouth, nose, or ears ■ Battle's sign ■ Lack of response to oculocephalic and oculovestibular stimulation ■ Possible motor and sensory deficits along with altered respirations	Head trauma
■ Partial and generalized seizures ■ Café-au-lait spots ■ Multiple skin tumors ■ Scoliosis ■ Kyphoscoliosis ■ Dizziness ■ Ataxia ■ Monocular blindness ■ Nystagmus	Neurofibromatosis
Tremors	
■ Intention tremor ■ Ataxia ■ Nystagmus ■ Incoordination ■ Muscle weakness and atrophy ■ Hypoactive or absent DTRs	Cerebellar tumor
Tremors *(continued)*	
■ Tremors beginning in the fingers and possibly affecting foot, eyelids, jaw, lips, and tongue ■ Slow, rhythmic resting tremor in the form of flexion-extension or abduction-adduction of the fingers or hand or pronation-supination of the hand — characteristic pill-rolling tremor ■ Cogwheel rigidity ■ Bradykinesia ■ Propulsive gait with forward leaning posture ■ Monotone voice ■ Masklike facies ■ Drooling ■ Dysphagia ■ Dysarthria ■ Occasionally, oculogyric crisis	Parkinson's disease
■ Mild cases with fever, headache, and body aches accompanied by rash and swollen lymph nodes ■ More severe cases with headache, high fever, neck stiffness, stupor, disorientation, coma, tremors, occasional seizures, paralysis	West Nile encephalitis

Aphasia

Aphasia is the impaired expression or comprehension of written or spoken language. It reflects disease or injury of the brain's language centers. Depending on its severity, it may slightly impede communication or may make it impossible.

History

If the patient doesn't display signs of increased intracranial pressure (ICP), or if aphasia has developed gradually, perform a thorough neurologic examination, starting with the patient history. If necessary, obtain this history from the patient's family because of the patient's impairment. Ask about a history of headaches, hypertension, or seizure disorders and about drug use. Ask about the patient's ability to communicate and to perform routine activities before the aphasia began.

Physical assessment

Check for obvious signs of neurologic deficit, such as ptosis or fluid leakage from the nose and ears. Be aware that assessing the patient's LOC may be difficult because the patient's verbal responses may be unreliable. Also, recognize that dysarthria or speech apraxia may accompany aphasia, so speak slowly and distinctly, and allow the patient ample time to respond. Assess the patient's pupillary response, eye movements, and motor function, especially mouth and tongue movement, swallowing ability, and spontaneous movements and gestures. To best assess motor function, first demonstrate the motions, and then have the patient imitate them.

Analysis

Aphasia reflects damage to one or more of the brain's primary language centers, which are normally located in the left hemisphere. It can be classified as Broca's, Wernicke's, anomic, or global aphasia. Anomic aphasia eventually resolves in more than 50% of patients, but global aphasia is generally irreversible. Some causes include stroke, encephalitis, brain tumor or abscess, and head trauma.

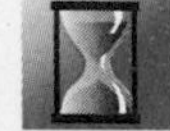

AGE ISSUE *The term "childhood aphasia" is sometimes mistakenly applied to children who fail to develop normal language skills but who aren't considered mentally retarded or developmentally delayed. Aphasia refers solely to loss of previously developed communication skills. Brain damage associated with aphasia in children usually follows anoxia, the result of near drowning or airway obstruction.*

Apraxia

Apraxia is the inability to perform purposeful movements in the absence of significant weakness, sensory loss, poor coordination, or lack of comprehension or motivation. Its onset, severity, and duration vary.

History

If apraxia is detected, ask about previous neurologic disease. Inquire about previous cerebrovascular disease, atherosclerosis, neoplastic disease, infection, or hepatic disease. Ask the patient if he has recently experienced headaches or dizziness. Then assess the apraxia further to help determine its type.

Physical assessment

If the patient fails to report such disease, begin a neurologic assessment. First, take the patient's vital signs and assess his LOC. Be alert for evidence of aphasia or dysarthria.

Test the patient's motor function, observing for weakness and tremors. Next, use a small pin or other pointed object to test sensory function. Check deep tendon reflexes for quality and symmetry. Finally, test the patient for visual field deficits.

CRITICAL POINT *Be alert for signs and symptoms of increased ICP, such as headache and vomiting. If present, elevate the head of the bed 30 degrees and monitor the patient closely for altered pupil size and reactivity, bradycardia, widened pulse pressure, and irregular respirations. Be prepared to perform emergency resuscitation measures.*

Analysis

Apraxia is a neurologic sign that usually indicates a lesion in the cerebral hemisphere. It's classified as ideational, ideomotor, or kinetic, depending on the stage at which voluntary movement is impaired. It can also be classified by type of motor or skill impairment. For example, facial and gait apraxia involve specific motor groups and are easily perceived. Constructional apraxia refers to the inability to copy simple drawings or patterns. Dressing apraxia refers to the inability to correctly dress oneself. Callosal apraxia refers to normal motor function on one side of the body accompanied by the inability to reproduce movements on the other side.

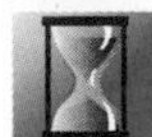

AGE ISSUE *In children, detecting apraxia can be difficult. However, any sudden inability to perform a previously accomplished movement warrants prompt neurologic evaluation because brain tumor—the most common cause of apraxia in children—can be treated effectively if detected early. Brain damage in a young child may cause developmental apraxia, which interferes with the ability to learn activities that require sequential movement, such as hopping, jumping, hitting or kicking a ball, or dancing.*

Babinski's reflex

Babinski's reflex—dorsiflexion of the great toe with extension and fanning of the other toes—is an abnormal reflex elicited by firmly stroking the lateral aspect of the sole with a blunt object.

History

Obtain a complete health history from the patient. Ask about previous neurologic disease. Inquire about previous cerebrovascular disease, atherosclerosis, neoplastic disease, infection, or hepatic disease. Ask the patient if he has recently experienced changes in mental status or consciousness.

Physical assessment

After eliciting a positive Babinski's reflex, evaluate the patient for other neurologic signs. Evaluate muscle strength in each extremity by having the patient push or pull against your resistance. Passively flex and extend the extremity to assess muscle tone. Intermittent resistance to flexion and extension indicates spasticity, and a lack of resistance indicates flaccidity.

Next, check for evidence of incoordination by asking the patient to perform a repetitive activity. Test DTRs in the patient's elbow, antecubital area, wrist, knee, and ankle by striking the tendon with a reflex hammer. An exaggerated muscle response indicates hyperactive DTRs; little or no muscle response indicates hypoactivity.

Evaluate pain sensation and proprioception in the feet. As you move the patient's toes up and down, ask him to identify the direction in which the toes have been moved without looking at his feet.

Analysis

In some patients, the Babinski's reflex can be triggered by noxious stimuli, such as pain, noise, or even bumping of the bed. An indicator of corticospinal damage, Babinski's reflex may occur unilaterally or bilaterally. It may also be temporary or permanent. A temporary Babinski's reflex commonly occurs during the postictal phase of a seizure, whereas a permanent Babinski's reflex occurs with corticospinal damage. A positive Babinski's reflex usually occurs with incoordination, weakness, and spasticity, all of which increase the patient's risk of injury.

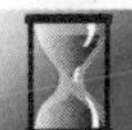

AGE ISSUE *Babinski's reflex occurs normally in infants up to 24 months old, reflecting immaturity of the corticospinal tract. After age 2, Babinski's reflex is pathologic and may result from hydrocephalus or any of the causes more commonly seen in adults.*

Brudzinski's sign

A positive Brudzinski's sign—flexion of the hips and knees in response to passive flexion of the neck—signals meningeal irritation. Passive flexion of the neck stretches the nerve roots, causing pain and involuntary flexion of the knees and hips.

History

If the patient is alert, ask him about headache, neck pain, nausea, and vision disturbances, such as blurred or double vision and photophobia—all indications of ICP. Next, observe the patient for signs and symptoms of increased ICP, such as an altered LOC, as evidenced by restlessness, irritability, confusion, lethargy, personality changes, and coma; pupillary changes; bradycardia; widened pulse pressure; irregular respiratory patterns such as Cheyne-Stokes or Kussmaul's respirations; vomiting, and moderate fever.

Ask the patient or his family, if necessary, about a history of hypertension, spinal arthritis, or recent head trauma. Also ask about dental work and abscessed teeth (a possible cause of meningitis), open-head injury, endocarditis, and I.V. drug abuse. Ask about sudden onset of headaches, which may be associated with subarachnoid hemorrhage.

Physical assessment

Continue the neurologic examination by evaluating the patient's cranial nerve function and noting any motor or sensory deficits. Be sure to look for Kernig's sign as evidenced by resistance to knee extension after flexion of the hip, which is a further indication of meningeal irritation. Also, look for signs of central nervous system (CNS) infection, such as fever and nuchal rigidity.

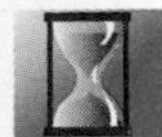

AGE ISSUE *In infants, Brudzinski's sign may not be a useful indicator of meningeal irritation because more reliable signs — such as bulging fontanels, a weak cry, fretfulness, vomiting, and poor feeding — appear early.*

Analysis

Brudzinski's sign is a common and important early indicator of life-threatening meningitis and subarachnoid hemorrhage. It can be elicited in children as well as adults, although more reliable indicators of meningeal irritation exist for infants. Testing for Brudzinski's sign isn't part of the routine examination, unless meningeal irritation is suspected.

Many patients with a positive Brudzinski's sign are critically ill. They need constant ICP monitoring and frequent neurologic checks, in addition to intensive assessment and monitoring of vital signs, intake and output, and cardiorespiratory status.

Corneal reflex, absent

The corneal reflex is tested bilaterally by drawing a fine-pointed wisp of sterile cotton from a corner of each eye to the cornea. Normally, even though only one eye is tested at a time, the patient blinks bilaterally each time either cornea is touched — this is the corneal reflex. When this reflex is absent, neither eyelid closes when the cornea of one is touched.

History

Because an absent corneal reflex may signify such progressive neurologic disorders as Guillain-Barré syndrome, ask the patient about associated symptoms — facial pain, dysphagia, and limb weakness. Obtain a thorough health history from the patient or family members.

Physical assessment

If you can't elicit the corneal reflex, look for other signs of trigeminal nerve dysfunction. To test the three sensory portions of the nerve, touch each side of the patient's face on the brow, cheek, and jaw with a cotton wisp, and ask him to compare the sensations.

If you suspect facial nerve involvement, note if both the upper face (the brow and eyes) and lower face (the cheek, mouth, and chin) are weak bilaterally. Lower-motor-neuron facial weakness affects the face on the same side as the lesion, whereas upper-motor-neuron weakness affects the side opposite the lesion — predominantly the lower facial muscles.

Analysis

The site of the afferent fibers for this reflex is in the ophthalmic branch of the trigeminal nerve (cranial nerve [CN] V); the efferent fibers are located in the facial nerve (CN VII). Unilateral or bilateral absence of the corneal reflex may result from damage to these nerves.

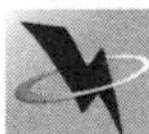

CRITICAL POINT *When the corneal reflex is absent, protect the patient's affected eye from injury by lubricating it with artificial tears to prevent drying.*

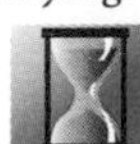

AGE ISSUE *In children, brain stem lesions and injuries are the most common causes of absent corneal reflexes; Guillain-Barré syndrome and trigeminal neuralgia occur less commonly. Infants, especially those born prematurely, may have an absent corneal reflex due to anoxic damage to the brain stem.*

Deep tendon reflexes, hyperactive

A hyperactive DTR is an abnormally brisk muscle contraction that occurs in response to a sudden stretch induced by sharply tapping the muscle's tendon of insertion. This elicited sign may be graded as brisk or pathologically hyperactive.

History

After eliciting hyperactive DTRs, take the patient's health history. Ask about spinal cord injury or other trauma and about prolonged exposure to cold, wind, or water. Find out if the patient could be pregnant. A positive response to any of these questions requires prompt evaluation to rule out life-threatening autonomic hyperreflexia, tetanus, preeclampsia, or hypothermia.

Ask about the onset and progression of associated signs and symptoms. Ask about vomiting or altered bladder habits.

Physical assessment

Perform a neurologic examination. Obtain vital signs. Evaluate LOC, and test motor and sensory function in the limbs. Ask about paresthesia. Check for ataxia or tremors and for speech and vision deficits. Test for Chvostek's sign, an abnormal spasm of the facial muscles elicited by light taps on the facial nerve in patients who have hypocalcemia. Also check for Trousseau's sign, a carpal spasm induced by inflating a sphygmomanometer cuff on the upper arm to a pressure exceeding systolic blood pressure for 3 minutes in patients who have hypocalcemia or hypomagnesemia. Finally, check for carpopedal spasm.

Analysis

Hyperactive DTRs are commonly accompanied by clonus. The corticospinal tract and other descending tracts govern the reflex arc — the relay cycle that produces any reflex response. A corticospinal lesion above the level of the reflex arc being tested may result in hyperactive DTRs. Abnormal neuromuscular transmission at the end of the reflex arc may also cause hyperactive DTRs. For example, a deficiency of calcium or magnesium may cause hyperactive DTRs because these electrolytes regulate neuromuscular excitability. Although hyperactive DTRs typically accompany other neurologic findings, they usually lack specific diagnostic value. For example, they're an early, cardinal sign of hypocalcemia.

AGE ISSUE *In neonates, hyperreflexia may be a normal sign. After age 6, reflex responses are similar to those of adults. When testing DTRs in small children, use distraction techniques to promote reliable results. In children, cerebral palsy commonly causes hyperactive DTRs. Reye's syndrome causes generalized hyperactive DTRs in stage II; in stage V, DTRs are absent. Adult causes of hyperactive DTRs may also appear in children.*

Deep tendon reflexes, hypoactive

A hypoactive DTR is an abnormally diminished muscle contraction that occurs in response to a sudden stretch induced by sharply tapping the muscle's tendon of insertion. It may be graded as minimal (+) or absent (0). Symmetrically reduced (+) reflexes may be normal.

History

After eliciting hypoactive DTRs, obtain a thorough history from the patient or a family member. Have him describe current signs and symptoms in detail. Ask about nausea, vomiting, constipation, and incontinence. Then take a family and drug history.

Physical assessment

Evaluate the patient's LOC. Test motor function in his limbs, and palpate for muscle atrophy or increased mass. Test sensory function, including pain, touch, temperature, and vibration sense. Ask about paresthesia. To observe gait and coordination, have the patient take several steps.

Check for Romberg's sign by asking him to stand with his feet together and his eyes closed. During conversation, evaluate speech. Check for signs of vision or hearing loss.

Look for autonomic nervous system effects by taking vital signs and monitoring for increased heart rate and blood pressure. Also, inspect the skin for pallor, dryness, flushing, or diaphoresis. Auscultate for hypoactive bowel sounds, and palpate for bladder distention.

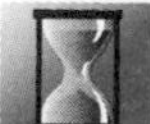

AGE ISSUE *In children, when assessing DTRs, use distraction techniques; to assess motor function watch the infant or child at play.*

Analysis

Normally, a DTR depends on an intact receptor, intact sensory-motor nerve fiber, an intact neuromuscular-glandular junction, and a functional synapse in the spinal cord. Hypoactive DTRs may result from damage to the reflex arc involving the specific muscle, the peripheral nerve, the nerve roots, or the spinal cord at that level. Hypoactive DTRs are an important sign of many disorders, especially when they appear with other neurologic signs and symptoms.

Abrupt onset of hypoactive DTRs accompanied by muscle weakness may occur with life-threatening Guillain-Barré syndrome, botulism, or spinal cord lesions with spinal shock. Drugs such as barbiturates and paralyzing drugs, such as pancuronium may cause hypoactive reflexes.

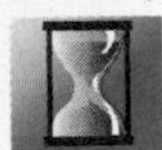

AGE ISSUE *Hypoactive DTRs commonly occur in patients with muscular dystrophy, Friedreich's ataxia, syringomyelia, and cord injury. They also accompany progressive muscular atrophy, which affects preschoolers and adolescents.*

Fasciculations

Fasciculations are local muscle contractions representing the spontaneous discharge of a muscle fiber bundle innervated by a single motor nerve filament. These contractions cause visible dimpling or wavelike twitching of the skin, but they aren't strong enough to cause a joint to move. They occur irregularly at frequencies ranging from once every several seconds to two or three times per second; less commonly, myokymia — continuous, rapid fasciculations that cause a rippling effect — may occur. Because fasciculations are brief and painless, they commonly go undetected or are ignored.

History

Begin by asking the patient about the nature, onset, and duration of the fasciculations. If the onset was sudden, ask about any precipitating events, such as exposure to pesticides.

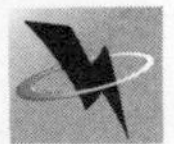

CRITICAL POINT *Pesticide poisoning, although uncommon, is a medical emergency requiring prompt and vigorous intervention.*

If the patient isn't in severe distress, find out if he has experienced any sensory changes, such as paresthesia, or any difficulty speaking, swallowing, breathing, or controlling bowel or bladder function. Ask him if he's in pain.

Explore the patient's medical history for neurologic disorders, cancer, and recent infections. Also, ask him about his lifestyle, especially stress at home, in his occupation, or at school. Ask the patient about his dietary habits and for a recall of his food and fluid intake in the recent past because electrolyte imbalances may also cause muscle twitching.

Physical assessment

Perform a physical examination, looking for fasciculations while the affected muscle is at rest. Observe and test for motor and sensory abnormalities, particularly muscle atrophy and weakness, and decreased deep tendon reflexes. If these signs and symptoms are noted, suspect motor neuron disease, and perform a comprehensive neurologic examination.

Analysis

Benign, nonpathologic fasciculations are common and normal. They commonly occur in tense, anxious, or overtired people and typically affect the eyelid, thumb, or calf. However, fasciculations may also indicate a severe neurologic disorder, most notably a diffuse motor neuron disorder that causes loss of control over muscle fiber discharge. They're also an early sign of pesticide poisoning.

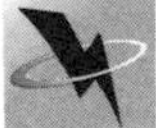

CRITICAL POINT *Fasciculations, particularly of the tongue, are an important early sign of Werdnig-Hoffmann disease.*

Headache

The most common neurologic symptom, headaches may be localized or generalized, producing mild to severe pain. About 90% of headaches are benign and can be described as vascular, muscle-contraction, or both.

History

Ask the patient to describe the headache's characteristics and location. Find out how often he gets a headache and how long it typically lasts. Try to identify precipitating factors, such as certain foods and exposure to bright lights. Ask the patient if he's under stress and if he has trouble sleeping. Take a drug history, and ask about head trauma within the last 4 weeks. Find out if the patient has recently experienced nausea, vomiting, photophobia, or vision changes. Ask him if he feels drowsy, confused, or dizzy.

Find out if he has recently developed seizures, or if he has a history of seizures.

Physical assessment

Begin the physical examination by evaluating the patient's LOC. While checking vital signs, be alert for signs of increased ICP — widened pulse pressure, bradycardia, altered respiratory pattern, and increased blood pressure. Check pupil size and response to light, and note any neck stiffness.

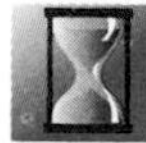

AGE ISSUE *If a child is too young to describe his symptom, suspect a headache if you see him banging or holding his head. In an infant, a shrill cry or bulging fontanels may indicate increased ICP and headache.*

Analysis

If not benign, headaches can indicate a severe neurologic disorder associated with intracranial inflammation, increased ICP, or meningeal irritation. They may also result from ocular or sinus disorders and the effects of drugs, tests, and treatments.

Other causes of headache include fever, eyestrain, dehydration, and systemic febrile illnesses. Headaches may occur with certain metabolic disturbances — such as hypoxemia, hypercapnia, hyperglycemia, and hypoglycemia — but they aren't a diagnostic or prominent symptom. Some individuals get headaches after seizures or from coughing, sneezing, heavy lifting, or stooping.

Kernig's sign

A reliable early indicator and tool used to diagnose meningeal irritation, Kernig's sign elicits both resistance and hamstring muscle pain when the health care provider attempts to extend the knee while the hip and knee are both flexed 90 degrees. However, when the patient's thigh isn't flexed on the abdomen, he can usually completely extend his leg.

History

If you don't suspect meningeal irritation, ask the patient if he feels back pain that radiates down one or both legs. Find out if he also feels leg numbness, tingling, or weakness. Ask about other signs and symptoms, and find out if he has a history of cancer or back injury.

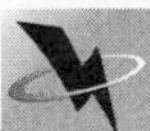

CRITICAL POINT *If a positive Kernig's sign is elicited, suspect life-threatening meningitis or subarachnoid hemorrhage and immediately prepare for emergency intervention.*

Physical assessment

Perform a physical examination, concentrating on motor and sensory function. Observe and test for motor and sensory abnormalities, particularly muscle atrophy and weakness, and decreased deep tendon reflexes.

Analysis

A positive Kernig's sign is usually elicited in meningitis or subarachnoid hemorrhage. With these potentially life-threatening disorders, hamstring muscle resistance results from stretching the blood- or exudate-irritated meninges surrounding spinal nerve roots.

Kernig's sign can also indicate a herniated disk or spinal tumor. With these disorders, sciatic pain results from disk or tumor pressure on spinal nerve roots.

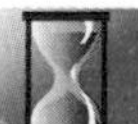

AGE ISSUE *In children, Kernig's sign is considered ominous because of their greater potential for rapid deterioration.*

Level of consciousness, decreased

A decrease in LOC can range from lethargy to stupor to coma. LOC can deteriorate suddenly or gradually and can remain altered temporarily or permanently.

The most sensitive indicator of decreased LOC is a change in the patient's mental status. The Glasgow Coma Scale, which measures ability to respond to verbal, sensory, and motor stimulation, can be used to quickly evaluate a patient's LOC.

History

Try to obtain health history information from the patient if he's lucid and from his family. Find out if the patient complained of headache, dizziness, nausea, vision or hearing disturbances, weakness, fatigue, or any other problems before his LOC decreased. Ask his family if they noticed changes in the patient's behavior, personality, memory, or temperament.

Ask about a history of neurologic disease, cancer, or recent trauma; drug and alcohol use; and the development of other signs and symptoms.

Physical assessment

Because decreased LOC can result from disorders that affect virtually every body system, tailor the remainder of the evaluation according to the patient's associated symptoms. Start by using the Glasgow Coma Scale.

Analysis

Decreased LOC usually results from a neurologic disorder and commonly signals life-threatening complications of hemorrhage, trauma, or cerebral edema. However, this sign can also result from a metabolic, GI, musculoskeletal, urologic, or cardiopulmonary disorder; severe nutritional deficiency; exposure to toxins; or use of certain drugs.

Consciousness is affected by the reticular activating system (RAS), an intricate network of neurons whose axons extend from the brain stem, thalamus, and hypothalamus to the cerebral cortex. A disturbance in any part of this integrated system prevents the intercommunication that makes consciousness possible. Loss of consciousness can result from a bilateral cerebral disturbance, an RAS disturbance, or both. Cerebral dysfunction characteristically produces the least dramatic decrease in a patient's LOC. In contrast, dysfunction of the RAS produces the most dramatic decrease in LOC—coma.

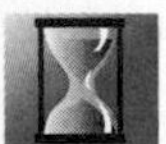

AGE ISSUE *In children, the primary cause of decreased LOC is head trauma, which commonly results from physical abuse or a motor vehicle accident. Other causes include accidental poisoning, hydrocephalus, and meningitis or brain abscess following an ear or respiratory tract infection.*

Muscle flaccidity

Flaccid muscles are profoundly weak and soft, with decreased resistance to movement, increased mobility, and greater than normal range of motion (ROM).

History

If the patient isn't in distress, ask about the onset and duration of muscle flaccidity and any precipitating factors. Ask about associated symptoms, notably weakness, other muscle changes, and sensory loss or paresthesia.

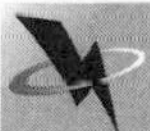

CRITICAL POINT *If the patient has experienced trauma resulting in muscle flaccidity, ensure that his cervical spine has been stabilized and quickly determine his respiratory status. Be prepared to institute emergency measures as necessary.*

Physical assessment

Perform a thorough neurologic examination, focusing on motor and sensory function. Examine the affected muscles for atrophy, which indicates a chronic problem. Test muscle strength, and check deep tendon reflexes in all limbs.

AGE ISSUE *When assessing an infant or young child, observe the positioning. An infant or young child with generalized flaccidity may lie in a froglike position, with his hips and knees abducted.*

Analysis

The result of disrupted muscle innervation, muscle flaccidity can be localized to a limb or muscle group or generalized over the entire body. Its onset may be acute, as in trauma, or chronic, as in neurologic disease.

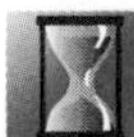

AGE ISSUE *Pediatric causes of muscle flaccidity include myelomeningocele, Lowe's disease, Werdnig-Hoffmann disease, and muscular dystrophy.*

Muscle spasticity

Spasticity is a state of excessive muscle tone manifested by increased resistance to stretching and heightened reflexes. It's commonly detected by evaluating a muscle's response to passive movement; a spastic muscle offers more resistance when the passive movement is performed quickly.

History

When you detect spasticity, ask the patient about its onset, duration, and progression. Find out what, if any, events precipitate the onset. Ask the patient if he has experienced other muscular changes or related symptoms. Find out if his medical history reveals any incidence of trauma or degenerative or vascular disease.

Physical assessment
Take the patient's vital signs, and perform a complete neurologic examination. Test reflexes and evaluate motor and sensory function in all limbs. Evaluate muscles for wasting contractures.

Analysis
Caused by an upper-motor-neuron lesion, spasticity usually occurs in the arm and leg muscles. Long-term spasticity results in muscle fibrosis and contractures.

CRITICAL POINT *Generalized spasticity and trismus in a patient with a recent skin puncture or laceration indicates tetanus.*

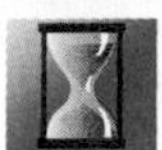

AGE ISSUE *In children, muscle spasticity may be a sign of cerebral palsy.*

Paralysis
Paralysis, the total loss of voluntary motor function, results from severe cortical or pyramidal tract damage. Paralysis can be local or widespread, symmetrical or asymmetrical, transient or permanent, and spastic or flaccid. It's usually classified according to location and severity as paraplegia, quadriplegia, or hemiplegia. Incomplete paralysis with profound weakness, or paresis, may precede total paralysis in some patients.

History
If the patient is in no immediate danger, perform a complete neurologic assessment. Start with the health history, relying on family members for information if necessary.

Ask about the onset, duration, intensity, and progression of paralysis and about the events leading up to it. Focus medical history questions on the incidence of degenerative neurologic or neuromuscular disease, recent infectious illness, sexually transmitted disease, cancer, or recent injury.

Explore related signs and symptoms, noting fever, headache, vision disturbances, dysphagia, nausea and vomiting, bowel or bladder dysfunction, muscle pain or weakness, and fatigue.

Physical assessment
Perform a complete neurologic examination, testing cranial nerve, motor, and sensory function and deep tendon reflexes. Assess strength in all major muscle groups, and note any muscle atrophy.

Analysis
Paralysis can occur in patients with a cerebrovascular disorder, degenerative neuromuscular disease, trauma, a tumor, or a CNS infection. Acute paralysis may be an early indicator of a life-threatening disorder such as Guillain-Barré syndrome.

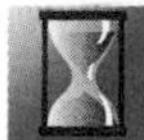

AGE ISSUE *Besides the obvious causes — trauma, infection, or tumors — paralysis may result from a hereditary or congenital disorder, such as Tay-Sachs disease, Werdnig-Hoffmann disease, spina bifida, or cerebral palsy.*

Pupils, nonreactive or sluggish
Nonreactive, or fixed, pupils fail to constrict in response to light or to dilate when the light is removed. A sluggish pupillary reaction is an abnormally slow pupillary response to light. It can occur in one pupil or both, unlike the normal reaction, which is always bilateral.

History
If the patient is conscious, obtain a brief health history. Ask him what type of eyedrops he's using, if any, and when they were last instilled. Also ask if he's experiencing pain and, if so, try to determine its location, intensity, and duration.

Physical assessment
Check the patient's visual acuity in both eyes. Then test the pupillary reaction to light. To evaluate pupillary reaction to light, first test the patient's direct light reflex. Darken the room, and cover one of the patient's eyes while you hold open the opposite eyelid. Using a bright penlight, bring the light toward the patient from the side and shine it directly into his opened eye. If normal, the pupil will promptly constrict. Next, test the consensual light reflex. Hold the patient's eyelids open and shine the light into one eye while watching the pupil of the opposite eye. If normal, both pupils will promptly constrict. Repeat both procedures in the opposite eye.

Also check the pupillary reaction to accommodation. Normally, both pupils constrict equally as the patient shifts his glance from a distant to a near object. Next, hold a penlight at the side of each eye and examine the cornea and iris for any abnormalities. Measure intraocular pressure (IOP) with a monometer, or estimate IOP by placing your second and third fingers over the patient's closed eyelid. If the eyeball feels rock-hard, suspect elevated IOP. Ophthalmoscopic and slit-lamp examinations of the eye will need to be performed.

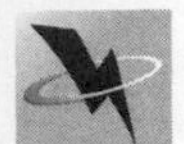

CRITICAL POINT *If the patient has experienced ocular trauma, don't manipulate the affected eye. After the examination, cover the affected eye with a protective metal shield, but don't let the shield rest on the globe.*

Analysis

The development of a unilateral or bilateral nonreactive response indicates an important change in the patient's condition and may signal a life-threatening emergency and possibly brain death. A unilateral or bilateral nonreactive response indicates dysfunction of cranial nerves II and III, which mediate the pupillary light reflex. It also occurs with the use of certain drugs. Instillation of a topical mydriatic and a cycloplegic may induce a temporarily nonreactive pupil in the affected eye. Opiates, such as heroin and morphine, cause pinpoint pupils with a minimal light response that can be seen only with a magnifying glass. Atropine poisoning produces widely dilated, nonreactive pupils.

A sluggish reaction accompanies degenerative disease of the CNS and diabetic neuropathy.

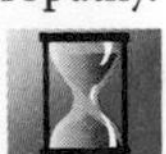

AGE ISSUE *Children have nonreactive or sluggish pupils for the same reasons as adults. The most common cause of nonreactive pupils in children is oculomotor nerve palsy from increased ICP. Sluggish pupils can occur normally in elderly people, whose pupils become smaller and less responsive with age.*

Romberg's sign

A positive Romberg's sign refers to a patient's inability to maintain balance when standing erect with his feet together and his eyes closed. Normally, a negative Romberg's sign, the patient should be able to stand with his feet together and his eyes closed with minimal swaying for about 20 seconds.

History

Obtain a thorough health history, focusing on areas of problems with coordination and balance. Question the patient about any problems involving dizziness or vertigo, and recent ear problems such as infection. Ask the patient if he can sit and stand without support. Note if he uses any assistive devices to maintain his balance or aid in walking.

Physical assessment

After you have detected a positive Romberg's sign, perform other neurologic screening tests. A positive Romberg's sign indicates only the presence of a defect; it doesn't pinpoint its cause or location. First, test proprioception. If the patient can't maintain his balance with his eyes open, ask him to hop on one foot and then on the other. Next, ask him to do a knee bend and to walk a straight line, placing heel to toe. Lastly, ask him to walk a short distance so you can evaluate his gait.

Test the patient's awareness of body part position by changing the position of one of his fingers, or any other joint, while his eyes are closed. Ask him to describe the change you've made.

Next, test the patient's direction of movement. Ask him to close his eyes and to touch his nose with the index finger of one hand and then with the other. Ask him to repeat this movement several times, gradually increasing his speed. Then test the accuracy of his movement by having him rapidly touch each finger of one hand to the thumb. Next, test sensation in all dermatomes, using a pin to assess differentiation between sharp and dull. Also test two-point discrimination by touching two pins, one in each hand, to his skin simultaneously. Ask him if he feels one or two pinpricks. Finally, test and characterize the patient's DTRs.

To test the patient's vibratory sense, ask him to close his eyes; then apply a mildly vibrating tuning fork to a bony prominence such as the medial malleolus. If the patient doesn't feel the stimulus initially, increase the vibration, and then test the knee or hip. This procedure can also be done to test the fingers, the elbow, and the shoulder. Record and compare all test results. Also, ask the patient if he has noticed sensory changes, such as numbness and tingling in his limbs. If so, find out when these changes began.

Analysis

If positive, Romberg's sign indicates a vestibular or proprioceptive disorder, or a disorder of the spinal tracts (the posterior columns) that carry proprioceptive information—the perception of one's position in space, of joint movements, and of pressure sensations—to the brain. Insufficient vestibular or proprioceptive information causes an inability to execute precise movements and maintain balance without visual cues. Difficulty performing this maneuver with eyes open or closed may indicate a cerebellar disorder.

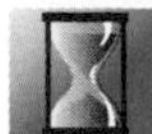

AGE ISSUE *In children, Romberg's sign can't be tested until they can stand without support and follow commands. However, a positive sign in children commonly results from spinal cord disease.*

Seizures, generalized tonic-clonic or simple partial

Like other types of seizures, generalized tonic-clonic seizures are caused by the paroxysmal, uncontrolled discharge of CNS neurons, leading to neurologic dysfunction. Unlike most other types of seizures, however, this cerebral hyperactivity isn't confined to the original focus or to a localized area but extends to the entire brain.

Generalized tonic-clonic seizures

A generalized tonic-clonic seizure may begin with or without an aura. As seizure activity spreads to the subcortical structures, the patient loses consciousness, falls to the ground, and may utter a loud cry that's precipitated by air rushing from the lungs through the vocal cords. His body stiffens in the tonic phase, then undergoes rapid, synchronous muscle jerking and hyperventilation in the clonic phase. Tongue biting, incontinence, diaphoresis, profuse salivation, and signs of respiratory distress may also occur. The seizure usually stops after 2 to 5 minutes. The patient then regains consciousness but displays confusion. He may complain of headache, fatigue, muscle soreness, and arm and leg weakness.

Simple partial seizures

Resulting from an irritable focus in the cerebral cortex, simple partial seizures typically last about 30 seconds and don't alter the patient's LOC. The type and pattern reflect the location of the irritable focus.

Simple partial seizures may be classified as motor, including both jacksonian seizures and epilepsia partialis continua, or somatosensory, including visual, olfactory, and auditory seizures.

A focal motor seizure is a series of unilateral clonic, or muscle jerking, and tonic, or muscle stiffening, movements of one part of the body. The patient's head and eyes characteristically turn away from the hemispheric focus—usually the frontal lobe near the motor strip. A tonic-clonic contraction of the trunk or extremities may follow.

A jacksonian motor seizure typically begins with a tonic contraction of a finger, the corner of the mouth, or one foot. Clonic movements follow, spreading to other muscles on the same side of the body, moving up the arm or leg, and eventually involving the whole side. Alternatively, clonic movements may spread to the opposite side, becoming generalized and leading to loss of consciousness. In the postictal phase, the patient may experience paralysis (Todd's paralysis) in the affected limbs, usually resolving within 24 hours.

Epilepsia partialis continua causes clonic twitching of one muscle group, usually in the face, arm, or leg. Twitching occurs every few seconds and persists for hours, days, or months without spreading. Spasms usually affect the distal arm and leg muscles more than the proximal ones; in the face, they affect the corner of the mouth, one or both eyelids and, occasionally, the neck or trunk muscles unilaterally.

A focal somatosensory seizure affects a localized body area on one side. Usually, this type of seizure initially causes numbness, tingling, or crawling or "electric" sensations; occasionally, it causes pain or burning sensations in the lips, fingers, or toes. A visual seizure involves sensations of darkness or of stationary or moving lights or spots, usually red at first, then blue, green, and yellow. It can affect both visual fields or the visual field on the side opposite the lesion. The irritable focus is in the occipital lobe. In contrast, the irritable focus in an auditory or olfactory seizure is in the temporal lobe.

History

If the patient isn't experiencing a generalized seizure at the moment or the seizure wasn't witnessed, obtain a description from the patient's companion. Ask when the seizure started and how long it lasted. Find out if the patient reported any unusual sensations before the seizure began. Ask the companion if the seizure started in one area of the body and spread, or if it affected the entire body right away. Find out if the patient fell on a hard surface and if his eyes or head turned. Find out if he turned blue and lost bladder control. Ask about any other seizures before he recovered.

If the patient may have sustained a head injury, observe him closely for loss of consciousness, unequal or nonreactive pupils, and focal neurologic signs. Ask the patient if he has a headache and muscle soreness. Note if he's increasingly difficult to arouse when you check on him at 20-minute intervals. Examine his arms, legs, and face, including tongue, for injury, residual paralysis, or limb weakness.

Next, obtain a health history. Find out if the patient has ever had generalized or focal seizures before. If so, find out if they occurred frequently. Ask him if other family members also have them. Find out if the patient is receiving drug therapy and if he's compliant. Also, ask about sleep deprivation and emotional or physical stress at time the seizure occurred.

For a partial seizure, note whether the patient turns his head and eyes. If so, note to which side he turns them. Observe where movement first starts and if it spreads. Because a partial seizure may become generalized, watch closely for loss of consciousness, bilateral tonicity and clonicity, cyanosis, tongue-biting, and urinary incontinence

After the seizure, ask the patient to describe exactly what he remembers, if anything, about the seizure. Check the patient's LOC. Ask the patient what happened before the seizure. Also ask him if he can describe an aura or if he recognized its onset. If so, find out how, such as if it was by a smell, a vision disturbance, or a sound or visceral phenomenon such as an unusual sensation in his stomach. Ask him how this seizure compares with others he has had. Also, explore fully any history, recent or remote, of head trauma. Check for a history of stroke or recent infection, especially with fever, headache, or a stiff neck.

Physical assessment

Perform a complete neurologic examination, focusing on the patient's mental status and LOC. Also observe for residual deficits, such as weakness in the involved extremity, and sensory disturbances.

Analysis

Generalized tonic-clonic seizures usually occur singly. The patient may be asleep or awake and active. Possible complications include respiratory arrest due to airway obstruction from secretions, status epilepticus (occurring in 5% to 8% of patients), head or spinal injuries and bruises, Todd's paralysis and, rarely, cardiac arrest. Life-threatening status epilepticus is marked by prolonged seizure activity or by rapidly recurring seizures with no intervening periods of recovery. It's most commonly triggered by abrupt discontinuation of anticonvulsant therapy.

Generalized seizures may be caused by a brain tumor, vascular disorder, head trauma, infection, metabolic defect, drug, such as a barbiturate, or alcohol withdrawal syndrome, exposure to toxins such as arsenic, or a genetic defect. Contrast agents used in radiologic tests may cause generalized seizures. Toxic blood levels of some drugs, such as theophylline, lidocaine, meperidine, penicillins, and cimetidine, may cause generalized seizures. Phenothiazines, tricyclic antidepressants, amphetamines, isoniazid, and vincristine may cause seizures in patients with preexisting epilepsy. Generalized seizures may also result from a focal seizure. With recurring seizures, or epilepsy, the cause may be unknown.

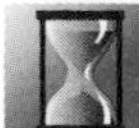

AGE ISSUE *In children, generalized seizures are common. In fact, between 75% and 90% of epileptic patients experience their first seizure before age 20. Many children between ages 3 months and 3 years experience generalized seizures associated with fever; some of these children later develop seizures without fever. Generalized seizures may also stem from inborn errors of metabolism, perinatal injury, brain infection, Reye's syndrome, Sturge-Weber syndrome, arteriovenous malformation, lead poisoning, hypoglycemia, and idiopathic*

causes. The pertussis component of the diphtheria and tetanus toxoids and pertussis vaccine also may cause seizures; although this is rare. Affecting more children than adults, focal seizures are likely to spread and become generalized. They typically cause the child's eyes, or his head and eyes, to turn to the side; in neonates, they cause mouth twitching, staring, or both. Focal seizures in children can result from hemiplegic cerebral palsy, head trauma, child abuse, arteriovenous malformation, or Sturge-Weber syndrome.

Tremors

The most common type of involuntary muscle movement, tremors are regular, rhythmic oscillations that result from alternating contraction of opposing muscle groups. Tremors can be characterized by their location, amplitude, and frequency.

History

Begin the patient history by asking him about the tremor's onset, sudden or gradual, and about its duration, progression, and any aggravating or alleviating factors. Find out if the tremor interferes with the patient's normal activities. Ask him if he has other symptoms. Find out if he has noticed behavioral changes or memory loss — the patient's family or friends may provide more accurate information on this.

Explore the patient's personal and family medical history for a neurologic (especially seizures), endocrine, or metabolic disorder. Obtain a complete drug history, noting especially the use of phenothiazines or herbal remedies. Also, ask about alcohol use.

Physical assessment

Assess the patient's overall appearance and demeanor, noting mental status. Test ROM and strength in all major muscle groups while observing for chorea, athetosis, dystonia, and other involuntary movements. Check DTRs and, if possible, observe the patient's gait.

Analysis

Tremors are classified as resting, intention, or postural. Resting tremors occur when an extremity is at rest and subside with movement. They include the classic pill-rolling tremor of Parkinson's disease. Conversely, intention tremors occur only with movement and subside with rest. Postural (or action) tremors appear when an extremity or the trunk is actively held in a particular posture or position. A common type of postural tremor is called an essential tremor.

Tremorlike movements may also be elicited, such as asterixis — the characteristic flapping tremor seen in hepatic failure. Stress or emotional upset tends to aggravate a tremor. Alcohol commonly diminishes postural tremors.

Tremors are typical signs of extrapyramidal or cerebellar disorders and can also result from certain drugs. Phenothiazines, particularly piperazine derivatives such as fluphenazine, and other antipsychotics may cause resting and pill-rolling tremors. Less commonly, metoclopramide and metyrosine also cause these tremors. Lithium toxicity, sympathomimetics, such as terbutaline and pseudoephedrine, amphetamines, and phenytoin can all cause tremors that disappear with dose reduction. Manganese toxicity and mercury poisoning also may cause tremors.

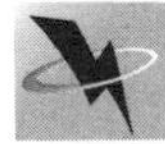

CRITICAL POINT *Herbal products, such as ephedra (ma huang), have been known to cause serious adverse reactions, which may include tremors.*

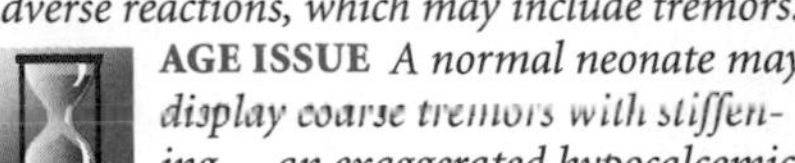

AGE ISSUE *A normal neonate may display coarse tremors with stiffening — an exaggerated hypocalcemic startle reflex — in response to noises and chills. Pediatric-specific causes of pathologic tremors include cerebral palsy, fetal alcohol syndrome, and maternal drug addiction.*

Assessing the pregnant patient

Assessing a pregnant patient can be a challenging and yet rewarding experience. A firm knowledge base as to how to thoroughly evaluate a woman's health during pregnancy allows development of an individualized care plan that will help secure a positive outcome for both mother and child.

Because pregnancy affects a woman's entire body, the assessment must be comprehensive. Performing a comprehensive assessment aids in determining if the woman is experiencing a common discomfort of pregnancy or a danger sign that requires immediate intervention. A complete assessment of each body system is essential. In addition, evaluation of the patient's emotional status, including her acceptance of the pregnancy, her preparation for parenthood, and the pregnancy's impact on the family is crucial.

Assessment of a pregnant patient must always be performed within the context of the maternal-fetal unit. Although mother and child have separate and distinct needs, their interdependent relationship means that factors influencing the mother's health may affect the health of the fetus, and alterations in fetal well-being may influence the mother's physical and emotional health.

Pregnancy

Pregnancy starts with fertilization of the ovum and ends with childbirth. On average, it lasts approximately 280 days or 38 to 40 weeks. During gestation the woman and fertilized ovum undergo numerous changes that ultimately lead to the birth of a full-term neonate.

Knowledge of the anatomy and physiology of the female reproductive system is cru-

HOW FERTILIZATION OCCURS

Fertilization begins when the spermatozoon activates upon contact with the ovum. This series of illustrations demonstrates the process of fertilization.

The spermatozoon, which has a covering called the *acrosome,* approaches the ovum.

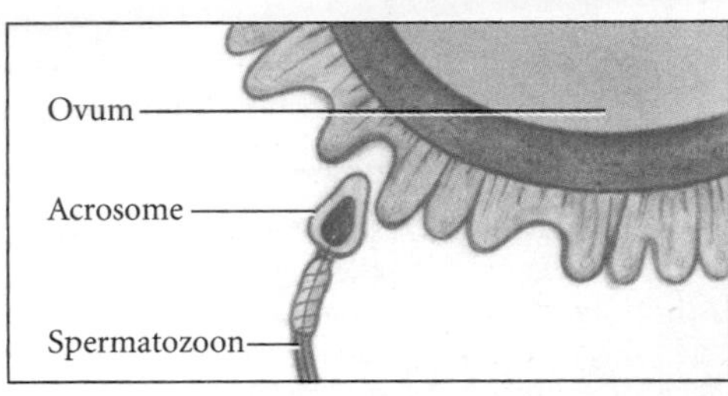

The acrosome develops small perforations through which it releases enzymes necessary for the sperm to penetrate the protective layers of the ovum before fertilization.

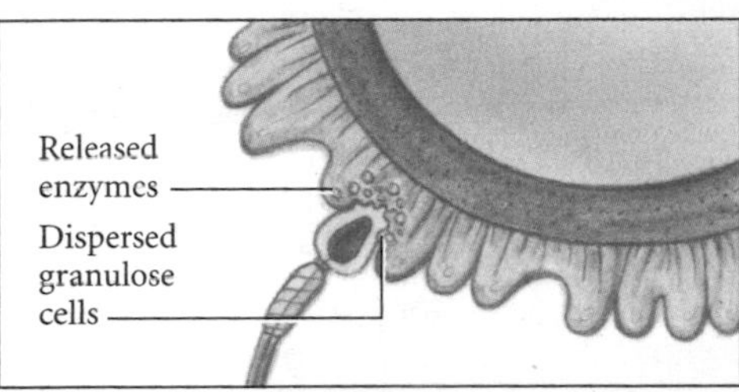

The spermatozoon then penetrates the zona pellucida, which is the inner membrane of the ovum. This triggers the ovum's second meiotic division, following meiosis, making the zona pellucida impenetrable to other spermatozoa.

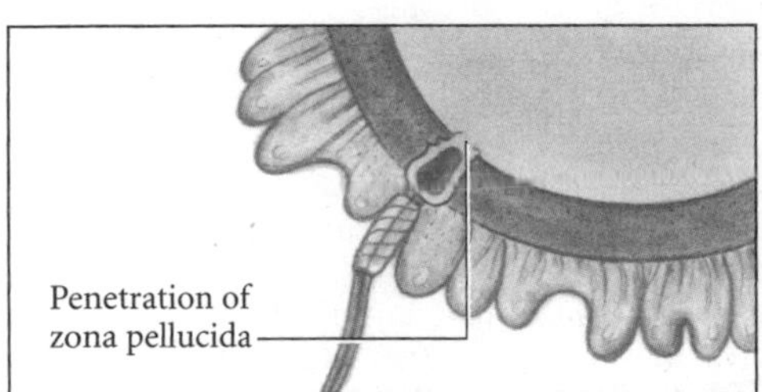

After the spermatozoon penetrates the ovum, its nucleus is released into the ovum, its tail degenerates, and its head enlarges and fuses with the ovum's nucleus. This fusion provides the fertilized ovum, called a *zygote,* with 46 chromosomes.

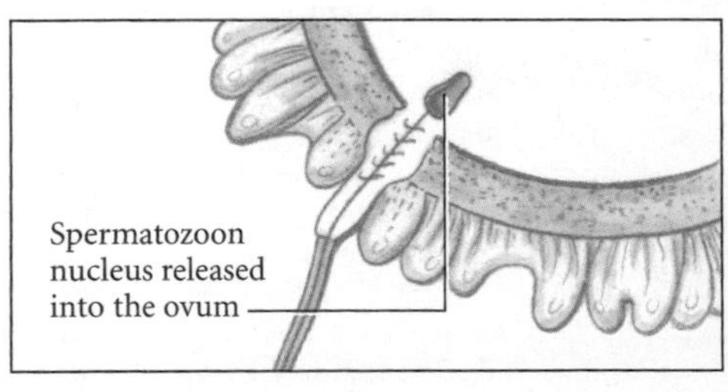

cial to understanding the changes that occur. (See chapter 14, Female genitourinary system, for a review.)

Fertilization

Production of a human being begins with fertilization, the union of a spermatozoon and an ovum to form a single new cell. After fertilization occurs, dramatic changes begin inside a woman's body. The cells of the fertilized ovum begin dividing as the ovum travels to the uterine cavity, where it implants itself in the uterine lining. (See *How fertilization occurs.*)

For fertilization to take place, however, the spermatozoon must first reach the ovum. Although a single ejaculation deposits several hundred million spermatozoa, many are destroyed by acidic vaginal secretions. The only spermatozoa that survive are those that enter the cervical canal, where cervical mucus protects them.

The ability of spermatozoa to penetrate the cervical mucus depends on the phase of the menstrual cycle at the time of transit. Early in the cycle, estrogen and progesterone levels cause the mucus to thicken, making it more difficult for spermatozoa to pass through the cervix. During midcycle, however, when the mucus is relatively thin, spermatozoa can pass readily through the cervix. Later in the cycle, the cervical mucus thickens again, hindering spermatozoa passage.

Spermatozoa travel through the female reproductive tract by means of flagellar movements, which are whiplike movements of the tail. After spermatozoa pass through the cervical mucus, however, the female reproductive system assists them on their journey with rhythmic contractions of the uterus that help the spermatozoa penetrate the fallopian tubes. Spermatozoa are typically viable to fertilize the ovum for up to 2 days after ejaculation; however, they can survive in the female reproductive tract for up to 4 days.

Before a spermatozoon can penetrate the ovum, it must disperse the granulosa cells and penetrate the zona pellucida, the thick, transparent layer surrounding the incompletely developed ovum. Enzymes in the acrosome, or the head cap, of the spermatozoon permit this penetration. After penetration, the ovum completes its second meiotic division and the zona pellucida prevents penetration by other spermatozoa.

The spermatozoon's head then fuses with the ovum nucleus, creating a cell nucleus with 46 chromosomes. The fertilized ovum is called a zygote. The zygote divides as it passes through the fallopian tube and attaches to the uterine lining by implantation. A complex sequence of preembryonic, embryonic, and fetal developments transforms the zygote into a full-term fetus.

Fetal development

During pregnancy, the fetus undergoes three major stages of development that include the preembryonic period (fertilization to week 3), the embryonic period (weeks 4 through 7), and the fetal period (week 8 through birth).

The preembryonic phase starts with ovum fertilization and lasts 3 weeks. As the zygote passes through the fallopian tube, it undergoes a series of mitotic divisions, or cleavage. (See *Preembryonic development.*)

During the embryonic period, which occurs from the fourth through the seventh week of gestation, the developing zygote starts to take on a human shape and is known as an embryo. Each germ layer — the ectoderm, mesoderm, and endoderm — eventually forms specific tissues in the embryo. For example, the ectoderm develops into the epidermis, nervous system, and hair; the mesoderm develops into the connective and supporting tissue and the kidneys and ureters; the endoderm develops into the pharynx and trachea, auditory canal, liver, pancreas, and bladder and urethra.

Organ systems form during the embryonic period. During this time, the embryo is particularly vulnerable to injury by maternal drug use, certain maternal infections, and other factors.

During the fetal stage of development, which extends from the eighth week until birth, the maturing fetus enlarges and grows heavier. For example, at the end of the second month, the fetus resembles a full-term neonate except for size. During the third month, the fetus grows 3" (7.6 cm) and weighs about 1 ounce (28.3 grams). Teeth and bones begin to appear and the kidneys start to function. At the end of the third month, sex can be discerned. Over the remaining 6 months, fetal growth continues as internal and external structures develop at a rapid rate. In the last 12 weeks, the fetus stores fats and minerals it will need to live outside the womb.

Two unusual features appear during the fetal stage. First, the fetus's head is disproportionately large compared with its body, which changes after birth as the infant grows. Second, the fetus lacks subcutaneous fat, but starts to accumulate it shortly after birth.

PREEMBRYONIC DEVELOPMENT

The preembryonic phase lasts from conception until approximately the end of the third week of development.

Zygote formation

As the fertilized ovum advances through the fallopian tube toward the uterus, it undergoes mitotic division, forming daughter cells, initially called *blastomeres,* that each contain the same number of chromosomes as the parent cell. The first cell division ends about 30 hours after fertilization; subsequent divisions occur rapidly.

The zygote then develops into a small mass of cells called a *morula,* which reaches the uterus around the third day after fertilization. Fluid that amasses in the center of the morula forms a central cavity.

Blastocyst formation

The structure, now a *blastocyst,* consists of a thin trophoblast layer, which includes the blastocyst cavity, and the inner cell mass. The trophoblast develops into fetal membranes and the placenta. The inner cell mass later forms the embryo (late blastocyst).

During the next phase, the blastocyst remains within the zona pellucida, unattached to the uterus. The zona pellucida degenerates and, by the end of the first week after fertilization, the blastocyst attaches to the endometrium. The part of the blastocyst adjacent to the inner cell mass is the first part to become attached.

The trophoblast, in contact with the endometrial lining, proliferates and invades the underlying endometrium by separating and dissolving endometrial cells.

Blastocyst penetration

During the next week, the invading blastocyst sinks below the endometrium's surface. The penetration site seals, restoring the continuity of the endometrial surface.

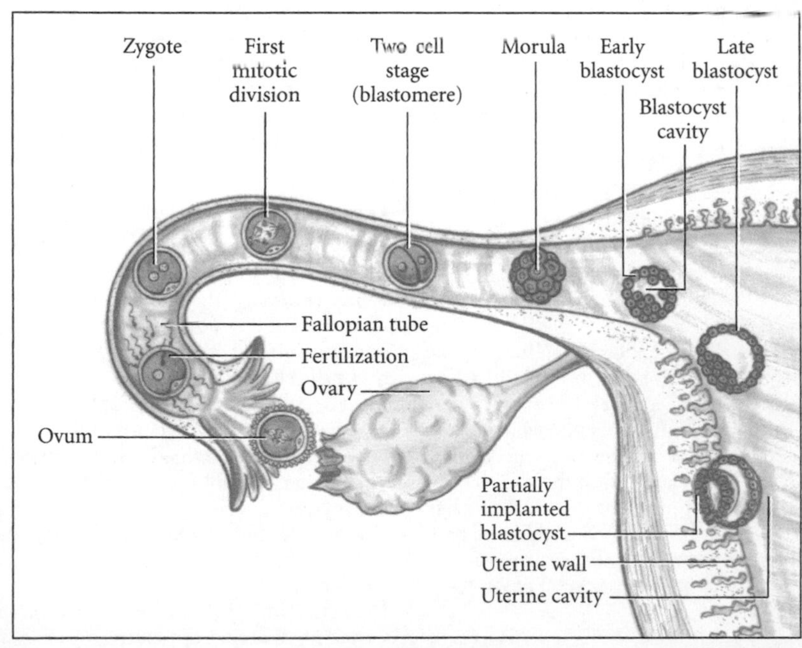

Structural changes in the ovaries and uterus

Pregnancy changes the normal development of the corpus luteum and results in the development of the decidua, amniotic sac and fluid, yolk sac, and placenta.

Corpus luteum

Normal functioning of the corpus luteum requires continuous stimulation by luteinizing hormone (LH). Progesterone produced by the corpus luteum suppresses LH release by the pituitary gland. If pregnancy occurs, the corpus luteum continues to produce progesterone until the placenta takes over. Otherwise, the corpus luteum atrophies 3 days before menstrual flow begins.

With age, the corpus luteum grows less responsive to LH. Therefore, the mature corpus luteum degenerates unless stimulated by progressively increasing amounts of LH. However, pregnancy stimulates the placental tissue to secrete large amounts of human chorionic gonadotropin (hCG), which resembles LH and follicle-stimulating hormone (FSH). hCG prevents corpus luteum degeneration, stimulating the corpus luteum to produce large amounts of estrogen and progesterone.

The corpus luteum, stimulated by the hormone hCG, produces the estrogen and progesterone needed to maintain the pregnancy during the first 3 months. hCG can be detected as early as 9 days after fertilization and can provide confirmation of pregnancy even before the woman has missed her first menses. The hCG level gradually increases during this time, peaks at about 10 weeks' gestation, and then gradually declines.

Decidua

The decidua is the endometrial lining of the uterus that undergoes hormone-induced changes during pregnancy. Decidual cells secrete the hormone prolactin, which promotes lactation; a peptide hormone, relaxin, which induces relaxation of the connective tissue of the symphysis pubis and pelvic ligaments and promotes cervical dilation; and a potent hormonelike fatty acid, prostaglandin, which mediates several physiologic functions.

Amniotic sac and fluid

The amniotic sac, enclosed within the chorion, gradually grows and surrounds the embryo. As it enlarges, the amniotic sac expands into the chorionic cavity, eventually filling the cavity and fusing with the chorion by the eighth week of gestation.

The amniotic sac and fluid serve the fetus in two important ways, one during gestation and the other during delivery. During gestation, the fluid gives the fetus a buoyant, temperature-controlled environment. Later, amniotic fluid serves as a fluid wedge that helps to open the cervix during birth.

Early in pregnancy, amniotic fluid comes chiefly from the fluid filtering into the amniotic sac from maternal blood as it passes through the uterus, the fluid filtering into the sac from fetal blood passing through the placenta, and the fluid diffusing into the amniotic sac from the fetal skin and respiratory tract.

Later in pregnancy, when the fetal kidneys begin to function, the fetus urinates into the amniotic fluid. Fetal urine then becomes the major source of amniotic fluid.

Production of amniotic fluid from maternal and fetal sources balances amniotic fluid that's lost through the fetal GI tract. Typically, the fetus swallows up to several hundred milliliters of amniotic fluid each day. The fluid is absorbed into the fetal circulation from the fetal GI tract; some is transferred from the fetal circulation to the maternal circulation and excreted in maternal urine.

Yolk sac

The yolk sac forms next to the endoderm of the germ disk; a portion of it is incorporated in the developing embryo and forms the GI tract. Another portion of the sac develops into primitive germ cells, which travel to the developing gonads and eventually form oocytes, the precursor of the ovum, or spermatocytes, the precursor of the spermatozoon, after gender has been determined.

During early embryonic development, the yolk sac also forms blood cells. Eventually, it undergoes atrophy and disintegrates.

Placenta

Using the umbilical cord as its conduit, the flattened, disk-shaped placenta provides nutrients to and removes wastes from the fetus from the third month of pregnancy until birth. The placenta is formed from the chorion, its chorionic villi, and the adjacent decidua basalis.

The umbilical cord contains two arteries and one vein and links the fetus to the placenta. The umbilical arteries, which transport blood from the fetus to the placenta, take a spiral course on the cord, divide on the placental surface, and branch off to the chorionic villi.

The placenta is a highly vascular organ. Large veins on its surface gather blood returning from the villi and join to form the single umbilical vein, which enters the cord, returning blood to the fetus.

The placenta contains two highly specialized circulatory systems. The first of which is the uteroplacental circulation that carries oxygenated arterial blood from the maternal circulation to the intervillous spaces—large spaces separating chorionic villi in the placenta. Blood enters the intervillous spaces from uterine arteries that penetrate the basal part of the placenta; it leaves the intervillous spaces and flows back into the maternal circulation through veins in the basal part of the placenta near the arteries. The second system is the fetoplacental circulation that transports oxygen-depleted blood from the fetus to the chorionic villi by the umbilical arteries and returns oxygenated blood to the fetus through the umbilical vein.

For the first 3 months of pregnancy, the corpus luteum is the main source of estrogen and progesterone—hormones required during pregnancy. By the end of the third month, however, the placenta produces most of the hormones; the corpus luteum persists but is no longer needed to maintain the pregnancy.

The levels of estrogen and progesterone increase progressively throughout pregnancy. Estrogen stimulates uterine development to provide a suitable environment for the fetus. Progesterone, synthesized by the placenta from maternal cholesterol, reduces uterine muscle irritability and prevents spontaneous abortion of the fetus.

The placenta also produces human placental lactogen (HPL), which resembles growth hormone. HPL stimulates maternal protein and fat metabolism to ensure a sufficient supply of amino acids and fatty acids for the mother and fetus. HPL also stimulates breast growth in preparation for lactation. Throughout pregnancy, HPL levels rise progressively.

Maternal responses to pregnancy

During pregnancy, a woman undergoes many physiologic and psychosocial changes. Her body adapts in response to the demands of the growing fetus while her mind prepares for the responsibilities that accompany becoming a parent. Physiologic changes initially indicate pregnancy and continue to affect the body throughout pregnancy as the fetus grows and develops. Psychosocial changes occur in both the mother and father and may vary from trimester to trimester.

Signs of pregnancy

Pregnancy produces several types of physiologic changes that must be evaluated before a definitive diagnosis of pregnancy is made. The changes can be presumptive (subjective), probable (objective), or positive.

Neither presumptive nor probable signs confirm pregnancy because both can be caused by other medical conditions. They simply suggest pregnancy, especially when several are present at the same time. (See *Evaluating pregnancy signs,* pages 526 and 527.)

Presumptive signs. Presumptive signs of pregnancy are those that can be assumed to indicate pregnancy until more concrete signs develop. These signs include breast changes, nausea and vomiting, amenorrhea, urinary frequency, fatigue, uterine enlargement, quickening, and skin changes. A pregnant patient typically reports some presumptive signs.

Probable signs. Probable signs of pregnancy strongly suggest pregnancy. They're more reliable indicators of pregnancy than presumptive signs, but they can also be explained by other medical conditions. Probable signs include positive laboratory tests, such as serum and urine tests; positive results on a home pregnancy test; Chadwick's sign; Goodell's sign; Hegar's sign; sonographic evidence of a gestational sac; ballottement; and Braxton Hicks contractions.

(Text continues on page 528.)

EVALUATING PREGNANCY SIGNS

This chart evaluates the signs of pregnancy by dividing them into three categories: presumptive, probable, and positive.

Sign	Weeks from implantation	Other possible causes
Presumptive		
Breast changes, including feelings of tenderness, fullness, or tingling and enlargement or darkening of areolae	2	▪ Hyperprolactinemia induced by tranquilizers ▪ Infection ▪ Prolactin-secreting pituitary tumor ▪ Pseudocyesis ▪ Premenstrual syndrome
Feeling of nausea or vomiting upon arising	2	▪ Gastric disorders ▪ Infections ▪ Psychological disorders, such as pseudocyesis and anorexia nervosa
Amenorrhea	2	▪ Anovulation ▪ Blocked endometrial cavity ▪ Endocrine changes ▪ Medications (phenothiazines) ▪ Metabolic changes
Frequent urination	3	▪ Emotional stress ▪ Pelvic tumor ▪ Renal disease ▪ Urinary tract infection
Fatigue	12	▪ Anemia ▪ Chronic illness
Uterine enlargement in which the uterus can be palpated over the symphysis pubis	12	▪ Ascites ▪ Obesity ▪ Uterine or pelvic tumor
Quickening (fetal movement felt by the woman)	18	▪ Excessive flatus ▪ Increased peristalsis
Linea nigra (line of dark pigment on the abdomen)	24	▪ Cardiopulmonary disorders ▪ Estrogen-progestin hormonal contraceptives ▪ Obesity ▪ Pelvic tumor
Melasma (dark pigment on the face)	24	▪ Cardiopulmonary disorders ▪ Estrogen-progestin hormonal contraceptives ▪ Obesity ▪ Pelvic tumor

EVALUATING PREGNANCY SIGNS *(continued)*

Sign	Weeks from implantation	Other possible causes
Presumptive *(continued)*		
Striae gravidarum (red streaks on the abdomen)	24	■ Cardiopulmonary disorders ■ Estrogen-progestin hormonal contraceptives ■ Obesity ■ Pelvic tumor
Probable		
Serum laboratory tests revealing the presence of human chorionic gonadotropin (hCG) hormone	1	■ Cross-reaction of luteinizing hormone (similar to hCG)
Chadwick's sign (vagina changes color from pink to violet)	6	■ Hyperemia of cervix, vagina, or vulva
Goodell's sign (cervix softens)	6	■ Estrogen-progestin hormonal contraceptives
Hegar's sign (lower uterine segment softens)	6	■ Excessively soft uterine walls
Sonographic evidence of gestational sac in which characteristic ring is evident	6	None
Ballottement (fetus can be felt to rise against abdominal wall when lower uterine segment is tapped on during bimanual examination)	16	■ Ascites ■ Uterine tumor or polyps
Braxton Hicks contractions (periodic uterine tightening)	20	■ Hematometra ■ Uterine tumor
Palpation of fetal outline through abdomen	20	■ Subserous uterine myoma
Positive		
Sonographic evidence of fetal outline	8	None
Fetal heart audible by Doppler ultrasound	10 to 12	None
Palpation of fetal movement through abdomen	20	None

Positive signs. Positive signs of pregnancy include sonographic evidence of the fetal outline, an audible fetal heart rate, and fetal movement that's felt by the health care provider. These signs confirm pregnancy because they can't be attributed to other conditions.

Physiologic changes

As the fetus grows and hormones shift during pregnancy, physiologic adaptations occur in every body system to accommodate the fetus.

Physiologic changes help a pregnant woman maintain health throughout the pregnancy and physically prepare for childbirth. These changes also create a safe and nurturing environment for the fetus and some take place even before the woman finds out that she's pregnant. Although changes occur in every body system, the reproductive and endocrine system changes are detailed here. (See *How the body responds to pregnancy.*)

Reproductive system changes. In addition to the physical changes that initially indicate pregnancy, such as Hegar's sign and Goodell's sign, the reproductive system undergoes significant changes throughout pregnancy.

External reproductive structures affected by pregnancy include the labia majora, labia minora, clitoris, and vaginal introitus. These structures enlarge because of increased vascularity. Fat deposits also contribute to the enlargement of the labia majora and labia minora. These structures reduce in size after childbirth, but they may not return to their prepregnant state because of loss of muscle tone or perineal injury, such as an episiotomy or a vaginal tear. For example, in many patients, the labia majora remain separated and gape after childbirth. In addition, varices may be caused by pressure on vessels in the perineal and perianal areas.

Internal reproductive structures, including the ovaries, uterus, and other structures, change dramatically to accommodate the developing fetus. These internal structures may not regain their prepregnant states after childbirth.

OVARIES. When fertilization occurs, ovarian follicles cease to mature and ovulation stops. The chorionic villi, which develop from the fertilized ovum, begin to produce hCG to maintain the ovarian corpus luteum. The corpus luteum produces estrogen and progesterone until the placenta is formed and functioning. At 8 to 10 weeks' gestation, the placenta assumes production of these hormones. The corpus luteum, which is no longer needed, then involutes due to a reduction in cell size.

UTERUS. In a nonpregnant woman, the uterus is smaller than the size of a fist, measuring approximately 7.5 cm × 5 cm × 2.5 cm (3″ × 2″ × 1″). It can weigh 60 to 70 g in a nulliparous patient and 100 g in a parous patient. In a nonpregnant state, a woman's uterus can hold up to 10 ml of fluid. Its walls are composed of several overlapping layers of muscle fibers that adapt to the developing fetus and help in expulsion of the fetus and placenta during labor and childbirth.

After conception, the uterus retains the developing fetus for approximately 280 days, or 9 calendar months. During this time, the uterus undergoes progressive changes in size, shape, and position in the abdominal cavity. In the first trimester, the pear-shaped uterus lengthens and enlarges in response to elevated levels of estrogen and progesterone. This hormonal stimulation primarily causes an increase in the size of myometrial cells, called hypertrophy, although a small increase in cell number, called hyperplasia, also occurs. These changes increase the amount of fibrous and elastic tissue to more than 20 times that of the nonpregnant uterus. Uterine walls become stronger and more elastic.

During the first few weeks of pregnancy, the uterine walls remain thick and the fundus rests low in the abdomen. The uterus can't be palpated through the abdominal wall. After 12 weeks of pregnancy, however, the uterus typically reaches the level of the symphysis pubis and then may be palpated through the abdominal wall.

In the second trimester, the corpus and fundus become globe-shaped. As pregnancy progresses, the uterus lengthens and becomes oval in shape. The uterine walls thin as the muscles stretch; the uterus rises out of the pelvis, shifts to the right, and rests against the anterior abdominal wall. At 20 weeks' gestation, the uterus is palpable just

HOW THE BODY RESPONDS TO PREGNANCY

Pregnancy affects not only the reproductive and endocrine systems but several other body systems as well.

Cardiovascular system

Blood pressure, systolic and diastolic, tends to fall slightly in midpregnancy and then rise to the woman's normal level during the third trimester. Consider a rise above 30 mm Hg systolic or 15 mm Hg diastolic from her normal pressure abnormal. Normally, the woman's heart rate increases by 10 to 15 beats/minute during pregnancy; exaggerated splitting of the first heart sounds, murmurs in the jugular and breast areas, and cardiac enlargement with displacement upward and to the left are also normal findings. Palpitations may also occur. White blood cell (WBC) count, which varies during pregnancy, is usually within a range of 5,000 to 12,000/µl.

Blood volume — red blood cells (RBCs) and plasma — increases during pregnancy by as much as 1,500 ml. As plasma volume expands, the concentration of RBCs falls, stimulating the bone marrow to increase RBC production and causing a hemodilution effect, because the rise in plasma volume exceeds the compensatory increase in RBCs. This condition is referred to as physiologic anemia or pseudoanemia.

Venous pressure in legs and feet increases during pregnancy because the enlarging uterus compresses the pelvic veins and impedes venous return. Venous compression also contributes to dependent edema and varicose veins in the legs and vulva.

GI system

Morning sickness may be among the first signs the pregnant patient experiences. Nausea and vomiting result from high levels of gonadotropins. Increased progesterone levels during pregnancy cause relaxation of the smooth muscles of the GI and biliary tracts, resulting in decreased colon motility, which predisposes the woman to constipation and — because constipation can lead to increased pressure in veins below the enlarged uterus — hemorrhoids. Decreased stomach emptying time and reflux of stomach contents, resulting in heartburn (pyrosis), may also result from relaxation of the smooth muscle of the GI tract.

The high estrogen level characteristic of pregnancy promotes increased excretion of cholesterol in the bile. The resulting cholesterol-supersaturated bile, coupled with stasis of bile in the gallbladder, caused by relaxation of the smooth muscle of the gallbladder, leads to the precipitation of cholesterol crystals from the bile and may predispose the patient to gallstones.

Integumentary system

Increased secretion of melanocyte-stimulating hormone from the pituitary gland causes a generalized increase in skin pigment during pregnancy. The most conspicuous early manifestation of this change is darkening of the areolae. Sometimes the woman's facial skin develops irregular areas of dark pigmentation, called *chloasma.* Pigmented skin nevi also become darker and more prominent. High estrogen levels may cause small hemangiomas on the skin over the chest and arms; these disappear after delivery. Stretch marks, or striae gravidarum, occur in 50% to 90% of all pregnant women during the second half of pregnancy. They appear on the abdomen and usually fade after birth; however, they never completely disappear.

Musculoskeletal system

A pregnant woman's enlarging uterus displaces her center of gravity forward, causing an increased lumbar lordosis, necessary to maintain balance. Enlarging

(continued)

HOW THE BODY RESPONDS TO PREGNANCY *(continued)*

breasts may cause kyphosis. Increased elasticity of connective and collagen tissue — caused by the increase in circulating steroid sex hormones during pregnancy — results in slight relaxation of the pelvic joints.

Respiratory system

The growing uterus displaces the diaphragm upward, which tends to hinder the mother's respiration. However, vital capacity doesn't change significantly, because the transverse diameter of the thorax increases and provides compensation. Thoracic size increases because of hormone-mediated relaxation of the ligaments connecting the ribs to the spinal column and sternum.

Urinary system

During the first trimester, the enlarging uterus puts pressure on the bladder, resulting in urinary frequency. Pressure is relieved in the second trimester, when the uterus becomes an abdominal organ. Late in pregnancy, engagement of the presenting part exerts pressure on the bladder. The bladder becomes concave, and its capacity is greatly reduced.

Some dilation of the ureters and the renal calices and pelves is common in pregnancy. It most likely occurs because the enlarged uterus compresses the ureter against the pelvic brim. Urine drainage is commonly impeded, which can lead to urine stasis and predispose the woman to urinary tract infections. These are relatively more common on the right side because the uterus tips to the right as it rises from the pelvis, putting pressure on the right ureter.

Hematologic system

Pregnancy affects iron demands and absorption as well as RBC, WBC, and fibrinogen levels. In addition, bone marrow becomes more active during pregnancy, producing up to a 30% excess of RBCs.

During pregnancy, the body's demand for iron increases. Not only does the developing fetus require approximately 350 to 400 mg of iron per day for healthy growth, but also the mother's iron requirement increases by 400 mg per day. This iron increase is necessary to promote RBC production and accommodate the increased blood volume that occurs during pregnancy. The total daily iron requirements of a woman and her fetus amount to roughly 800 mg. Because the average woman's store of iron is only about 500 mg, a pregnant woman should take iron supplements.

Iron supplements may also be necessary to accommodate for impaired iron absorption. Absorption of iron may be hindered during pregnancy as a result of decreased gastric acidity (iron is absorbed best from an acid medium). In addition, increased plasma volume (from 2,600 ml in a nonpregnant woman to 3,600 ml in a pregnant woman) is disproportionately greater than the increase in RBCs, which lowers the patient's hematocrit (the percentage of RBCs in whole blood) and causes anemia. The hemoglobin level also decreases. A hematocrit below 35% and hemoglobin level below 11.5 g/dl indicate pregnancy-related anemia. Iron supplements are commonly prescribed during pregnancy to reduce the risk of this complication.

The WBC count rises from 7,000 ml before pregnancy to 20,500 ml during pregnancy. The reason for this is unknown. The count may increase to 25,000 ml or more during labor, childbirth, and the early postpartum period.

Fibrinogen, a protein in blood plasma, is converted to fibrin by thrombin and is known as coagulation factor I. In a nonpregnant patient, levels average 250 mg/dl. In a pregnant patient, levels average 450 mg/dl, increasing as much as 50% by term. This increase in the coagulation factor plays an important role

HOW THE BODY RESPONDS TO PREGNANCY *(continued)*

in preventing maternal hemorrhage during childbirth.

Immune system

Immunologic competency naturally decreases during pregnancy, most likely to prevent the woman's body from rejecting the fetus. The immune system recognizes the fetus as a foreign object. In most cases, the immune system responds to foreign objects by sending defense cells that attempt to destroy them. For certain types of foreign objects, such as a cold virus, this immune response is necessary to protect the body. In a situation such as organ transplantation, however, the patient must be given medications to reduce the immune system response so that the body doesn't attack the transplant.

A similar process occurs naturally in a pregnant woman, whereby her immune system response decreases, allowing the fetus to remain. In particular, immunoglobulin G (IgG) production is decreased, which increases the risk of infection during pregnancy. A simultaneous increase in the WBC count may help to counteract the decrease in IgG response.

Neurologic system

Changes in the neurologic system during pregnancy are poorly defined and aren't completely understood. For most patients, neurologic changes are temporary and revert back to normal postpartum.

Functional disturbances called entrapment neuropathies occur in the peripheral nervous system as a result of mechanical pressure. In other words, nerves become trapped and pinched by the enlarging uterus and enlarged edematous vessels, making them less functional. For example, the patient may experience meralgia paresthetica, a tingling and numbness in the anterolateral portion of the thigh that results when the lateral femoral cutaneous nerve becomes entrapped in the area of the inguinal ligaments. This feeling is more pronounced in late pregnancy, as the gravid uterus presses on the nerves and as vascular stasis occurs.

below the umbilicus and reaches the umbilicus at 22 weeks' gestation. As uterine muscles stretch, Braxton Hicks contractions may occur, helping to move blood more quickly through the intervillous spaces of the placenta.

In the third trimester, the fundus reaches nearly to the xiphoid process, the lower tip of the breastbone. Between weeks 38 and 40, the fetus begins its descent into the pelvis, called lightening, which causes fundal height to gradually drop. The uterus remains oval in shape. Its muscular walls become progressively thinner as it enlarges, finally reaching a muscle wail thickness of 5 mm (¼″) or less. At term (40 weeks), the uterus typically weighs approximately 1,100 g, holds 5 to 10 L of fluid, and has stretched to approximately 28 cm × 24 cm × 21 cm (11″ × 9½″ × 8¼″).

ENDOMETRIAL DEVELOPMENT. During the menstrual cycle, progesterone stimulates increased thickening and vascularity of the endometrium, preparing the uterine lining for implantation and nourishment of a fertilized ovum. After implantation, menstruation stops. The endometrium then becomes the decidua, which is divided into three layers that include the decidua capsularis, which covers the blastocyst (fertilized ovum); the decidua basalis, which lies directly under the blastocyst and forms part of the placenta; and the decidua vera, which lines the rest of the uterus.

VASCULAR GROWTH. As the fetus grows and the placenta develops, uterine blood vessels and lymphatics increase in number and size. Vessels must enlarge to accommodate the increased blood flow to the uterus and placenta. By the end of pregnancy, an average of 500 ml of blood may flow through the maternal side of the placenta each minute. Maternal arterial pressure, uterine contractions, and maternal position affect uterine blood flow throughout pregnancy.

Because one-sixth of the body's blood supply is circulating through the uterus at any given time, uterine bleeding in pregnancy is always potentially serious and can result in major blood loss.

CERVICAL CHANGES. The cervix consists of connective tissue, elastic fibers, and endocervical folds. This composition allows it to stretch during childbirth. During pregnancy, the cervix softens. It also takes on a bluish color during the second month due to increased vasculature. It becomes edematous and may bleed easily on examination or sexual activity.

During pregnancy, hormonal stimulation causes the glandular cervical tissue to increase in cell number and become hyperactive, secreting thick, tenacious mucus. This mucus thickens into a mucoid weblike structure, eventually forming a mucus plug that blocks the cervical canal. This creates a protective barrier against bacteria and other substances attempting to enter the uterus.

VAGINA. During pregnancy, estrogen stimulates vascularity, tissue growth, and hypertrophy in the vaginal epithelial tissue. White, thick, odorless, and acidic vaginal secretions increase. The acidity of these secretions helps prevent bacterial infections but can also foster yeast infections, a common occurrence during pregnancy.

Other vaginal changes include development of a bluish color due to increased vascularity; hypertrophy of the smooth muscles and relaxation of connective tissues, which allow the vagina to stretch during childbirth; lengthening of the vaginal vault; and possible heightened sexual sensitivity.

BREASTS. In addition to the presumptive signs that occur in the breasts during pregnancy, such as tenderness, tingling, darkening of the areolae, and appearance of Montgomery's tubercles, the nipples enlarge, become more erectile, and darken. The areolae widen from a diameter of less than 1¼″ (3 cm) to 2″ or 3″ (5 or 6 cm) in the primigravid patient.

Rarely, patches of brownish discoloration appear on the skin adjacent to the areolae. These patches, known as secondary areolae, may indicate pregnancy if the patient has never breast-fed an infant.

The breasts also undergo several changes in preparation for lactation. As blood vessels enlarge, veins beneath the skin of the breasts become more visible and may appear as intertwining patterns over the anterior chest wall. Breasts become fuller and heavier as lactation approaches and may throb causing discomfort.

Increasing hormones cause the secretion of colostrum, which is a yellowish, viscous fluid, from the nipples. High in protein, antibodies, and minerals—but low in fat and sugar relative to mature human milk—colostrum may be secreted as early as the 16th week of pregnancy, but it's most common during the last trimester. It continues until 2 to 4 days after delivery and is followed by mature milk production.

Breast changes are more pronounced in a primigravida patient than in a multigravida patient. In a multigravida patient, changes are even less significant if the patient has breast-fed an infant within the past year because her areolae are still dark and her breasts enlarged.

Endocrine system changes. The endocrine system undergoes many fluctuations during pregnancy. Changes in hormone levels and protein production help support fetal growth and maintain body functions.

PLACENTA. The most striking change in the endocrine system during pregnancy is the addition of the placenta. The placenta is an endocrine organ that produces large amounts of estrogen, progesterone, hCG, HPL, relaxin, and prostaglandins.

The estrogen produced by the placenta causes breast and uterine enlargement as well as palmar erythema, redness in the palm of the hand. Progesterone helps maintain the endometrium by inhibiting uterine contractility. It also prepares the breasts for lactation by stimulating breast tissue development.

Secreted by the trophoblast cells of the placenta in early pregnancy, hCG stimulates progesterone and estrogen synthesis until the placenta assumes this role.

Also called human chorionic somatotroopin, the hormone HPL is secreted by the placenta. It promotes fat breakdown (lipolysis), providing the patient with an alternate source of energy so that glucose is available for fetal growth. This hormone, however, has a complicating effect. Along with estrogen, progesterone, and cortisol, HPL inhibits the action of insulin, resulting in an increased insulin need throughout pregnancy.

Relaxin, secreted primarily by the corpus luteum, helps inhibit uterine activity and helps soften the cervix, which allows for dilation at delivery. It also helps soften the collagen in body joints, allowing for laxness in the lower spine, and helps enlarge the birth canal.

PROSTAGLANDINS. Prostaglandins are found in high concentration in the female reproductive tract and the decidua during pregnancy. They affect smooth-muscle contractility to such an extent that they may trigger labor at the pregnancy's term.

PITUITARY GLAND. The pituitary gland undergoes various changes during pregnancy. High estrogen and progesterone levels in the placenta stop the pituitary gland from producing FSH and LH. Increased production of growth hormone and melanocyte-stimulating hormone causes skin pigment changes.

Late in pregnancy, the posterior pituitary gland begins to produce oxytocin, which stimulates uterine contractions during labor. Prolactin production also starts late in pregnancy as the breasts prepare for lactation after birth.

THYROID GLAND. As early as the second month of pregnancy, the thyroid gland's production of thyroxine-binding protein increases, causing total thyroxine (T_4) levels to rise. Because the amount of unbound T_4 doesn't increase, these thyroid changes don't cause hyperthyroidism; however, they increase basal metabolic rate (BMR), cardiac output, pulse rate, vasodilation, and heat intolerance. BMR increases by about 20% during the second and third trimesters as the growing fetus places additional demands for energy on the woman's system. By term, the woman's BMR may increase by 25%, but returns to the prepregnant level within 1 week after childbirth.

In addition to T_4 level changes, increased estrogen levels augment the circulating amounts of triiodothyronine (T_3). Like the elevation of T_4 the elevation of T_3 levels doesn't lead to a hyperthyroid condition during pregnancy because much of this hormone is bound to proteins and, therefore, nonfunctional.

PARATHYROID GLANDS. As pregnancy progresses, fetal demands for calcium and phosphorus increase. The parathyroid gland responds by increasing hormone production during the third trimester to as much as twice the prepregnancy level.

ADRENAL GLANDS. Adrenal gland activity increases during pregnancy as production of corticosteroids and aldosterone escalates.

Some researchers believe that increased corticosteroid levels suppress inflammatory reactions and help to reduce the possibility of the woman's body rejecting the foreign protein of the fetus. Corticosteroids also help to regulate glucose metabolism in the woman.

Increased aldosterone levels help to promote sodium reabsorption and maintain the osmolarity of retained fluid. This indirectly helps to safeguard the blood volume and provide adequate perfusion pressure across the placenta.

PANCREAS. Although the pancreas itself doesn't change during pregnancy, maternal insulin, glucose, and glucagon production do. In response to the additional glucocorticoids produced by the adrenal glands, the pancreas increases insulin production. Insulin is less effective than normal, however, because estrogen, progesterone, and HPL act as antagonists to it. Despite insulin's diminished action and increased fetal demands for glucose, maternal glucose levels remain fairly stable because the mother's fat stores are used for energy.

Psychosocial changes

Pregnancy and childbirth are events that deeply affect the lives of parents, partners, and families. Psychological, social, economic, and cultural factors as well as family and individual influences toward sex-specific and family roles, affect the parents' response to pregnancy and childbirth. All of these aspects of childbearing affect the health of the parents and the child.

Phases of acceptance. A mother's acceptance of the pregnancy can progress through different phases. During the first stage, called *full embodiment*, a woman may become dependent on her partner or significant others and may be introspective and calm. The woman, especially if she's a new mother, may initially feel some ambivalence about finding out that she's pregnant. She may spend the first few weeks imagining how the pregnancy will change her life. As the pregnancy progresses, however, the mother incorporates the fetus into her body image.

The next phase is the *developmental* stage of fetal distinction. In this stage, the woman starts to view her fetus as a separate individual. She begins to accept her new body image and may even characterize it as being "full of life." She may become closer or more dependent on her mother at this stage.

During the final, or *transition*, stage, the woman prepares to separate from and give up her attachment to the fetus. She may become anxious about labor and delivery. Discomfort and frustration over the awkwardness of her body may lead her to become impatient about the impending delivery. During this stage, the patient also begins to get ready for the baby and to mentally prepare for her role as mother.

Factors affecting acceptance. Such factors as cultural background, family influences, and individual temperaments can affect a mother's acceptance of the pregnancy.

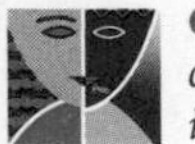

CULTURAL INSIGHT *A woman's cultural background may strongly influence how she progresses through the stages of acceptance. They may also guide how actively the woman participates in her pregnancy. Certain beliefs and taboos may place restrictions on her behavior and activities. For example, Native Americans may not seek prenatal care as soon as other pregnant women because they view pregnancy as a normal condition.*

The home in which a woman was raised can also influence her beliefs about and her acceptance of pregnancy. If a woman was raised in a home in which children were loved and viewed as pleasant additions to a happy family, she'll probably have a more positive attitude toward pregnancy. If she was raised in a home in which children were considered intruders or were blamed for the breakup of a marriage, the woman's view of pregnancy may be negative.

More specifically, the views of the pregnant patient's mother commonly influence the patient's attitudes about pregnancy. If her mother disliked being pregnant and always reminded her that she was a burden and that children weren't always wanted, she may view her pregnancy in the same way.

A woman's temperament and ability to cope with or adapt to stress plays a role in how she resolves conflict and adapts to her new life after childbirth. How she accepts her pregnancy depends on her self-image and the support that's given to her. For example, a woman may view pregnancy as a situation that robs her of her career, looks, and freedom.

A woman's relationship with the child's father also influences her acceptance of the pregnancy. If the father is there to provide emotional support, acceptance of the pregnancy is likely to be easier than if he isn't a part of the pregnancy. Whether the father of the child can accept the pregnancy depends on the same factors that affect the mother, including cultural background, past experiences, and relationship with family members.

Changes during the first trimester. During the first trimester, the family's key psychosocial challenge is to resolve any ambivalence. The mother copes with the common discomforts and changes of the first trimester; the father begins to accept the reality of the pregnancy.

Many women have unrealistic ideas about maternal instincts, expecting to feel only loving, happy thoughts about the fetus and motherhood. In fact, most women feel some ambivalence about pregnancy and motherhood. Pregnancy involves stressful changes that force women to think and behave differently from they way they behaved in the past. During this time, both partners also may experience vivid dreams about the impending birth. The woman may recall her dreams with greater intensity, however, because she typically is awakened more often at night by heartburn, fetal activity, and the need to urinate. Dreams tend to follow a predictable pattern during pregnancy. Other psychosocial challenges that the parents face include maternal acceptance of physical changes and paternal acceptance of and preparation for fatherhood.

In the early weeks of the first trimester, the woman watches for body changes that confirm her pregnancy. Her body image, the mental image of how her body looks, feels, and moves and how others see her, changes as her breasts enlarge, her menses cease, and she begins to experience nausea, fatigue, waist thickening, and general weight gain. Depending on her acceptance of the pregnancy, the woman may enjoy or dread these changes.

During the first trimester, the father typically finds the pregnancy unreal and intangible. The idea of the fetus may be abstract to him because he can't observe physical changes in his partner Accepting the reality of pregnancy is the father's main psychological task in the first trimester.

Changes during the second trimester. During the second trimester, psychosocial tasks include mother-image development, father-image development, coping with body image and sexuality changes, and development of prenatal attachment. Parents may experience various fears. Feeling dependent and vulnerable, the woman may fear for her partner's safety. In touch with mortality, the man may consider how his death would affect his family. He may recall risks he has taken, such as driving recklessly, and, as a result, he may commit to being more careful to avoid the risk of abandoning his partner and fetus.

During the second trimester, the parents' dreams may reflect concerns about the normalcy of the fetus, parental abilities, divided loyalties, and related subjects. To help alleviate these concerns, the couple may examine their dreams and fears.

Changes during the third trimester. As the third trimester begins, the woman feels a sense of accomplishment because her fetus has reached the age of viability. She may feel sentimental about the approaching end of her pregnancy, when the mother-child relationship replaces the mother-fetus relationship. At the same time, however, she may look forward to giving birth because the last months of pregnancy involve bulkiness, insomnia, childbirth anxieties, and concern about the neonate's normalcy.

During the third trimester, the woman and her partner must adapt to activity changes, prepare for parenting, provide partner support, accept body image and sexuality changes, develop birth plans, and prepare for labor. At this time, the woman needs to overcome any fears she may have about the unknown, labor pain, loss of self-esteem, loss of control, and death.

Health history

Assessment begins with the pregnant patient's first prenatal visit and continues throughout labor and delivery and the postpartum period. It includes evaluation of fetal and neonatal well-being.

Throughout each assessment stage, keep in mind the interdependence of the mother and fetus. Changes in the mother's health may affect fetal health, and changes in fetal health may affect the mother's physical and emotional health.

The first prenatal visit is the best time to establish baseline data for the pregnant patient. A thorough assessment of the reproductive system should be included. As with other body systems, this assessment depends on an accurate history (see *Conducting a successful interview,* page 536) and a thorough physical examination.

Remember to keep the patient informed about assessment findings. Sharing this information with her may help promote compliance with health care recommendations and encourage her to seek additional information about problems or questions that she has later in the pregnancy.

During the patient's first prenatal visit, expect to obtain biographic data and information about her nutritional, medical, family, gynecologic, and obstetric history. After this initial assessment, plan to perform intermittent evaluations during subsequent visits throughout the pregnancy.

Biographic data

When obtaining biographic data, assure the patient that the information remains confidential. Topics to discuss include age; cul-

EXPERT TECHNIQUE

CONDUCTING A SUCCESSFUL INTERVIEW

When conducting your assessment of the pregnant patient, following these steps can help you obtain an accurate and thorough patient history and ensure a successful interview.

Interview setting

Pregnancy is a private matter; therefore, make every effort to interview your patient in a private, quiet setting. Attempting to talk to a pregnant woman in a crowded area, such as a busy waiting room in a clinic, is rarely effective. Remember patient confidentiality and respect the patient's privacy, especially when discussing intimate topics.

Patient history

To ensure that your history is complete, make sure you ask about the patient's:

- overall patterns of health and illness
- medical and surgical history
- history of pregnancy or abortion
- date of last menses and whether it was regular or irregular
- sexual history, including number of partners, frequency, current method of birth control, and satisfaction with chosen method of birth control
- patient's family history
- allergies
- health-related habits, such as smoking and alcohol use.

tural considerations, such as race and religion; marital status; occupation; and education.

Age

The patient's age is an important factor in pregnancy because reproductive risks increase among adolescents younger than age 15 and women older than age 35. For example, pregnant adolescents are more likely to have pregnancy-induced hypertension. Expectant mothers older than age 35 are at risk for other problematic conditions, including placenta previa; hydatidiform mole; and vascular, neoplastic, and degenerative diseases. (See *Recognizing abnormal findings during pregnancy.*)

Race and religion

The patient's race and religion as well as other cultural considerations may also impact a pregnancy. Obtaining information from the patient about these topics aids in planning the patient's care. It also provides greater insight into and an understanding of the patient's behavior, potential problems in health promotion and maintenance, and the patient's ways of coping with illness.

Make sure that you familiarize yourself with the cultural communities in the area and investigate and become knowledgeable about their cultural practices.

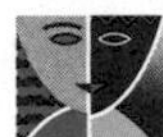

CULTURAL INSIGHT *Encourage the patient to discuss her cultural beliefs regarding health, illness, and health care. Be considerate of the patient's cultural background. Also be aware that members of many cultures are reluctant to talk about sexual matters, and in some cultures, they aren't discussed freely with members of the opposite sex.*

Many women from Southeast Asia (Cambodia, Laos, and Vietnam) don't seek care during pregnancy because they don't believe it's a time when medical intervention is necessary. In many cases, they're extremely modest and may find pelvic examinations embarrassing. They may rely on folk or herbal remedies to manage common discomforts of pregnancy. In addition, they may hold the belief that blood isn't replaceable, which may prevent them from agreeing to laboratory blood studies. Interpreters, classes in prenatal health, and explanations of how health promotion regimens can fit within their cultural belief systems may be necessary.

Because some diseases are more common among certain cultural groups, asking the patient about her race can be an important part of the assessment. For example, a pregnant black woman should be screened for sickle cell trait because this trait primarily occurs in people of African or Mediterranean descent. On the other hand, a Jewish woman of East-

RECOGNIZING ABNORMAL FINDINGS DURING PREGNANCY

When performing a health history and assessment, look for the following abnormal findings to determine if a pregnant patient is at risk for complications.

Obstetric history
- History of infertility
- Grandmultiparity
- Incompetent cervix
- Uterine or cervical anomaly
- Previous preterm labor or preterm birth
- Previous cesarean birth
- Previous infant with macrosomia
- Two or more spontaneous or elective abortions
- Previous hydatidiform mole or choriocarcinoma
- Previous ectopic pregnancy
- Previous stillborn neonate or neonatal death
- Previous multiple gestation
- Previous prolonged labor
- Previous low-birth-weight infant
- Previous midforceps delivery
- Diethylstilbestrol exposure in utero
- Previous infant with neurologic deficit, birth injury, or congenital anomaly
- Less than 1 year since last pregnancy

Medical history
- Cardiac disease
- Metabolic disease
- Renal disease
- Recent urinary tract infection or bacteriuria
- GI disorders
- Seizure disorders
- Family history of severe inherited disorders
- Surgery during pregnancy
- Emotional disorders or mental retardation
- Previous surgeries, particularly those involving the reproductive organs
- Pulmonary disease
- Endocrine disorders
- Hemoglobinopathies
- Sexually transmitted disease (STD)
- Chronic hypertension
- History of abnormal Papanicolaou smear
- Malignancy
- Reproductive tract anomalies

Current obstetric status
- Inadequate prenatal care
- Intrauterine growth restricted fetus
- Large-for-gestational-age fetus
- Preeclampsia
- Abnormal fetal surveillance tests
- Polyhydramnios
- Placenta previa
- Abnormal presentation
- Maternal anemia
- Weight gain of less than 10 lb (4.5 kg)
- Weight loss of more than 5 lb (2.3 kg)
- Overweight or underweight status
- Fetal or placenta malformation
- Rh sensitization
- Preterm labor
- Multiple gestation
- Premature rupture of membranes
- Abruptio placentae
- Postdate pregnancy
- Fibroid tumors
- Fetal manipulation
- Cervical cerclage (purse string suture placed around incompetent cervix to prevent premature opening and subsequent spontaneous abortion)
- STD
- Maternal infection
- Poor immunization status

Psychosocial factors
- Inadequate finances
- Social problems
- Adolescent
- Poor nutrition
- More than two children at home with no additional support
- Lack of acceptance of pregnancy
- Attempt at or ideation of suicide
- Poor housing
- Lack of involvement of baby's father
- Minority status
- Parental occupation
- Inadequate support systems
- Dysfunctional grieving

Demographic factors
- Maternal age younger than 16 or older than 35
- Fewer than 11 years of education

Lifestyle
- Smoking (more than 10 cigarettes per day)
- Substance abuse
- Long commute to work
- Refusal to use seatbelts
- Alcohol consumption
- Heavy lifting or long periods of standing
- Unusual stress
- Lack of smoke detectors in the home

ern European ancestry should be screened for Tay-Sachs disease.

Religious beliefs and practices can also affect the patient's health during pregnancy and can predispose her to complications. For example, Amish women may not be immunized against rubella, putting them at risk. In addition, Seventh-Day Adventists traditionally exclude dairy products from their diets, and Jehovah's Witnesses refuse blood transfusions. Each of these practices could impact prenatal care and the patient's risk of complications.

Marital status

Knowing the patient's marital status may help identify whether family support systems are available. Marital status can also provide information on the size of the patient's home, her sexual practices, and possible stress factors.

Occupation

Ask about the patient's occupation and work environment to assess possible risk factors. If the patient works in a high-risk environment that exposes her to such hazards as chemicals, inhalants, or radiation, inform her of the dangers of these substances as well as the possible effects on her pregnancy. Knowing the patient's occupation can also help to identify such risks as working long hours, lifting heavy objects, and standing for prolonged periods.

Education

The patient's formal education and her life experiences may influence several aspects of the pregnancy, including her attitude toward the pregnancy, her willingness to seek prenatal care, the adequacy of her at-home prenatal care and nutritional status, her knowledge of infant care, and her emotional response to childbirth and the responsibilities of parenting. Information about the patient's education can provide clues to areas requiring patient teaching.

Nutritional history

Adequate nutrition is especially vital during pregnancy. During the prenatal assessment, take a 24-hour diet history, or recall. For more information, see chapter 4, Nutrition.

Medical history

When taking a medical history, find out whether the patient is taking any prescription or over-the-counter drugs. Also ask about her smoking practices, alcohol consumption, and use of illegal drugs.

Many drugs — except drugs with molecules that are too large, such as insulin and heparin — can cross the placenta and affect the fetus. All of the medications the patient is currently taking must be carefully evaluated, and the benefits of each medication should be weighed against the risk to the fetus.

Ask the patient about previous and current medical conditions that may jeopardize the pregnancy. Diabetes can worsen during pregnancy and harm the mother and fetus. Even a woman who has been successfully managing her diabetes may find it challenging during pregnancy because the glucose-insulin regulatory system changes during pregnancy. Every woman appears to develop insulin resistance during pregnancy. In addition, the fetus uses maternal glucose, which may lead to hypoglycemia in the mother. When glucose regulation is poor, the mother is at risk for pregnancy induced hypertension and infection, especially monilial infection. The fetus is at risk for asphyxia and stillbirth. Macrosomia, an abnormally large body, may also occur, resulting in an increased risk of birth complications.

Maternal hypertension, which is more common in women with essential hypertension, renal disease, or diabetes, increases the risk of abruptio placentae. Rubella infection during the first trimester can cause malformation in the developing fetus. Genital herpes can be transmitted to the neonate during birth. A woman with a history of this disease should have cultures done throughout her pregnancy and may require a cesarean delivery to reduce the risk of transmission.

Specific problems that require investigation with the pregnant patient include cardiac disorders, respiratory disorders such as tuberculosis; reproductive disorders, such as sexually transmitted diseases and endometriosis; phlebitis; epilepsy; and gallbladder disorders. Also, ask the patient if she has a history of urinary tract infections, cancer, alcoholism, smoking, drug addiction, or psychiatric problems.

Family history

Knowing the medical histories of the patient's family members can also help plan and guide the assessment by identifying complications for which the patient may be at greater risk. For example, if the patient has a family history of varicose veins, she may inherit a weakness in blood vessel walls that becomes evident when she develops varicosities during pregnancy. Pregnancy induced hypertension has also been shown to have a familial tendency, so a history of this complication in the patient's family members puts her at greater risk. Be sure to ask whether there's a family history of multiple births, congenital diseases or deformities, or mental disability.

When possible, obtain a medical history from the child's father as well. Note that some fetal congenital anomalies may be traced to the father's exposure to environmental hazards.

Gynecologic history

The gynecologic portion of the assessment should include a menstrual history and contraceptive history.

Menstrual history

When obtaining a menstrual history, be sure to ask the patient at what age she began menstruating.

CRITICAL POINT *Age of menarche is important when determining pregnancy risks in adolescents. Pregnancy that occurs within 3 years of menarche indicates an increased risk of maternal and fetal mortality; such a pregnancy also places the patient at risk for delivering a neonate who's small for gestational age. Pregnancy can also occur before regular menses are established.*

Next, ask the patient when her last menses began and how many days there are between the start of one and the start of her next. Find out if her last menses was normal and if the one before that was normal. Ask her what the usual amount and duration of her menstrual flow is. Find out if she has had bleeding or spotting since her last normal menses.

Ask the patient to describe the intensity of her menstrual cramps. If she indicates that her cramps are very painful, anticipatory counseling to prepare for labor may be needed.

Contraceptive history

To obtain a contraceptive history, ask the patient what form of contraception she used before her pregnancy and find out how long she used it. Ask her if she was satisfied with the method and if she experienced any complications while on this type of birth control.

If the patient's method of birth control before becoming pregnant was oral contraceptives, also inquire about how long it was between when the patient ceased taking oral contraceptives and when she became pregnant. A woman whose pregnancy results from contraceptive failure needs special attention to ensure her medical and emotional well-being. Because the pregnancy wasn't planned, the woman may have emotional and financial issues.

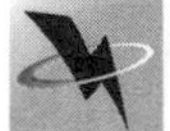

CRITICAL POINT *If the patient has an intrauterine device (IUD) in place, be aware of the risk of spontaneous abortion or preterm labor and delivery. If she becomes pregnant with an IUD in place, the device should be removed immediately by a health care provider.*

Obstetric history

Obtaining an obstetric history is another important part of the assessment. The obstetric history gives important information about the patient's past pregnancies. No matter how old the patient is, don't assume that this is her first pregnancy. (See *Pregnancy classification system,* page 540.)

The obstetric history should include specific details about past pregnancies, including whether the patient had difficult or long labors and whether she experienced complications. Make sure you document each child's sex and the location and date of birth. Always record the patient's obstetric history chronologically. For a list of the types of information you should include in a complete obstetric history, see *Taking an obstetric history,* page 540.

In addition to asking about pregnancy history, ask the woman if she knows her blood type. If the woman's blood type is

PREGNANCY CLASSIFICATION SYSTEM

When referring to a patient's obstetric and pregnancy history, use these terms:
- Primigravida — a woman who's pregnant for the first time
- Primipara — a woman who has delivered one child past the age of viability
- Multigravida — a woman who has been pregnant before but didn't necessarily carry to term
- Multipara — a woman who has carried two or more pregnancies to viability
- Nulligravida — a woman who has never been and isn't currently pregnant

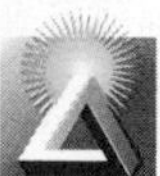

EXPERT TECHNIQUE

TAKING AN OBSTETRIC HISTORY

When taking the pregnant patient's obstetric history, make sure you ask her about:
- genital tract anomalies
- medications used during this pregnancy
- history of hepatitis, pelvic inflammatory disease, acquired immunodeficiency syndrome, blood transfusions, and herpes or other sexually transmitted diseases (STDs)
- partner's history of STDs
- previous abortions
- history of infertility.

Pregnancy history

Also ask the patient about past pregnancies. Make sure you note the number of past full-term and preterm pregnancies and obtain the following information about each of the patient's past pregnancies, if applicable:
- Planned pregnancies
- Complications, such as spotting, swelling of the hands and feet, surgery, or falls
- Medications (type, duration, and reason for taking)
- Prenatal care and when it began
- Pregnancy's duration
- Overall experience of pregnancy

Birth and postpartum history

Also obtain the following information about the birth and postpartum condition of previous pregnancies:
- Labor's duration
- Type of birth
- Type of anesthesia, if any
- Complications during pregnancy or labor
- Birthplace, condition, sex, weight, and Rh factor of the neonate
- Labor expectations and if labor was better or worse than expected
- Stitches after birth
- Condition of the infant after birth
- Infant's Apgar score
- Special care for the infant, if needed and, if so, what type
- Neonate problems during the first several days after birth
- Child's present state of health
- Infant's discharge from the heath care facility and if it was with the mother
- Postpartum problems

Rh-negative, ask if she received Rh immune globulin (RhoGAM) after miscarriages, abortions, or previous births to determine if Rh sensitization occurred. If she didn't receive RhoGAM after any of these situations, her present pregnancy may be at risk for Rh sensitization. Also ask if she has ever had a blood transfusion to establish possible risk of hepatitis B and human immunodeficiency virus exposure.

GRAVIDA AND PARA CLASSIFICATION SYSTEMS

Various classification systems have been developed to provide accurate information about a woman's obstetric history. Three of the most common systems—TPAL, GTPAL, and GTPALM—are described here.

TPAL

In TPAL, the most basic of the three systems, the patient is assigned a four-digit number as follows:

- T is the number of full-term infants born (those born at 37 weeks or later).
- P is the number of preterm infants born (those born before 37 weeks).
- A is the number of spontaneous or induced abortions.
- L is the number of living children.

Note that the patient's gravida number remains the same, but the TPAL system allows subclassification of the patient's para status. In most cases, a health care provider includes the patient's gravida status in addition to her TPAL number. Here are some examples:

- A woman who has had two previous pregnancies, has delivered two term children, and is pregnant again is a gravida 3 and is assigned a TPAL of 2-0-0-2.
- A woman who has had two abortions at 12 weeks (under the age of viability) and is pregnant again is a gravida 3 and is assigned a TPAL of 0-0-2-0.
- A woman who's pregnant for the sixth time, has delivered four term children and one preterm child, and has had one spontaneous abortion and one elective abortion is a gravida 6 and is assigned a TPAL of 4-1-2-5.

GTPAL and GTPALM

More comprehensive systems for classifying pregnancy status include the GTPAL and GTPALM systems. In the GTPAL system, the patient's gravida status is incorporated into her TPAL number. In GTPALM, a number is added to the GTPAL to represent the number of multiple pregnancies the patient has experienced (M). Note that a patient who hasn't given birth to multiple pregnancies doesn't receive a number to represent M. These classification tools provide greater detail about the patient's pregnancy history. For example:

- If a woman has had two previous pregnancies, has delivered two term children, and is currently pregnant, she's assigned a GTPAL of 3-2-0-0-2.
- If a woman who's pregnant with twins delivers at 35 weeks' gestation and both of the neonates survive, she's classified as a gravida 1, para 0-2-0-2 and is assigned a GTPAL of 1-0-2-0-2. Using the GTPALM system, the same woman would be identified as 1-0-2-0-2-1.

Two important components of a patient's obstetric history are her gravida and para status. Gravida represents the number of times the patient has been pregnant. Para refers to the number of children above the age of viability the patient has delivered. The age of viability is the earliest time at which a fetus can survive outside the womb, generally at age 24 weeks or a weight of more than 400 g. These two pieces of information are important but provide only the most rudimentary information about the patient's obstetric history.

A slightly more informative system reflects the gravida and para numbers and includes the number of abortions in the patient's history. For example, G-3, P-2, Ab-1 describes a patient who has been pregnant three times, has had two deliveries after 20 weeks' gestation, and has had one abortion. In an attempt to provide more detailed information about the patient's obstetric history, many facilities now use one of the following classification systems: TPAL, GTPAL, or GTPALM. These systems involve the assignment of numbers to various aspects of a patient's obstetric past. They offer health care providers a way to quickly obtain fairly comprehensive information about obstetric history. In particular, these systems offer more detailed information about the patient's para history. (See *Gravida and para classification systems.*)

If the patient is a multigravida, ask about complications that affected her previous pregnancies. A woman who has delivered one or more large neonates (more than 9 lb [4.1 kg]) or who has a history of recurrent Candida infections or unexplained unsuccessful pregnancies should be screened for obesity and a family history of diabetes. A history of recurrent second-trimester abortions may indicate an incompetent cervix.

Estimating date of delivery

Based on the information obtained in the patient's menstrual history, calculate the patient's estimated date of delivery using Nägele's rule: first day of last normal menses, minus 3 months, plus 7 days.

Because Nägele's rule is based on a 28-day cycle, you may need to vary the calculation for a woman whose menstrual cycle is irregular, prolonged, or shortened.

Physical assessment

Physical assessment should occur throughout pregnancy, starting with the pregnant patient's first prenatal visit and continuing through labor, delivery, and the postpartum period. Physical assessment includes evaluation of maternal and fetal well-being. At each assessment stage, keep in mind the interdependence of the mother and fetus. Changes in the mother's health may affect fetal health, and changes in fetal health may affect the mother's physical and emotional health.

At the first prenatal visit, measurements of height and weight establish baselines for the patient and allow comparison with expected values throughout the pregnancy. Vital signs, including blood pressure, respiratory rate, and pulse rate, are also measured for baseline assessment.

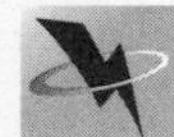

CRITICAL POINT *Monitoring vital signs, especially blood pressure, during each prenatal visit is a key aspect of prenatal assessment. A sudden increase in blood pressure is a danger sign of gestational hypertension or pregnancy-induced hypertension (PIH). Likewise a sudden decrease in pulse or respiratory rate may suggest bleeding, such as in an early placenta previa or an abruption.*

Prenatal care visits are usually scheduled every 4 weeks for the first 28 weeks of pregnancy, every 2 weeks until the 36th week, and then weekly until delivery, which usually occurs between weeks 38 and 42. Women who have known risk factors for complications and those who develop complications during the pregnancy require more frequent visits. (See *Assessing pregnancy by trimester.*)

Regular prenatal visits usually consist of weight measurements, vital sign checks, palpation of the abdomen, and fundal height checks. You should also assess the patient for preterm labor symptoms, fetal heart tones, and edema. Also, be sure to ask her if she has felt her baby move.

Before beginning the physical assessment, have the patient undress, put on a gown, and empty her bladder. Emptying the bladder makes the pelvic examination more comfortable, allows for easier identification of pelvic organs, and provides a urine specimen for laboratory testing.

Head-to-toe assessment

A thorough physical assessment should include evaluation of the patient's general appearance, head and scalp, eyes, nose, ears, mouth, neck, breasts, heart, lungs, back, rectum, and extremities and skin.

General appearance

Inspect the patient's general appearance. This helps form an impression of her overall health and well-being. The manner in which a patient dresses and speaks, in addition to her body posture, can reveal how she feels about herself. Also inspect for signs of spousal abuse.

Head and scalp

Examine the head and scalp for symmetry, normal contour, and tenderness. Check the hair for distribution, thickness, dryness or oiliness, and use of hair dye. Look for chloasma, an extra pigment on the face that may accompany pregnancy. Dryness or sparseness of hair suggests poor nutrition. Lack of cleanliness suggests fatigue.

Eyes

Carefully inspect the eyes. Look for edema in the eyelids. Ask the patient if she ever sees spots before her eyes or has diplopia (double vision) or other vision problems. These

ASSESSING PREGNANCY BY TRIMESTER

The first trimester includes weeks 1 to 12; the second trimester, weeks 13 to 27. The third trimester begins at week 28.

Weeks 1 to 4
- Amenorrhea occurs.
- Breasts begin to change.
- Immunologic pregnancy tests become positive: Radioimmunoassay test results are positive a few days after implantation; urine human chorionic gonadotropin test results are positive 10 to 14 days after amenorrhea occurs.
- Nausea and vomiting begin between the fourth and sixth weeks.

Weeks 5 to 8
- Goodell's sign occurs, involving the softening of cervix and vagina.
- Ladin's sign occurs, involving the softening of uterine isthmus.
- Hegar's sign occurs, involving the softening of lower uterine segment.
- Chadwick's sign appears with purple-blue coloration of the vagina, cervix, and vulva.
- McDonald's sign appears with easy flexion of the fundus toward the cervix.
- Braun von Fernwald's sign occurs with irregular softening and enlargement of the uterine fundus at the site of implantation.
- Piskacek's sign may occur with asymmetrical softening and enlargement of the uterus.
- The cervical mucus plug forms.
- Uterus changes from pear shape to globular.
- Urinary frequency and urgency occur.

Weeks 9 to 12
- Fetal heartbeat detected using ultrasonic stethoscope.
- Nausea, vomiting, and urinary frequency and urgency lessen.
- By the 12th week, the uterus is palpable just above the symphysis pubis.

Weeks 13 to 17
- Pregnant patient gains 10 to 12 lb (4.5 to 5.5 kg) during the second trimester.
- Uterine soufflé is heard on auscultation.
- Pregnant patient's heartbeat increases by about 10 beats/minute between 14 and 30 weeks' gestation. Rate is maintained until 40 weeks' gestation.
- By the 16th week, the pregnant patient's thyroid gland enlarges by about 25%, and the uterine fundus is palpable halfway between the symphysis pubis and the umbilicus.
- Maternal recognition of fetal movements, or quickening, occurs between 16 and 20 weeks' gestation.

Weeks 18 to 22
- Uterine fundus is palpable just below the umbilicus.
- Fetal heartbeats are heard with fetoscope at 20 weeks' gestation.
- Fetal rebound or ballottement is possible.

Weeks 23 to 27
- Umbilicus appears to be level with abdominal skin.
- Striae gravidarum are usually apparent.
- Uterine fundus is palpable at the umbilicus.
- Shape of uterus changes from globular to ovoid.
- Braxton Hicks contractions begin.

Weeks 28 to 31
- Pregnant patient gains 8 to 10 lb (3.5 to 4.5 kg) in third trimester.
- The uterine wall feels soft and yielding.
- The uterine fundus is halfway between the umbilicus and xiphoid process.
- Fetal outline is palpable.
- The fetus is mobile and may be found in any position.

(continued)

ASSESSING PREGNANCY BY TRIMESTER *(continued)*

Weeks 32 to 35
- The pregnant patient may experience heartburn.
- Striae gravidarum become more evident.
- The uterine fundus is palpable just below the xiphoid process.
- Braxton Hicks contractions increase in frequency and intensity.
- The pregnant patient may experience shortness of breath.

Weeks 36 to 40
- The umbilicus protrudes.
- Varicosities, if present, become very pronounced.
- Ankle edema is evident.
- Urinary frequency recurs.
- Engagement, or lightening, occurs.
- The mucus plug is expelled.
- Cervical effacement and dilation begin.

assessment findings may indicate PIH. Also perform an ophthalmoscopic examination, which may reveal that the optic disk appears swollen from edema associated with this condition.

Nose
Inspect the nose for nasal congestion and nasal membrane swelling, which may result from increased estrogen levels. If these conditions occur, advise the patient to avoid using topical medicines and nose sprays for relief. These medications can be absorbed into the bloodstream and may harm the fetus.

Ears
During early pregnancy, nasal stuffiness may lead to blocked eustachian tubes, which can cause a feeling of fullness and dampening of sound. This disappears as the body adjusts to the new estrogen level.

Mouth
Examine the inside and outside of the mouth. Cracked corners may reveal a vitamin A deficiency. Pinpoint lesions with an erythematous base on the lips suggest herpes infection. Gingival hypertrophy may result from estrogen stimulation during pregnancy; the gums may be slightly swollen and tender to the touch.

Neck
Inspect and palpate the neck. Palpate the thyroid gland. Slight thyroid hypertrophy may occur during pregnancy because overall metabolic rate is increased. Lymph nodes normally aren't palpable and, if enlarged, may indicate an infection.

Breasts
Inspect and palpate the breasts, noting any changes in skin color or appearance or evidence of nodules or lumps. During pregnancy, the areolae may darken, breast size increases, and breasts become firmer. Blue streaking of veins may occur on the breasts. Colostrum may be expressed as early as 16 weeks' gestation. Montgomery's tubercles may become more prominent.

Heart
Assess the patient's heart rate, which should range from 70 to 80 beats per minute. Occasionally, a benign functional heart murmur that's caused by increased vascular volume may be auscultated. If this occurs, the patient needs further evaluation to ensure that the condition is only a physiologic change related to the pregnancy and not a previously undetected heart condition.

Lungs
Assess respiratory rate and rhythm. Vital capacity, the amount of air that can be exhaled after maximum inspiration, shouldn't be reduced despite the fact that lung tissue assumes a more horizontal appearance as the growing uterus pushes up on the diaphragm. Auscultate breath sounds for changes. Assess diaphragmatic excursion. Late in pregnancy, diaphragmatic excursion, or diaphragm movement, is reduced because the diaphragm can't descend as fully as usual because of the distended uterus.

Back

When examining the patient's back, assess for scoliosis. If she has scoliosis, refer her to an orthopedic surgeon to make sure the condition doesn't worsen during pregnancy. Typically, the lumbar curve is accentuated when standing so the patient can maintain body posture in the face of increasing abdominal size. If she has scoliosis, however, the added pressure of the growing fetus on the back may be more bothersome and painful.

Rectum

Assess the rectum for hemorrhoidal tissue, which commonly results from pelvic pressure that prevents venous return.

Extremities and skin

Assess for palmar erythema, an itchy redness in the palms that occurs early in pregnancy as a result of high estrogen levels. Assess for varicose veins and check the filling time of nail beds. Observe for edema, and assess the patient's gait. Proper posture and walking are important to prevent musculoskeletal and gait problems later in pregnancy.

Pelvic examination

A pelvic examination provides information on the health of internal and external reproductive organs and is valuable in assessment.

Take these steps to prepare the patient for the pelvic examination:

- Ask the patient if she has douched within the past 24 hours. Explain that douching can wash away cells and organisms that the examination is designed to evaluate.
- For the patient's comfort, instruct her to empty her bladder before the examination. Provide a urine specimen container if needed.
- To help the patient relax, which is essential for a thorough pelvic examination, explain what the examination entails and why it's necessary. The patient may desire to have a person in the room with her for support. It may also be beneficial to review some relaxation techniques with the patient such as deep breathing.
- If the patient is scheduled for a Papanicolaou (Pap) test, inform her that she may have to return later for another test if the findings of the first test aren't conclusive. Reassure her that this is done to confirm the results of the first test. If she has never had a Pap test, tell her that the test shouldn't hurt.
- Explain to the patient that a bimanual examination is performed to assess the size and location of the ovaries and uterus.

After the examination, offer the patient premoistened tissues to clean the vulva. See chapter 14, Female genitourinary system, for more information about pelvic examination.

Fundal assessment

At about 12 to 14 weeks' gestation, the uterus is palpable over the symphysis pubis as a firm globular sphere. It reaches the umbilicus at 20 to 22 weeks, the xiphoid at 36 weeks, and then, in many cases, returns to about 4 cm below the xiphoid due to lightening at 40 weeks. (See *Measuring fundal height,* page 546.)

If the woman is past 12 weeks of pregnancy, palpate fundus location, measure fundal height from the notch above the symphysis pubis to the superior aspect of the uterine fundus, and plot the height on a graph. This information helps detect variations in fetal growth. If an abnormality is detected, further investigation with ultrasound can determine the cause.

During the pelvic examination, record the patient's uterine fundal height and fetal heart sounds. Compare the new fundal height findings with the information obtained in the patient's history. In other words, make sure that the information obtained about the patient's last menses and her estimated date of delivery correlate with the current fundal height.

Estimation of pelvic size

The size and shape of a woman's pelvis can affect her ability to deliver her neonate vaginally. It's impossible to predict from a woman's outward appearance if her pelvis is adequate for the passage of a fetus. For example, a woman may look as if she has a wide pelvis, but she may only have a wide iliac crest and a normal, or smaller than normal, internal ring. (See *Pelvic shape and potential problems,* page 547.)

Internal pelvic measurements give diameters of the inlet and outlet through which the fetus passes. The internal pelvis must be

(Text continues on page 548.)

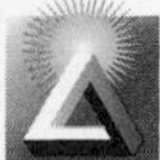

EXPERT TECHNIQUE

MEASURING FUNDAL HEIGHT

The height of the uterus above the symphysis pubis reflects the progress of fetal growth, provides a gross estimate of the duration of pregnancy, and may indicate intrauterine growth retardation. Excessive increase in fundal height could mean multiple pregnancy or hydramnios, an excess of amniotic fluid.

To measure fundal height, use a pliable tape measure or pelvimeter to measure from the notch of the symphysis pubis to the top of the fundus, without tipping back the corpus. During the second and third trimesters, make the measurement more precise by using the following calculation, known as McDonald's rule:

height of fundus (in centimeters) × 8/7
= duration of pregnancy in weeks.

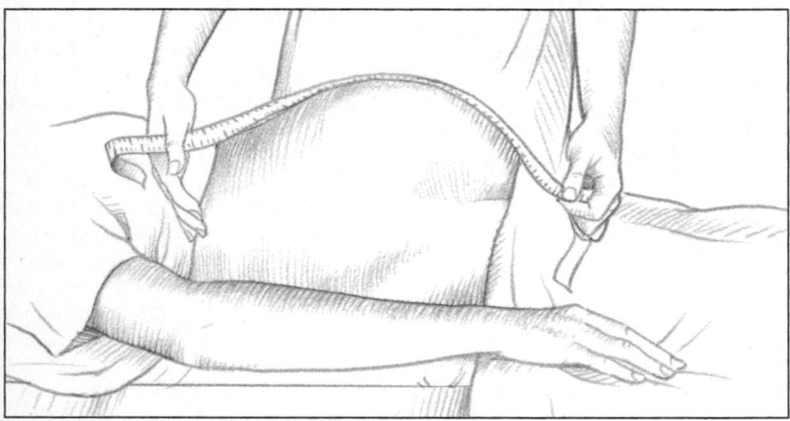

The illustration here shows the approximate fundal heights at various times, indicated by weeks, during pregnancy. Note that between weeks 38 and 40, the fetus begins to descend into the pelvis.

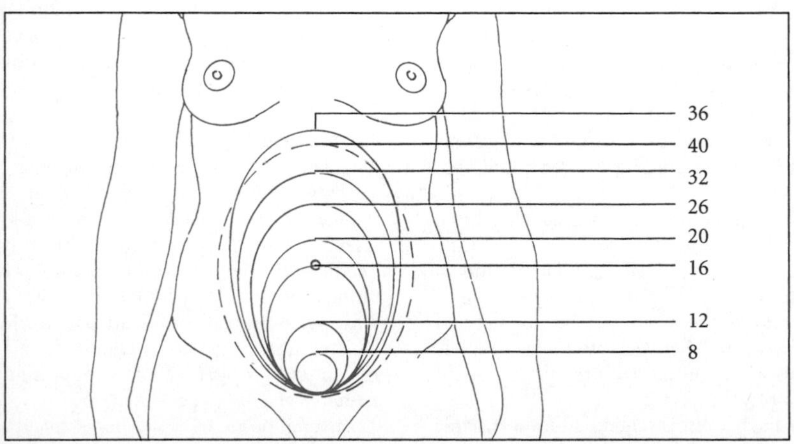

PELVIC SHAPE AND POTENTIAL PROBLEMS

The shape of a woman's pelvis can affect the delivery of her fetus. Four types of pelvic shapes along with the problems that can arise are described here.

Android pelvis
In an android pelvis, the pelvic arch forms an acute triangle, making the lower dimensions of the pelvis extremely narrow. A pelvis of this shape is typically associated with males, but can also occur in women. A pregnant woman with this pelvic shape may experience difficulty delivering the fetus because the narrow shape makes it difficult for the fetus to exit.

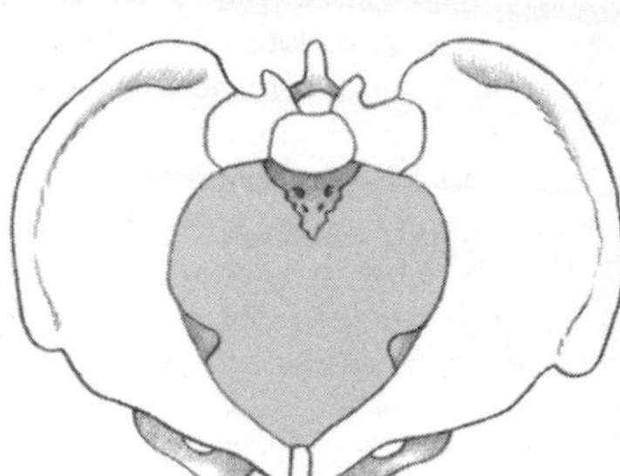

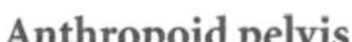

Anthropoid pelvis
In an anthropoid pelvis, also known as an apelike pelvis, the transverse diameter is narrow and the inlet's anteroposterior diameter is larger than normal. This pelvic shape doesn't accommodate a fetal head as well as a gynecoid pelvis because the transverse diameter is narrow.

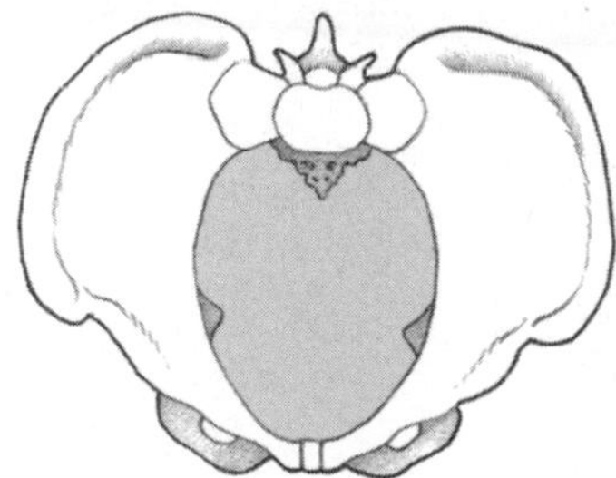

Gynecoid pelvis
In a gynecoid pelvis, the inlets are well rounded in the forward and backward diameters and the pubic arch is wide. This type of pelvis is ideal for childbirth.

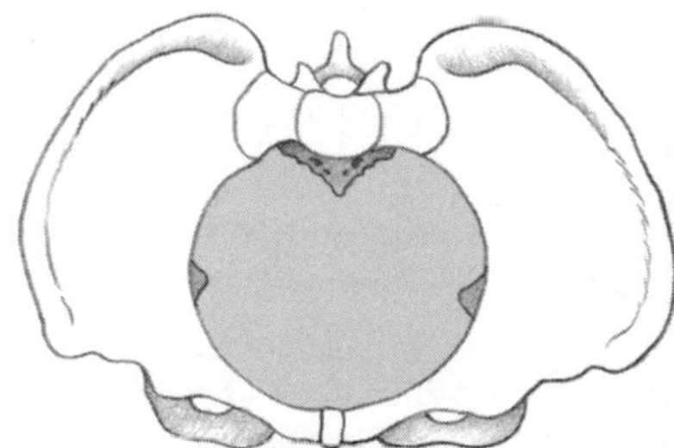

Platypelloid pelvis
In a platypelloid, or flattened, pelvis, the inlet is oval and smoothly curved but the anteroposterior diameter is shallow. Problems may occur during childbirth for a patient with this pelvic shape if the fetal head can't rotate to match the spine's curves because the anteroposterior diameter is shallow and the pelvis is flat.

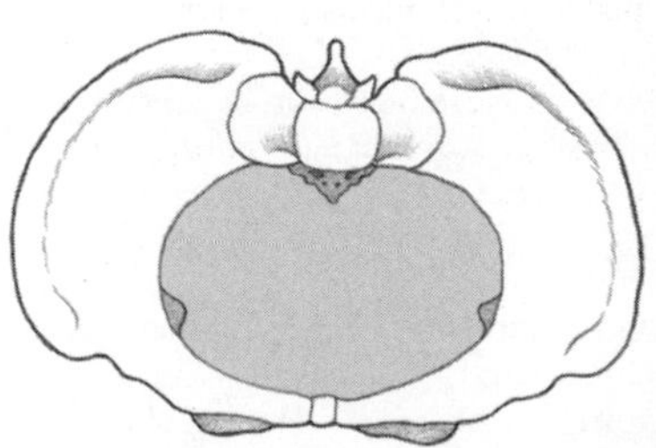

EXPERT TECHNIQUE

MEASURING DIAGONAL CONJUGATE

Measure the diagonal conjugate while the female patient is in the lithotomy position. Place two fingers of your examining hand in the vagina and press inward and upward until the middle finger touches the sacral prominence. (The woman may feel the pressure of the examining finger.) Use your other hand to mark the location where your examining hand touches the symphysis pubis. After withdrawing your examining hand, measure the distance between the tip of the middle finger and the marked point with a ruler or a pelvimeter.

If your examining hand is small with short fingers, the fingers may not reach the sacral prominence, making manual pelvic measurements impossible.

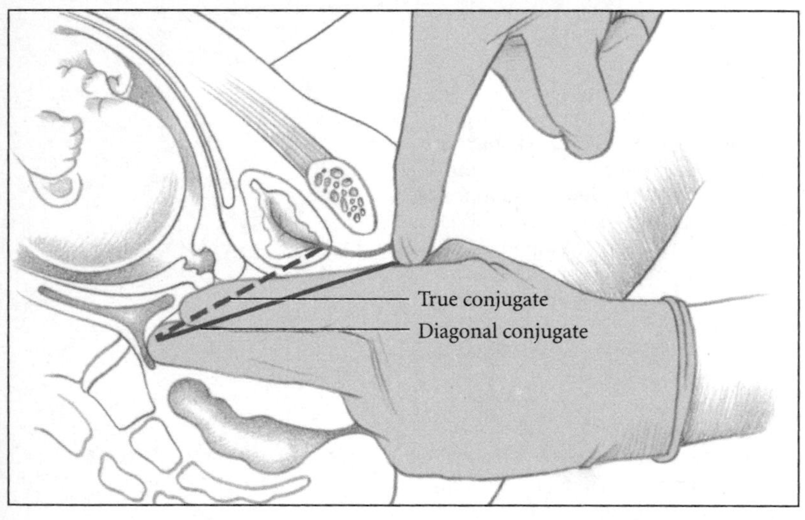

large enough to allow a patient to give birth vaginally without difficulty. Differences in pelvic contour develop mainly because of heredity factors. However, such diseases as rickets may cause contraction of the pelvis, and pelvic injury may also be responsible for pelvic distortion.

Pelvic measurements can be taken at the initial visit or at a visit later in pregnancy, when the woman's pelvic muscles are more relaxed. If a routine ultrasound is scheduled, estimations of pelvic size may be made through a combination of pelvimetry and fetal ultrasound.

Estimation of pelvic adequacy should be done by the 24th week of pregnancy because, by this time, a danger exists that the fetal head will reach a size that interferes with safe passage and birth if the pelvic measurements are small. In this case, the woman should be advised that she may not be able to deliver her fetus vaginally and may require a cesarean delivery. If a woman has already given birth vaginally, her pelvis has proven to be adequate. Measuring the pelvis again isn't necessary unless trauma occurred to the pelvis after her last vaginal birth.

Diagonal conjugate. The diagonal conjugate is the distance between the anterior surface of the sacral prominence and the anterior surface of the inferior margin of the symphysis pubis. It's the most useful gauge of pelvic size because it indicates the anteroposterior diameter of the pelvic inlet,

EXPERT TECHNIQUE

MEASURING SUBPUBIC ARCH AND TRANSVERSE DIAMETER

Measuring the subpubic arch and pelvic outlet provides additional information to determine the adequacy of the pelvis for vaginal delivery.

Measuring the subpubic arch

To measure the subpubic arch, place both hands with the thumbs up at the inferior margin of the symphysis pubis in the perineum. The thumbs should be touching. Both hands should fit comfortably and form an angle that's greater than 90 degrees.

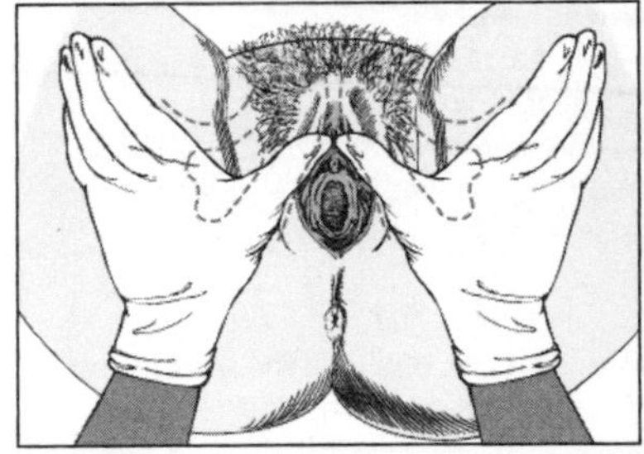

Measuring the transverse diameter

To measure the transverse diameter with a clenched fist, first measure the width of the knuckles (span of the fist) to provide an approximate baseline measurement for comparison. Next, insert the fist between the ischial tuberosities at the level of the anus. If the knuckles are a width of 10 cm or more, and they fit adequately, then the pelvic outlet is considered to be adequate. Typically, a diameter of 10 to 11 cm is considered adequate to allow the widest part of the fetal head to pass through the outlet.

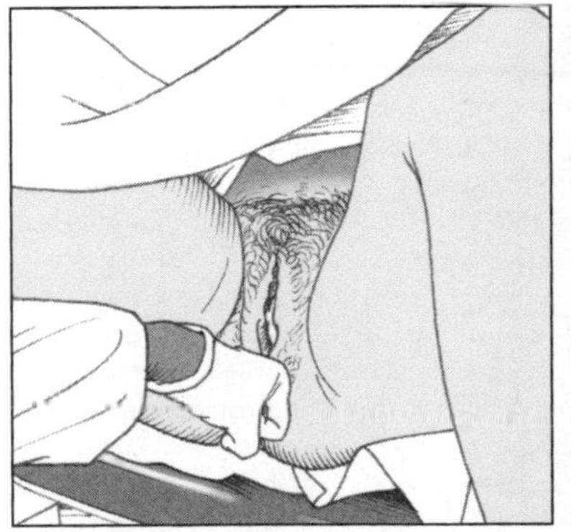

the narrower diameter. (See *Measuring diagonal conjugate.*)

If the measurement obtained is more than 12.7 cm, the pelvic inlet is considered adequate for childbirth (the diameter of the fetal head that must pass that point averages 9 cm).

True conjugate. The true conjugate, also known as the *conjugate vera,* is the measurement between the anterior surface of the sacral prominence and the posterior surface of the inferior margin of the symphysis pubis. The true conjugate reflects the diameter of the pelvic inlet through which the fetal head must pass. This measurement can't be made directly but is estimated from the measurement of the diagonal conjugate and an assumed measurement of the depth of the symphysis pubis, assumed to be 1 to 2 cm.

To determine the true conjugate, subtract the depth of the symphysis pubis from the diagonal conjugate measurement. On average, the true conjugate diameter ranges from 10.5 to 11 cm.

Angle of subpubic arch. The subpubic arch refers to the inferior margin of the symphysis pubis. Estimating the angle also aids in determining the pelvic adequacy for a vaginal birth. (See *Measuring subpubic arch and transverse diameter.*)

Transverse diameter. The transverse diameter, also known as the *ischial tuberosity di-*

ameter is the distance between the ischial tuberosities. It's the narrowest diameter at that point and the one diameter that commonly leads to problems with delivery. A pelvimeter can be used to obtain an accurate measurement. However, the diameter can be estimated by using a ruler or your clenched fist or hand for which the measurement is known.

CRITICAL POINT *When using the clenched fist to estimate the transverse diameter, measure the span of the fist before using it to obtain the transverse diameter.*

Fetal assessment

Fetal assessment typically involves monitoring fetal heart rate (FHR) and fetal activity.

Fetal heart rate

Obtain an FHR by placing a fetoscope or Doppler stethoscope on the mother's abdomen and counting fetal heartbeats. Simultaneously palpating the mother's pulse helps to avoid confusion between maternal and fetal heartbeats. A fetoscope can detect fetal heartbeats as early as 20 weeks' gestation. The Doppler ultrasound stethoscope, a more sensitive instrument, can detect fetal heartbeats as early as 10 weeks' gestation and remains a useful tool throughout labor. (See *Evaluating FHR.*)

To determine the FHR of a fetus who's less than 20 weeks old, place the head of the Doppler stethoscope at the midline of the patient's abdomen above the pubic hairline. After the 20th week of pregnancy, when fetal position can be determined, palpate for the back of the fetal thorax and position the instrument directly over it. Locate the loudest heartbeats and palpate the maternal pulse. Count fetal heartbeats for at least 15 seconds while monitoring maternal pulse. Use Leopold's maneuvers to determine fetal position, presentation, and attitude. (See *Performing Leopold's maneuvers,* pages 552 and 553.)

Because FHR usually ranges from 120 to 160 beats per minute, auscultation yields only an average rate at best. It can detect gross, but commonly late, signs of fetal distress, such as tachycardia and bradycardia, and is thus recommended only for a patient with an uncomplicated pregnancy. For a patient with a high-risk pregnancy, indirect or direct fetal monitoring provides more accurate information on fetal status.

Fetal activity

The activity of the fetus, or kick counts, determines its condition in utero. Daily evaluation of movement by the mother provides an inexpensive, noninvasive way of assessing fetal well-being. Decreased activity in a previously active fetus may reflect a disturbance in placental function.

As early as 7 weeks' gestation, the embryo can produce spontaneous movements; however, these movements don't become apparent to the mother until sometime between the 14th and 26th weeks, but generally between weeks 18 and 22. The first fetal movement noticeable by the mother is called quickening. The acknowledgment of fetal movements may be delayed if the due date is miscalculated or if the mother doesn't recognize the sensation. A patient who has had a baby before is likely to recognize movement earlier. If the mother hasn't felt any movements by the 22nd week, an ultrasound may be necessary to assess the fetus's condition.

Fetal movements may be elicited by having the patient lie down for about an hour after having a glass of milk or another snack. The jolt of energy produced by a light snack commonly produces fetal movement. After the 28th week, patients are usually asked to monitor fetal movements twice daily—once in the morning, when activity tends to be sparser, and once in the more-active evening hours. Instruct the patient to check the clock when she's ready to start counting fetal movements. She should count movements of any kind including kicks, flutters, swishes, and rolls. After she counts 10 movements, she should note the time again.

CRITICAL POINT *If the patient doesn't feel 10 movements after 30 minutes, she should eat another snack and then count for another 30 minutes. If the patient feels no movement or less than 10 movements after the second 30-minute period, she should contact the health care provider. The closer the patient is to her due date, the more important regular checking of fetal movements becomes.*

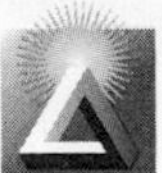

EXPERT TECHNIQUE

EVALUATING FHR

To evaluate fetal heart rate (FHR), position the fetoscope or Doppler ultrasound stethoscope on the patient's abdomen, midway between the umbilicus and symphysis pubis for cephalic presentation, or above or at the level of the umbilicus for breech presentation. Locate the loudest heartbeats, and palpate the maternal pulse. Monitor maternal pulse and count fetal heartbeats for 60 seconds.

Fetoscope
A fetoscope is a modified stethoscope attached to a headpiece. A fetoscope can detect fetal heartbeats as early as 20 weeks' gestation.

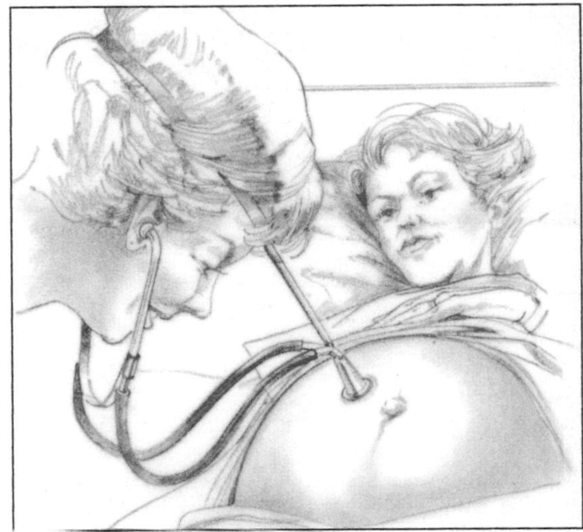

Doppler stethoscope
A Doppler stethoscope uses ultrasound waves that bounce off the fetal heart to produce echoes or a clicking noise that reflect the rate of the fetal heartbeat. Detecting fetal heartbeats as early as 10 weeks' gestation, the Doppler stethoscope has greater sensitivity than the fetoscope.

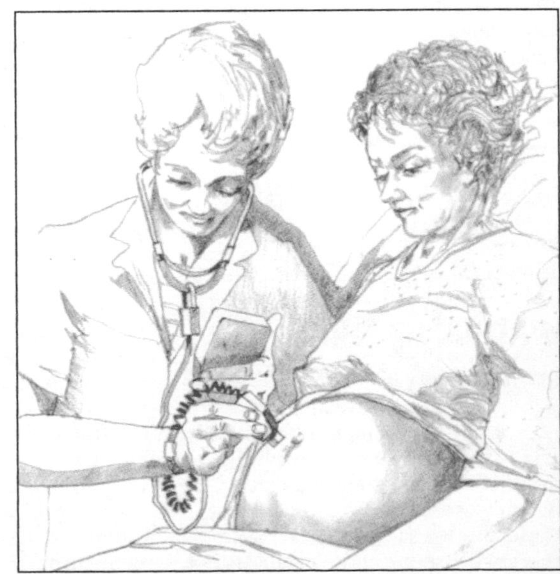

EXPERT TECHNIQUE

PERFORMING LEOPOLD'S MANEUVERS

You can determine fetal position, presentation, and attitude by performing Leopold's maneuvers. Ask the patient to empty her bladder, assist her to a supine position, and expose her abdomen. Then perform the following four maneuvers in order.

First maneuver

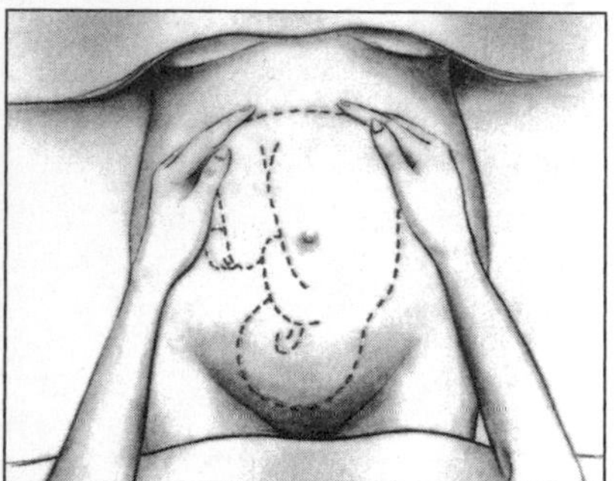

Face the patient and warm your hands. Place your hands on the patient's abdomen to determine fetal position in the uterine fundus. Curl your fingers around the fundus. When the fetus is in the vertex position, with the head first, the buttocks should feel irregularly shaped and firm. When the fetus is in breech position, the head should feel hard, round, and movable.

Second maneuver

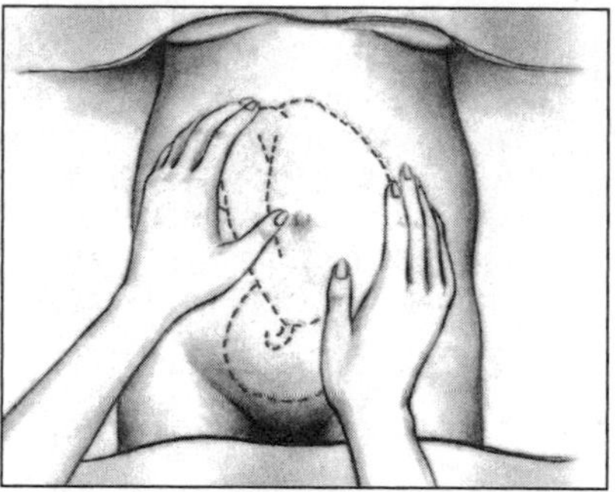

Move your hands down the side of the abdomen, applying gentle pressure. If the fetus is in the vertex position, you'll feel a smooth, hard surface on one side — the fetal back. Opposite, you'll feel lumps and knobs — the knees, hands, feet, and elbows. If the fetus is in the breech position, you may not feel the back at all.

Abnormal findings

Although pregnancy is considered a state of wellness, problems can develop that place the patient at risk for complications. While assessing a pregnant patient, carefully listen to what the patient is saying. A pregnant woman may not mention her concerns or discomforts unless she's specifically asked because she isn't aware of the significance of her problems or she's reluctant to take up a lot of time during a prenatal visit. Encourage the patient to discuss whatever concerns she has at her visits.

Common discomforts during the first trimester associated with pregnancy include nausea and vomiting, urinary frequency, breast tenderness, fatigue, and increased vaginal discharge that's white.

During the second and third trimesters, common discomforts include indigestion, ankle edema, varicose veins, hemorrhoids, constipation, backache, leg cramps, short-

Third maneuver

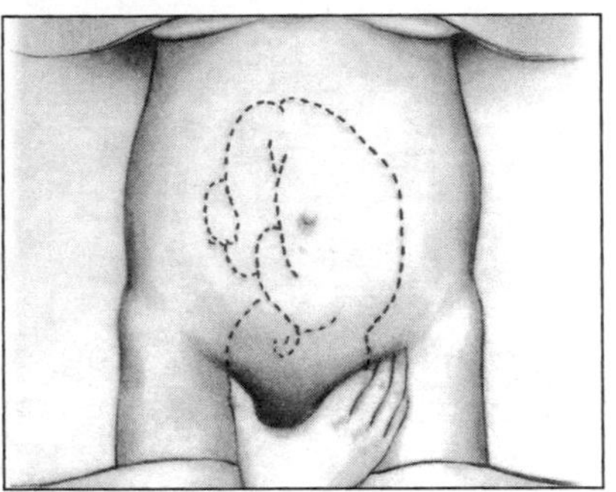

Spread apart your thumb and fingers of one hand. Place them just above the patient's symphysis pubis. Bring your fingers together. If the fetus is in the vertex position and hasn't descended, you'll feel the head. If the fetus is in the vertex position and has descended, you'll feel a less distinct mass. If the fetus is in the breech position, you'll also feel a less distinct mass, which could be the feet or knees.

Fourth maneuver

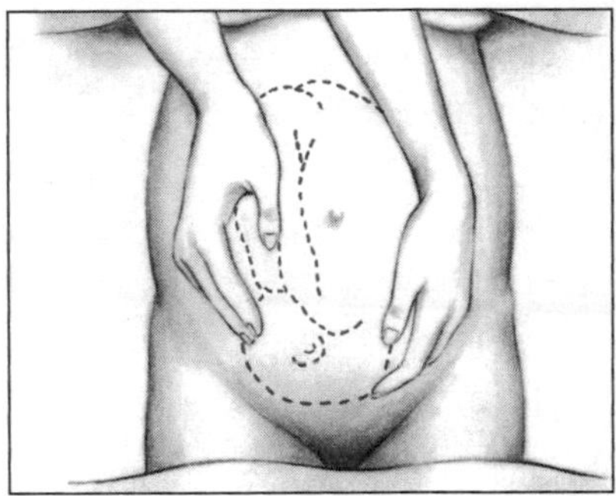

The fourth maneuver can determine flexion or extension of the fetal head and neck. Place your hands on both sides of the lower abdomen. Apply gentle pressure with your fingers as you slide your hands downward, toward the symphysis pubis. If the head is the presenting fetal part (rather than the feet or a shoulder), one of your hands is stopped by the cephalic prominence. The other hand descends unobstructed more deeply. If the fetus is in the vertex position, you'll feel the cephalic prominence on the same side as the small parts; if it's in the face position, on the same side as the back. If the fetus is engaged, you won't be able to feel the cephalic prominence.

ness of breath, insomnia, and abdominal discomfort and Braxton Hicks contractions.

Although the common discomforts are associated with normal pregnancy, others may be early indicators of potential problems. The patient may seek care for several signs and symptoms related to the pregnancy that are considered danger signs. The most significant findings are bleeding, vaginal; blood pressure, elevated; fetal movement, decreased; fever; pain, abdominal or chest; sudden gush of clear vaginal fluid; and vomiting, persistent. The following history, physical assessment, and analysis summaries will help you assess each one quickly and accurately. After obtaining further information, begin to interpret the findings. (See *The pregnant patient: Interpreting your findings,* pages 554 to 557.)

Bleeding, vaginal

Vaginal bleeding at any time during a pregnancy is a potential danger sign that requires further investigation. The bleeding

(Text continues on page 557.)

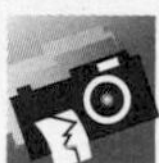

CLINICAL PICTURE

THE PREGNANT PATIENT: INTERPRETING YOUR FINDINGS

After you assess the pregnant patient, a group of findings may lead you to suspect a particular disorder. The chart below shows some common groups of findings for major signs and symptoms related to pregnancy, along with their probable causes.

Sign or symptom and findings	Probable cause
Bleeding, vaginal	
Marginal separation ▪ Mild to moderate vaginal bleeding ▪ Vague abdominal discomfort ▪ Mild to moderate abdominal tenderness ▪ Uterine irritability ***Moderate abruption*** ▪ Gradual or abrupt onset of moderate dark-red vaginal bleeding ▪ Continuous abdominal pain ▪ Tender uterus remaining firm between contractions ▪ Barely audible or irregular and bradycardic fetal heart tones ***Severe abruption*** ▪ Abrupt onset of moderate vaginal bleeding ▪ Agonizing, unremitting uterine pain that's knifelike or tearing ▪ Boardlike tender uterus ▪ Absence of fetal heart tones ▪ Rapidly progressing shock	Abruptio placentae
***Bleeding, vaginal** (continued)*	
▪ Amenorrhea or abnormal menses followed by slight vaginal bleeding ▪ Unilateral pelvic pain with extreme pain during cervical movement and palpation of adnexa ▪ Lower abdominal pain precipitated by activities that increase abdominal pressure ▪ Boggy tender uterus ▪ Sharp lower abdominal pain possibly radiating to shoulder and neck with rupture	Ectopic pregnancy
▪ Painless bright-red vaginal bleeding after 20th week of pregnancy; episodic ▪ Soft nontender uterus ▪ Fetal malpresentation ▪ Minimal descent of fetal presenting part ▪ Strong audible fetal heart tones	Placenta previa

THE PREGNANT PATIENT: INTERPRETING YOUR FINDINGS *(continued)*

Sign or symptom and findings	Probable cause
Bleeding, vaginal *(continued)*	
▪ Pink vaginal discharge for several days or scant brown discharge for several weeks before onset of cramps and increased vaginal bleeding ▪ Intensification of cramps with increased frequency ▪ Cervical dilation	Spontaneous abortion
Blood pressure, elevated	
▪ Elevated blood pressure with sudden weight gain of more than 3 lb per week in the second trimester and more than 1 lb per week during the third trimester ▪ Generalized edema of face; pitting edema of legs and feet ▪ Hyperreflexia ▪ Possible oliguria ▪ Severe frontal headache ▪ Proteinuria ▪ Blurred vision in severe preeclampsia ▪ Liver dysfunction and epigastric pain in severe preeclampsia	Preeclampsia
▪ Seizure or coma	Eclampsia
Blood pressure, elevated *(continued)*	
▪ Right upper quadrant, epigastric, or lower chest pain ▪ Nausea and vomiting ▪ General malaise ▪ Severe edema ▪ Right upper quadrant tenderness on palpation	HELLP
Fetal movement, decreased	
▪ Absence of fetal movement ▪ Absence of fetal heart tones ▪ Absence of fetal heartbeat on ultrasound	Fetal demise
▪ Decreased fetal movement ▪ Changes in fetal heart rate	Fetal distress
Fever	
▪ Abrupt onset of fever above 101° F (38.3° C) and chills ▪ Pleuritic chest pain ▪ Productive cough ▪ Rust-colored sputum	Bacterial pneumonia
▪ Low-grade fever ▪ Painful small vesicles with erythematous base on vulva or vagina rupturing within 1 to 7 days to form ulcers ▪ Dyspareunia ▪ Positive viral culture of vesicle fluid ▪ Positive ELISA	Genital herpes

(continued)

THE PREGNANT PATIENT: INTERPRETING YOUR FINDINGS *(continued)*

Sign or symptom and findings	Probable cause
Fever *(continued)*	
▪ Fever, slight elevation possibly up to 103° F (39.4° C) ▪ Urinary frequency and urgency ▪ Dysuria ▪ Pain in lumbar region radiating downward; area tender on palpation ▪ Nausea and vomiting ▪ Malaise	Pyelonephritis
Pain, abdominal or chest	
Marginal separation ▪ Mild to moderate vaginal bleeding ▪ Vague abdominal discomfort ▪ Mild to moderate abdominal tenderness ▪ Uterine irritability ***Moderate abruption*** ▪ Gradual or abrupt onset of moderate dark-red vaginal bleeding ▪ Continuous abdominal pain ▪ Tender uterus remaining firm between contractions ▪ Barely audible or irregular and bradycardic fetal heart tones	Abruptio placentae
Pain, abdominal or chest *(continued)*	
Severe abruption ▪ Abrupt onset of moderate vaginal bleeding ▪ Agonizing, unremitting uterine pain that's knifelike or tearing ▪ Boardlike tender uterus ▪ Absence of fetal heart tones ▪ Rapidly progressing shock	Abruptio placentae
▪ Unilateral pelvic pain with extreme pain during cervical movement and palpation of adnexa ▪ Lower abdominal pain precipitated by activities that increase abdominal pressure ▪ Sharp lower abdominal pain possibly radiating to shoulder and neck with rupture ▪ Amenorrhea or abnormal menses followed by slight vaginal bleeding ▪ Boggy tender uterus	Ectopic pregnancy
▪ Onset of rhythmic uterine contractions; at least 4 every 20 minutes ▪ Possible rupture of membranes ▪ Passage of cervical mucus plug ▪ Pregnancy gestation less than 37 weeks ▪ Cervical effacement >80% and dilation >1 cm	Preterm labor

THE PREGNANT PATIENT: INTERPRETING YOUR FINDINGS *(continued)*

Sign or symptom and findings	Probable cause
Pain, abdominal or chest *(continued)*	
▪ Acute onset of chest pain or choking sensation ▪ Sudden dyspnea with intense angina-like pain aggravated by deep breathing ▪ Tachycardia, tachypnea ▪ Cough ▪ Low-grade fever ▪ Restlessness ▪ Diaphoresis ▪ Crackles, pleural friction rub ▪ Paradoxical pulse ▪ Hemoptysis ▪ Cerebral ischemia	Pulmonary embolism
Sudden gush of clear vaginal fluid	
▪ Abrupt onset of clear vaginal fluid expulsion with continued leakage ▪ Nitrazine testing revealing color change to blue	Preterm rupture of membranes
Vomiting, persistent	
▪ Unremitting nausea and vomiting beyond first trimester ▪ Vomitus containing undigested food, mucus, and small amounts of bile early in the disorder; changing to coffee-ground appearance ▪ Weight loss, emaciation ▪ Headache ▪ Oliguria ▪ Dry coated tongue ▪ Delirium, stupor, coma ▪ Thyroid dysfunction ▪ Fetid, fruity breath	Hyperemesis gravidarum

can range from slight spotting to frank bleeding. It can occur with or without pain.

History

Ascertain information about the current bleeding episode, including events befor the bleeding, measures to control the bleeding, and duration of the bleeding episode. Ask the patient what she was doing before the bleeding started. Find out how long the bleeding lasted or if it's still continuing. If the bleeding has occurred before, ask the patient how long the episode lasted and if it was intermittent or steady.

Question the patient about the appearance and amount of bleeding. Have her describe the color of the bleeding, such as if it was bright red, pink, or brown. Ask the patient if she noticed any tissue fragments or clots. Find out if there was any clear mucus or clear drainage mixed with the blood and if it had an odor. Ask the patient to estimate the amount, using common household measurements, such as teaspoon, tablespoon, or cup. Find out how many pads she used in a 1- to 2-hour period and if the pads were damp, wet, or saturated.

Inquire about accompanying symptoms. Ask the patient if she experienced abdominal cramping or sharp or dull abdominal pain. Depending on the gestational age, ask the patient about any changes in fetal movement.

In addition, obtain an obstetric history to determine if the patient has had similar problems, such as spontaneous abortions or placenta previa or abruption, in previous pregnancies. Also ask about a history of ectopic pregnancies or genetic disorders. Gather additional information about possible exposure to teratogens such as in the environment or at work. Also inquire about the use of any medications or drugs, such as cocaine or nicotine. Question the patient about any recent history of infections, including urinary tract infections, cytomegalovirus, rubella, or syphilis. Cocaine and nicotine use are risk factors for abruptio placentae. Abnormal fetal formations from exposure to teratogens and infections are risk factors for spontaneous abortions.

Physical assessment

Obtain the patient's vital signs to establish a baseline. Then perform a complete physical examination. Inspect the perineum for bleeding and note the color and amount of the bleeding. Palpate the fundus and assess the fetal status, checking fetal heart rate if indicated. Perform a pelvic examination.

CRITICAL POINT *A pelvic examination is contraindicated in a woman with painless vaginal bleeding late in pregnancy when placenta previa is suspected because of the risk of massive hemorrhage secondary to further disruption of the placenta.*

Analysis

Vaginal bleeding during pregnancy isn't a typical or normal finding. Although it may not be a serious problem, the potential for life-threatening hemorrhage is always a risk. In the first trimester, vaginal bleeding is most commonly associated with spontaneous abortion and ectopic pregnancy. In the second trimester, vaginal bleeding commonly indicates gestational trophoblastic disease or premature cervical dilation, also known as an *incompetent cervix.* In the third trimester, spotting may be the result of minor trauma or coitus, neither of which indicates a serious problem. However, placenta previa and abruptio placentae are two serious causes of vaginal bleeding in the third trimester.

Blood pressure, elevated

In the pregnant patient, elevated blood pressure is evidenced by systolic blood pressure readings greater than 140 mm Hg or an increase of 30 mm Hg or more about the patient's normal systolic blood pressure and a diastolic blood pressure of 90 mm Hg or more or an increase of 15 mm Hg or more above the patient's normal baseline diastolic pressure. These readings are measured on two occasions, 6 hours apart.

History

Obtain a complete health history, including a menstrual and obstetrical history. Ask the patient about the number of previous pregnancies, multiple gestations, and problems with previous pregnancies such as hydramnios. Identify the patient's estimated date of delivery.

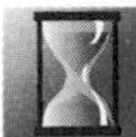

AGE ISSUE *Elevated blood pressure during pregnancy suggesting pregnancy induced hypertension is more common in adolescents and primiparas older than age 35.*

Also, inquire about underlying medical conditions, such as cardiac disease, diabetes with vascular involvement, or a history of hypertension.

Question the patient about any complaints of swelling, including edema of the face, eyes, hands, and ankles. Ask the patient if she has noticed her rings getting tight or her ankles swelling more than usual. Find out if she has gained a lot of weight recently, for example, over the past week or two.

Also ask the patient about complaints of headache, blurred vision, or problems with urinating. Additionally, question the patient about seizures.

Physical assessment

Obtain vital signs and compare them with baseline readings. Also weigh the patient and compare the results with the baseline.

CRITICAL POINT *A weight gain of 2 lb per week or 1 lb per week in the second or third trimesters, respectively, indicates abnormal fluid retention.*

Inspect the face, eyelids, hands, and extremities for edema. Palpate for pitting edema in the legs and feet. Check deep tendon reflexes, noting any hyperreflexia. Perform an ophthalmoscopic examination, noting any papilledema, retinal edema, or arteriovenous nicking.

Additionally, assess the patient's fundus and fetal heart rate and activity. Obtain a urine specimen to test for protein.

Analysis

Elevated blood pressure during pregnancy is suggestive of pregnancy induced hypertension. Also called hypertension of pregnancy, this is a potentially life-threatening condition that usually develops after the 20th week of pregnancy. Typically it's classified as preeclampsia or eclampsia depending on the associated findings.

Fetal movement, decreased

A fetus typically moves approximately the same amount everyday. This movement indicates that the fetus is responding to the need for additional oxygen. A decrease in fetal movement suggests a problem with the fetus.

History

In addition to obtaining a complete health history, ask the patient when she first noticed a change in fetal movements and whether the change has continued or if fetal movements have resumed their normal pattern. Question the patient about any measures used to attempt to increase fetal movement, such as sitting, lying down, or eating a snack. Ask her if she has experienced vaginal spotting or bleeding. If so, ask her if she noticed the passage of tissue. Also determine the patient's estimated date of delivery.

Physical assessment

In addition to completing a thorough physical examination, perform a pelvic examination, noting any evidence of bleeding at the perineum. Also palpate the patient's fundus and auscultate fetal heart sounds.

Analysis

Fetal movements may be elicited by having the patient lie down for about an hour after having a glass of milk or another snack. The jolt of energy produced by a light snack commonly produces fetal movement. A decrease in fetal movement may suggest fetal distress. Absence of fetal movement may indicate fetal demise.

Fever

Fever is a common sign that can arise from any one of several disorders. Because these disorders can affect virtually any body system, fever in the absence of other signs usually has little diagnostic significance. A persistent high fever, though, indicates an emergency.

History

If the patient's fever is mild to moderate, ask her when it began and how high her temperature reached. Find out if the fever disappeared, only to reappear later. Ask her if she experienced other symptoms, such as chills, fatigue, or pain.

Obtain a complete history, noting especially any history of sexually transmitted diseases (STDs) or infections such as urinary tract infection (UTI) or pyelonephritis, and use of medications.

Physical assessment

Let the history findings direct the physical examination. Because fever can accompany diverse disorders, the examination may range from a brief evaluation of one body system to a comprehensive review of all systems.

Inspect the perineum for evidence of lesions or vaginal discharge. Note any vaginal discharge that's malodorous or not clear and white. Obtain a culture of any discharge. Perform a pelvic examination if indicated.

Also assess the patient's fundus and fetal heart rate and activity.

Analysis

Fever during pregnancy indicates a serious complication for the mother and fetus. Most commonly, it suggests an intrauterine infection. However, other infections, such as STDs, UTI, pyelonephritis, or bacterial pneumonia may also be the cause.

Pain, abdominal or chest

Abdominal pain arises from the abdominopelvic viscera, the parietal peritoneum, or the capsules of the liver, kidney, or spleen. It may be acute or chronic, diffuse or localized. Visceral pain develops slowly into a deep, dull, aching pain that's poorly localized in the epigastric, periumbilical, or lower midabdominal (hypogastric) region. In contrast, somatic (parietal, peritoneal) pain produces a sharp, more intense, and well-localized discomfort that rapidly follows the insult. Movement or coughing aggravates this pain.

Pain may also be referred to the abdomen from another site with the same or similar nerve supply. This sharp, well-localized, referred pain is felt in skin or deeper tissues and may coexist with skin hyperesthesia and muscle hyperalgesia.

Mechanisms that produce abdominal pain include stretching or tension of the gut wall, traction on the peritoneum or mesentery, vigorous intestinal contraction, inflammation, ischemia, and sensory nerve irritation. With the reproductive organs, visceral pain is noted at the hypogastrium and groin; parietal pain occurs over the affected site; and referred pain typically is noted in the inner thighs.

Chest pain can arise suddenly or gradually, and its cause may be difficult to ascertain initially. The pain can radiate to the arms, neck, jaw, or back. It can be steady or intermittent, mild or acute. It can range in character from a sharp, shooting sensation to a feeling of heaviness, fullness, or even indigestion. It can be provoked or aggravated by stress, anxiety, exertion, deep breathing, or eating certain foods.

History

If the patient's complaint isn't severe, obtain a health history, including a menstrual and obstetric history. Determine her estimated date of delivery. Question the patient about any past history of illnesses, including heart disease or thrombophlebitis.

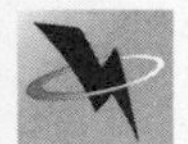

CRITICAL POINT *If the patient is experiencing sudden and severe abdominal pain, quickly take her vital signs and palpate pulses below the waist. Be alert for signs of hypovolemic shock, such as tachycardia and hypotension. Initiate emergency measures if indicated. If the patient is experiencing sudden and severe chest pain, ask the patient when her chest pain began and if it developed suddenly or gradually. Find out if it's more severe or frequent now than when it first started. Ask the patient what measures relieve the pain or aggravate it. Ask the patient about associated symptoms. Sudden, severe chest pain requires prompt evaluation and treatment because it may herald a life-threatening disorder.*

Ask her if she has had this type of pain before. Have her describe the pain — for example if it's dull, sharp, stabbing, or burning. Ask about measures that relieve the pain or make it worse. Ask the patient if the pain is constant or intermittent and when the pain began. If pain is intermittent, find out the duration.

In addition, ask the patient where the pain is located and if it radiates to other areas, such as the back or thighs. Also question the patient about any complaints of perineal pressure, bearing down, or sudden leakage of fluid from the vagina.

Physical assessment

Obtain the patient's vital signs and compare them with the baseline. In addition to assessing the mother and fetus, perform a focused assessment of the patient's abdomen or chest.

When assessing the abdomen, assess skin turgor and mucous membranes. Inspect the abdomen for possible distention or visible peristaltic waves and, if indicated, measure abdominal girth.

Auscultate for bowel sounds and characterize their motility. Percuss all quadrants, noting the percussion sounds. Palpate the entire abdomen for masses, rigidity, and tenderness. Check for costovertebral angle tenderness, abdominal tenderness with guarding, and rebound tenderness.

When assessing the chest and lungs, note any pallor or cyanosis, tachypnea, fever, tachycardia, oxygen saturation, paradoxical pulse, and hypertension or hypotension. Observe the patient's breathing pattern, and inspect the chest for asymmetrical expansion. Auscultate the lungs for pleural friction rub, crackles, rhonchi, wheezing, or diminished or absent breath sounds. Next, auscultate murmurs, clicks, gallops, or pericardial friction rub. Palpate for lifts, heaves, thrills, gallops, tactile fremitus, and abdominal masses or tenderness.

Inspect the lower extremities for redness, warmth, swelling, or pain. If indicated, measure the calf circumference in each extremity and compare findings.

Analysis

In addition to the wide range of disorders associated with abdominal pain in a nonpregnant patient (see chapter 11, Gastrointestinal system), abdominal pain in a pregnant woman can suggest serious complications, including rupture of an ectopic pregnancy, preterm labor, or abruptio placentae. Chest pain in the pregnant woman may suggest a pulmonary embolus secondary to thrombophlebitis as well as other problems typically seen in a nonpregnant patient (see chapter 9, Cardiovascular system).

Sudden gush of clear vaginal fluid

During pregnancy, a woman may experience leukorrhea, a white viscous vaginal discharge, secondary to hormonal changes associated with pregnancy. However, a sudden gush of clear fluid from the vagina is a sign that suggests a problem when it occurs before term.

History

Ask the patient to describe the fluid leakage, including onset, duration, color, and amount. Also question the patient about any signs and symptoms of labor such as abdominal cramping or the onset of contractions, or lower abdominal pressure.

Obtain an obstetrical history, noting any previous episodes of early rupture of the membranes or history of infections, such as chorioamnionitis. Determine her estimated date of delivery. Assess vital signs to establish a baseline.

Also question the patient about any problems with stress incontinence.

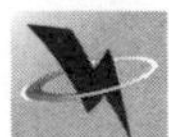

CRITICAL POINT *Some woman may mistake fluid leakage for stress incontinence. Amniotic fluid can't be differentiated from urine by inspection.*

Physical examination

In addition to performing a maternal and fetal assessment, including fundal palpation, fundal height measurement, and fetal heart rate assessment, inspect the perineum and perform a sterile pelvic examination. Observe the vaginal floor for pooling of fluid. Inspect for possible prolapse of the umbilical cord. Test any fluid with nitrazine paper to establish if fluid is amniotic fluid. Check for cervical dilation and effacement. Auscultate fetal heart rate for changes.

Analysis

A sudden gush of clear vaginal fluid suggests rupture of the membranes and the onset of labor. This typically occurs at term. However, if this occurs earlier in the pregnancy, the woman is experiencing preterm rupture of membranes (PROM) which predisposes her and her fetus to possible infection. Additionally, PROM can lead to inadequate nutritional supply to the fetus and possible prolapse of the umbilical cord.

Vomiting, persistent

Vomiting is the forceful expulsion of gastric contents through the mouth. Characteristically preceded by nausea, vomiting results from a coordinated sequence of abdominal muscle contractions and reverse esophageal peristalsis.

History

Ask your patient to describe the onset, duration, and intensity of her vomiting. Find out what started it, what makes it subside and, if possible, collect, measure, and inspect the character of the vomitus.

Explore any associated complaints, particularly nausea, abdominal pain, anorexia and weight loss, changes in bowel habits or stools, excessive belching or flatus, and bloating or fullness.

Obtain a history of disorders, noting GI, endocrine, and metabolic disorders; recent infections; and cancer, including any history of treatment with chemotherapy or radiation therapy. Ask about current medication use and alcohol consumption.

Physical assessment

Obtain the patient's weight and note any changes from baseline. Measure the fundal height and compare it with the expected height for gestational age. Auscultate maternal and fetal heart rates.

Assess skin turgor and texture; check mucous membranes for color and moistness. Palpate peripheral pulses.

Inspect the abdomen for distention, and wauscultate for bowel sounds and bruits. Palpate for rigidity and tenderness. Next, palpate and percuss the liver for enlargement. Assess other body systems as appropriate.

Analysis

A common sign of GI disorders, vomiting also occurs with fluid and electrolyte imbalances; infections; and metabolic, endocrine, labyrinthine, central nervous system, and cardiac disorders. It can also result from drug therapy, surgery, radiation, stress, anxiety, pain, alcohol intoxication, overeating, or ingestion of distasteful foods or liquids.

Vomiting is a common discomfort during the first trimester of pregnancy. It typically occurs with nausea. Although it's commonly referred to as morning sickness, it can last all day for some women. Nausea and vomiting rarely interfere with proper nutrition enough to harm the developing fetus.

Vomiting during pregnancy is considered abnormal if:

- the patient is losing weight instead of gaining it
- the patient hasn't gained the projected amount of weight for a particular week of pregnancy
- lost meals can't be made up for during the day
- signs of dehydration, such as little urine output, are present
- nausea lasts past the 12th week of pregnancy
- the patient vomits more than once daily.

Persistent, severe vomiting that continues past the first trimester may signal hyperemesis gravidarum.

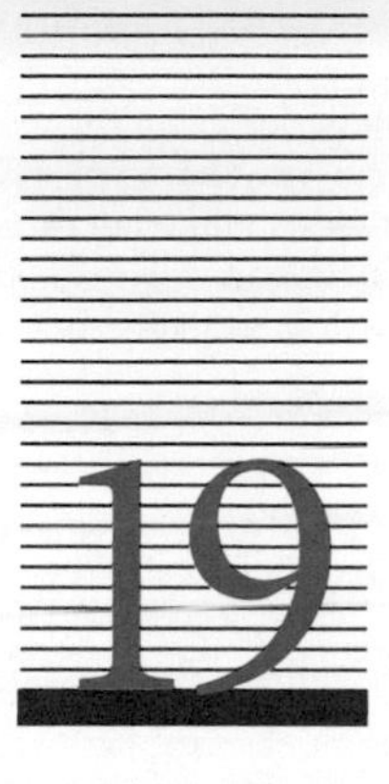

Assessing the neonate

Neonatal assessment is an ongoing process that begins immediately after delivery, continues until the neonate's discharge from the health care facility, and progresses through the neonate's first 28 days of life.

To conduct the neonatal assessment, the health care provider must know how to calculate an Apgar score and how to make general — but crucial — observations about the neonate's appearance and behavior. This information, coupled with pertinent maternal and fetal history data, provides an initial database for use during subsequent examinations.

Transition to extrauterine life

After birth, a neonate must quickly adapt to extrauterine life, even though many of the neonate's body systems are still developing. During this time of adaptation, knowledge of normal neonatal physiologic characteristics and assessment findings is essential to detect possible problems so that appropriate interventions can be initiated. (See *Physiology of the neonate,* page 564.)

Respiratory system

The major adaptation for the neonate is that he must breathe on his own rather than depend on fetal circulation. At birth, air is substituted for the fluid that filled the neonate's respiratory tract in the alveoli during gestation. In a normal vaginal delivery, some of this fluid is forced out during birth. After delivery, the fluid is absorbed across the alveolar membrane into the capillaries.

The onset of the neonate's breathing is stimulated by several factors including low blood oxygen levels, increased blood carbon

PHYSIOLOGY OF THE NEONATE

This chart provides a summary of the physiologic characteristics of a neonate after birth, including adaptations the neonate must make to cope with extrauterine life.

Body system	Physiology after birth
Respiratory	▪ Onset of breathing occurs as air replaces the fluid that filled the lungs before birth.
Cardiovascular	▪ Functional closure of fetal shunts occurs. ▪ Transition from fetal to postnatal circulation occurs.
Renal	▪ System doesn't mature fully until after the first year of life; fluid imbalances may occur.
Gastrointestinal	▪ System continues to develop. ▪ Uncoordinated peristalsis of the esophagus occurs. ▪ The neonate has a limited ability to digest fats. ▪ The neonate may exhibit jaundice.
Immune	▪ The inflammatory response of the tissues to localize infection is immature.
Hematopoietic	▪ Coagulation time is prolonged.
Neurologic	▪ Presence of primitive reflexes and time in which they appear and disappear indicate the maturity of the developing nervous system.
Integumentary	▪ The epidermis and dermis are thin and bound loosely to each other. ▪ Sebaceous glands are active.
Musculoskeletal	▪ More cartilage is present than ossified bone.
Reproductive	▪ Females may have a mucoid vaginal discharge and pseudomenstruation due to maternal estrogen levels. ▪ In males, testes descend into the scrotum. ▪ Small, white, firm cysts called *epithelial pearls* may be visible at the tip of the prepuce. ▪ Genitals may be edematous if the neonate presented in breech position.
Thermogenic	▪ The neonate is more susceptible to rapid heat loss due to acute change in environment and thin layer of subcutaneous fat. ▪ Nonshivering thermogenesis occurs. ▪ The presence of brown fat (more in mature neonate; less in premature neonate) warms the neonate by increasing heat production.

dioxide levels, low blood pH, and temperature change from the warm uterine environment to the cooler extrauterine environment. Noise, light, and other sensations related to the birth process may also influence the neonate's initial breathing.

Although the neonate can breathe on his own, his respiratory system isn't as developed as an adult's system. The neonate is an obligatory nose breather. In addition, the neonate has a relatively large tongue whereas the trachea and glottis are small.

Other significant differences between a neonate's respiratory system and an adult's system include airway lumens that are narrower and collapse more easily, respiratory tract secretions that are more abundant, mucous membranes that are more delicate and susceptible to trauma, alveoli that are more sensitive to pressure changes, a capillary network that's less developed, and a rib cage and respiratory musculature that are less developed.

Cardiovascular system

The neonate's first breath triggers the start of several cardiopulmonary changes that help him transition from fetal circulation to postnatal circulation. During this transition, the foramen ovale, ductus arteriosis, and ductus venosus close. These closures allow blood to start flowing to the lungs.

When the neonate takes his first breath, the lungs inflate. When the lungs are inflated, pulmonary vascular resistance to blood flow is reduced and pulmonary artery pressure drops. Pressure in the right atrium decreases, and the increased blood flow to the left side of the heart increases the pressure in the left atrium. This change in pressure causes the foramen ovale, the fetal shunt between the left and right atria, to close. Increased blood oxygen levels then influence other fetal shunts to close.

The ductus arteriosus, located between the aorta and pulmonary artery, eventually closes and becomes a ligament. The ductus venosus, between the left umbilical vein and the inferior vena cava, closes because of vasoconstriction and lack of blood flow; then it also becomes a ligament. The umbilical arteries and vein and the hepatic arteries also constrict and become ligaments.

Renal system

After birth, the renal system is called into action because the neonate can no longer depend on the placenta to excrete waste products. However, the renal system function doesn't fully mature until after the first year, which means that the neonate is at risk for chemical imbalances. The neonate's limited ability to excrete drugs because of renal immaturity, coupled with excessive neonatal fluid loss, can rapidly lead to acidosis and fluid imbalances.

GI system

At birth, the neonate's GI system isn't fully developed because normal bacteria aren't present in the GI tract. The lower intestine contains meconium, which usually starts to pass within 24 hours. It appears greenish black and viscous.

As the GI system begins to develop, audible bowel sounds appear 1 hour after birth, uncoordinated peristaltic activity appears in the esophagus for the first few days of life, limited ability to digest fats appears because amylase and lipase are absent at birth, and frequent regurgitation occurs because of an immature cardiac sphincter.

Additionally, liver function is immature at birth. Jaundice, or yellowing of the skin, is a major concern. It's caused by hyperbilirubinemia, a condition that occurs when serum levels of unconjugated bilirubin increase because of increased red blood cell lysis, altered bilirubin conjugation, or increased bilirubin reabsorption from the GI tract.

Immune system

The neonatal immune system depends largely on three immunoglobulins: immunoglobulin (Ig) A, IgG, and IgM.

IgG, which can be detected in the fetus at 3 months' gestation, is an immunoglobulin consisting of bacterial and viral antibodies. It's the most abundant immunoglobulin and is found in all body fluids. In utero, IgG crosses from the placenta to the fetus. After birth, the neonate produces his own IgG during the first 3 months while the leftover maternal antibodies in the neonate break down.

IgA, an immunoglobulin that limits bacterial growth in the GI tract, is produced gradually. Maximum levels of IgA are reached during childhood. The neonate obtains IgA from maternal colostrum and breast milk.

IgM, found in blood and lymph fluid, is the first immunoglobulin to respond to infection. It's produced at birth, and by age 9 months the IgM level in the neonate reaches the level found in adults. Although these immunoglobulins are present in the neonate, the inflammatory response of the tissues to localized infection is still immature. All neonates, especially those born prematurely, are at high risk for infection during the first several months of life.

Hematopoietic system

In the neonatal hematopoietic system, blood volume accounts for 80 to 85 ml/kg of body weight. Immediately after birth, the neonatal blood volume averages 300 ml; however, it can drop as low as 100 ml depending on how long the neonate remains attached to the placenta via the umbilical cord. In addition, neonatal blood has a prolonged coagulation time because of decreased levels of vitamin K.

Neurologic system

At birth, the neurologic system isn't completely integrated, but it's developed enough to sustain extrauterine life. Most functions of this system are primitive reflexes. The full-term neonate's neurologic system should produce equal strength and symmetry in responses and reflexes. Diminished or absent reflexes may indicate a serious neurologic problem, and asymmetrical responses may indicate that trauma, such as nerve damage, paralysis, or fracture, occurred during birth.

Integumentary system

All of the structures of the integumentary system are present at birth, but many of their functions are immature. The epidermis and dermis are bound loosely to each other and are extremely thin. In addition, the sebaceous glands are active in early infancy because of maternal hormones.

Musculoskeletal system

The skeletal system, at birth, contains more cartilage than ossified bone. The process of ossification occurs rapidly during the first year of life. The muscular system is almost completely formed at birth.

Reproductive system

The ovaries of the female neonate contain thousands of primitive germ cells. These germ cells represent the full potential for ova. The number of ova decreases from birth to maturity by about 90%. After birth, the uterus undergoes involution and decreases in size and weight because, in utero, the fetal uterus enlarges from the effects of maternal hormones.

For 90% of male neonates, the testes descend into the scrotum after birth. However, spermatogenesis doesn't occur until puberty.

Thermogenesis

Among the many adaptations that occur after birth, the neonate must regulate his body temperature by producing and conserving heat. Because he has a thin layer of subcutaneous fat and his blood vessels are closer to the skin's surface, this regulation can be difficult for the neonate. In addition, the neonate's vasomotor control is less developed, his body surface area to weight ratio is high, and his sweat glands have minimal thermogenic function until he's age 4 weeks or older.

The neonate's body also has to work against four routes of heat loss:

- convection — the flow of heat from the body to cooler air
- radiation — the loss of body heat to cooler, solid surfaces near but not in direct contact with the neonate
- evaporation — heat loss that occurs when liquid is converted to a vapor
- conduction — the loss of body heat to cooler substances in direct contact with the neonate.

To maintain body temperature, the neonate must produce heat through a process called nonshivering thermogenesis. This involves an increase in the neonate's metabolism and oxygen consumption. Thermogenesis mainly occurs in the heart, liver, and brain. Brown adipose tissue, also called *brown fat,* is another source of thermogenesis that's unique to the neonate.

Neonatal assessment

Neonatal assessment includes initial and ongoing assessments, a head-to-toe physical examination, and neurologic and behavioral assessments.

Initial assessment

The initial neonatal assessment involves draining secretions, assessing abnormalities, and keeping accurate records. To complete an initial assessment, follow these steps:

RECORDING THE APGAR SCORE

Use this chart to determine the neonatal Apgar score at 1 minute and 5 minutes after birth. For each category listed, assign a score of 0 to 2, as shown. A total score of 7 to 10 indicates that the neonate is in good condition; 4 to 6, fair condition, the neonate may have moderate central nervous system depression, muscle flaccidity, cyanosis, and poor respirations; 0 to 3, danger, the neonate needs immediate resuscitation, as ordered.

Sign	Apgar score		
	0	1	2
Heart rate	Absent	Less than 100 beats/minute	More than 100 beats/minute
Respiratory effort	Absent	Slow, irregular	Good crying
Muscle tone	Flaccid	Some flexion and resistance to extension of extremities	Active motion
Reflex irritability	No response	Grimace or weak cry	Vigorous cry
Color	Pallor, cyanosis	Pink body, blue extremities	Completely pink

- For infection control purposes, wear gloves when assessing a neonate until after his initial bath.
- Ensure a proper airway by suctioning, and administer oxygen as needed.
- Dry the neonate under the warmer while keeping his head lower than his trunk to promote the drainage of secretions.
- Apply a cord clamp, and monitor the neonate for abnormal bleeding from the cord; check the number of cord vessels.
- Observe the neonate for voiding and meconium; document the first void and stools.
- Assess the neonate for gross abnormalities and clinical manifestations of suspected abnormalities.
- Continue to assess the neonate by using the Apgar score criteria even after the 5-minute score is received.
- Obtain clear footprints and fingerprints. (In some health care facilities, the neonate's footprints are kept on a record that also includes the mother's fingerprints.)
- Apply identification bands with matching numbers to the mother (one band) and the neonate (two bands) before they leave the delivery room. Some health care facilities also give the father or partner an identification band.
- Put the neonate to the mother's breast or have the mother and neonate engage in skin to skin contact.

Apgar scoring

During the initial examination of a neonate, expect to calculate an Apgar score and make general observations about the neonate's appearance and behavior. Developed by anesthesiologist Dr. Virginia Apgar in 1952, Apgar scoring evaluates neonatal heart rate, respiratory effort, muscle tone, reflex irritability, and color. Evaluation of each category is performed 1 minute after birth and again at 5 minutes after birth. Each item has a maximum score of 2 and a minimum score of 0. The final Apgar score is the sum total of the five items; a maximum score is 10.

Evaluation at 1 minute quickly indicates the neonate's initial adaptation to extrauterine life and whether resuscitation is necessary. The 5-minute score gives a more accurate picture of his overall status. (See *Recording the Apgar score.*)

Heart rate. Assess heart rate first. If the umbilical cord still pulsates, palpate the neonate's heart rate by placing the fingertips at the junction of the umbilical cord and the skin. The neonate's cord stump continues to pulsate for several hours and is a good, easy place, in addition to the abdomen, to check heart rate. You can also place two fingers or a stethoscope over the neonate's chest at the fifth intercostal space to obtain an apical pulse. For accuracy, the heart rate should be counted for 1 full minute.

Respiratory effort. Next, check the neonate's respiratory effort, the second most important Apgar sign. Assess the neonate's cry, noting its volume and vigor. Then auscultate his lungs using a stethoscope. Assess his respirations for depth and regularity. If the neonate exhibits abnormal respiratory responses, begin neonatal resuscitation according to the guidelines of the American Heart Association and the American Academy of Pediatrics. Then use the Apgar score to judge the progress and success of resuscitation efforts.

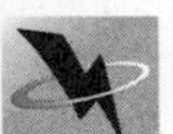

CRITICAL POINT *Closely observe a neonate whose mother received heavy sedation just before delivery. Even if he has a high Apgar score at birth, he may exhibit secondary effects of sedation later. Watch for respiratory depression or unresponsiveness.*

Muscle tone. Determine muscle tone by evaluating the degree of flexion in the neonate's arms and legs and their resistance to straightening. This can be done by extending the limbs and observing their rapid return to flexion — the neonate's normal state.

Reflex irritability. Assess reflex irritability by evaluating the neonate's cry for presence, vigor, and pitch. Initially he may not cry, but you should be able to elicit a cry by flicking his soles. The usual response is a loud, angry cry. A high-pitched or shrill cry is abnormal.

Color. Finally, observe skin color for cyanosis. A white neonate usually has a pink body with blue extremities. This condition, called acrocyanosis, appears in about 85% of normal neonates 1 minute after birth. Acrocyanosis results from decreased peripheral oxygenation caused by the transition from fetal to independent circulation.

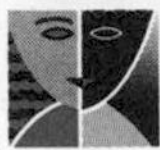

CULTURAL INSIGHT *When assessing a nonwhite neonate, observe for color changes in the mucous membranes of the mouth, conjunctivae, lips, palms, and soles.*

Gestational age and birth weight

Perinatal mortality and morbidity are related to gestational age and birth weight. Classifying a neonate by both weight and gestational age provides a more accurate method for assessing mortality risk and offers guidelines for treatment. The neonate's age and weight classifications should also be considered during future assessments.

Gestational age. The clinical assessment of gestational age classifies a neonate as preterm (less than 37 weeks' gestation), term (37 to 42 weeks' gestation), or postterm (42 weeks' gestation or longer). The Ballard scoring system uses physical and neurologic findings to estimate a neonate's gestational age within 1 week, even in extremely premature neonates. This evaluation can be done at any time between birth and 42 hours after birth, but the greatest reliability is when the evaluation is done between 30 and 42 hours after birth. (See *Ballard gestational-age assessment tool.*)

Birth weight. Normal birth weight is 2,500 g (5 lb, 8 oz) or greater. A neonate is considered to have a low birth weight if he weighs between 1,500 g (3 lb, 5 oz) and 2,499 g. A neonate of very low birth weight ranges between 1,000 g (2 lb, 3 oz) and 1,499 g. A neonate weighing less than 1,000 g has an extremely low birth weight.

Postnatal growth charts are used to assess the neonate based on head circumference, weight, length, and gestational age. Neonates who are small for gestational age have a birth weight less than the 10th percentile on postnatal growth charts; weight appropriate for gestational age signifies a birth weight within the 10th and 90th percentiles; and weight large for gestational age means a birth weight greater than the 90th percentile.

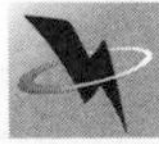

CRITICAL POINT *When assessing a preterm neonate, be alert for problems even if the neonate is of*

(Text continues on page 572.)

EXPERT TECHNIQUE

BALLARD GESTATIONAL-AGE ASSESSMENT TOOL

To use this assessment tool, evaluate and score the neuromuscular and physical maturity criteria, total the score, and then plot the sum in the maturity rating box to determine the neonate's corresponding gestational age.

Posture
With the neonate supine and quiet, score as follows:
- Arms and legs extended = 0
- Slight or moderate flexion of hips and knees = 1
- Moderate to strong flexion of hips and knees = 2
- Legs flexed and abducted, arms slightly flexed = 3
- Full flexion of arms and legs = 4

Square window
Flex the hand at the wrist. Measure the angle between the base of the thumb and the forearm. Score as follows:
- > 90 degrees = –1
- 90 degrees = 0
- 60 degrees = 1
- 45 degrees = 2
- 30 degrees = 3
- 0 degrees = 4

Arm recoil
With the neonate supine, fully flex the forearm for 5 seconds, then fully extend by pulling the hands and releasing. Observe and score the reaction according to this criteria:
- Remains extended 180 degrees or random movements = 0
- Minimal flexion (140 to 180 degrees) = 1
- Small amount of flexion (110 to 140 degrees) = 2
- Moderate flexion (90 to 110 degrees) = 3
- Brisk return to full flexion (< 90 degrees) = 4

Popliteal angle
With the neonate supine and the pelvis flat on the examination surface, use one hand to flex the leg and then the thigh. Then use the other hand to extend the leg. Score the angle attained:
- 180 degrees = –1
- 160 degrees = 0
- 140 degrees = 1
- 120 degrees = 2
- 100 degrees = 3
- 90 degrees = 4
- < 90 degrees = 5

Scarf sign
With the neonate supine, take his hand and draw it across the neck and as far across the opposite shoulder as possible. You may assist the elbow by lifting it across the body. Score according to the location of the elbow:
- Elbow reaches or nears level of opposite shoulder = –1
- Elbow crosses opposite anterior axillary line = 0
- Elbow reaches opposite anterior axillary line = 1
- Elbow at midline = 2
- Elbow doesn't reach midline = 3
- Elbow doesn't cross proximate axillary line = 4

Heel to ear
With the neonate supine, hold his foot with one hand and move it as near to the head as possible without forcing it. Keep the pelvis flat on the examination surface. Score as shown in the chart.

(continued)

BALLARD GESTATIONAL-AGE ASSESSMENT TOOL *(continued)*

Neuromuscular maturity

Neuromuscular maturity sign	Score −1	0	1	2	3	4	5	Record score here
Posture	—	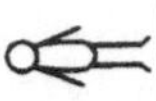	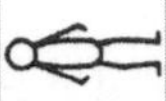	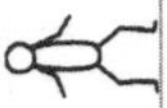	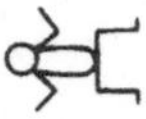	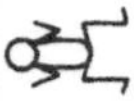	—	
Square window (wrist)	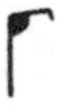 > 90°	90°	60°	45°	30°	0°	—	
Arm recoil	—	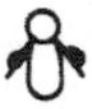 180°	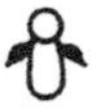 140° to 180°	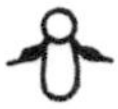 110° to 140°	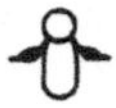 90° to 100°	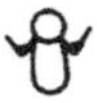 < 90°	—	
Popliteal angle	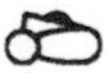 180°	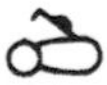 160°	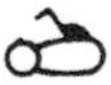 140°	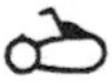 120°	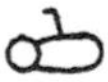 100°	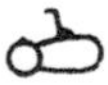 90°	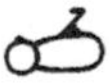 < 90°	
Scarf sign	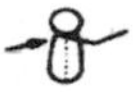	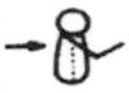	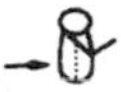	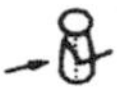	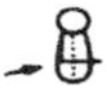	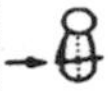	—	
Heel to ear	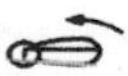	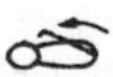	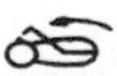	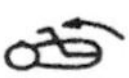	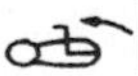	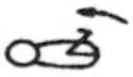	—	

Total neuromuscular maturity score

BALLARD GESTATIONAL-AGE ASSESSMENT TOOL *(continued)*

Physical maturity

Physical maturity sign	Score −1	0	1	2	3	4	5	Record score here
Skin	Sticky, friable, transparent	Gelatinous, red, translucent	Smooth, pink; visible vessels	Superficial peeling or rash; few visible vessels	Cracking; pale areas; rare visible vessels	Parchment-like; deep cracking; no visible vessels	Leathery, cracked, wrinkled	
Lanugo	None	Sparse	Abundant	Thinning	Bald areas	Mostly bald	—	
Plantar surface	Heel-to-toe 40 to 50 mm: −1; < 40 mm: −2	> 50 mm; no crease	Faint red marks	Anterior transverse crease only	Creases over anterior two-thirds	Creases over entire sole	—	
Breast	Imperceptible	Barely perceptible	Flat areola; no bud	Stippled areola; 1- to 2-mm bud	Raised areola; 3- to 4-mm bud	Full areola; 5- to 10-mm bud	—	
Eye and ear	Lids fused, loosely: −1; tightly: −2	Lids open; pinna flat, stays folded	Slightly curved pinna; soft, slow, recoil	Well-curved pinna; soft but ready recoil	Formed and firm; instant recoil	Thick cartilage; ear stiff	—	
Genitalia (male)	Scrotum flat, smooth	Scrotum empty; faint rugae	Testes in upper canal; rare rugae	Testes descending; few rugae	Testes down; good rugae	Testes pendulous; deep rugae	—	
Genitalia (female)	Clitoris prominent; labia flat	Prominent clitoris; small labia minora	Prominent clitoris; enlarging minora	Majora and minora equally prominent	Majora large; minora small	Majora cover clitoris and minora	—	
							Total physical maturity score	

(continued)

BALLARD GESTATIONAL-AGE ASSESSMENT TOOL *(continued)*

Score
*Neuromuscular:*____________
*Physical:*____________
Total maturity score:

Gestational age (weeks)
*By dates:*____________
*By ultrasound:*____________
By score: ____________

Total maturity score	−10	−5	0	5	10	15	20	25	30	35	40	45	50
Gestational age (weeks)	20	22	24	26	28	30	32	34	36	38	40	42	44

Adapted with permission from Ballard, J.L., et al. "New Ballad Score, expanded to include extremely premature infants," *Journal of Pediatrics* 119(3):417-23, 1991. Used with permission from Mosby–Year Book, Inc.

average size. A preterm neonate who's an appropriate weight for his gestational age is more prone to respiratory distress syndrome, apnea, patent ductus arteriosus, with left to right shunt, and infection. A preterm neonate who's small for his gestational age is more likely to experience asphyxia, hypoglycemia, and hypocalcemia.

Ongoing assessment

Ongoing neonatal physical assessment includes observing and recording vital signs and administering prescribed medications. To perform ongoing assessment, follow these steps:

- Assess the neonate's vital signs.
- Measure and record the neonate's vital statistics.
- Administer prescribed medications such as vitamin K, or phytonadione (AquaMEPHYTON), which is a prophylactic to the transient deficiency of coagulation factors II, VII, IX, and X.
- Administer erythromycin ointment (Ilotycin), the drug of choice for neonatal eye prophylaxis, to prevent damage and blindness from conjunctivitis caused by *Neisseria gonorrhoeae* and Chlamydia; treatment is required by law.
- Perform laboratory tests.
- Monitor glucose levels and hematocrit test results, which aid in assessing for hypoglycemia and anemia.

Vital signs

Measuring vital signs establishes the baseline of any neonatal assessment. Vital signs include the respiratory rate, heart rate (taken apically), and the first neonatal temperature, which is taken rectally to verify rectal patency. Subsequent temperature readings are axillary to avoid injuring the rectal mucosa. Blood pressure readings may be assessed by sphygmomanometer or by palpation or auscultation. An electronic vital signs monitor may be used. (See *Reviewing normal neonatal vital signs.*)

Respiratory rate. Observe respirations first, before the neonate becomes active or agitated. Watch and count respiratory movements for 1 minute and record the result. A normal respiratory rate is usually between 30 and 50 breaths per minute. Also, note any signs of respiratory distress, such as cyanosis, tachypnea, sternal retractions, grunting, nasal flaring, or periods of apnea. Short periods of apnea, less than 15 seconds, are characteristic in the neonate. (See *Counting neonatal respirations,* page 574.)

Heart rate. Use a pediatric stethoscope to determine the neonate's apical heart rate. Place the stethoscope over the apical impulse on the fourth or fifth intercostal space at the left midclavicular line over the cardiac apex. To ensure an accurate measurement, count the beats for 1 minute. A normal heart rate ranges from 110 to 160 beats per minute. Variations during sleeping and waking states are normal.

Temperature. The technique for taking a rectal temperature in a neonate is relatively simple. With the neonate lying in a supine position, place a diaper over the penis, if applicable, and firmly grasp his ankles with your index finger between them. Then insert a lubricated thermometer into the rectum, no more than ½″ (1.3 cm). Place your palm on his buttocks and hold the thermometer between your index and middle fingers. If resistance is met while inserting the thermometer, withdraw the thermometer and notify the primary care provider.

Hold a mercury thermometer in place for 3 minutes and an electronic thermometer in place until the temperature registers. Remove the thermometer and record the result. Body temperature in neonates is less constant than in adults and can fluctuate during the course of a day, without reason. The normal range for a rectal temperature is 96° to 99.5° F (35.6° to 37.5° C). To take an axillary temperature, make sure that the axillary skin is dry. Place the thermometer in the axilla and hold it along the outer aspect of the neonate's chest between the axillary line and the arm. Hold the thermometer in place until the temperature registers. Normal axillary temperature is 97.5° to 99° F (36.4° to 37.2° C).

Reassess axillary temperature in 15 to 30 minutes if the first measurement registers outside the normal range. If the temperature remains abnormal, notify the primary care provider.

Decreased temperatures by either the rectal or axillary route could suggest prematurity, infection, low environmental temperature, inadequate clothing, or dehydration. Possible reasons for increased temperatures include infection, high environmental temperature, excessive clothing, proximity to heating unit or direct sunlight, drug addiction, and diarrhea and dehydration.

REVIEWING NORMAL NEONATAL VITAL SIGNS

The list below includes the normal ranges for neonatal vital signs.

Respiration
- 30 to 50 breaths/minute

Heart rate (apical)
- 110 to 160 beats/minute

Temperature
- Rectal: 96° to 99.5° F (35.6° to 37.5° C)
- Axillary: 97.5° to 99° F (36.4° to 37.2° C)

Blood pressure
- Systolic: 60 to 80 mm Hg
- Diastolic: 40 to 50 mm Hg

Blood pressure. If possible, measure a neonate's blood pressure when he's in a quiet or relaxed state. Make sure that the blood pressure cuff is small enough for the neonate—cuff width should be about one-half of the circumference of the neonate's arm. Then wrap the cuff one or two fingerbreadths above the antecubital or popliteal area. With the stethoscope held directly over the chosen artery, hold the cuffed extremity firmly to keep it extended and inflate the cuff no faster than 5 mm Hg per second.

Normal neonatal systolic readings are 60 to 80 mm Hg; normal diastolic readings are 40 to 50 mm Hg. A drop in systolic blood pressure (about 15 mm Hg) during the first hour after birth is common. Crying and movement result in blood pressure changes.

Compare blood pressures in the upper and lower extremities at least once to detect abnormalities. Remember that blood pressure readings from the thigh will be approximately 10 mm Hg higher than the arm. If the blood pressure reading in the thigh is the same or lower than the arm, notify the

EXPERT TECHNIQUE

COUNTING NEONATAL RESPIRATIONS

When counting a neonate's respirations, observe abdominal excursions rather than chest excursions. You can also count respirations by auscultating the chest or by placing the stethoscope in front of the mouth and nares.

primary care provider. This could indicate coarctation of the aorta, a congenital heart defect, and should be investigated further.

Size and weight

Size and weight measurements establish the baseline for monitoring growth. Size and weight measurements can also be used to detect such disorders as failure to thrive and hydrocephalus. (See *Obtaining anthropometric measurements*).

Head circumference. Head circumference reflects the rate of growth of the head and its contents. To measure head circumference, slide the tape measure under the neonate's head at the occiput and draw the tape around snugly, just above the eyebrows. Normal neonatal head circumference is 13″ to 14″ (33 to 35.5 cm). Cranial molding or caput succedaneum from a vaginal delivery may affect this measurement.

Chest circumference. Measure the neonate's chest circumference by placing the tape under the back, wrapping it snugly around the chest at the nipple line, and keeping the back and front of the tape level. Take the measurement after the neonate inspires and before he begins to exhale. Normal neonatal chest circumference is 12″ to 13″ (30.5 to 33 cm).

Head-to-heel length. Fully extend the neonate's legs with the toes pointing up. Measure the distance from the heel to the top of the head. A length board may be used, if available. Normal length is 18″ to 21″ (46 to 53 cm).

Weight. Weigh a neonate before a feeding, using a scale that has been balanced. Remove the diaper and place the neonate in the middle of the scale tray. Keep one hand poised over the neonate at all times. Average weight is 2,500 to 4,000 g (5 lb, 8 oz to 8lb, 13 oz).

Return the neonate to the crib or examination table. Be sure to document if the neonate had any clothing or equipment on him, such as an I.V. Take the neonate's weight at the same time each day, if possible. Use measures to minimize heat loss.

Head-to-toe assessment

The neonate should receive a thorough physical examination of each body part. However, before each body part is examined, assess the neonate's general appearance and posture. Neonates usually lie in a symmetrical, flexed position — the characteristic fetal position — as a result of their position while in utero.

Skin

The term neonate has beefy red skin for a few hours after birth. Then the skin turns to its normal color. It commonly appears mottled or blotchy, especially on the extremities.

Common findings in a neonatal assessment may include:

- acrocyanosis, caused by vasomotor instability, capillary stasis, and high hemoglobin level, for the first 24 hours after birth
- milia, or clogged sebaceous glands, on the nose or chin
- lanugo, which is fine, downy hair, appearing after 20 weeks of gestation on the entire body, except the palms and soles
- vernix caseosa, which is a white, cheesy protective coating composed of desquamated epithelial cells and sebum
- erythema toxicum neonatorum, a transient, maculopapular rash
- telangiectasia, which are flat, reddened vascular areas, appearing on the neck, upper eyelid, or upper lip
- port-wine stain, also called nevus flammeus, a capillary angioma located below the dermis and commonly found on the face
- strawberry hemangioma, also called *nevus vasculosus,* a capillary angioma located

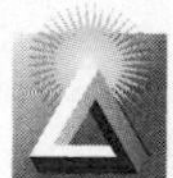

EXPERT TECHNIQUE

OBTAINING ANTHROPOMETRIC MEASUREMENTS

Anthropometric measurements include head and chest circumference, head-to-heel length, and weight. These measurements serve as a baseline and show whether neonatal size is within normal ranges or whether there may be a significant problem or anomaly—especially if values stray far from the mean.

Measurement		Average initial anthrompometric range
Head circumference Place measuring tape around the neonate's head at the occiput and encircle the head to the front at eyebrow level.	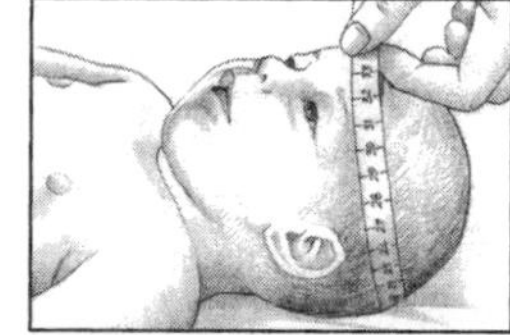	13″ to 14″ (33 to 35.5 cm)
Chest circumference Place a measuring tape under the neonate's back and wrap it snugly around the chest at the nipple line.	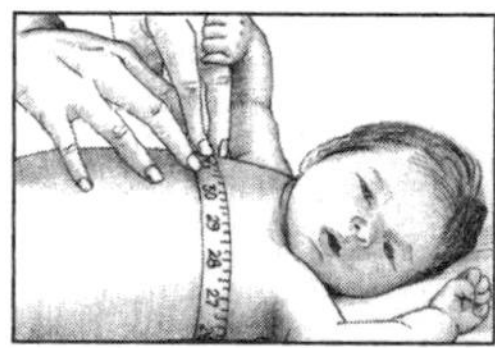	12″ to 13″ (30.5 to 33 cm)
Head-to-heel length Place the neonate in the supine position with the legs fully extended and measure the distance from the top of the head to the heel.	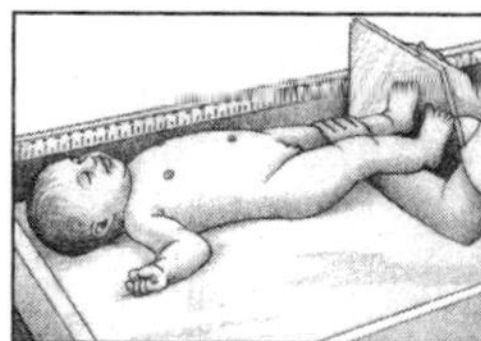	18″ to 21″ (46 to 53 cm)
Weight Place the neonate in the middle of the scale tray on a prebalanced scale. Maintain one hand over the neonate without touching the neonate or the scale.	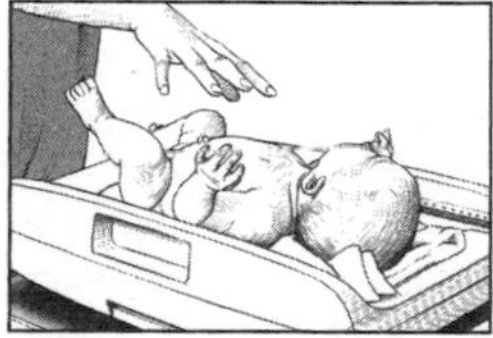	2,500 g to 4,000 g (5 lb, 8 oz to 8 lb, 13 oz)

in the dermal and subdermal skin layers indicated by a rough, raised, sharply demarcated birthmark

- sudamina or miliaria, or distended sweat glands, causing minute vesicles on the skin surface, especially on the face
- Mongolian spots, bluish black areas of pigmentation more commonly noted on the back and buttocks of dark-skinned neonates, regardless of race.

Make general observations about the appearance of the neonate's skin in relationship to his activity, position, and temperature. Usually, the neonate is redder when crying or hot. He may also have transient episodes of cyanosis with crying. Cutis marmorata is transient mottling when the neonate is exposed to cooler temperatures.

Palpate the skin to assess turgor. To do this, roll a fold of skin on the neonate's abdomen between the thumb and forefinger. Assess consistency, amount of subcutaneous tissue, and degree of hydration. A well-hydrated neonate's skin returns to normal immediately upon release.

Head

The neonate's head is about one-fourth of its body size. Six bones make up the cranium: the frontal bone, the occipital bone, two parietal bones, and two temporal bones.

Bands of connective tissue, called sutures, lie between the junctures of these bones. Inspect and palpate the sutures. Suture lines should be separated, but not widely. Occasionally, suture lines may override. This occurs as a result of the extreme pressure exerted on the sutures during a vaginal birth.

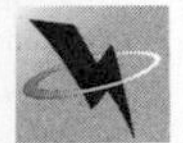

CRITICAL POINT *Widely separated suture lines suggest increased intracranial pressure (ICP) and require further evaluation.*

At the junction of the sutures are wider spaces of membranous tissues, called fontanels. The neonatal skull has two fontanels. The anterior fontanel is diamond-shaped and located at the juncture of the frontal and parietal bones. It measures 1⅛″ to 1⅝″ (3 to 4 cm) long and ¾″ to 1⅛″ (2 to 3 cm) wide. The anterior fontanel closes in about 18 months. The posterior fontanel is triangular. It's located at the juncture of the occipital and parietal bones and measures about ¾″ across. The posterior fontanel closes in 8 to 12 weeks.

Palpate the fontanels. The fontanels should feel soft to the touch but shouldn't be depressed. A depressed fontanel indicates dehydration. In addition, fontanels shouldn't bulge. Pulsations in the fontanels reflect the peripheral pulse.

CRITICAL POINT *Bulging fontanels require immediate attention because they may indicate increased ICP.*

Inspect the shape of the neonate's head. Occasionally, molding may be noted where the portion of the head that presented to the cervix appears asymmetric and highly prominent, giving the neonate's head a cone-shaped appearance.

Two other types of cranial abnormalities may be noted and include cephalohematoma and caput succedaneum. Cephalohematoma occurs when blood collects between a skull bone and the periosteum. It's caused by pressure during delivery and tends to spontaneously resolve in 3 to 6 weeks. A cephalohematoma doesn't cross cranial suture lines. Caput succedaneum is a localized edematous area of the presenting part of the scalp. It's also caused by pressure during delivery, but disappears spontaneously in 3 to 4 days and can cross cranial suture lines. (See *Cephalohematoma and caput succedaneum.*)

Also assess the degree of head control in the neonate. If neonates are placed down on a firm surface, they'll turn their heads to the side to maintain an open airway. They also attempt to keep their heads in line with their body when raised by their arms. Although head lag is normal in the neonate, marked head lag is seen in neonates with Down syndrome or brain damage and hypoxic infants.

Eyes

Neonates tend to keep their eyes tightly shut. Observe the lids for edema, which is normally present for the first few days of life. The eyes should also be assessed for symmetry in size and shape.

Common findings of neonatal eye examination include:

- The neonate's eyes are usually blue or gray because of scleral thinness. Permanent eye color is established within 3 to 12 months.
- Lacrimal glands are immature at birth, resulting in tearless crying for up to 2 months.
- The neonate may demonstrate transient strabismus.
- The doll's eye reflex — when the head is rotated laterally, the eyes deviate in the opposite direction — may persist for up to 10 days.
- Subconjunctival hemorrhages may appear from vascular tension changes during birth.
- The corneal reflex is present but generally isn't elicited unless a problem is suspected.
- The pupillary reflex and the red reflex are present.

CEPHALOHEMATOMA AND CAPUT SUCCEDANEUM

Two distinct swellings may be observed when assessing the neonate's head.

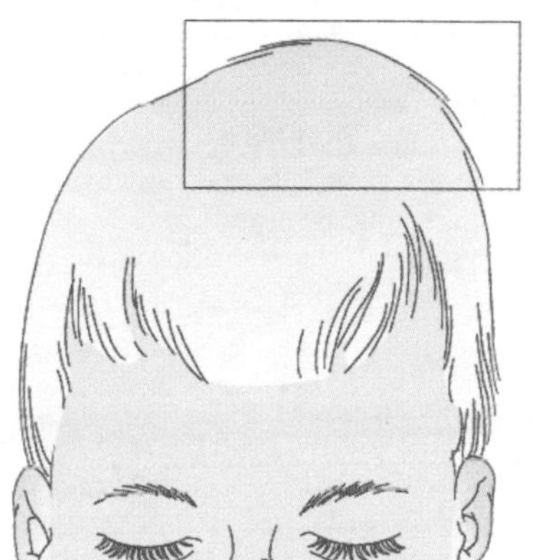

A cephalohematoma occurs when blood collects between a skull bone and the periosteum. The swelling doesn't cross the suture lines.

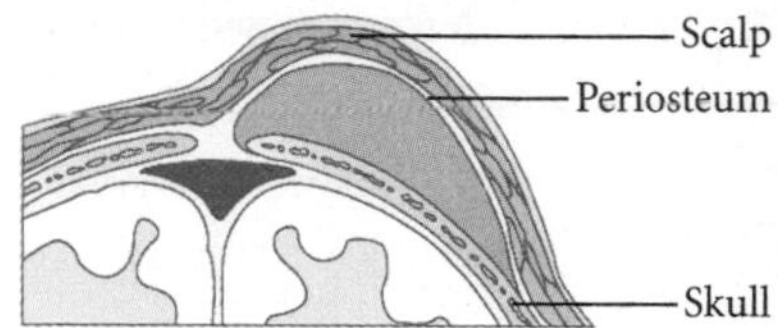

Caput succedaneum is a localized edematous area of the presenting part of the scalp. It can cross the suture lines.

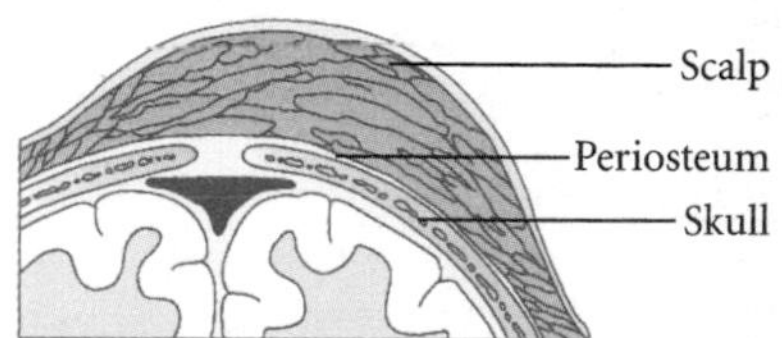

Adapted with permission from Pillitteri, A. *Maternal & Child Health Nursing: Care of the Childbearing & Childrearing Family,* 4th ed. Philadelphia: Lippincott Williams & Wilkins, 2003.

Nose

Observe the neonate's nose for shape, placement, patency, and bridge configuration. Because neonates are obligatory nose breathers for the first few months of life, nasal passages must be kept clear to ensure adequate respiration. Neonates instinctively sneeze to remove obstruction. Test the patency of the nasal passages by occluding each naris alternately while holding the neonate's mouth closed. Observe closely for nasal flaring.

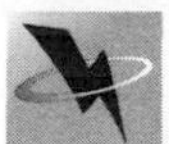

CRITICAL POINT *In the neonate, nasal flaring is a serious sign of air hunger from respiratory distress. Nasal flaring, seesaw respirations, pale, gray skin, periods of apnea, or bradycardia may indicate respiratory distress syndrome.*

Mouth and pharynx

Inspect the neonate's mouth and pharynx. The neonate's mouth usually has scant saliva and pink lips. Inspect the mouth for its existing structures. The palate is usually narrow and highly arched. Inspect the hard and soft palates for clefts.

Epstein's pearls, which are pinhead-size, white or yellow, rounded elevations, may be found on the gums or hard palate. These are caused by retained secretions and disappear within a few weeks or months. The frenulum of the upper lip may be quite thick. Precocious teeth may also be apparent. The pharynx can be best assessed when the neonate is crying. Tonsillar tissue generally isn't visible.

Ears

Assess the neonate's ears for placement on head, amount of cartilage, open auditory canal, and hearing.

The neonate's ears are characterized by incurving of the pinna and cartilage deposition. The pinna is usually flattened against the side of the head from pressure in utero. The top of the ear should be above or parallel to an imaginary line from the inner to the outer canthus of the eye. Low-set ears are associated with several syndromes, including chromosomal abnormalities.

Procedures to screen for hearing in neonates have become common practice before a neonate leaves the health care or birthing facility. Testing can detect permanent bilateral or unilateral sensory or conductive hearing loss.

Auditory assessment is performed by noninvasive, objective, physiologic measures that include otoacoustic emissions or auditory brain stem response. Both testing methods are painless and can be performed while the neonate rests. If the neonate doesn't pass the screening test, the test is usually repeated at age 3 months.

Neck

The neonate's neck is typically short and weak with deep folds of skin. Observe for range of motion (ROM), shape, and abnormal masses.

Also, palpate each clavicle and sternocleidomastoid muscle. Note the trachea's position. The thyroid gland generally isn't palpable.

Chest

Inspect and palpate the chest, noting its shape, clavicles, ribs, nipples, breast tissue, respiratory movements, and amount of cartilage in the rib cage.

The neonatal chest is characterized by a cylindrical thorax, because the anteroposterior and lateral diameters are equal, and flexible ribs. Slight intercostal retractions are usually seen on inspiration. The sternum is raised and slightly rounded, and the xiphoid process is usually visible as a small protrusion at the end of the sternum.

Breast engorgement from maternal hormones may be apparent, and the secretion of "witch's milk" may occur. Supernumerary nipples may be located below and medial to the true nipples.

Lungs

The neonate's normal respirations are abdominal with a rate between 30 and 50 breaths per minute. After the first breaths to initiate respiration, subsequent breaths should be easy and fairly regular. Occasional irregularities may occur with crying, sleeping, and feeding.

Auscultate the lung fields when the neonate is quiet. Bilateral bronchial breath sounds should be heard. Crackles soon after birth represent the transition of the lungs to extrauterine life.

Heart

The neonate's heart rate is normally between 110 and 160 beats per minute. Because neonates have a fast heart rate, it's difficult to auscultate the specific components of the cardiac cycle. Heart sounds during the neonatal period are generally of higher pitch, shorter duration, and greater intensity than in later life. The first sound is usually louder and duller than the second, which is sharp in quality. Murmurs are commonly heard, especially over the base of the heart or at the third or fourth intercostal space at the left sternal border, due to incomplete functional closure of the fetal shunts.

Note the location of the apical impulse, the point of maximal impulse. It's at the fourth intercostal space and to the left of the midclavicular line.

Abdomen

Neonatal abdominal assessment should include inspection and palpation of the umbilical cord, evaluation of the size and contour of the abdomen, auscultation of bowel sounds, assessment of skin color, observation of movement with respirations, and palpation of internal organs.

The neonatal abdomen is usually cylindrical with some protrusion. Bowel sounds are heard a few hours after birth. A scaphoid appearance indicates a diaphragmatic hernia. Inspect the umbilical cord which should appear white and gelatinous with two arteries and one vein. It begins to dry 1 to 2 hours after delivery.

Palpate the liver. The liver is normally palpable 1″ (2.5 cm) below the right costal margin. Sometimes the tip of the spleen can be felt, but a spleen that's palpable more than ³⁄₈″ (1 cm) below the left costal margin warrants further investigation.

Also palpate the kidneys. Both kidneys should be palpable; this is easiest done soon after delivery, when muscle tone is lowest. The suprapubic area should be palpated for a distended bladder. Check for voiding. The neonate should void within the first 24 hours of birth.

Femoral pulses should also be palpated at this point in the examination. Inability to palpate femoral pulses could signify coarctation of the aorta.

Genitalia

Characteristics of a male neonate's genitalia include rugae on the scrotum and testes descended into the scrotum. Scrotal edema may be present for several days after birth due to the effects of maternal hormones. Note the location of the urinary meatus. It may be found in one of three places: at the penile tip (normal), on the dorsal surface (epispadias), or on the ventral surface (hypospadias).

In the female neonate, the labia majora cover the labia minora and clitoris. These structures may be prominent due to maternal hormones. Vaginal discharge may also occur and the hymenal tag is present.

Extremities

Assess the extremities for ROM, symmetry, and signs of trauma. All neonates are bowlegged and have flat feet. The hips should be assessed for dislocation. (See *Eliciting Ortolani's sign,* pages 580 and 581.)

Hyperflexibility of joints is characteristic of Down syndrome. Some neonates may have abnormal extremities. They may be polydactyl, with more than five digits on an extremity, or syndactyl, with two or more digits fused together.

The nail beds should be pink, although they may appear slightly blue due to acrocyanosis. Persistent cyanosis indicates hypoxia or vasoconstriction. The palms should have the usual creases. A transverse palmar crease, called a simian crease, suggests Down syndrome.

Assess muscle tone. Extension of any extremity is usually met with resistance and, upon release, returns to its previously flexed position.

Spine

Inspect the spine and alignment of other structures. The neonatal spine should be straight and flat, and the anus should be patent without any fissure. Dimpling at the base of the spine is commonly associated with spina bifida. The shoulders, scapulae, and iliac crests should line up in the same plane.

Neurologic assessment

An examination of the reflexes provides useful information about the neonate's nervous system and his state of neurologic maturation. Some reflexive behaviors in the neonate are necessary for survival whereas other reflexive behaviors act as safety mechanisms.

Neonatal reflexes

Normal neonates display several types of reflexes. Abnormalities are indicated by absence, asymmetry persistence, or weakness in these reflexes:

- sucking — begins when a nipple is placed in the neonate's mouth
- Moro's reflex — when the neonate is lifted above the crib and suddenly lowered; the arms and legs symmetrically extend and then abduct while the fingers spread to form a "C"
- rooting — when the neonate's cheek is stroked, the neonate turns his head in the direction of the stroke
- tonic neck or fencing position — when the neonate's head is turned while he's lying in a supine position, the extremities on same side straighten and those on the opposite side flex
- Babinski's reflex — when the sole on the side of the neonate's small toe is stroked and the toes fan upward
- grasping — when a finger is placed in each of the neonate's hands, the neonate's fingers grasp tightly enough to be pulled to a sitting position
- stepping — when the neonate is held upright with the feet touching a flat surface, he responds with dancing or stepping movements
- startle — when a loud noise such as a hand clap elicits neonatal arm abduction

(Text continues on page 582.)

EXPERT TECHNIQUE

ELICITING ORTOLANI'S SIGN

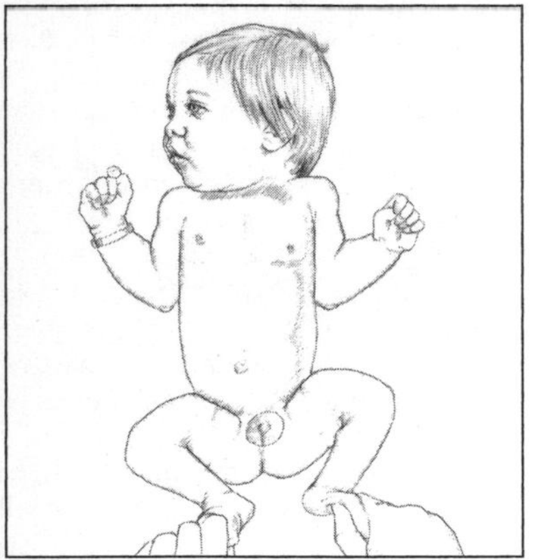

When assessing the neonate, attempt to elicit Ortolani's sign to detect developmental dysplasia of the hip (DDH). Begin by placing the infant in a supine position with his knees and hips flexed. Observe for symmetry.

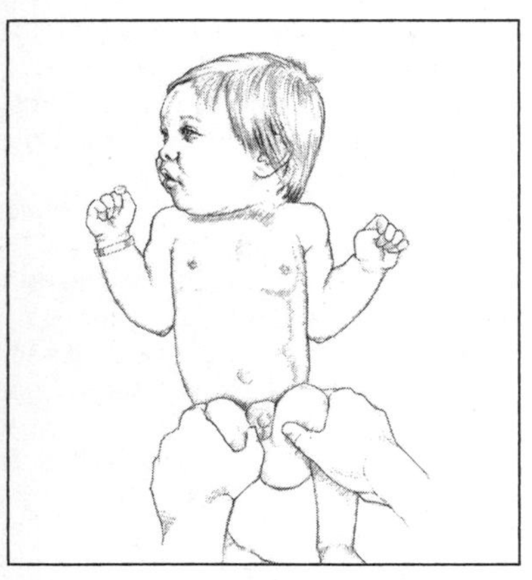

Place your hands on the infant's knees, with your index fingers along his lateral thighs on the greater trochanter. Then raise his knees to a 90-degree angle with his back.

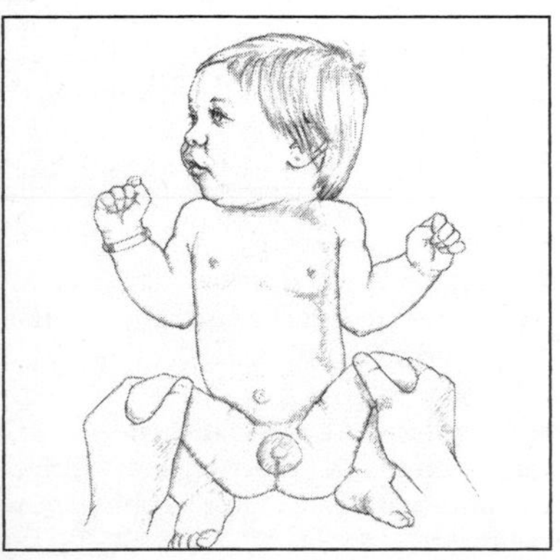

Abduct the infant's thighs so that the lateral aspect of his knees lies almost flat on the table. If the infant has a dislocated hip, you'll feel and usually hear a click, clunk, or popping sensation (Ortolani's sign) as the head of the femur moves out of the acetabulum. The infant may also give a sudden cry of pain. Be sure to distinguish a positive Ortolani's sign from the normal clicks due to rotation of the hip, that don't elicit the sensation of instability, or simultaneous movement of the knee.

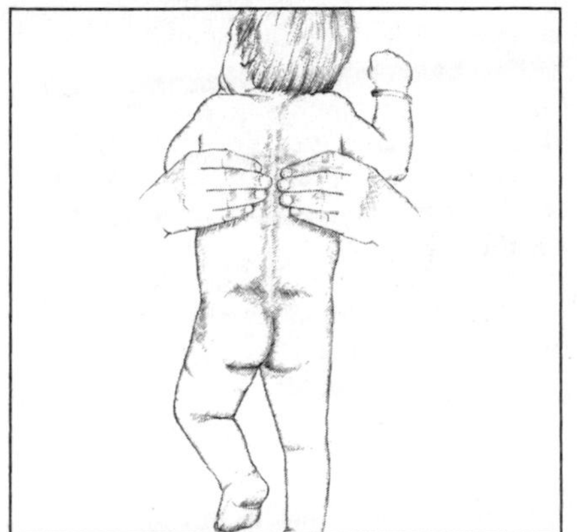

If you elicit a positive Ortolani's sign, look for other signs of DDH.

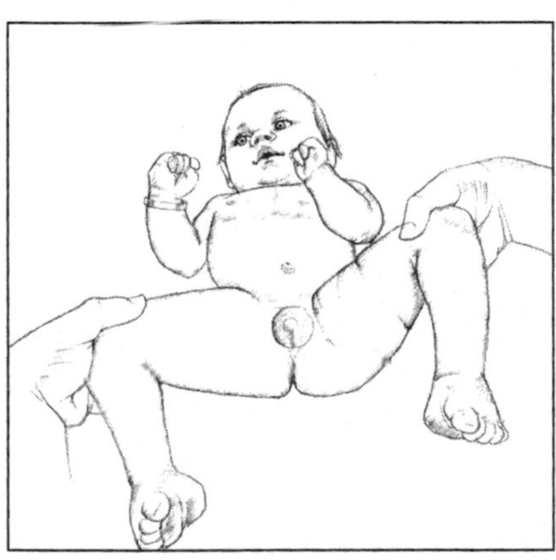

Flex the infant's hips to detect limited abduction.

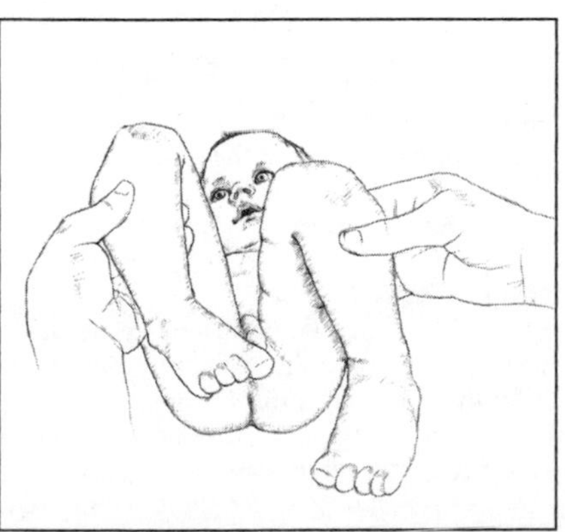

Flex the infant's knees, and observe for apparent shortening of the femur.

and elbow flexion and the neonate's hands stay clenched

- trunk incurvature — when a finger is run laterally down the neonate's spine, the trunk flexes and the pelvis swings toward the stimulated side
- blinking — when the neonate's eyelids close in response to bright light
- acoustic blinking — when both of the neonate's eyes blink in response to a loud noise
- Perez reflex — when the neonate is suspended prone in one of the health care provider's hands and the thumb of the other hand is moved firmly up the neonate's spine from the sacrum, the neonate's head and spine extend, the knees flex, the neonate cries, and he may empty his bladder. (See *Assessing neonatal reflexes,* pages 584 and 585.)

Behavioral assessment

Behavioral characteristics are an important part of neonatal development. To assess whether a neonate is exhibiting normal behavior, be aware of the neonate's principle behaviors of sleep, wakefulness, and activity, such as crying, as well as his social capabilities and ability to adapt to certain stimuli.

Factors that affect behavioral responses include gestational age, time of day, stimuli, and medication. Other factors that affect behaviors include consolability, the ability of the neonate to console himself or be consoled; cuddliness, the neonate's response to being held; irritability, how easily a neonate is upset; and crying, the ability of the neonate to communicate different needs with his cry.

Cry

Assess the neonate's cry, including strength and pitch. A neonate should begin life with a strong, lusty cry. Variations in this initial cry can indicate abnormalities. For example, a weak, groaning cry or grunt during expiration usually signifies respiratory disturbances. Absent, weak, or constant crying suggests brain damage. A high-pitched shrill cry may be a sign of increased ICP.

Sleep-wake cycles

Observe the neonate's sleep-wake cycles, the variations in the neonate's consciousness. Note how the neonate handles transitions from one state in the cycle to the next.

Six specific neonatal sleep-activity states have been defined:

- deep sleep — regular breathing, eyes closed, no spontaneous activity
- light sleep — eyes closed, rapid eye movement, random movements and startles, irregular breathing, sucking movements
- drowsy — eyes open, dull, heavy eyelids, variable activity, delayed response to stimuli
- alert — bright, seems focused, minimal motor activity
- active — eyes open, considerable motor activity, thrusting movements, briefly fussy
- crying — high motor activity.

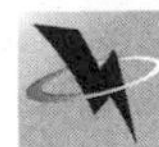

CRITICAL POINT *In neonates, the sleep-wake cycles are highly influenced by the environment.*

Readiness for social interaction

Neonates possess sensory capabilities that indicate their readiness for social interaction. Assess the neonate for these behavioral responses:

- sensitivity to light — a neonate opens his eyes when the lights are dim and his responses to movement are noticeable
- selective listening — a neonate tends to exhibit selective listening to his mother's voice stimuli
- response to touch — a neonate responds to touch, such as calming when touched softly, suggesting that he's ready to receive tactile messages
- taste preferences — a series of studies have demonstrated that neonates prefer sweet fluids to those that are sour or bitter
- sense of smell — studies have shown that neonates prefer pleasant smells and that they have the ability to learn and remember odors.

An absence of any of these behavioral responses is cause for concern and requires further investigation.

Habituation

Each neonate has a unique temperament and varies in his ability to handle stimuli from the external world. Through habituation, the neonate can control the type and amount of stimuli processed, which decreases his response to constant or repeated stimuli. The ability to habituate depends on the neonate's state of consciousness, hunger, fatigue, and temperament.

Observe the neonate's response to stimuli. A neonate presented with new stimuli becomes wide-eyed and alert but eventually shows decreased interest. Habituation enables the neonate to respond to select stimuli, such as human voices, that encourage continued learning about the social world.

Follow-up assessment and adaptations

Follow-up assessment may be necessary if the neonate has been discharged from the health care facility and then returns with a problem. In these cases, adaptations are necessary. Although vital signs, anthropometric measurements, head-to-toe examination, and neurologic assessment would be performed, information would need to be obtained about the neonate's problem. In addition, obtaining a health history from parents also would be important.

Common problems associated with neonates include skin color changes such as pallor or jaundice; neurologic changes, such as lethargy, irritability, or tremors; respiratory problems, such as apnea, grunting respirations, retractions, or nasal flaring; and GI problems such as abdominal distention, vomiting, and feeding difficulties.

Ask the parents about the onset of the problem, including if it occurred suddenly or gradually, and how frequently it occurs. Find out what seems to cause the problem and if they have noticed any measures that make it better or worse. Ask the parents how the neonate appears when the problem occurs. Also find out if it interferes with the neonate's activities, such as feeding or sleeping.

Obtain information about the past health history. A neonate's past history includes information about his health status before the examination. Inquire about the neonate's feeding and elimination patterns, including the amount and frequency of feedings, ease of feedings, and the number of voidings and stools per day. In addition, obtain information from family members about any known congenital anomalies and other problems.

The neonate's past health history, especially during the first few critical days of life, also includes these maternal history aspects:

- Maternal age. The mother's age, the outcome of the pregnancy, and the neonate's health can be directly related. Adolescents and mothers older than age 35 are at higher risk for problems.
- Drug and alcohol use. Both over-the-counter and prescription drugs taken during pregnancy may be passed to the fetus transplacentally. Additionally, neonates born to mothers who use substances are at greater risk for the development of substance withdrawal and congenital malformations. Consumption of alcohol is associated with fetal alcohol syndrome. Use of nicotine during pregnancy may lead to growth retardation and an increased risk of sudden infant death syndrome.
- Infections. Infections in the mother may be transmitted via the placenta causing infection in the neonate.
- Diseases and disorders. Many pathologic maternal conditions, such as diabetes mellitus, chronic hypertension, cardiac disease, and pregnancy induced hypertension, can cause numerous problems for the neonate, such as hypoglycemia or congenital malformations.
- Prenatal care. Neonates born to mothers who didn't have adequate prenatal care are more likely to have complications.

Information about the events of labor and delivery also is important to address. Labor and delivery is stressful for every neonate. Uterine contractions exert extreme pressure on the fetus at the same time that the fetus meets resistance from pelvic structures. The fetus must also withstand brief periods of hypoxia, caused by decreased circulation during uterine contractions. This traumatic process occurs in all vaginal deliveries. For some neonates, vaginal birth may be even more dangerous, so cesarean delivery may be necessary to reduce the risk.

When assessing a neonate's prenatal history related to labor and delivery, ask the mother about the duration and progress of labor, use of medications such as oxytocin or analgesics, and any problems that may have occurred with her or the fetus during labor or delivery. Specifically ask about problems such as premature labor, preterm rupture of membranes, dysfunctional labor pattern, or abnormal fetal presentation.

Obtain the neonate's family history. Ask the parents about any family history of con-

(Text continues on page 586.)

EXPERT TECHNIQUE

ASSESSING NEONATAL REFLEXES

Some of the more common reflexes are depicted here as well as how to assess them in the neonate.

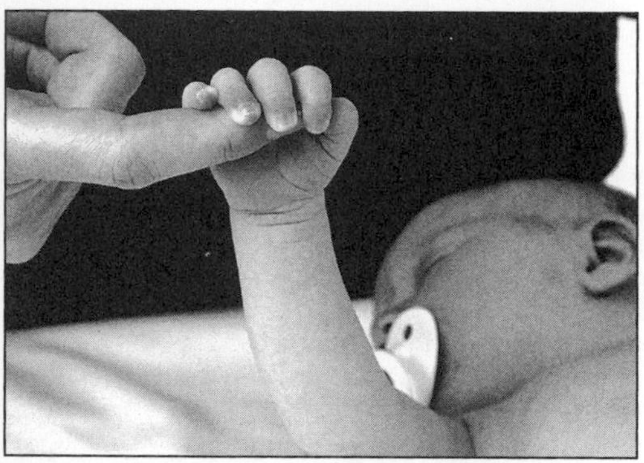

Palmar grasp reflex
Place a finger in the palm of the neonate's hand. The neonate will close his fingers around the examiner's fingers.

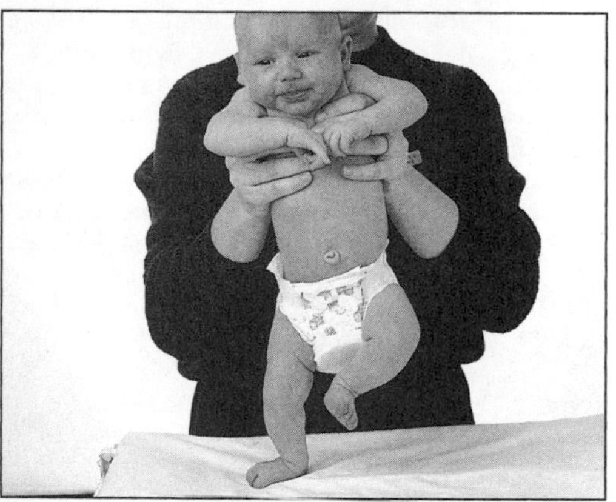

Stepping reflex
Place one hand under each of the neonate's axillae and hold the neonate upright. The neonate's feet should be touching a flat surface. The neonate responds by making stepping motions.

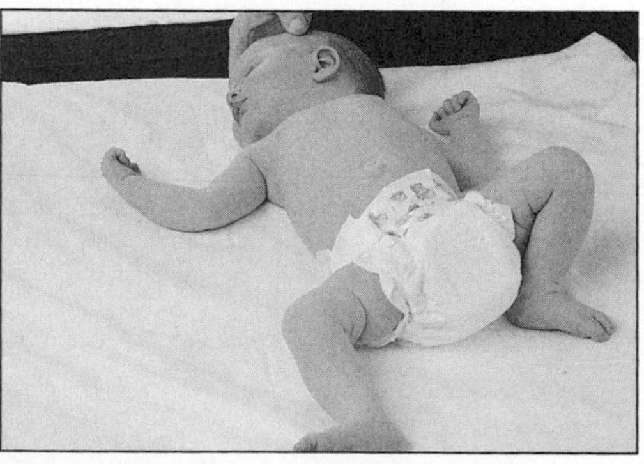

Tonic neck reflex
Place the neonate in a supine position on a flat surface. Then turn the neonate's head to one side so that his jaw is at the shoulder. The neonate responds by extending the extremities on the side to which the head is turned and flexing the opposite side extremities, giving the appearance that the neonate is in a "fencing" position.

Adapted with permission from Weber, J., and Kelley, J. *Health Assessment in Nursing.* Philadelphia: Lippincott-Raven Publishers, 1998.

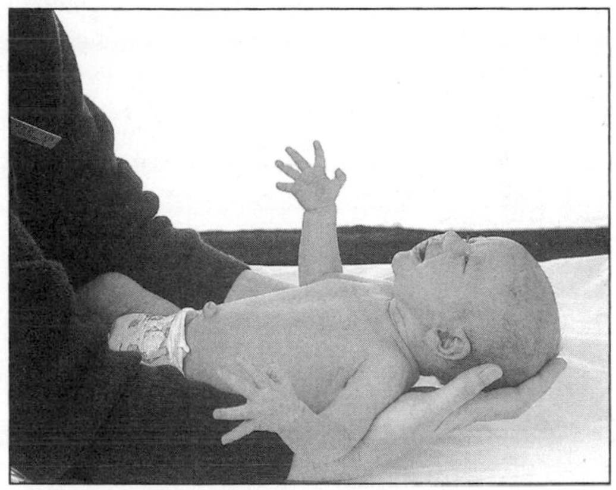

Moro reflex
Place the neonate in the supine position on a flat surface. Hit the table surface or clap your hands loudly to startle the neonate. The neonate responds by slightly flexing and abducting the legs, laterally extending and abducting the arms, making a "C" with the thumb and fingers of one hand and fanning out the fingers of the other hand.

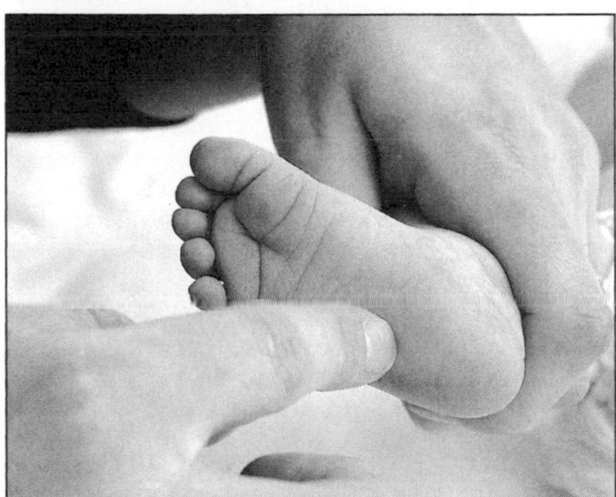

Babinski's reflex
While holding the neonate's foot, apply slight pressure with a fingertip, running the finger up the lateral side of the sole of the foot. The neonate responds by fanning the toes.

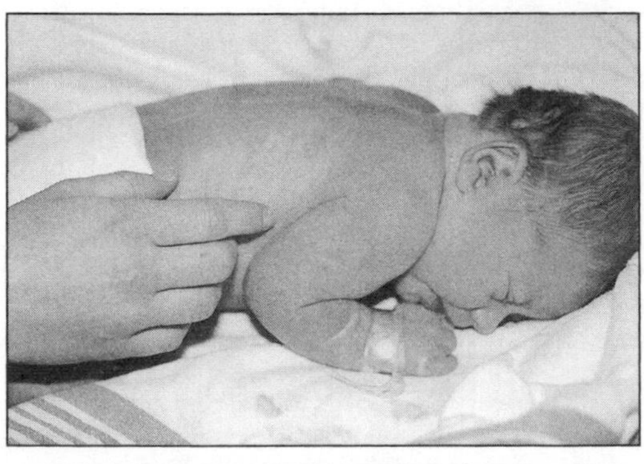

Trunk incurvature reflex
Place the neonate in the prone position. Apply gentle pressure using a finger to the paravertebral area, the lateral aspect of the spine. The neonate responds by flexing the trunk and moving the pelvis toward the location of the stimulus. (Photo courtesy of Caroline Brown, RNC, MS, DEd.)

genital defects or genetically transmitted diseases, previous multiple births, infant deaths, including stillbirths and abortions, and family members' general health. Ask about such diseases as diabetes or seizures.

Inquire about the neonate's family. Areas to address include: arrangements at home for the neonate's care; siblings and their adjustment to the neonate; financial and occupational situation, such as whether the mother will be returning to work; other family members available for support or assistance; possible lifestyle conflicts; and health practices and beliefs.

Abnormal findings

Although birth of a child typically is considered an exciting and happy event, problems can develop. A neonate may require care for several signs and symptoms that indicate complications. The most significant findings are fontanel bulging or depression; low birth weight; jaundice; meconium-stained amniotic fluid; nasal flaring; Ortolani's sign; respirations, grunting; retractions, costal and sternal; and tachypnea. The following history, physical assessment, and analysis summaries will help you assess each one quickly and accurately. After obtaining further information, begin to interpret the findings. (See *The neonate: Interpreting your findings.*)

Fontanel bulging

In a normal neonate, the anterior fontanel, or "soft spot," is a flat, soft yet firm, and well demarcated area against surrounding skull bones. The posterior fontanel shouldn't be fused at birth, but may be overriding following the birthing process. The fontanel usually closes by age 3 months. Subtle pulsations may be visible, reflecting the arterial pulse.

History

Obtain the neonate's history from a parent or caregiver, paying particular attention to any recent infection or trauma, including birth trauma. Ask the parents or caregiver if the neonate or any family member has had a recent rash or fever. Find out about any changes in the neonate's behavior, such as frequent vomiting, lethargy, or disinterest in feeding.

Physical assessment

Measure the neonate's fontanel size and head circumference, and note the overall shape of the head. Take vital signs, and determine level of consciousness by observing spontaneous activity, postural reflex activity, and sensory responses. Note whether the neonate assumes a normal, flexed posture or one of extreme extension, opisthotonos, or hypotonia. Observe arm and leg movements; excessive tremulousness or frequent twitching may herald the onset of a seizure. Observe for other signs of increased intracranial pressure (ICP) such as abnormal respiratory patterns and a distinctive, high-pitched cry.

Analysis

A bulging fontanel—widened, tense, and with marked pulsations—is a cardinal sign of meningitis associated with increased ICP, a medical emergency. It can also be an indication of encephalitis or fluid overload.

CRITICAL POINT *Because prolonged coughing, crying, or lying down can cause transient, physiologic bulging, the neonate's head should be observed and palpated while he's upright and relaxed to detect pathologic bulging.*

Fontanel depression

In a normal neonate, the anterior fontanel, or "soft spot," is a flat, soft yet firm, and well demarcated area against surrounding skull bones. The posterior fontanel shouldn't be fused at birth, but may be overriding after the birthing process. Normally closed by age 3 months, this fontanel is characterized by subtle pulsations that may be visible, reflecting the arterial pulse.

History

Obtain a thorough history from a parent or caregiver, focusing on recent fever, vomiting, diarrhea, and behavioral changes. Inquire about the neonate's fluid intake and urine output over the last 24 hours, including the number of wet diapers during that time. Ask about the neonate's pre-illness weight, and compare it with his current weight. Weight loss in a neonate reflects water loss.

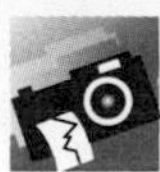

CLINICAL PICTURE

THE NEONATE: INTERPRETING YOUR FINDINGS

After you assess the neonate, a group of findings may lead you to suspect a particular disorder. The chart below shows some common groups of findings for major signs and symptoms related to the neonate, along with their probable causes.

Sign or symptom and findings	Probable cause
Fontanel bulging	
▪ Bulging with increased head circumference ▪ Behavioral changes ▪ Irritability ▪ Fatigue ▪ Vomiting ▪ Pupillary dilation with increasing pressure ▪ Drowsiness progressing to coma with increasing pressure	Increased intracranial pressure
▪ Widened suture lines with tense bulging fontanels ▪ Shiny scalp with visible scalp veins ▪ Bulging brow ▪ Sunset eyes ▪ Irritability or lethargy ▪ Shrill high-pitched cry	Hydrocephalus
Fontanel depression	
▪ Fontanel depression slight to prominent depending on degree of dehydration ▪ Weight loss ▪ Pale dry skin and mucous membranes ▪ Decreased urine output ▪ Normal or elevated pulse rate ▪ Irritability	Dehydration
Low birth weight	
▪ Low birth weight associated with prematurity or small for gestational age ▪ Petechiae and ecchymoses ▪ Jaundice ▪ Hepatosplenomegaly ▪ High fever ▪ Lymphadenopathy ▪ Tachypnea ▪ Prolonged bleeding at puncture site	Cytomegalovirus infection
▪ Low birth weight associated with prematurity or small for gestational age ▪ Hydrocephalus or microcephalus ▪ Fever ▪ Seizures ▪ Lymphadenopathy ▪ Jaundice ▪ Rash ▪ Strabismus, blindness, and mental retardation occurring months to years later	Congenital toxoplasmosis
Jaundice	
▪ Yellowish skin discoloration including the sclerae ▪ History of Rh incompatibility or ABO incompatibility ▪ Pallor ▪ Hepatosplenomegaly	Hyperbilirubinemia

(continued)

THE NEONATE: INTERPRETING YOUR FINDINGS *(continued)*

Sign or symptom and findings	Probable cause
Meconium-stained amniotic fluid	
▪ Dark greenish staining or streaking of amniotic fluid or greenish stain to skin ▪ Limp appearance at birth ▪ Cyanosis ▪ Rapid labored breathing and apnea ▪ Signs of postmaturity including dry peeling skin, long nails ▪ Low Apgar score ▪ Hypothermia ▪ Hypoglycemia ▪ Hypocalcemia	Meconium aspiration syndrome
Nasal flaring	
▪ Nasal flaring accompanied by tachypnea ▪ Labored respirations ▪ Expiratory grunting ▪ Retractions ▪ Cyanosis	Transient tachypnea of the neonate
▪ Nasal flaring with progressively increasing respiratory rate ▪ Retractions becoming progressively more pronounced ▪ Fine crackles on lung auscultation ▪ Expiratory grunting ▪ Cyanosis ▪ Flaccidity ▪ Apneic episodes ▪ Diminished breath sounds ▪ Unresponsiveness	Respiratory distress syndrome
Ortolani's sign	
▪ Positive Ortolani's sign ▪ Affected extremity appearing shorter than unaffected extremity ▪ Unequal number of gluteal folds posteriorly	Developmental dysplasia of the hip
Respirations, grunting	
▪ Grunting respirations with fever ▪ Diminished breath sounds ▪ Scattered crackles ▪ Retractions ▪ Nasal flaring ▪ Cyanosis ▪ Increasing lethargy ▪ Possible vomiting, diarrhea, and abdominal distention	Pneumonia
▪ Audible grunting accompanied by intercostal, subcostal, or substernal retractions ▪ Tachycardia ▪ Tachypnea ▪ Low birth weight ▪ Apnea or irregular respiratory patterns with progression of illness ▪ Severe respiratory distress including cyanosis, frothy sputum, dramatic nasal flaring, lethargy, bradycardia, and hypotension	Respiratory distress syndrome

THE NEONATE: INTERPRETING YOUR FINDINGS *(continued)*

Sign or symptom and findings	Probable cause
Retractions, costal and sternal	
■ Intercostal and substernal retractions ■ Nasal flaring ■ Progressive tachypnea ■ Grunting respirations, edema and cyanosis (if severe) ■ Productive cough ■ Crackles ■ Tachycardia	Heart failure
■ Substernal and subcostal retractions, most commonly in premature neonate ■ Low birth weight ■ Tachypnea ■ Tachycardia ■ Expiratory grunting ■ Apnea or irregular respiratory patterns with progression of illness ■ Severe respiratory distress including cyanosis, frothy sputum, dramatic nasal flaring, lethargy, bradycardia, and hypotension	Respiratory distress syndrome
Tachypnea	
■ Tachypnea accompanied by nasal flaring ■ Labored respirations ■ Expiratory grunting ■ Retractions ■ Cyanosis	Transient tachypnea of the neonate
■ Tachypnea with audible grunting accompanied by intercostal, subcostal, or substernal retractions ■ Tachycardia ■ Low birth weight ■ Apnea or irregular respiratory patterns with progression of illness ■ Severe respiratory distress including cyanosis, frothy sputum, dramatic nasal flaring, lethargy, bradycardia, and hypotension	Respiratory distress syndrome

Physical assessment
Obtain vital signs, weigh the neonate, and check for signs of shock — tachycardia, tachypnea, and cool, clammy skin. Check skin turgor and mucous membranes for moisture. Assess urine color and check urine output by weighing the wet diapers.

Analysis
Depression of the anterior fontanel below the surrounding bony ridges of the skull is a sign of dehydration. A common disorder of infancy and early childhood, dehydration can result from insufficient fluid intake, but typically reflects excessive fluid loss from severe vomiting or diarrhea. It may also reflect insensible water loss, pyloric stenosis, or tracheoesophageal fistula.

Jaundice
A yellow discoloration of the skin, mucous membranes, or sclera of the eyes, jaundice indicates excessive levels of conjugated or unconjugated bilirubin in the blood.

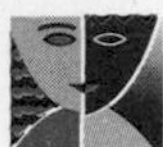

CULTURAL INSIGHT *In fair-skinned neonates, jaundice is most evident on the face, trunk, and sclera. In dark-skinned neonates, it's noticeable on the hard palate, sclera, and conjunctiva.*

Jaundice is most apparent in natural sunlight. In fact, it may be undetectable in artificial or poor light. It's commonly accompanied by pruritus, because bile pigment damages sensory nerves; dark urine; and clay-colored stools.

History

Begin taking the neonate's history by asking the parents or caregiver when they first noticed the jaundice. Ask if the neonate has clay-colored stools or dark urine. Determine if the neonate is being breast-fed or bottle-fed. Question the mother about Rh status and administration of Rh immune globulin. Ask about past episodes or a family history of jaundice. Find out about other signs or symptoms, such as fever or vomiting.

Physical assessment

Perform the physical examination in a room with natural light. Make sure that the orange-yellow hue is jaundice and not due to hypercarotenemia, which is more prominent on the palms and soles and doesn't affect the sclera.

Inspect the neonate's skin for texture and dryness and for hyperpigmentation.

CRITICAL POINT *To verify jaundice in the neonate, press the skin on the cheek or abdomen lightly with one finger, then release pressure and observe skin color immediately.*

Auscultate for crackles and abnormal bowel sounds. Palpate the lymph nodes for swelling and the abdomen for tenderness, pain, and swelling. Palpate and percuss the liver and spleen for enlargement. Obtain baseline data on the patient's neurologic status.

Analysis

Jaundice resulting from physiologic hyperbilirubinemia occurs in 50% of full-term neonates and 80% of preterm neonates. It's a mild form of jaundice that appears after the first 24 hours of extrauterine life and usually disappears in 7 days (9 or 10 days in preterm neonates). However, if bilirubin levels rise, pathologic conditions such as kernicterus may develop.

Jaundice resulting from pathologic hyperbilirubinemia is evident at birth or within the first 24 hours of extrauterine life. It may be caused by hemolytic disease, liver disease, or severe infection. Prognosis varies depending on the cause.

Low birth weight

Two groups of neonates are born weighing less than the normal minimum birth weight of 5 lb, 8 oz (2,500 g) — those who are born prematurely, before the 37th week of gestation, and those who are small for gestational age. The premature neonate weighs an appropriate amount for his gestational age and probably would have matured normally if carried to full term. Conversely, the small for gestational age neonate weighs less than the normal amount for his age; however, his organs are mature. Differentiating between the two groups can help you to direct the search for a cause.

History

Obtain the neonate's complete health history from the parents or caregiver. Inquire specifically about the prenatal history and events of labor and delivery.

Physical assessment

Because low birth weight may be associated with poorly developed body systems, particularly the respiratory system, assess the neonate's respiratory status. Note any signs of distress, such as apnea, grunting respirations, intercostal or xiphoid retractions, or a respiratory rate exceeding 60 breaths per minute after the first hour of life. Assess vital signs including axillary temperature. Decreased fat reserves may keep the neonate from maintaining normal body temperature, and a drop below 97.8° F (36.5° C) exacerbates respiratory distress by increasing oxygen consumption.

Evaluate the neonate's neuromuscular and physical maturity to determine gestational age. Perform a head-to-toe neonatal assessment.

Analysis

In the premature neonate, low birth weight usually results from a disorder that prevents the uterus from retaining the fetus, interferes with the normal course of pregnancy, causes premature separation of the placenta, or stimulates uterine contractions before term. In the small for gestational age neonate, intrauterine growth may be retarded by a disorder that interferes with placental circulation, fetal development, or maternal health.

Regardless of the cause, low birth weight is associated with higher neonate morbidity and mortality; in fact, low birth weight neonates are 20 times more likely to die within the first month of life. Low birth weight can also signal a life-threatening emergency.

Meconium-stained amniotic fluid

Meconium is a thick, sticky, greenish-black substance that constitutes the neonate's first feces. It's present in the bowel of the fetus as early as 10 weeks' gestation.

History

Obtain a complete prenatal history from the neonate's mother. Note any risk factors such as a history of maternal diabetes or hypertension. Also inquire about the neonate's gestational age and weight when born.

Review the labor and delivery history. Focus on events during labor and delivery. Find out how far along in the pregnancy the mother was when she delivered. Find out how long her labor was and if any problems arose during labor. If so, find out what types of problems arose, such as if the fetus was distressed.

Physical assessment

Assess the amniotic fluid, if possible, for color. Meconium-stained fluid appears dark greenish or may be streaked with green. Assess the neonate's skin color. The skin may have a greenish stain. Observe for cyanosis.

Assess the neonate's respiratory status closely. Note respiratory rate and rhythm. Auscultate breath sounds for coarse crackles. Inspect the neonate's vocal cords for a greenish stain. Continue with a complete head-to-toe neonatal assessment.

Analysis

Meconium-stained amniotic fluid suggests meconium aspiration syndrome. This syndrome results when the neonate inhales meconium that's mixed with amniotic fluid. It typically occurs while the neonate is in utero or with the neonate's first breath. Meconium in the amniotic fluid may result with fetal distress, when a fetus becomes hypoxic in utero. Subsequently, peristalsis increases and the anal sphincter relaxes. Occasionally, healthy neonates pass meconium before birth. In either case, if the neonate gasps or inhales the meconium it can partially or completely block his airways so that air becomes trapped during exhalation. The meconium also irritates the neonate's airways, making breathing difficult. The resulting lack of oxygen may lead to brain damage.

Nasal flaring

Nasal flaring is the abnormal dilation of the nostrils. Usually occurring during inspiration, nasal flaring may occasionally occur during expiration or throughout the respiratory cycle. It indicates respiratory dysfunction, ranging from mild difficulty to potentially life-threatening respiratory distress.

History

Obtain the neonate's complete health history from the parents or caregiver. Ask about any underlying cardiac and pulmonary problems. Ask if the neonate has experienced a recent illness, such as a respiratory tract infection, or trauma. Find out if the parents or caregiver smoke near the neonate. Obtain a drug history including a prenatal maternal drug history.

Physical assessment

Perform a complete head-to-toe neonatal assessment. Focus on inspection of the skin for color, noting any pallor or cyanosis. Inspect the nose for redness, drainage, or obstruction. Assess vital signs, including respiratory rate, depth, and character. Observe for apnea. Auscultate breath sounds for changes including crackles or decreased breath sounds. Inspect the chest for retractions and labored breathing.

Assess the neonate's neurologic status for changes, such as decreasing or lack of responsiveness and lethargy. Inspect the extremities and positioning of the neonate. Note muscle flaccidity.

Analysis

Nasal flaring is an important sign of respiratory distress in neonates, infants, and young children, who can't verbalize their discomfort. Common causes include airway obstruction, respiratory distress syndrome, croup, and acute epiglottiditis.

Ortolani's sign

Ortolani's sign refers to a click, clunk, or popping sensation that's felt and usually heard when a neonate's hip is flexed 90 degrees and abducted.

History

Obtain a complete health history, including maternal, prenatal, and labor and delivery history. Investigate if the neonate was born in a vertex or breech position.

Physical examination

Perform a complete head-to-toe neonatal assessment with a focus on the lower extremities. Test the neonate for Ortolani's sign (see *Eliciting Ortolani's sign,* pages 580 and 581). If positive, evaluate the neonate for asymmetrical gluteal folds, limited hip abduction, and unequal leg length.

Analysis

Ortolani's sign is an indication of developmental dysplasia of the hip (DDH); it results when the femoral head enters or exits the acetabulum.

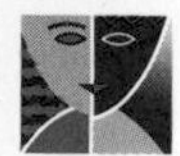

CULTURAL INSIGHT *DDH is most common in female neonates. A strong relationship between hip dysplasia and methods of handling the infant has been demonstrated. For instance, Inuit and Navajo Indians have a high incidence of DDH, which may be related to their practice of wrapping neonates in blankets or strapping them to cradle-boards. In cultures where mothers carry infants on their backs or hips, such as in the Far East and Africa, hip dysplasia is rarely seen.*

Screening for Ortolani's sign is an important part of neonatal care because early detection and treatment of DDH improves the infant's chances of growing with a correctly formed, functional joint.

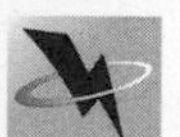

CRITICAL POINT *Ortolani's sign can be elicited only during the first 4 to 6 weeks of life; this is also the optimum time for effective corrective treatment. If treatment is delayed, DDH may cause degenerative hip changes, lordosis, joint malformation, and soft-tissue damage.*

Respirations, grunting

Grunting respirations are characterized by a deep, low-pitched grunting sound at the end of each breath. They may be soft and heard only on auscultation, or loud and clearly audible without a stethoscope.

History

Ask the neonate's parents or caregiver when the grunting respirations began. If the patient is a premature neonate, find out his gestational age. Ask the parents if anyone in the home has recently had an upper respiratory tract infection. Find out if the neonate has had signs and symptoms of infection, such as a runny nose, cough, low-grade fever, or anorexia. Ask about a history of frequent colds or upper respiratory tract infections. Find out if the neonate has a history of respiratory syncytial virus. Ask the parents to describe changes in the neonate's activity level or feeding pattern to determine if he's lethargic or less alert than usual.

Physical assessment

Begin the physical examination by auscultating the lungs, especially the lower lobes. Note diminished or abnormal sounds, such as crackles or sibilant rhonchi, which may indicate mucus or fluid buildup. Also, characterize the color, amount, and consistency of any discharge or sputum. Note the characteristics of the cough, if any.

Assess for signs of respiratory distress: wheezing; tachypnea with a minimum respiratory rate of 60 breaths per minute; accessory muscle use; substernal, subcostal, or intercostal retractions; nasal flaring; tachycardia; cyanotic lips or nail beds; hypotension (less than 80/40 mm Hg in neonates); and decreased level of consciousness.

Complete the physical assessment when the neonate's condition has stabilized.

Analysis

Grunting respirations are a chief sign of respiratory distress in neonates, infants, and children. Grunting respirations indicate intrathoracic disease with lower respiratory involvement. Typically, the intensity of grunting respirations reflects the severity of respiratory distress. The grunting sound coincides with closure of the glottis, an effort to increase end-expiratory pressure in the lungs and prolong alveolar gas exchange, thereby enhancing ventilation and perfusion.

Retractions, costal and sternal

Retractions are visible indentations of the soft tissue covering the chest wall. They may be suprasternal, appearing directly above the sternum and clavicles; intercostal, located between the ribs; subcostal, located below the lower costal margin of the rib cage; or substernal, located just below the xiphoid process. Retractions may be mild or severe, producing barely visible to deep indentations.

Normally, neonates, infants, and young children use abdominal muscles for breathing, unlike older children and adults, who use the diaphragm. When breathing requires extra effort, accessory muscles assist respiration, especially inspiration. Retractions typically accompany accessory muscle use.

History

If the neonate's condition permits, ask the parents or caregiver about his medical history. Find out if he was born prematurely and with a low birth weight. Find out about any delivery complications. Ask about recent signs of an upper respiratory tract infection, such as a runny nose, cough, and a low-grade fever. Find out if the neonate has had contact with anyone who has had a cold, the flu, or other respiratory ailments. Ask if he ever had respiratory syncytial virus. Find out if the neonate aspirated any food, liquid, or foreign body. Inquire about any personal or family history of allergies or asthma.

Physical assessment

If retractions are noted, assess quickly for other signs of respiratory distress, such as cyanosis, tachypnea, and tachycardia. Observe the depth and location of retractions. Also, note the rate, depth, and quality of respirations. Look for accessory muscle use, nasal flaring during inspiration, or grunting during expiration. If the neonate has a cough, record the color, consistency, and odor of any sputum. Note whether the neonate appears restless or lethargic. Finally, auscultate the lungs to detect abnormal breath sounds.

Complete the physical assessment when the neonate's condition has stabilized.

Analysis

Retractions may occur with any respiratory problem, including respiratory distress syndrome and pneumonia.

CRITICAL POINT *In neonates, infants, and children, retractions are a cardinal sign of respiratory distress.*

Tachypnea

Tachypnea is an abnormally fast respiratory rate — greater than 20 or more breaths per minute in an adult, and greater than 60 breaths per minute in a neonate.

History

If the neonate's condition permits, obtain a health history from the parents or caregiver. Find out when the tachypnea began and if it followed activity. Find out if the neonate had had tachypnea before. Also obtain a prenatal and labor and delivery history from the mother. Ask about any maternal history of diabetes or smoking during pregnancy. Find out if the neonate was born vaginally or via cesarean delivery.

Physical assessment

Begin the physical examination by taking the neonate's vital signs, including oxygen saturation, and observing his overall behavior. Observe the neonate for restlessness, irritability, or lethargy. Then auscultate the chest for abnormal heart and breath sounds. If the neonate has a productive cough, record the color, amount, and consistency of sputum. Examine the skin for pallor, cyanosis, edema, and warmth or coolness.

Analysis

Tachypnea may reflect the need to increase minute volume — the amount of air breathed each minute. Under these circumstances, it may be accompanied by an increase in tidal volume — the volume of air inhaled or exhaled per breath — resulting in hyperventilation. Tachypnea, however, may also reflect stiff lungs or overloaded ventilatory muscles, in which case tidal volume may be reduced.

Tachypnea may result from reduced arterial oxygen tension or arterial oxygen content, decreased perfusion, or increased oxygen demand. Heightened oxygen demand, for example, may result from fever (generally, respirations increase by 4 breaths per minute for every 1° F [0.5° C] increase in body temperature), exertion, anxiety, and pain. It may also occur as a compensatory response to metabolic acidosis or may result from pulmonary irritation, stretch receptor stimulation, or a neurologic disorder that upsets medullary respiratory control.

Some causes of tachypnea include transient tachypnea of the neonate, congenital heart defects, meningitis, metabolic acidosis, and cystic fibrosis. Hunger and anxiety may also cause tachypnea in the neonate.

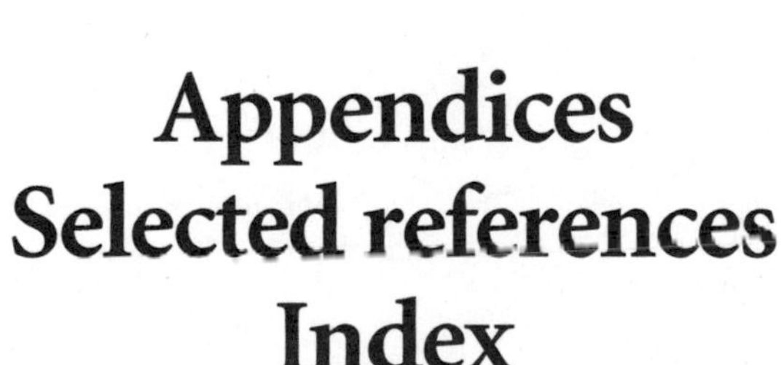

Appendices
Selected references
Index

Quick-reference guide to laboratory test results

A

Acetylcholine receptor antibodies, serum
Negative

Acid mucopolysaccharides, urine
Adults: < 13.3 μg glucuronic acid/mg/creatinine/24 hours

Acid phosphatase, serum
0 to 3.7 U/L (SI, 0 to 3.7 U/L)

Adrenocorticotropic hormone, plasma
<120 pg/ml (SI, < 26.4 pmol/L)

Alanine aminotransferase
8 to 50 IU/L (SI, 0.14 to 0.85 μkat/L)

Aldosterone, serum
- Supine individuals: 3 to 16 ng/dl (SI, 80 to 440 pmol/L)
- Upright individuals: 7 to 30 ng/dl (SI, 190 to 832 pmol/L)

Aldosterone, urine
3 to 19 mcg/24 hours (SI, 8 to 51 nmol/d)

Alkaline phosphatase, peritoneal fluid
- Males > 18 years: 90 to 239 U/L (SI, 90 to 239 U/L)
- Females < 45 years: 76 to 196 U/L (SI, 76 to 196 U/L); > 45 years: 87 to 250 U/L (87 to 250 U/L)

Alkaline phosphatase, serum
45 to 115 U/L (SI, 45 to 115 U/L)

Alpha-fetoprotein serum
Males and nonpregnant, females: < 15 ng/ml (SI, < 15 mg/L)

Ammonia, peritoneal fluid
< 50 ng/dl (SI, < 29 μmol/L)

Amniotic fluid analysis
- Lecithin-sphingomyelin ratio: > 2
- Meconium: absent (except in breech presentation)
- Phosphatidylglycerol: present

Amylase, peritoneal fluid
138 to 404 U/L (SI, 138 to 404 U/L)

Amylase, serum
Adults: ≥ 18 years: 26 to 102 U/L (SI, 0.4 to 1.74 μkat/L)

Amylase, urine
1 to 17 U/hour (SI, 0.017 to 0.29 μkat/h)

Androstenedione (radioimmunoassay)
- Males: 75 to 205 ng/dl (SI, 2.6 to 7.2 nmol/L)
- Females: 85 to 275 ng/dl (SI, 3.0 to 9.6 nmol/L)

Angiotensin-converting enzyme
Adults ≥ 20 years: 8 to 52 U/L (SI, 0.14 to 0.88 μkat/L)

Anion gap
8 to 14 mEq/L (SI, 8 to 14 mmol/L)

Antibody screening, serum
Negative

Antidiuretic hormone, serum
1 to 5 pg/ml (SI, 1 to 5 ng/L)

Antiglobulin test, direct
Negative

Antimitochondrial antibodies, serum
Negative

Anti-smooth-muscle antibodies, serum
Negative

Antistreptolysin-O, serum
- Preschoolers and adults: 85 Todd units/ml
- School-age children: 170 Todd units/ml

Antithrombin III
80% to 120% of normal control values

Antithyroid antibodies, serum
Normal titer < 1:100

Arginine test
- Human growth hormone levels
  - Males: increase to > 10 ng/ml (SI, >10 mcg/L)
  - Females: increase to > 15 ng/ml (SI, > 15 mcg/L)
  - Children: increase to > 48 ng/ml (SI, > 48 mcg/L)

Arterial blood gases
- pH: 7.35 to 7.45 (SI, 7.35 to 7.45)
- PaO_2: 80 to 100 mm Hg (SI, 10.6 to 13.3 kPa)
- $PaCO_2$: 35 to 45 mm Hg (SI, 4.7 to 5.3 kPa)
- O_2 CT: 15% to 23% (SI, 0.15 to 0.23)
- SaO_2: 94% to 100% (SI, 0.94 to 1.00)
- HCO_3^-: 22 to 25 mEq/L (SI, 22 to 25 mmol/L)

Arylsulfatase A, urine
- Random: 16 to 42 μ/g creatinine
- 24-hour: 0.37 to 3.60 μ/day creatinine
- 1-hour test: 2 to 19 μ/1 hour (SI, 2 to 19 μ/h)
- 2-hour test: 4 to 37 μ/2 hours (SI, 4 to 37 μ/h)
- 24-hour test: 170 to 2,000 μ/24 hours (SI, 2.89 to 34.0 μkat/L)

Aspartate aminotransferase
- 12 to 31 U/L (SI, 0.21 to 0.53 μkat/L)

Aspergillosis antibody, serum
Normal titer < 1:8

Atrial natriuretic factor, plasma
20 to 77 pg/ml

B

Bacterial meningitis antigen
Negative

Bence Jones protein, urine
Negative

Beta-hydroxybutyrate
< 0.4 mmol/L (SI, 0.4 mmol/L)

Bilirubin, amniotic fluid
- Early: < 0.075 μg/dl (SI, < 1.3 μmol/L)
- Term: < 0.025 μg/dl (SI, < 0.41 μmol/L)

Bilirubin, serum
- Adults
  - Direct: < 0.5 mg/dl (SI, < 6.8 μmol/L)
  - Indirect: 1.1 mg/dl (SI, 19 μmol/L)
- Neonates
  - Total: 1 to 12 mg/dl (SI, 34 to 205 μmol/L)

Bilirubin, urine
Negative

Blastomycosis antibody, serum
Normal titer < 1:8

Bleeding time
- Template: 3 to 6 minutes (SI, 3 to 6 m)
- Ivy: 3 to 6 minutes (SI, 3 to 6 m)
- Duke: 1 to 3 minutes (SI, 1 to 3 m)

Blood urea nitrogen
8 to 20 mg/dl (SI, 2.9 to 7.5 mmol/L)

B-lymphocyte count
270 to 640/μl

C

Calcitonin, plasma
- Baseline
  - Males: < 16 pg/ml (SI, < 16 ng/L)
  - Females: < 8 pg/ml (SI, < 8 ng/L)

Calcium, serum
- Adults: 8.2 to 10.2 mg/dl (SI, 2.05 to 2.54 mmol/L)
- Children: 8.6 to 11.2 mg/dl (SI, 2.15 to 2.79 mmol/L)
- Ionized: 4.65 to 5.28 mg/dl (SI, 1.1 to 1.25 mmol/L)

Calcium, urine
100 to 300 mg/24 hours (SI, 2.50 to 7.50 mmol/d)

Candida antibodies, serum
Negative

Capillary fragility

Petechiae per 5 cm:	Score:
11 to 20	2+
21 to 50	3+
over 50	4+

Carbon dioxide, total, blood
22 to 26 mEq/L (SI, 22 to 26 mmol/L)

Carcinoembryonic antigen, serum
< 5 ng/ml (SI, < 5 mg/L)

Catecholamines, plasma
- Supine
  - Epinephrine: undetectable to 110 pg/ml (SI, undetectable to 600 pmol/L)
  - Norepinephrine: 70 to 750 pg/ml (SI, 413 to 4,432 pmol/L)
- Standing
  - Epinephrine: undetectable to 140 pg/ml (SI, undetectable to 764 pmol/L)
  - Norepinephrine: 200 to 1,700 pg/ml (SI, 1182 to 10,047 pmol/L)

Catecholamines, urine
- Epinephrine: 0 to 20 μg/24 hours (SI, 0 to 109 nmol/24 h)
- Norepinephrine: 15 to 80 μg/24 hours (SI, 89 to 473 nmol/24 h)
- Dopamine: 65 to 400 μg/24 hours (SI, 425 to 2,610 nmol/24 h)

Cerebrospinal fluid
- Pressure: 50 to 180 mm H_2O
- Appearance: clear, colorless
- Gram stain: no organisms

Ceruloplasmin, serum
22.9 to 43.1 mg/dl (SI, 0.22 to 0.43 g/L)

Chloride, cerebrospinal fluid
118 to 130 mEq/L (SI, 118 to 130 mmol/L)

Chloride, serum
100 to 108 mEq/L (SI, 100 to 108 mmol/L)

Chloride, urine
- Adults: 110 to 250 mmol/24 hours (SI, 110 to 250 mmol/d)
- Children: 15 to 40 mmol/24 hours (SI, 15 to 40 mmol/d)
- Infants: 2 to 10 mmol/24 hours (SI, 2 to 10 mmol/d)

Cholinesterase (pseudocholinesterase)
204 to 532 IU/dl (SI, 2.04 to 5.32 kU/L)

Coccidioidomycosis antibody, serum
Normal titer < 1:2

Cold agglutinins, serum
Normal titer < 1:64

Complement, serum
■ Total
– 40 to 90 U/ml (SI, 0.4 to 0.9 g/L)
■ C3
– Males: 80 to 180 mg/dl (SI, 0.8 to 1.8 g/L)
– Females: 76 to 120 mg/dl (SI, 0.76 to 1.2 g/L)
■ C4
– Males: 15 to 60 mg/dl (SI, 0.15 to 0.6 g/L)
– Females: 15 to 52 mg/dl (SI, 0.15 to 0.52 g/L)

Copper, urine
3 to 35 μg/24 hours (SI, 0.05 to 0.55 μmol/d)

Cortisol, free, urine
< 50 μg/24 hours (SI, < 138 nmol/d)

Cortisol, plasma
■ Morning: 7 to 25 mcg/dl (SI, 0.2 to 0.7 μmol/L)
■ Afternoon: 2 to 14 mcg/dl (SI, 0.06 to 0.39 μmol/L)

C-reactive protein, serum
< 0.8 mg/dl (SI, < 8 mg/L)

Creatine kinase
■ Total
– Males: 55 to 170 U/L (SI, 0.94 to 2.89 μkat/L)
– Females: 30 to 135 U/L (SI, 0.51 to 2.3 μkat/L)

Creatinine clearance
■ Males: 94 to 140 ml/min/1.73 m^2 (SI, 0.91 to 1.35 ml/s/m^2)
■ Females: 72 to 110 ml/min/1.73 m^2 (SI, 0.69 to 1.06 ml/s/m^2)

Creatinine, serum
■ Males: 0.8 to 1.2 mg/dl (SI, 62 to 115 μmol/L)
■ Females: 0.6 to 0.9 mg/dl (SI, 53 to 97 μmol/L)

Creatinine, urine
■ Males: 14 to 26 mg/kg body weight/24 hours (SI, 124 to 230 μmol/kg body weight/d)
■ Females: 11 to 20 mg/kg body weight/24 hours (SI, 97 to 177 μmol/kg body weight/d)

Cryoglobulins, serum
Negative

Cyclic adenosine monophosphate, urine
■ 0.3 to 3.6 mg/day (SI, 100 to 723 μmol/d)
or
■ 0.29 to 2.1 mg/g creatinine (SI, 100 to 723 μmol/mol creatinine)

Cytomegalovirus antibodies, serum
Negative

D

D-xylose absorption
■ Blood
– Adults: 25 to 40 mg/dl in 2 hours
– Children: > 30 mg/dl in 1 hour
■ Urine
– Adults: > 3.5 g excreted in 5 hours (age 65 of older, > 5 g in 24 hours)
– Children: 16% to 33% excreted in 5 hours

E

Epstein-Barr virus antibodies
Negative

Erythrocyte sedimentation rate
■ Males: 0 to 10 mm/hour (SI, 0 to 10 mm/h)
■ Females: 0 to 20 mm/hour (SI, 0 to 20 mm/h)

Esophageal acidity
pH > 5.0

Estrogens, serum
- Females
– Menstruating: 26 to 149 pg/ml (SI, 90 to 550 pmol/L)
– Postmenopausal: 0 to 34 pg/ml (SI, 0 to 125 pmol/L)
- Males
– 12 to 34 pg/ml (SI, 40 to 125 pmol/L)
- Children
– < 6 years: 3 to 10 pg/ml (SI, 10 to 36 pmol/L)

Euglobulin lysis time
2 to 4 hours (SI, 2 to 4 h)

F

Factor assay, one-stage
50% to 150% of normal activity (SI, 0.50 to 1.50)

Febrile agglutination, serum
- Salmonella antibody: < 1:80
- Brucellosis antibody: < 1:80
- Tularemia antibody: < 1:40
- Rickettsial antibody: < 1:40

Ferritin, serum
- Males
– 20 to 300 ng/ml (SI, 20 to 300 μg/L)
- Females
– 20 to 120 ng/ml (SI, 20 to 120 μg/L)
- Infants
– 1 month: 200 to 600 ng/ml (SI, 200 to 600 μg/L)
– 2 to 5 months: 50 to 200 ng/ml (SI, 50 to 200 μg/L)
– 6 months to 15 years: 7 to 140 ng/ml (SI, 7 to 140 μg/L)
- Neonates
– 25 to 200 ng/ml (SI, 25 to 200 μg/L)

Fibrinogen, plasma
200 to 400 mg/dl (SI, 2 to 4 g/L)

Fibrin split products
- Screening assay: < 10 mcg/ml (SI, < 10 mg/L)
- Quantitative assay: < 3 mcg/ml (SI, < 3 mg/L)

Fluorescent treponemal antibody absorption, serum
Negative

Folic acid, serum
1.8 to 20 ng/ml (SI, 4 to 45.3 nmol/L)

Follicle-stimulating hormone, serum
- Menstruating females
– Follicular phase: 5 to 20 mIU/ml (SI, 5 to 20 IU/L)
– Ovulatory phase: 15 to 30 mIU/ml (SI, 15 to 30 IU/L)
– Luteal phase: 5 to 15 mIU/ml (SI, 5 to 15 IU/L)
- Menopausal females
– 5 to 100 mIU/ml (SI, 50 to 100 IU/L)
- Males
– 5 to 20 mlU/ml (5 to 20 IU/L)

Free thyroxine, serum
0.9 to 2.3 ng/dl (SI, 10 to 30 nmol/L)

Free triiodothyronine
0.2 to 0.6 ng/dl (SI, 0.003 to 0.009 nmol/L)

G

Galactose 1-phosphate uridyl transferase
- Qualitative: negative
- Quantitative: 18.5 to 28.5 U/g of hemoglobin

Gamma-glutamyl transferase
- Males ≥ 16 years: 6 to 38 U/L (SI, 0.10 to 0.63 μkat/L)
- Females 16 to 45 years: 4 to 27 U/L (SI, 0.08 to 0.46 μkat/L); > 45 years: 6 to 38 U/L (SI, 0.10 to 0.63 μkat/L)
- Children: 3 to 30 U/L (SI, 0.05 to 0.51 μkat)

Gastric acid stimulation
- Males: 18 to 28 mEq/hour
- Females: 11 to 21 mEq/hour

Gastric secretion, basal
- Males: 1 to 5 mEq/hour
- Females: 0.2 to 3.3 mEq/hour

Gastrin, serum
50 to 150 pg/ml (SI, 50 to 150 ng/L)

Globulin, peritoneal fluid
30% to 45% of total protein

Glucose, amniotic fluid
< 45 mg/dl (SI, < 2.3 mmol/L)

Glucose, cerebrospinal fluid
50 to 80 mg/dl (SI, 2.8 to 4.4 mmol/L)

Glucose, peritoneal fluid
70 to 100 mg/dl (SI, 3.5 to 5 mmol/L)

Glucose, plasma, fasting
70 to 100 mg/dl (SI, 3.9 to 6.1 mmol/L)

Glucose-6-phosphate dehydrogenase
4.3 to 11.8 U/g (SI, 0.28 to 0.76 mU/mol) of hemoglobin

Glucose tolerance, oral
Peak at 160 to 180 mg/dl (SI, 8.8 to 9.9 mmol/L) 30 to 60 minutes after challenge dose

Growth hormone suppression
Undetectable to 3 ng/ml (SI, undetectable to 3 μg/L) after 30 minutes to 2 hours

H

Ham test
Negative

Haptoglobin, serum
40 to 180 mg/dl (SI, 0.4 to 1.8 g/L)

Heinz bodies
Negative

Hematocrit
- Males
  - 42% to 52% (SI, 0.42 to 0.52)
- Females
  - 36% to 48% (SI, 0.36 to 0.48)
- Children
  - 10 years: 36% to 40% (SI, 0.36 to 0.40)
- Infants
  - 3 months: 30% to 36% (SI, 0.30 to 0.36)
  - 1 year: 29% to 41% (SI, 0.29 to 0.41)
- Neonates
  - At birth: 55% to 68% (SI, 0.55 to 0.68)
  - 1 week: 47% to 65% (SI, 0.47 to 0.65)
  - 1 month: 37% to 49% (SI, 0.37 to 0.49)

Hemoglobin (Hb) electrophoresis
- Hb A: 95% (SI, 0.95)
- Hb A_2: 1.5% to 3% (SI, 0.015 to 0.03)
- Hb F: < 2% (SI, < 0.02)

Hemoglobin, unstable
- Heat stability: negative
- Isopropanol: stable

Hemoglobin, urine
Negative

Hemosiderin, urine
Negative

Hepatitis B surface antigen, serum
Negative

Herpes simplex antibodies, serum
Negative

Heterophil agglutination, serum
Normal titer < 1:56

Hexosaminidase A and B, serum
Total: 5 to 12.9 U/L (hexosaminidase A constitutes 55% to 76% of total)

Histoplasmosis antibody, serum
Normal titer < 1:8

Homovanillic acid, urine
< 10 mg/24 hours (SI, < 55 μmol/d)

Human chorionic gonadotropin, serum
< 4 IU/L

Human chorionic gonadotropin, urine
- Pregnant women
- – First trimester: 500,000 IU/24 hours
- – Second trimester: 10,000 to 25,000 IU/24 hours
- – Third trimester: 5,000 to 15,000 IU/24 hours

Human growth hormone, serum
- Males: undetectable to 5 ng/ml (SI, undetectable to 5 μg/L)
- Females: undetectable to 10 ng/ml (SI, undetectable to 10 μg/L)
- Children: undetectable to 16 ng/ml (SI, undetectable to 16 μg/L)

Human immunodeficiency virus antibody, serum
Negative

Human placental lactogen, serum
- Males and nonpregnant females: < 0.5 mcg/ml
- Pregnant females at term: 9 to 11 mcg/ml

17-hydroxycorticosteroids, urine
- Males
- – 4.5 to 12 mg/24 hours (SI, 12.4 to 33.1 μmol/d)
- Females
- – 2.5 to 10 mg/24 hours (SI, 6.9 to 27.6 μmol/d)
- Children
- – 8 to 12 years: < 4.5 mg/24 hours (SI, < 12.4 μmol/d)
- – < 8 years: < 1.5 mg/24 hours (SI, < 4.14 μmol/d)

5-hydroxyindoleacetic acid, urine
2 to 7 mg/24 hours (SI, 10.4 to 36.6 μmol/d)

Hydroxyproline, total, urine
1 to 9 mg/24 hours (SI, 1.0 to 3.4 IU/d)

IJ

Immune complex, serum
Negative

Immunoglobulins (Ig), serum
- IgG: 800 to 1,800 mg/dl (SI, 8 to 18 g/L)
- IgA: 100 to 400 mg/dl (SI, 1 to 4 g/L)
- IgM: 55 to 150 mg/dl (SI, 0.55 to 1.5 g/L)

Insulin, serum
0 to 35 μU/ml (SI, 144 to 243 pmol/L)

Insulin tolerance test
10- to 20-ng/dl (SI, 10- to 20-μg/L) increase over baseline levels of human growth hormone and adrenocorticotropic hormone

Iron, serum
- Males: 65 to 175 mcg/dl (SI, 11.6 to 31.3 μmol/L)
- Females: 50 to 170 mcg/dl (SI, 9 to 30.4 μmol/L)

Iron, total binding capacity, serum
300 to 360 mcg/dl (SI, 54 to 64 μmol/L)

K

17-ketogenic steroids, urine
- Males: 4 to 14 mg/24 hours (SI, 13 to 49 μmol/d)
- Females: 2 to 12 mg/24 hours (SI, 7 to 42 μmol/d)
- Children
- – Infants to 11 years: 0.1 to 4 mg/24 hours (SI, 0.3 to 14 μmol/d)
- – 11 to 14 years: 2 to 9 mg/24 hours (SI, 7 to 31 μmol/d)

Ketones, urine
Negative

17-ketosteroids, urine
- Males: 10 to 25 mg/24 hours (SI, 35 to 87 μmol/d)
- Females: 4 to 6 mg/24 hours (SI, 4 to 21 μmol/d)
- Children
- – Infants to 10 years: < 3 mg/24 hours (SI, < 10 μmol/d)
- – 10 to 14 years: 1 to 6 mg/24 hours (SI, 2 to 21 μmol/d)

L

Lactate dehydrogenase (LD)
- Total: 71 to 207 IU/L (SI, 1.2 to 3.52 μkat/L)
- LD_1: 14% to 26% (SI, 0.14 to 0.26)
- LD_2: 29% to 39% (SI, 0.29 to 0.39)
- LD_3: 20% to 26% (SI, 0.20 to 0.26)
- LD_4: 8% to 16% (SI, 0.08 to 0.16)
- LD_5: 6% to 16% (SI, 0.06 to 0.16)

Lactic acid, blood
0.5 to 2.2 mEq/L (SI, 0.5 to 2.2 mmol/L)

Leucine aminopeptidase
- Males: 80 to 200 U/ml (SI, 80 to 200 kU/L)
- Females: 75 to 185 U/ml (SI, 75 to 185 kU/L)

Leukoagglutinins
Negative

Lipase, serum
10 to 73 U/L (SI, 0.17 to 1.24 μkat/L)

Lipids, fecal
Constitute < 20% of excreted solids; < 7 g excreted in 24 hours

Lipoproteins, serum
- High-density lipoprotein cholesterol
  - Males: 37 to 70 mg/dl (SI, 0.96 to 1.8 mmol/L)
  - Females: 40 to 85 mg/dl (SI, 1.03 to 2.2 mmol/L)
- Low-density lipoprotein cholesterol:
  - In individuals who don't have coronary artery disease: < 130 mg/dl (SI, < 3.36 mmol/L)

Long-acting thyroid stimulator, serum
Negative

Lupus erythematosus cell preparation
Negative

Luteinizing hormone, serum
- Menstruating women
  - Follicular phase: 5 to 15 mIU/ml (SI, 5 to 15 IU/L)
  - Ovulatory phase: 30 to 60 mIU/ml (SI, 30 to 60 IU/L)
  - Luteal phase: 5 to 15 mIU/ml (SI, 5 to 15 IU/L)
- Postmenopausal women
  - 50 to 100 mIU/ml (SI, 50 to 100 IU/L)
- Males
  - 5 to 20 mIU/ml (SI, 5 to 20 IU/L)
- Children
  - 4 to 20 mIU/ml (SI, 4 to 20 IU/L)

Lyme disease serology
Nonreactive

Lysozyme, urine
0 to 3 mg/24 hours

M

Magnesium, serum
1.3 to 2.1 mg/dl (SI, 0.65 to 1.05 mmol/L)

Magnesium, urine
6 to 10 mEq/24 hours (SI, 3 to 5 mmol/d)

Manganese, serum
0.4 to 1.4 μg/ml

Melanin, urine
Negative

Myoglobin, urine
Negative

N

5′-nucleotidase
2 to 17 U/L (SI, 0.034 to 0.29 μkat/L)

O

Occult blood, fecal
< 2.5 ml

Oxalate, urine
≤40 mg/24 hours (SI, ≤456 μmol/d)

PQ

Parathyroid hormone, serum
- Intact: 10 to 50 pg/ml (SI, 1.1 to 5.3 pmol/L)
- N-terminal fraction: 8 to 24 pg/ml (SI, 0.8 to 2.5 pmol/L)
- C-terminal fraction: 0 to 340 pg/ml (SI, 0 to 35.8 pmol/L)

Partial thromboplastin time
21 to 35 seconds (SI, 21 to 35 s)

Pericardial fluid
- Amount: 10 to 50 ml
- Appearance: clear, straw-colored
- White blood cell count: < 1,000/μl (SI, < 1.0 × 10⁹/L)
- Glucose: approximately whole blood level

Peritoneal fluid
- Amount: < 50 ml
- Appearance: clear, straw-colored

Phenylalanine, serum
< 2 mg/dl (SI, < 121 μmol/L)

Phosphates, serum
- Adults: 2.7 to 4.5 mEq/L (SI, 0.87 to 1.45 mmol/L)
- Children: 4.5 to 6.7 mEq/L (SI, 1.45 to 1.78 mmol/L)

Phosphates, urine
< 1,000 mg/24 hours

Phospholipids, plasma
180 to 320 mg/dl (SI, 1.8 to 3.2 g/L)

Plasma renin activity
- Normal sodium diet: 1.1 to 4.1 ng/ml/hour (SI, 0.30 to 1.14 ng LS)
- Restricted sodium diet: 6.2 to 12.4 ng/ml/hour (SI, 1.72 to 3.44 ng LS)

Phosphate, tubular reabsorption, urine and plasma
80% reabsorption

Plasminogen, plasma
80% to 130%

Platelet aggregation
3 to 5 minutes (SI, 3 to 5 m)

Platelet count
- Adults: 140,000 to 400,000/μl (SI, 140 to 400 × 10^9/L)
- Children: 150,000 to 450,000/μl (SI, 150 to 450 × 10^9/L)

Potassium, serum
3.5 to 5 mEq/L (SI, 3.5 to 5 mmol/L)

Potassium, urine
- Adults: 25 to 125 mmol/24 hours (SI, 25 to 125 mmol/d)
- Children: 22 to 57 mmol/24 hours (SI, 22 to 57 mmol/d)

Pregnanediol, urine
- Nonpregnant females
  - 0.5 to 1.5 mg/24 hours (during the follicular phase of the menstrual cycle)
- Pregnant females
  - First trimester: 10 to 30 mg/24 hours
  - Second trimester: 35 to 70 mg/24 hours
  - Third trimester: 70 to 100 mg/24 hours
- Postmenopausal females
  - 0.2 to 1 mg/24 hours
- Males
  - 0 to 1 mg/24 hours

Pregnanetriol, urine
- Males ≥ 16 years: 0.4 to 2.5 mg/24 hours (SI, 1.2 to 7.5 μmol/d)
- Females ≥ 16 years: 0 to 1.8 mg/24 hours (SI, 0.3 to 5.3 μmol/d)

Progesterone, plasma
- Menstruating females
  - Follicular phase: < 150 ng/dl (SI, < 5 nmol/L)
  - Luteal phase: 300 to 1,200 ng/dl (SI, 10 to 40 nmol/L)
- Pregnant women
  - First trimester: 1,500 to 5,000 ng/dl (SI, 50 to 160 nmol/L)
  - Second and third trimesters: 8,000 to 20,000 ng/dl (SI, 250 to 650 nmol/L)

Prolactin, serum
Undetectable to 23 ng/ml (SI, undetectable to 23 mcg/L)

Prostate-specific antigen
- 40 to 50 years: 2 to 2.8 ng/ml (SI, 2 to 2.8 μg/L)
- 51 to 60 years: 2.9 to 3.8 ng/ml (SI, 2.9 to 3.8 μg/L)
- 61 to 70 years: 4 to 5.3 ng/ml (SI, 4 to 5.3 μg/L)
- ≥ 71 years: 5.6 to 7.2 ng/ml (SI, 5.6 to 7.2 μg/L)

Protein, cerebrospinal fluid
15 to 50 mg/dl (SI, 0.15 to 0.5 g/L)

Protein C, plasma
70% to 140% (SI, 0.70 to 1.40)

Protein, total, peritoneal fluid
0.3 to 4.1 g/dl (SI, 3 to 41 g/L)

Protein, urine
50 to 80 mg/24 hours (SI, 50 to 80 mg/d)

Prothrombin time
10 to 14 seconds (10 to 14 s)

Pulmonary artery pressures
- Right atrial: 1 to 6 mm Hg
- Left atrial: approximately 10 mm Hg
- Systolic: 20 to 30 mm Hg
- Systolic right ventricular: 20 to 30 mm Hg
- Diastolic: 10 to 15 mm Hg
- End-diastolic right ventricular: < 5 mm Hg
- Mean: < 20 mm Hg
- Pulmonary artery wedge pressure: 6 to 12 mm Hg

Pyruvate kinase
- Ultraviolet: 9 to 22 U/g of hemoglobin
- Low substrate assay: 1.7 to 6.8 U/g of hemoglobin

Pyruvic acid, blood
0.08 to 0.16 mEq/L (SI, 0.08 to 0.16 mmol/L)

R

Red blood cell count
- Males: 4.2 to 5.4 × 10^6/mm^3 (SI, 4.2 to 5.4 × 10^{12}/L)
- Females: 3.6 to 5 × 10^6/mm^3 (SI, 3.6 to 5 × 10^{12}/L)
- Neonates: 4.4 to 5.8 million/μl (SI, 4.4 to 5.8 × 10^{12}/L)
- 2 months: 3 to 3.8 million/μl (SI, 3 to 3.8 × 10^{12}/L) (increasing slowly)
- Children: 4.6 to 4.8 million/μl (SI, 4.6 to 4.8 × 10^{12}/L)

Red blood cell survival time
25 to 35 days

Red blood cells, urine
0 to 3 per high-power field

Red cell indices
- Mean corpuscular volume: 84 to 99 μm^3 (SI, 84 to 99 fL)
- Mean corpuscular hemoglobin: 26 to 32 pg/cell (SI, 0.40 to 0.53 fmol/cell)
- Mean corpuscular hemoglobin concentration: 30 to 36 g/dl (SI, 300 to 360 g/L)

Respiratory syncytial virus antibodies, serum
Negative

Reticulocyte count
- Adults: 0.5% to 2.5% (SI, 0.005 to 0.025)
- Infants (at birth): 2% to 6% (SI, 0.02 to 0.06), decreasing to adult levels in 1 to 2 weeks

Rheumatoid factor, serum
Negative or titer < 1:20

Ribonucleoprotein antibodies
Negative

Rubella antibodies, serum
Titer of 1:8 or less indicates little or no immunity; titer more than 1:10 indicates adequate protection against rubella

S

Semen analysis
- Volume: 0.7 to 6.5 ml
- pH: 7.3 to 7.9
- Liquefaction: within 20 minutes
- Sperm count: 20 to 150 million/ml

Sickle cell test
Negative

Sjögren's antibodies
Negative

Sodium chloride, urine
110 to 250 mEq/L (SI, 100 to 250 mmol/d)

Sodium, serum
135 to 145 mEq/L (SI, 135 to 145 mmol/L)

Sodium, urine
- Adults: 40 to 220 mEq/L/24 hours (SI, 40 to 220 mmol/d)
- Children: 41 to 115 mEq/L/24 hours (SI, 41 to 115 mmol/d)

Sporotrichosis antibody, serum
Normal titers < 1:40

T

Terminal deoxynucleotidyl transferase, serum
- Bone marrow: < 2%
- Blood: undetectable

Testosterone, plasma or serum
- Males: 300 to 1,200 ng/dl (SI, 10.4 to 41.6 nmol/L)
- Females: 20 to 80 ng/dl (SI, 0.7 to 2.8 nmol/L)

Thrombin time, plasma
10 to 15 seconds (10 to 15 s)

Thyroid-stimulating hormone, neonatal
- ≤ 2 days: 25 to 30 μIU/ml (SI, 25 to 30 mU/L)
- > 2 days: < 25 μIU/ml (SI, < 25 mU/L)

Thyroid-stimulating hormone, serum
Undetectable to 15 μIU/ml (SI, undetectable to 15 mU/L)

Thyroid-stimulating immunoglobulin, serum
Negative

Thyroxine, total, serum
5 to 13.5 μg/dl (SI, 60 to 165 nmol/L)

T-lymphocyte count
1,500 to 3,000/μl

Transferrin, serum
200 to 400 mg/dl (SI, 2 to 4 g/L)

Triglycerides, serum
- Males: 44 to 180 mg/dl (SI, 0.44 to 2.01 mmol/L)
- Females: 11 to 190 mg/dl (SI, 0.11 to 2.21 mmol/L)

Triiodothyronine, serum
80 to 200 ng/dl (SI, 1.2 to 3 nmol/L)

U

Uric acid, serum
- Males: 3.4 to 7 mg/dl (SI, 202 to 416 μmol/L)
- Females: 2.3 to 6 mg/dl (SI, 143 to 357 μmol/L)

Uric acid, urine
250 to 750 mg/24 hours (SI, 1.48 to 4.43 mmol/d)

Urinalysis, routine
- Color: straw to dark yellow
- Appearance: clear
- Specific gravity: 1.005 to 1.035
- pH: 4.5 to 8.0
- Epithelial cells: 0 to 5 per high-power field
- Casts: none, except 1 to 2 hyaline casts per low-power field
- Crystals: present

Urine osmolality
- 24-hour urine: 300 to 900 mOsm/kg
- Random urine: 50 to 1,400 mOsm/kg

Urobilinogen, fecal
50 to 300 mg/24 hours (SI, 100 to 400 EU/100 g)

Urobilinogen, urine
- 0.1 to 0.8 EU/2 hours (SI 0.1 to 0.8 EU/2 h)

or

- 0.5 to 4.0 EU/24 hours (SI, 0.5 to 4.0 EU/d)

Uroporphyrinogen I synthase
≥7 nmol/second/L

V

Vanillylmandelic acid, urine
1.4 to 6.5 mg/24 hours (SI, 7 to 33 μmol/d)

Venereal Disease Research Laboratory test, cerebrospinal fluid
Negative

Venereal Disease Research Laboratory test, serum
Negative

Vitamin A, serum
30 to 80 μg/dl (SI, 1.05 to 2.8 μmol/L)

Vitamin B_2, serum
3 to 15 μg/dl

Vitamin B_{12}, serum
200 to 900 pg/ml (SI, 148 to 664 pmol/L)

Vitamin C, plasma
0.2 to 2 mg/dl (SI, 11 to 114 μmol/L)

Vitamin C, urine
30 mg/24 hours

Vitamin D_3, serum
10 to 60 ng/ml (SI, 25 to 150 nmol/L)

WXY

White blood cell count, blood
4,000 to 10,000/μl (SI, 4 to 10 × 10^9/L)

White blood cell count, peritoneal fluid
< 300/μl (SI, < 300 × 10^9/L)

White blood cell count, urine
0 to 4 per high-power field

White blood cell differential, blood
- Adults
- – Neutrophils: 54% to 75% (SI, 0.54 to 0.75)
- – Lymphocytes: 25% to 40% (SI, 0.25 to 0.40)
- – Monocytes: 2% to 8% (SI, 0.02 to 0.08)
- – Eosinophils: 1% to 4% (SI, 0.01 to 0.04)
- – Basophils: 0 to 1% (SI, 0 to 0.01)

Z

Zinc, serum
70 to 120 μg/dl (SI, 10.7 to 18.4 μmol/L)

Quick guide to head-to-toe assessment

The chart on the following pages provides guidelines for a systematic head-to-toe assessment. It groups assessment techniques by body region and practitioner-patient positioning to make the assessment as efficient as possible and to avoid tiring the patient. The first column describes the assessment technique to use for each body system or region. The second column lists normal findings for adults. The third column reviews special considerations, including the purpose of the technique as well as nursing and developmental considerations.

Technique	Normal findings	Special considerations
Head and neck		
Inspect the patient's head. Note hair color, texture, and distribution. Palpate from the forehead to the posterior triangle of the neck for the posterior cervical lymph nodes.	Symmetrical, rounded normocephalic head positioned at midline and erect with no lumps or ridges	■ This technique can detect asymmetry, size changes, enlarged lymph nodes, and tenderness. ■ Wear gloves for palpation if the patient has scalp lesions. ■ Inspect and gently palpate the fontanels and sutures in an infant.
Palpate in front of and behind the ears, under the chin, and in the anterior triangle for the anterior cervical lymph nodes.	Nonpalpable lymph nodes or small, round, soft, mobile, nontender lymph nodes	■ This technique can detect enlarged lymph nodes. ■ Palpable lymph nodes may be normal in a patient under age 12.
Palpate the left and then the right carotid artery.	Bilateral equality in pulse amplitude and rhythm	■ This technique evaluates circulation through the carotid pulse.
Auscultate the carotid arteries.	No bruit on auscultation	■ Auscultation in this area can detect a bruit, a sign of turbulent blood flow.

Technique	Normal findings	Special considerations
Head and neck *(continued)*		
Palpate the trachea.	Straight, midline trachea	▪ This technique evaluates trachea position.
Palpate the suprasternal notch.	Palpable pulsations with an even rhythm	▪ Palpation in this area allows evaluation of aortic arch pulsations.
Palpate the supraclavicular area.	Nonpalpable lymph nodes	▪ This technique can detect enlarged lymph nodes.
Palpate the thyroid gland and auscultate for bruits.	Thin, mobile thyroid isthmus; nonpalpable thyroid lobes	▪ Palpation detects thyroid enlargement, tenderness, or nodules.
Have the patient touch his chin to his chest and to each shoulder, each ear to the corresponding shoulder, then tip his head back as far as possible.	Symmetrical strength and movement of neck muscles	▪ These maneuvers evaluate range of motion (ROM) in the neck.
Place your hands on the patient's shoulders while the patient shrugs them against resistance. Then place your hand on the patient's left cheek, then the right, and have the patient push against it.	Symmetrical strength and movement of neck muscles	▪ This procedure checks cranial nerve XI (accessory nerve) functioning and trapezius and sternocleidomastoid muscle strength.
Have the patient smile, frown, wrinkle his forehead, and puff out his cheeks.	Symmetrical smile, frown, and forehead wrinkles; equal puffing out of the cheeks	▪ This maneuver evaluates the motor portion of cranial nerve VII (facial nerve).
Occlude one nostril externally with your finger while the patient breathes through the other. Repeat on the other nostril.	Patent nostrils	▪ This technique checks the patency of the nasal passages.
Inspect the internal nostrils using a nasal speculum or an ophthalmoscope handle with a nasal attachment.	Moist, pink to red nasal mucosa without deviated septum, lesions, or polyps	▪ This technique can detect edema, inflammation, and excessive drainage. ▪ Use only a flashlight to inspect an infant's or toddler's nostrils; a nasal speculum is too sharp.

Technique	Normal findings	Special considerations
Head and neck *(continued)*		
Palpate the nose.	No bumps, lesions, edema, or tenderness	▪ This technique assesses for structural abnormalities in the nose. ▪ An infant's nose usually is slightly flattened.
Palpate and percuss the frontal and maxillary sinuses. If palpation and percussion elicit tenderness, assess further by transilluminating the sinuses.	No tenderness on palpation or percussion	▪ These techniques are used to elicit tenderness, which may indicate sinus congestion or infection. ▪ In a child under age 8, frontal sinuses commonly are too small to assess.
Palpate the temporomandibular joints as the patient opens and closes his jaws.	Smooth joint movement without pain; correct approximation	▪ This action assesses the temporomandibular joints and the motor portion of cranial nerve V (trigeminal nerve).
Inspect the oral mucosa, gingivae, teeth, and salivary gland openings, using a tongue blade and a penlight.	Pink, moist, smooth oral mucosa without lesions or inflammation; pink, moist slightly irregular gingivae without sponginess or edema; 32 teeth with correct occlusion	▪ This technique evaluates the condition of several oral structures. ▪ A child may have up to 20 temporary (baby) teeth. ▪ Slight gingival swelling may be normal during pregnancy.
Observe the tongue and the hard and soft palates.	Pink, slightly rough tongue with a midline depression; pink to light red palates with symmetrical lines	▪ Observation provides information about the patient's hydration status and the condition of these oral structures.
Ask the patient to stick out his tongue.	Midline tongue without tremors	▪ This procedure tests cranial nerve XII (hypoglossal nerve).
Ask the patient to say "Ahh" while sticking out his tongue. Inspect the visible oral structures.	Symmetrical rise in soft palate and uvula during phonation; pink, midline, cone-shaped uvula; +1 tonsils (both tonsils behind the pillars)	▪ Phonation ("Ahh"') checks portions of cranial nerves IX and X (glossopharyngeal and vagus nerves). Lowering the tongue aids viewing.
Test the gag reflex using a tongue blade.	Gagging	▪ Gagging during this procedure indicates that cranial nerves IX and X are intact.

Technique	Normal findings	Special considerations
Head and neck (continued)		
Place the tongue blade at the side of the tongue while the patient pushes it to the left and right with his tongue.	Symmetrical ability to push tongue blade to left and right	▪ This action tests cranial nerve XII.
Test the sense of smell using a test tube of coffee, chocolate, or another familiar substance.	Correct identification of smells in both nostrils	▪ This action tests cranial nerve I (olfactory nerve). ▪ Make sure the patient keeps both eyes closed during the test.
Eyes and ears		
Perform a visual acuity test using the standard Snellen eye chart or another visual acuity chart, with the patient wearing corrective lenses if needed.	20/20 vision	▪ This test assesses the patient's distance vision (central vision) and evaluates cranial nerve II (optic nerve).
Ask the patient to identify the pattern in a specially prepared page of color dots or plates.	Correct identification of pattern	▪ This test assesses the patient's color perception.
Test the six cardinal positions of gaze.	Bilaterally equal eye movement without nystagmus	▪ This test evaluates the function of each of the six extraocular muscles and tests cranial nerves III, IV, and VI (oculomotor, trochlear, and abducens nerves).
Inspect the external structures of the eyeball (eyelids, eyelashes, and lacrimal apparatus).	Bright, clear, symmetrical eyes free of nystagmus; eyelids close completely; no lesions, scaling, or inflammation	▪ This inspection allows detection of such problems as ptosis, ectropion (outward-turning eyelids), entropion (inward-turning eyelids), and styes.
Inspect the conjunctiva and sclera.	Pink palpebral conjunctiva and clear bulbar conjunctiva without swelling, drainage, or hyperemic blood vessels; white, clear sclera	▪ Inspection detects conjunctivitis and the scleral color changes that may occur with systemic disorders.

Technique	Normal findings	Special considerations
***Eyes and ears** (continued)*		
Inspect the cornea, iris, and anterior chamber by shining a penlight tangentially across the eye.	Clear, transparent cornea and anterior chamber; illumination of total iris	▪ This technique assesses anterior chamber depth and the condition of the cornea and iris. ▪ An elderly patient may exhibit a thin, grayish ring in the cornea (called *arcus senilis*).
Examine the pupils for equality of size, shape, reaction to light, and accommodation.	Pupils equal, round, reactive to light and accommodation (PERRLA), directly and consensually	▪ Testing the pupillary response to light and accommodation assesses cranial nerves III, IV, and VI.
Observe the red reflex using an ophthalmoscope.	Sharp, distinct orange-red glow	▪ Presence of the red reflex indicates that the cornea, anterior chamber, and lens are free from opacity and clouding.
Inspect the ear. Perform an otoscopic examination if indicated.	Nearly vertically positioned ears that line up with the eye, match the facial color, are similarly shaped, and are in proportion to the face; no drainage, nodules, or lesions	▪ A dark-skinned patient may have darker orange or brown cerumen (earwax); a fair-skinned patient typically will have yellow cerumen.
Palpate the ear and mastoid process.	No pain, swelling, nodules, or lesions	▪ This assessment technique can detect inflammation or infection. It may also uncover other abnormalities, such as nodules or lesions.
Perform the whispered voice test or the watch-tick test on one ear at a time.	Whispered voice heard at a distance of 1′ to 2′ (30 to 61 cm); watch-tick heard at a distance of 5″ (13 cm)	▪ This test provides a gross assessment of cranial nerve VIII (acoustic nerve).
Perform Weber's test using a 512 or 1024 hertz (Hz) tuning fork.	Tuning fork vibrations heard equally in both ears or in the middle of the head	▪ This test differentiates conductive from sensorineural hearing loss. ▪ The sound is heard best in the ear with a conductive loss.
Perform the Rinne test using a 512 or 1024 Hz tuning fork.	Tuning fork vibrations heard in front of the ear for as long as they are heard on the mastoid process	▪ This test helps differentiate conductive from sensorineural hearing loss.

Technique	Normal findings	Special considerations
Posterior thorax		
Observe the skin, bones, and muscles of the spine, shoulder blades, and back as well as symmetry of expansion and accessory muscle use.	Even skin tone; symmetrical placement of all structures; bilaterally equal shoulder height; symmetrical expansion with inhalation; no accessory muscle use	▪ Observation provides information about lung expansion and accessory muscle use during respiration. It may also detect a deformity that can alter ventilation, such as scoliosis.
Assess the anteroposterior and lateral diameters of the thorax.	Lateral diameter up to twice the anteroposterior diameter (2:1)	▪ This assessment may detect abnormalities, such as an increased anteroposterior diameter (barrel chest may be as low as 1:1). ▪ Normal anteroposterior diameters vary with age. ▪ Measure an infant's chest circumference at the nipple line.
Palpate down the spine.	Properly aligned spinous processes without lesions or tenderness; firm, symmetrical, evenly spaced muscles	▪ This technique detects pain in the spine and paraspinous muscles. It also evaluates the muscles' consistency.
Palpate over the posterior thorax.	Smooth surface; no lesions, lumps, or pain	▪ This technique helps detect musculoskeletal inflammation.
Assess respiratory excursion.	Symmetrical expansion and contraction of the thorax	▪ This technique checks for equal expansion of the lungs.
Palpate for tactile fremitus as the patient repeats the words "ninety-nine."	Equally intense vibrations of both sides of the chest	▪ Palpation provides information about the content of the lungs; vibrations increase over consolidated or fluid-filled areas and decrease over gas-filled areas.
Percuss over the posterior and lateral lung fields.	Resonant percussion note over the lungs that changes to a dull note at the diaphragm	▪ This technique helps identify the density and location of the lungs, diaphragm, and other anatomic structures. ▪ Percussion may produce hyperresonant sounds in a patient with chronic obstructive pulmonary disease or an elderly patient because of hyperinflation of lung tissue.

Technique	Normal findings	Special considerations
Posterior thorax *(continued)*		
Percuss for diaphragmatic excursion on each side of the posterior thorax.	Excursion from 1¼″ to 2¼″ (3 to 6 cm)	▪ This technique evaluates diaphragm movement during respiration.
Auscultate the lungs through the posterior thorax as the patient breathes slowly and deeply through the mouth. Also auscultate lateral areas.	Bronchovesicular sounds (soft, breezy sounds) between the scapulae; vesicular sounds (soft, swishy sounds about two notes lower than bronchovesicular sounds) in the lung periphery	▪ Lung auscultation helps detect abnormal fluid or mucus accumulation as well as obstructed passages. ▪ Auscultate a child's lungs before performing other assessment techniques that may cause crying, which increases the respiratory rate and interferes with clear auscultation. ▪ A child's breath sounds are normally harsher or more bronchial than an adult's.
Anterior thorax		
Observe the skin, bones, and muscles of the anterior thoracic structures as well as symmetry of expansion and accessory muscle use during respiration.	Even skin tone; symmetrical placement of all structures; symmetrical costal angle of less than 90 degrees; symmetrical expansion with inhalation; no accessory muscle use	▪ Observation provides information about lung expansion and accessory muscle use. It may also detect a deformity that can prevent full lung expansion, such as pigeon chest.
Inspect the anterior thorax for lifts, heaves, or thrusts. Also check for the apical impulse.	No lifts, heaves, or thrusts; apical impulse not usually visible	▪ Apical impulse may be visible in a thin or young patient.
Palpate over the anterior thorax.	Smooth surface; no lesions, lumps, or pain	▪ This technique helps detect musculoskeletal inflammation.
Assess respiratory excursion.	Symmetrical expansion and contraction of the thorax	▪ This technique checks for equal expansion of the lungs.
Palpate for tactile fremitus as the patient repeats the words "ninety-nine."	Equally intense vibrations of both sides of the chest, with more vibrations in the upper chest than in the lower chest	▪ Palpation provides information about the content of the lungs.

Technique	Normal findings	Special considerations
***Anterior thorax** (continued)*		
Percuss over the anterior thorax.	Resonant percussion note over lung fields that changes to a dull note over ribs and other bones	▪ This technique helps identify the density and location of the lungs, diaphragm, and other anatomic structures. ▪ Percussion is unreliable in an infant because of the infant's small chest size. ▪ Percussion may produce hyperresonant sounds in an elderly patient because of hyperinflation of lung tissue.
Auscultate the lungs through the anterior thorax as the patient breathes slowly and deeply through the mouth. Also auscultate lateral areas.	Bronchovesicular sounds (soft, breezy sounds) between the scapulae; vesicular sounds (soft, swishy sounds about two notes lower than bronchovesicular sounds) in the lung periphery	▪ Lung auscultation helps detect abnormal fluid or mucus accumulation. ▪ Auscultate a child's lungs before performing other assessment techniques that may cause crying. ▪ Breath sounds are normally harsher or more bronchial in a child.
Inspect the breasts and axillae with the patient's hands resting at the sides of her body, placed on her hips, and raised above her head.	Symmetrical, convex, similar-looking breasts with soft, smooth skin and bilaterally similar venous patterns; symmetrical axillae with varying amounts of hair, but no lesions; nipples at same level on chest and of same color	▪ This technique evaluates the general condition of the breasts and axillae and detects such abnormalities as retraction, dimpling, and flattening. ▪ Expect to see enlarged breasts with darkened nipples and areolae and purplish linear streaks if the patient is pregnant.
Palpate the axillae with the patient's arms resting against the sides of the body.	Nonpalpable nodes	▪ This technique detects nodular enlargements and other abnormalities.

Technique	Normal findings	Special considerations
Anterior thorax *(continued)*		
Palpate the breasts and nipples with the patient lying supine.	Smooth, relatively elastic tissue without masses, cracks, fissures, areas of induration (hardness), or discharge	▪ This technique evaluates the consistency and elasticity of the breasts and nipples and may detect nipple discharge. ▪ The premenstrual patient may exhibit breast tenderness, nodularity, and fullness. ▪ A pregnant patient may discharge colostrum from the nipple and may exhibit nodular breasts with prominent venous patterns.
Inspect the neck for jugular vein distention with the patient lying supine at a 45-degree angle.	No visible pulsations	▪ This technique assesses right-sided heart pressure.
Palpate the precordium for the apical impulse.	Apical impulse present in the apical area (fifth intercostal space at the midclavicular line)	▪ This action evaluates the size and location of the left ventricle.
Auscultate the aortic, pulmonic, tricuspid, and mitral areas for heart sounds.	S_1 and S_2 heart sounds with a regular rhythm and an age-appropriate rate	▪ Auscultation over the precordium evaluates the heart rate and rhythm and can detect other abnormal heart sounds. ▪ A child or a pregnant woman in the third trimester may have functional (innocent) heart murmurs.
Abdomen		
Observe the abdominal contour.	Symmetrical flat or rounded contour	▪ This technique determines whether the abdomen is distended or scaphoid. ▪ An infant or a toddler will have a rounded abdomen.
Inspect the abdomen for skin characteristics, symmetry, contour, peristalsis, and pulsations.	Symmetrical contour with no lesions, striae, rash, or visible peristaltic waves	▪ Inspection can detect an incisional or umbilical hernia, or an abnormality caused by bowel obstruction.
Auscultate all four quadrants of the abdomen.	Normal bowel sounds in all four quadrants; no bruits	▪ Abdominal auscultation can detect abnormal bowel sounds.

Technique	Normal findings	Special considerations
***Abdomen** (continued)*		
Percuss from below the right breast to the inguinal area down the right midclavicular line.	Dull percussion note over the liver; tympanic note over the rest of the abdomen	▪ Percussion in this area helps evaluate the size of the liver.
Percuss from below the left breast to the inguinal area down the left midclavicular line.	Tympanic percussion note	▪ Percussion that elicits a dull note in this area can detect an enlarged spleen.
Palpate all four abdominal quadrants.	Nontender organs without masses	▪ Palpation provides information about the location, size, and condition of the underlying structures.
Palpate for the kidneys on each side of the abdomen.	Nonpalpable kidneys or solid, firm, smooth kidneys (if palpable)	▪ This technique evaluates the general condition of the kidneys.
Palpate the liver at the right costal border.	Nonpalpable liver or smooth, firm, nontender liver with a rounded, regular edge (if palpable)	▪ This technique evaluates the general condition of the liver.
Palpate for the spleen at the left costal border.	Nonpalpable spleen	▪ This procedure detects splenomegaly (spleen enlargement).
Palpate the femoral pulses in the groin.	Strong, regular pulse	▪ Palpation assesses vascular patency.
Upper extremities		
Observe the skin and muscle mass of the arms and hands.	Uniform color and texture with no lesions; elastic turgor; bilaterally equal muscle mass	▪ The skin provides information about hydration and circulation. Muscle mass provides information about injuries and neuromuscular disease.
Ask the patient to extend his arms forward and then rapidly turn his palms up and down.	Steady hands with no tremor or pronator drift	▪ This maneuver tests proprioception and cerebellar function.

Technique	Normal findings	Special considerations
Upper extremities *(continued)*		
Place your hands on the patient's upturned forearms while the patient pushes up against resistance. Then place your hands under the forearms while the patient pushes down.	Symmetrical strength and ability to push up and down against resistance	▪ This procedure checks the muscle strength of the arms.
Inspect and palpate the fingers, wrists, and elbow joints.	Smooth, freely movable joints with no swelling	▪ An elderly patient may exhibit osteoarthritic changes.
Palpate the patient's hands to assess skin temperature.	Warm, moist skin with bilaterally even temperature	▪ Skin temperature assessment provides data about circulation to the area.
Palpate the radial and brachial pulses.	Bilaterally equal rate and rhythm	▪ Palpation of pulses helps evaluate peripheral vascular status.
Inspect the color, shape, and condition of the patient's fingernails, and test for capillary refill.	Pink nail beds with smooth, rounded nails; brisk capillary refill; no clubbing	▪ Nail assessment provides data about the integumentary, cardiovascular, and respiratory systems.
Place two fingers in each of the patient's palms while the patient squeezes your fingers.	Bilaterally equal hand strength	▪ This maneuver tests muscle strength in the hands.
Lower extremities		
Inspect the legs and feet for color, lesions, varicosities, hair growth, nail growth, edema, and muscle mass.	Even skin color; symmetrical hair and nail growth; no lesions, varicosities, or edema; bilaterally equal muscle mass	▪ Inspection assesses adequate circulatory function.
Test for pitting edema in the pretibial area.	No pitting edema	▪ This test assesses for excess interstitial fluid.
Palpate for pulses and skin temperature in the posterior tibial, dorsalis pedis, and popliteal areas. Perform the straight leg test on one leg at a time.	Bilaterally even pulse rate, rhythm, and skin temperature	▪ Palpation of pulses and temperature in these areas evaluates the patient's peripheral vascular status.
Perform the straight leg test on one leg at a time	Painless leg lifting	▪ This test checks for vertebral disk problems.

Technique	Normal findings	Special considerations
Lower extremities (continued)		
Palpate for crepitus as the patient abducts and adducts the hip. Repeat on the opposite leg.	No crepitus; full ROM without pain	▪ Perform Ortolani's maneuver on an infant to assess hip abduction and adduction.
Ask the patient to raise his thigh against the resistance of your hands. Repeat this procedure on the opposite thigh.	Each thigh lifts easily against resistance	▪ This maneuver tests the motor strength of the upper legs.
Ask the patient to push outward against the resistance of your hands.	Each leg pushes easily against resistance	▪ This maneuver tests the motor strength of the lower legs.
Ask the patient to pull backward against the resistance of your hands.	Each leg pulls easily against resistance	▪ This maneuver tests the motor strength of the lower legs.
Nervous system		
Lightly touch the ophthalmic, maxillary, and mandibular areas on each side of the patient's face with a cotton-tipped applicator and a pin.	Correct identification of sensation and location	▪ This test evaluates the function of cranial nerve V (trigeminal nerve).
Touch the dorsal and palmar surfaces of the arms, hands, and fingers with a cotton-tipped applicator and a pin.	Correct identification of sensation and location	▪ This test evaluates the function of the ulnar, radial, and medial nerves.
Touch several nerve distribution areas on the legs, feet, and toes with a cotton-tipped applicator and a pin.	Correct identification of sensation and location	▪ This test evaluates the function of the dermatome areas randomly.
Place your fingers above the patient's wrist and tap them with a reflex hammer. Repeat on the other arm.	Normal reflex reaction	▪ This procedure elicits the brachioradialis deep tendon reflex (DTR).
Place your fingers over the antecubital fossa and tap them with a reflex hammer. Repeat on the other arm.	Normal reflex reaction	▪ This procedure elicits the biceps DTR.

Technique	Normal findings	Special considerations
Nervous system (continued)		
Place your fingers over the triceps tendon area and tap them with a reflex hammer. Repeat on the other arm.	Normal reflex reaction	■ This procedure elicits the triceps DTR.
Tap just below the patella with a reflex hammer. Repeat this procedure on the opposite patella.	Normal reflex reaction	■ This procedure elicits the patellar DTR.
Tap over the Achilles tendon area with a reflex hammer. Repeat this procedure on the opposite ankle.	Normal reflex reaction	■ This procedure elicits the Achilles DTR.
Stroke the sole of the patient's foot with the end of the reflex hammer handle.	Plantar reflex	■ This procedure elicits plantar flexion of all toes. ■ Expect Babinski's sign in children age 2 and under.
Ask the patient to demonstrate dorsiflexion by bending both feet upward against resistance.	Both feet lift easily against resistance	■ This procedure tests foot strength and ROM.
Ask the patient to demonstrate plantar flexion by bending both feet downward against resistance.	Both feet push down easily against resistance	■ This procedure tests foot strength and ROM.
Using your finger, trace a one-digit number in the palm of the patient's hand.	Correct identification of traced number	■ This procedure evaluates the patient's tactile discrimination through graphesthesia.
Place a familiar object, such as a key or a coin, in the patient's hand.	Correct identification of object	■ This procedure evaluates the patient's tactile discrimination.
Observe the patient while he walks with a regular gait, on the toes, on the heels, and heel-to-toe.	Steady gait, good balance, and no signs of muscle weakness or pain in any style of walking	■ This technique evaluates the cerebellum and motor system and checks for vertebral disk problems.
Inspect the scapulae, spine, back, and hips as the patient bends forward, backward, and from side to side.	Full ROM, easy flexibility, and no signs of scoliosis or varicosities	■ Inspection evaluates the patient's ROM and detects musculoskeletal abnormalities such as scoliosis.

Technique	Normal findings	Special considerations
Nervous system *(continued)*		
Perform the Romberg test. Ask the patient to stand straight with both eyes closed and both arms extended, with hands palms up.	Steady stance with minimal weaving	▪ This test checks cerebellar functioning and evaluates balance and coordination.

Normal laboratory value changes in elderly patients

Test values ages 20 to 40	Age-related changes	Considerations
Serum		
Albumin 3.5 to 5 g/dl (SI, 35 to 50 g/L)	▪ Younger than age 65: Higher in males ▪ Older than age 65: Equal levels that then decrease at same rate	Increased dietary protein intake needed in older patients if liver function is normal; edema — a sign of low albumin level
Alkaline phosphatase 30 to 85 IU/L (SI, 42 to 128 U/L)	Increases 8 to 10 IU/L	May reflect liver function decline or vitamin D malabsorption and bone demineralization
Beta globulin 0.7 to 1.1 g/dl (SI, 7 to 11 g/L)	Increases slightly	Increases in response to decrease in albumin if liver function is normal; increased dietary protein intake needed
Blood urea nitrogen ▪ Men: 10 to 25 mg/dl (SI, 3.6 to 9.3 mmol/L) ▪ Women: 8 to 20 mg/dl (SI, 2.9 to 7.5 mmol/L)	Increases, possibly to 69 mg/dl (SI, 25.8 mmol/L)	Slight increase acceptable in absence of stressors, such as infection or surgery

Test values ages 20 to 40	Age-related changes	Considerations
Serum *(continued)*		
Cholesterol ▪ Men: < 205 mg/dl (SI,< 5.30 mmol/L) ▪ Women: < 190 mg/dl (SI, < 4.90 mmol/L)	▪ Men: Increases to age 50, then decreases ▪ Women: Lower than men until age 50, increases to age 70, then decreases	Rise in cholesterol level (and increased cardiovascular risk) in women as a result of postmenopausal estrogen decline; dietary changes, weight loss, and exercise needed
Creatine kinase 55 to 170 U/L (SI, 0.94 to 2.89 μkat/L)	Increases slightly	May reflect decreasing muscle mass and liver function
Creatinine 0.6 to 1.3 mg/dl (SI, 53 to 115 μmol/L)	Increases, possibly to 1.9 mg/dl (SI, 168 μmol/L) in men	Important factor to prevent toxicity when giving drugs excreted in urine
Creatinine clearance ▪ Men: 94 to 140 ml/min/1.73 m^2 (SI, 0.91 to 1.35 ml/s/m^2) ▪ Women: 72 to 110 ml/min/1.73 m^2 (SI, 0.69 to 1.06 ml/s/m^2)	▪ Men: Decreases; formula: ([140 – age]) × kg body weight)/(72 × serum creatinine) ▪ Women: 85% of men's rate	Reflects reduced glomerular filtration rate; important factor to prevent toxicity when giving drugs excreted in urine
Hematocrit ▪ Men: 45% to 52% (SI, 0.45 to 0.52) ▪ Women: 37% to 48% (SI, 0.37 to 0.48)	May decrease slightly (unproven)	Reflects decreased bone marrow and hematopoiesis, increased risk of infection (because of fewer and weaker lymphocytes and immune system changes that diminish antigen-antibody response)
Hemoglobin ▪ Men: 14 to 18 g/dl (SI, 140 to 180 g/L) ▪ Women: 12 to 16 g/dl (SI, 120 to 160 g/L)	▪ Men: Decreases by 1 to 2 g/dl ▪ Women: Unknown	Reflects decreased bone marrow, hematopoiesis, and (for men) androgen levels
High-density lipoprotein ▪ Men: 37 to 70 mg/dl (SI, 0.96 to 1.8 mmol/L) ▪ Women: 40 to 85 mg/dl (SI, 1.03 to 2.2 mmol/L)	Levels higher in women than in men but equalize with age	Compliance with dietary restrictions required for accurate interpretation of test results

Test values ages 20 to 40	Age-related changes	Considerations
Serum *(continued)*		
Lactate dehydrogenase		
71 to 207 U/L (SI, 1.2 to 3.52 μkat/L)	Increases slightly	May reflect declining muscle mass and liver function
Leukocyte count		
4,000 to 10,0000/μl (SI, 4 to 10 × 10^9/L)	Decreases to 3,100 to 9,000/μl (SI, 3.1 to 9 × 10^9/L)	Decrease proportionate to lymphocyte count
Lymphocyte count		
25% to 40% (SI, 0.25 to 0.4)	Decreases	Decrease proportionate to leukocyte count
Platelet count		
140,000 to 400,000/μl (SI, 140 to 400 × 10^9/L)	Change in characteristics; decreased granular constituents, increased platelet-release factors	May reflect diminished bone marrow and increased fibrinogen levels
Potassium		
3.5 to 5.5 mEq/L (SI, 3.5 to 5.5 mmol/L)	Increases slightly	Requires avoidance of salt substitutes composed of potassium, vigilance in reading food labels, and knowledge of hyperkalemia's signs and symptoms
Thyroid-stimulating hormone		
0 to 15 μIU/ml (SI, 15 mU/L)	Increases slightly	Suggests primary hypothyroidism or endemic goiter at much higher levels
Thyroxine		
5 to 13.5 mcg/dl (SI, 60 to 165 mmol/L)	Decreases 25%	Reflects declining thyroid function
Triglycerides		
▪ Men: 44 to 180 mg/dl (SI, 0.44 to 2.01 mmol/L) ▪ Women: 10 to 190 mg/dl (SI, 0.11 to 2.21 mmol/L)	Increases slightly	Suggests abnormalities at any other levels, requiring additional tests such as serum cholesterol
Triiodothyronine		
80 to 220 ng/dl (SI, 1.2 to 3 nmol/L)	Decreases 25%	Reflects declining thyroid function

Test values ages 20 to 40	Age-related changes	Considerations
Urine		
Glucose 0 to 15 mg/dl (SI, 0 to 8 mmol/L)	Decreases slightly	May reflect renal disease or urinary tract infection (UTI); unreliable check for older diabetics because glucosuria may not occur until plasma glucose level exceeds 300 mg/dl
Protein 50 to 80 mg/24 hours (SI, 50 to 80 mg/d)	Increases slightly	May reflect renal disease or UTI
Specific gravity 1.032 (SI, 1.032)	Decreases to 1.024 (SI, 1.024) by age 80	Reflects 30% to 50% decrease in number of nephrons available to concentrate urine

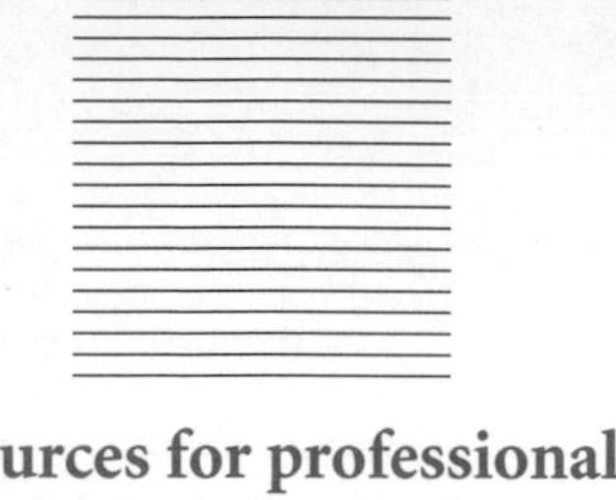

Resources for professionals, patients, and caregivers

General health care Web sites

■ *www.healthfinder.gov*—from the U.S. government; searchable database with links to Web sites, support groups, government agencies, and not-for-profit organizations that provide health care information for patients

■ *www.healthweb.org*—from a group of librarians and information professionals at academic medical centers in the midwestern United States; offers a searchable database of evaluated Web sites for patients and health care professionals

■ *www.medmatrix.org*—includes journal articles, abstracts, reviews, conference highlights, and links to other major sources for health care professionals

■ *www.mwsearch.com*—named Medical World Search, this site searches thousands of selected medical sites

Organizations

■ American Academy of Family Physicians—offers handouts and other resources to patients and health care professionals, plus links to other sites: *www.aafp.org*

■ Joint Commission on Accreditation of Healthcare Organizations: *www.jcaho.org*

Government agencies

■ Agency for Healthcare Research and Quality: *www.ahcpr.gov*

■ Centers for Disease Control and Prevention: *www.cdc.gov*

■ Centers for Medicare & Medicaid Services: *www.cms.hss.gov*

■ National Center for Complementary and Alternative Medicine: *www.nccam.nih.gov*

■ National Guideline Clearinghouse: *www.guideline.com*

■ National Library of Medicine, Specialized Information Services (information resources and services in toxicology, environmental health, chemistry, HIV/AIDS, and specialized topics in minority health): *www.sis.nlm.nih.gov*

■ U.S. Department of Health & Human Services: *www.dhhs.gov*

■ U.S. Food and Drug Administration: *www.fda.gov*

Spanish-language sites

■ Agency for Healthcare Research and Quality: *www.ahcpr.gov* (click on "Información en español")

■ CANCERCare, Inc.: *www.cancercare.org* (click on "En español")

■ Healthfinder: *www.healthfinder.gov* (click on "Español")

■ National Cancer Institute: *www.cancer.gov/espanol*

Condition-specific sites

Aging

■ American Society on Aging: *www.asaging.org*

■ National Institute on Aging: *www.nia.nih.gov;* 301-496-1752

■ U.S. Administration on Aging: *www.aoa.dhhs.gov*

AIDS/HIV/STDs

■ Centers for Disease Control and Prevention, National Prevention Information Network: *www.cdcnpin.org/scripts/index.asp*

■ HIV/AIDS Treatment Information Service: *www.sis.nlm.nih.gov/aids/aidstrea.html;* 800-448-0440 (Spanish available); TTY, 800-243-7012

■ National AIDS Hotline (24 hours): 800-342-AIDS; Spanish, 800-344-7432; TTY, 800-243-7889

■ Office of AIDS Research: *www.sis.nlm.nih.gov/aids/oar.html*

Allergies and asthma

■ Allergy & Asthma Disease Management Center: *www.aaaai.org/aadmc*

■ Allergy & Asthma Network—Mothers of Asthmatics: *www.aanma.org;* 800-878-4403

■ Allergy, Asthma & Immunology Online: *www.allergy.mcg.edu*

■ American Academy of Allergy Asthma & Immunology: *www.aaaai.org;* 800-822-2762

■ Global Initiative For Asthma: *www.ginasthma.com*

■ Joint Council of Allergy, Asthma and Immunology: *www.jcaai.org*

■ National Asthma Education and Prevention Program: *www.nhlbi.nih.gov/about/naepp*

■ National Institute of Allergy and Infectious Diseases: *www.niaid.nih.gov*

Alzheimer's disease

■ Agency for Healthcare Research and Quality (AHRQ) Early Alzheimer's Disease Clinical Practice Guideline—Patient and Family Guide: *www.ahcpr.gov/clinic/alzcons.htm*

■ AHRQ's Recognition and Assessment Guideline: *www.ahcpr.gov/clinic/alzover.htm*

■ Alzheimer's Association: *www.alz.org;* 800-272-3900

■ Alzheimer's Disease Education & Referral Center: *www.alzheimers.org;* 800-438-4380

■ Alzheimer Europe: *www.alzheimer-europe.org*

■ AlzWell Caregiver Page: *www.alzwell.com*

Arthritis

■ American Autoimmune Related Diseases Association, Inc.: *www.aarda.org*

■ American College of Rheumatology: *www.rheumatology.org*

■ Arthritis Foundation: *www.arthritis.org;* 800-283-7800

■ National Institute of Arthritis and Musculoskeletal and Skin Diseases: *www.nih.gov/niams*

Attention deficit disorder/hyperactivity

■ National Attention Deficit Disorder Association: *www.add.org*

Cancer

■ American Cancer Society: *www.cancer.org*; 800-ACS-2345

■ CANCERCare, Inc.: *www.cancercare.org*

■ Cancer News on the Net: *www.cancernews.com*

■ National Breast Cancer Awareness Month: *www.nbcam.org*

■ National Cancer Institute: *www.cancer.gov*

■ National Cancer Institute, Cancer Information Service: 800-4-CANCER

- National Cancer Institute, Cancer Literature Search: *www.cancer.gov/search/pubmed*
- National Cancer Institute, Cancer Trials: *www.cancer.gov/clinicaltrials*
- National Center for Chronic Disease Prevention and Health Promotion: *www.cdc.gov/nccdphp*
- National Comprehensive Cancer Network: *www.nccn.org*
- Susan G. Komen Breast Cancer Foundation: *www.komen.org*
- Y-Me National Breast Cancer Organization: *www.y-me.org;* 800-221-2141; 800-986-9505 (Español)

Cardiac

- American Heart Association: *www.americanheart.org;* 800-242-8721
- Mayo Heart Center: *www.mayohealth.org* (click on "Heart")
- National Heart, Lung, and Blood Institute: *www.nhlbi.nih.gov*
- National Stroke Association: *www.stroke.org*

Diabetes

- American Association of Diabetes Educators: *www.aadenet.org;* 800-338-3633
- American Diabetes Association: *www.diabetes.org*
- Diabetes self-care equipment for the visually impaired: Palco Labs, Inc.: *www.palcolabs.com;* 800-346-4488
- Joslin Diabetes Center: *www.joslin.harvard.edu*
- National Institute of Diabetes & Digestive & Kidney Diseases: *www.niddk.nih.gov*

Disabilities

- University of Virginia: General Resources About Disabilities: *www.curry.edschool.virginia.edu/go/cise/ose/resources/general.html;* Assistive Technology Resources: *www.curry.edschool.virginia.edu/go/cise/ose/resources/asst_tech.html*

Elder abuse

- National Center for Victims of Crime: *www.ncvc.org*
- National Center on Elder Abuse: *www.elderabusecenter.org*

Gastrointestinal

- American Liver Foundation: *www.liverfoundation.org*
- National Institute of Diabetes & Digestive & Kidney Diseases: *www.niddk.nih.gov*
- National Kidney Foundation: *www.kidney.org;* 800-622-9010

Musculoskeletal

- American College of Foot and Ankle Surgeons: *www.acfas.org*
- Amputee Coalition of America: *www.amputee-coalition.org;* 888-AMP-KNOW (267-5669)
- National Institute of Arthritis and Musculoskeletal and Skin Disorders: *www.niams.nih.gov*
- National Osteoporosis Foundation: *www.nof.org*

Neurology

- ALS Association: *www.alsa.org;* 818-880-9007
- American Brain Tumor Association: *www.abta.org;* 800-886-2282
- Association of Late-Deafened Adults, Inc.: *www.alda.org*
- EAR Foundation/Ménière's Network: *www.theearfoundation.org*
- National Association of the Deaf: *www.nad.org*
- National Federation of the Blind: *www.nfb.org*
- National Institute of Neurological Disorders and Stroke: *www.ninds.nih.gov*
- National Institute on Deafness and Other Communication Disorders: *www.nidcd.nih.gov*

Pediatrics

- Children with Diabetes: *www.childrenwithdiabetes.com*
- Cystic Fibrosis Foundation: *www.cff.org;* 800-FIGHT CF (344-4823)

- Cystic Fibrosis Mutation Data Base: *www.genet.sickkids.on.ca/cftr*
- Cystic Fibrosis USA: *www.cfusa.org*
- Down's Heart Group: *www.downs-heart.downsnet.org*
- Emory University Sickle Cell Information Center: *www.emory.edu/PEDS/SICKLE/newweb.htm*
- Families of Spinal Muscular Atrophy: *www.fsma.org;* 800-886-1762
- Growth Charts for Children with Down Syndrome: *www.growthcharts.com*
- Internet Resource for Special Children: *www.irsc.org*
- National Down Syndrome Society: *www.ndss.org*
- National Institute of Child Health & Human Development: *www.nichd.nih.gov*
- National Pediatric AIDS Network: *www.npan.org*
- Spina Bifida Association of America: *www.sbaa.org;* 800-621-3141
- United Cerebral Palsy: *www.ucpa.org;* 800-872-5827

Psychiatry

- American Psychological Association: *www.apa.org;* 800-374-2721
- Depressive and Bipolar Support Alliance: *www.dbsalliance.org*
- National Alliance for the Mentally Ill: *www.nami.org;* 800-950-NAMI (950-6264)
- National Mental Health Association: *www.nmha.org;* 800-969-6642

Respiratory

- American Heart Association (smoking cessation information): 800-242-8721
- American Lung Association: *www.lungusa.org;* 800-LUNG-USA (local affiliates answer)
- National Emphysema Foundation: *www.emphysemafoundation.org*

Skin

- National Pressure Ulcer Advisory Panel: *www.npuap.org*
- Wound Care Information Network: *www.medicaledu.com*
- Wound Care Institute, Inc.: *www.woundcare.org;* 305-919-9192
- Wound, Ostomy and Continence Nurses Society: *www.wocn.org;* 888224-WOCN

Substance abuse

- Al-Anon & Alateen (including Spanish and French language options): *www.al-anon.alateen.org*
- Alcoholics Anonymous (including Spanish and French language options): *www.alcoholics-anonymous.org*
- Narcotics Anonymous World Services: *www.wsoinc.com*
- National Centers for Disease Control and Prevention, Tobacco Information and Prevention Source: *www.cdc.gov/tobacco*
- National Council on Alcoholism and Drug Dependence: *www.ncadd.org;* 800-NCA-CALL (622-2255)
- National Institute on Alcohol Abuse and Alcoholism: *www.niaaa.nih.gov*
- Substance Abuse & Mental Health Services Administration: *www.samhsa.gov*

Women's health

- American College of Cardiology: *www.acc.org*
- American Heart Association: *www.women.americanheart.org*
- American Medical Women's Association: *www.amwa-doc.org*
- JAMA Women's Health Information Center: *www.amaassn.org/special/womh/womh.htm*
- Johns Hopkins Intelihealth: *www.intelihealth.com* (click on "Women's health")
- Office on Women's Health (U.S. Department of Health & Human Services): *www.4women.gov/owh*
- Womens' Health Initiative: *www.nhlbi.nih.gov/wh*

Selected references

Alcentius, M. "Successfully Meet Pain Assessment Standards," *Nursing Management* 35(3):12, March 2004.

Assessment Made Incredibly Easy! 3rd ed. Philadelphia: Lippincott Williams & Wilkins, 2005.

Assessment: A 2-in-1 Reference for Nurses, Philadelphia: Lippincott Williams & Wilkins, 2004.

Bickley, L.S. *Bate's Guide to Physical Examination and History Taking*, 8th ed. Philadelphia: Lippincott Williams & Wilkins, 2004.

Braunwald, E., et al. *Harrison's Principles of Internal Medicine,* 15th ed. New York: McGraw-Hill Book Co., 2001.

Coviello, J.S. "Cardiac Assessment 101: A New Look at the Guidelines for Cardiac Homecare Patients," *Home Healthcare Nurse* 22(2):116-23, February 2004.

Davis, S.L. "How the Heart Failure Picture has Changed," *Nursing2002* 32(11):36-44, November 2002.

DeVon, H.A., and Zerwic, J.J. "The Symptoms of Unstable Angina: Do Women and Men Differ?" *Nursing Research* 52(2):108-18, March-April 2003.

Doughty, D.B. "Wound Assessment: Tips and Techniques," *Home Healthcare Nurse* 22(3):192-95, March 2004.

Eliopoulos, C. *Gerontological Nursing,* 5th ed. Philadelphia: Lippincott Williams & Wilkins, 2001.

Erickson, B.A. *Heart Sounds and Murmurs Across the Lifespan with Audiotape*, 4th ed. St. Louis: Mosby–Year Book, Inc., 2003.

Habif, T.P. *Clinical Dermatology,* 4th ed. St. Louis: Mosby–Year Book, Inc., 2003.

Hatchett, R.G. and Thompson, D.R. *Cardiac Nursing: A Comprehensive Guide.* St. Louis: Mosby–Year Book, Inc., 2002.

Hickey, J. *The Clinical Practice of Neurological and Neurosurgical Nursing,* 5th ed. Philadelphia: Lippincott Williams & Wilkins, 2003.

Ignatavicius, D.D., and Workman, M.L. *Medical-Surgical Nursing: Critical Thinking for Collaborative Care,* 4th ed. Philadelphia: W.B. Saunders Co., 2002.

Giger, N.J., and Davidhizar, R.E. *Transcultural Nursing: Assessment and Intervention,* 4th ed. St. Louis: Mosby-Year Book, Inc., 2004.

Mandell, G.L., et al. *Principles and Practice of Infectious Diseases,* 6th ed. New York: Churchill Livingstone, Inc., 2004.

Middelton, C. "The Assessment and Treatment of Patients with Chronic Pain," *Nursing Times* 100(18):40-44, May 2004.

Nursing2004 Herbal Medicine Handbook, 2nd ed. Philadelphia: Lippincott Williams & Wilkins, 2004.

Porth, C.M. *Pathophysiology Concepts of Altered Health States,* 7th ed. Philadelphia: Lippincott Williams & Wilkins, 2005.

Potter, P.A., and Perry, A.G. *Fundamentals of Nursing,* 6th ed. St. Louis: Mosby–Year Book, Inc. 2005.

Professional Guide Diseases, 7th ed. Philadelphia: Lippincott Williams & Wilkins. 2001.

Professional Guide to Signs and Symptoms, 4th ed. Philadelphia: Lippincott Williams & Wilkins, 2003.

Woodrow, P. "Assessing Blood Pressure in Older People," *Nursing Older People* 16(1)29-31, March 2004.

Woods, S., et al. *Cardiac Nursing,* 5th ed. Philadelphia: Lippincott Williams & Wilkins, 2005.

Color photo credits

Pages C1 to C4
Squamous cell carcinoma, Psoriasis: Reprinted with permission from Bickley, L.S. *Bate's Guide to Physical Examination and History Taking,* 8th ed. Philadelphia: Lippincott Williams & Wilkins, 2003.

Malignant melanoma: Courtesy of The American Cancer Society; American Academy of Dermatology.

Kaposi's sarcoma: From Sanders, C.V. & Nesbitt, L.T., Jr. *The Skin and Infection: A Color Atlas and Text.* Baltimore: Williams and Wilkins, 1995.

Telangiectasia: From Willis, M.C., CMA-AC. *Medical Terminology: A Programmed Learning Approach to the Language of Health Care.* Baltimore: Lippincott Williams & Wilkins. 2002.

Basal cell carcinoma, Candidiasis, Contact dermatitis, Eczema, Herpes zoster, Impetigo, Systemic lupus erythematosus, Tinea corporis, Urticaria: Goodheart, H.P., M.D. *Goodheart's Photoguide of Common Skin Disorders,* 2nd ed. Philadelphia: Lippincott Williams & Wilkins, 2003.

Scabies, Vitiligo: Stedman's Medical Dictionary, 27th ed. Philadelphia: Lippincott Williams & Wilkins, 2000.

Pages C5 to C8
Assets provided by Anatomical Chart Company.

Index

A

i refers to an illustration; t refers to a table; **boldface** indicates color pages.

i refers to an illustration; t refers to a table; **boldface** indicates color pages.

B

i refers to an illustration; t refers to a table; **boldface** indicates color pages.

C

i refers to an illustration; t refers to a table; **boldface** indicates color pages.

i refers to an illustration; t refers to a table; **boldface** indicates color pages.

D

E

i refers to an illustration; t refers to a table; **boldface** indicates color pages.

F

i refers to an illustration; t refers to a table; **boldface** indicates color pages.

G

H

i refers to an illustration; t refers to a table; **boldface** indicates color pages.

i refers to an illustration; t refers to a table; **boldface** indicates color pages.

I

J

K

i refers to an illustration; t refers to a table; **boldface** indicates color pages.

L

M

i refers to an illustration; t refers to a table; **boldface** indicates color pages.

N

i refers to an illustration; t refers to a table; **boldface** indicates color pages.

i refers to an illustration; t refers to a table; **boldface** indicates color pages.

i refers to an illustration; t refers to a table; **boldface** indicates color pages.

i refers to an illustration; t refers to a table; **boldface** indicates color pages.

i refers to an illustration; t refers to a table; **boldface** indicates color pages.

Q

R

i refers to an illustration; t refers to a table; **boldface** indicates color pages.

i refers to an illustration; t refers to a table; **boldface** indicates color pages.

T

i refers to an illustration; t refers to a table; **boldface** indicates color pages.

U

i refers to an illustration; t refers to a table; **boldface** indicates color pages.

V

i refers to an illustration; t refers to a table; **boldface** indicates color pages.

W

X

Y

Z

i refers to an illustration; t refers to a table; **boldface** indicates color pages.